Advances in Parvovirus Research 2022

Advances in Parvovirus Research 2022

Editor

Giorgio Gallinella

MDPI

Basel • Beijing • Wuhan • Barcelona • Belgrade • Novi Sad • Cluj • Manchester

Editor
Giorgio Gallinella
University of Bologna
Bologna, Italy

Editorial Office
MDPI
St. Alban-Anlage 66
4052 Basel, Switzerland

This is a reprint of articles from the Special Issue published online in the open access journal *Viruses* (ISSN 1999-4915) (available at: https://www.mdpi.com/journal/viruses/special_issues/parvovirus_2022).

For citation purposes, cite each article independently as indicated on the article page online and as indicated below:

Lastname, A.A.; Lastname, B.B. Article Title. *Journal Name* **Year**, *Volume Number*, Page Range.

ISBN 978-3-0365-9448-4 (Hbk)
ISBN 978-3-0365-9449-1 (PDF)
doi.org/10.3390/books978-3-0365-9449-1

Contents

About the Editor vii

Preface ix

Giorgio Gallinella and Antonio Marchini
The XVIII International Parvovirus Workshop Rimini, Italy, 14–17 June 2022
Reprinted from: *Viruses* **2023**, *15*, 2129, doi:10.3390/v15102129 1

Angelica Bravo, Leandro Fernández-García, Rodrigo Ibarra-Karmy, Gonzalo A. Mardones, Luis Mercado, Fernando J. Bustos, et al.
Antiviral Activity of an Endogenous Parvoviral Element
Reprinted from: *Viruses* **2023**, *15*, 1420, doi:10.3390/v15071420 27

Marina I. Beloukhova, Alexander N. Lukashev, Pavel Y. Volchkov, Andrey A. Zamyatnin, Jr. and Andrei A. Deviatkin
Robust AAV Genotyping Based on Genetic Distances in Rep Gene That Are Maintained by Ubiquitous Recombination
Reprinted from: *Viruses* **2022**, *14*, 1038, doi:10.3390/v14051038 43

Stefania Leopardi, Adelaide Milani, Monia Cocchi, Marco Bregoli, Alessia Schivo, Sofia Leardini, et al.
Carnivore protoparvovirus 1 (CPV-2 and FPV) Circulating in Wild Carnivores and in Puppies Illegally Imported into North-Eastern Italy
Reprinted from: *Viruses* **2022**, *14*, 2612, doi:10.3390/v14122612 57

Giovanni Franzo, Francesco Mira, Giorgia Schirò and Marta Canuti
Not Asian Anymore: Reconstruction of the History, Evolution, and Dispersal of the "Asian" Lineage of CPV-2c
Reprinted from: *Viruses* **2023**, *15*, 1962, doi:10.3390/v15091962 69

Giovanni Franzo, Habibata Lamouni Zerbo, Bruno Lalidia Ouoba, Adama Drabo Dji-Tombo, Marietou Guitti Kindo, Rasablaga Sawadogo, et al.
A Phylogeographic Analysis of Porcine Parvovirus 1 in Africa
Reprinted from: *Viruses* **2023**, *15*, 207, doi:10.3390/v15010207 85

Federica Bichicchi, Niccolò Guglietta, Arthur Daniel Rocha Alves, Erika Fasano, Elisabetta Manaresi, Gloria Bua and Giorgio Gallinella
Next Generation Sequencing for the Analysis of Parvovirus B19 Genomic Diversity
Reprinted from: *Viruses* **2023**, *15*, 217, doi:10.3390/v15010217 95

Renuk Lakshmanan, Mario Mietzsch, Alberto Jimenez Ybargollin, Paul Chipman, Xiaofeng Fu, Jianming Qiu, et al.
Capsid Structure of Aleutian Mink Disease Virus and Human Parvovirus 4: New Faces in the Parvovirus Family Portrait
Reprinted from: *Viruses* **2022**, *14*, 2219, doi:10.3390/v14102219 109

Michael Velez, Mario Mietzsch, Jane Hsi, Logan Bell, Paul Chipman, Xiaofeng Fu and Robert McKenna
Structural Characterization of Canine Minute Virus, Rat and Porcine Bocavirus
Reprinted from: *Viruses* **2023**, *15*, 1799, doi:10.3390/v15091799 125

Cornelia Bircher, Jan Bieri, Ruben Assaraf, Remo Leisi and Carlos Ros
A Conserved Receptor-Binding Domain in the VP1u of Primate Erythroparvoviruses Determines the Marked Tropism for Erythroid Cells
Reprinted from: *Viruses* **2022**, *14*, 420, doi:10.3390/v14020420 . . . . **139**

Tiago Ferreira, Amit Kulkarni, Clemens Bretscher, Petr V. Nazarov, Jubayer A. Hossain, Lars A. R. Ystaas, et al.
Oncolytic H-1 Parvovirus Hijacks Galectin-1 to Enter Cancer Cells
Reprinted from: *Viruses* **2022**, *14*, 1018, doi:10.3390/v14051018 . . . . **155**

Alessandro Reggiani, Andrea Avati, Francesca Valenti, Erika Fasano, Gloria Bua, Elisabetta Manaresi and Giorgio Gallinella
A Functional Minigenome of Parvovirus B19
Reprinted from: *Viruses* **2022**, *14*, 84, doi:10.3390/v14010084 . . . . **181**

Patrick Hauswirth, Philipp Graber, Katarzyna Buczak, Riccardo Vincenzo Mancuso, Susanne Heidi Schenk, Jürg P. F. Nüesch and Jörg Huwyler
Design and Characterization of Mutated Variants of the Oncotoxic Parvoviral Protein NS1
Reprinted from: *Viruses* **2023**, *15*, 209, doi:10.3390/v15010209 . . . . **195**

Clairine I. S. Larsen and Kinjal Majumder
The Autonomous Parvovirus Minute Virus of Mice Localizes to Cellular Sites of DNA Damage Using ATR Signaling
Reprinted from: *Viruses* **2023**, *15*, 1243, doi:10.3390/v15061243 . . . . **215**

Yanfei Gao, Haiwei Wang, Shanghui Wang, Mingxia Sun, Zheng Fang, Xinran Liu, et al.
Self-Assembly of Porcine Parvovirus Virus-like Particles and Their Application in Serological Assay
Reprinted from: *Viruses* **2022**, *14*, 1828, doi:10.3390/v14081828 . . . . **231**

Arthur Daniel Rocha Alves, Barbara Barbosa Langella, Mariana Magaldi de Souza Lima, Wagner Luís da Costa Nunes Pimentel Coelho, Rita de Cássia Nasser Cubel Garcia, Claudete Aparecida Araújo Cardoso, et al.
Evaluation of Molecular Test for the Discrimination of "Naked" DNA from Infectious Parvovirus B19 Particles in Serum and Bone Marrow Samples
Reprinted from: *Viruses* **2022**, *14*, 843, doi:10.3390/v14040843 . . . . **243**

Daniela P. Mendes-de-Almeida, Joanna Paes Barreto Bokel, Arthur Daniel Rocha Alves, Alexandre G. Vizzoni, Isabel Cristina Ferreira Tavares, Mayara Secco Torres Silva, et al.
Clinical Presentation of Parvovirus B19 Infection in Adults Living with HIV/AIDS: A Case Series
Reprinted from: *Viruses* **2023**, *15*, 1124, doi:10.3390/v15051124 . . . . **257**

Franziska K. Kaiser, Madeleine de le Roi, Wendy K. Jo, Ingo Gerhauser, Viktor Molnár, Albert D. M. E. Osterhaus, et al.
First Report of Skunk Amdoparvovirus (Species *Carnivore amdoparvovirus 4*) in Europe in a Captive Striped Skunk (*Mephitis mephitis*)
Reprinted from: *Viruses* **2023**, *15*, 1087, doi:10.3390/v15051087 . . . . **267**

About the Editor

Giorgio Gallinella

Giorgio Gallinella, MD, PhD. Born on 20.06.1963. Full Professor of Microbiology at the Department of Pharmacy and Biotechnology at the University of Bologna, Italy. He is currently teaching Medical Microbiology in the Master Degree Program in Health Biology, and Microbiology and Vaccines in the Master Degree Program in Pharmaceutical Biotechnology. He obtained his Degree in Medicine and Surgery in 1989, a PhD in Microbiological Sciences in 1993, and a Medical Specialization Degree in Microbiology and Virology in 1997. In year 2000 he received the Abbott Murex Award, conferred by the European Society for Clinical Virology, for the original contribution in the field of virologic diagnosis. In his scientific activity, he has conducted research in the field of basic and clinical virology. A special interest has been devoted to the study of Parvovirus B19, both as a model system for research in basic virology, and also for its clinical implication as a human pathogenic virus. In this context, the research is mainly focused on the study of virus-cell interactions; the study of the pathogenesis and of the clinical and epidemiological aspects of infectious processes; the development of innovative methodologies and diagnostic assays; the development of novel antiviral drugs. He has organized the IX Parvovirus Workshop, Bologna, Italy, august 2002, and more recently, the XVIII Parvovirus Workshop, Rimini, Italy, June 2022.

Preface

This Special Issue entitled 'Advances in Parvovirus Research 2022' continues the series dedicated to research on viruses belonging to the *Parvoviridae* family following the successful Special Issues "New Insights into Parvovirus Research" and "Advances in Parvovirus Research 2020". As for the previous Special Issues, the aim was to offer a dedicated opportunity to bring together the latest contributions in the field of parvovirus research, providing advanced knowledge and new insights and addressing research on unresolved topics. Furthermore, this Special Issue was associated with the XVIII International Parvovirus Workshop, which took place in Rimini, Italy, from the 14th to the 17th of June 2022. The international workshops dedicated to parvoviruses started in 1985 and are continuously held every two years and are events strictly centered on all aspects of parvovirus research, providing excellent opportunities to focus on research topics in this area. The 2022 event continued the series, filling the gap in the original schedule in 2020 when the workshop had to be postponed due to the then-peaking COVID-19 pandemic, and fostering renewed research in the field. A conference report opens this collection, as a union thread gathering the scientific community involved in research on parvoviruses.

Evolution and phylogenetics have been the subject of many contributions to this Special Issue. Bravo et al. report on ancestral endogenous parvoviral elements in rodents and their possible adaptive role in conferring antiviral protection to hosts. Beloukhova et al. propose a genotype-based AAV classification as an alternative to the common serotype-based classification scheme. Leopardi et al and Franzo et al. provide information on the evolution and spatial and temporal distribution of CPV and PPV. Franzo et al. further report on the utility of the phylogenetic analysis of CPV to track the alien introduction of animals in a definite geographic scenario. Bichicchi et al. analyze sequence heterogeneity in B19V clinical isolates by means of NGS techniques and also provide innovative bioinformatic tools and an analytical frame for the interpretation of such diversity.

The portfolio of atomic-scale structural models in the family is now further expanded due to the contributions of Lakshmanan et al and Velez et al., now including viruses as diverse as AMDV, Human parvovirus 4, and members of the *Bocaparvovirus* genus. Virus-receptor interactions are the subject of contributions by Bircher et al., for members of the genus *Erythroparvovirus*, and Ferreira et al, for the oncolytic H-1 virus. Concerning replication and genetics, Reggiani et al. describe a functional replicating minigenome of B19V, Hauswirth et al. describe mutants of the NS1 protein of the H-1 virus, and Larsen et al. report on the characterization of interactions of MVM and cellular DNA damage repair pathways.

Finally, regarding translational issues, Gao et al. describe the generation of PPV viral-like particles and their application in serological assays; Alves et al. report on the evaluation of molecular test for the discrimination of DNA from infectious parvovirus B19 particles from clinical samples; Mendes-de-Almeida et al. describe the clinical presentation of B19V infection in cases of HIV-infected patients; and Kaiser et al. describe the first instances of the identification of Skunk *Amdoparvovirus* in Europe.

In the years these papers were submitted, the most critical phases of the COVID-19 pandemic were over, but the antecedent impact has been profound and critical, diverting substantial energies and resources. However, the pandemic also brought into focus not only the 'One Health' concept but also the key role viruses can play in it. In this regard, the wide diversity of viruses in the Parvoviridae family and their evolutionary potential is a topic of sure relevance and interest, adding to the well-established relevance in clinical and translational research.

Giorgio Gallinella
Editor

viruses

MDPI

Conference Report

The XVIII International Parvovirus Workshop Rimini, Italy, 14–17 June 2022

Giorgio Gallinella [1,*] and Antonio Marchini [2,†]

1 Department of Pharmacy and Biotechnology, University of Bologna, 40138 Bologna, Italy
2 Laboratory of Oncolytic Virus Immuno-Therapeutics, German Cancer Research Centre, 69120 Heidelberg, Germany; a.marchini@dkfz.de or antonio.marchini@ec.europa.eu
* Correspondence: giorgio.gallinella@unibo.it
† Current address: European Commission, Joint Research Centre (JRC), 2440 Geel, Belgium.

Abstract: The XVIII International Parvovirus Workshop took place in Rimini, Italy, from 14 to 17 June 2022 as an on-site event, continuing the series of meetings started in 1985 and continuously held every two years. The communications dealt with all aspects of research in the field, from evolution and structure to receptors, from replication to trafficking, from virus–host interactions to clinical and veterinarian virology, including translational issues related to viral vectors, gene therapy and oncolytic parvoviruses. The oral communications were complemented by a poster exhibition available for view and discussion during the whole meeting. The XVIII International Parvovirus Workshop was dedicated to the memory of our dearest colleague Mavis Agbandje-McKenna (1963–2021).

Keywords: Parvoviridae; international workshop; conference report

1. Introduction

The XVIII International Parvovirus Workshop took place in Rimini, Italy, from 14 to 17 June 2022 as an on-site event—this following a gap in the original schedule in 2020, when the workshop had to be postponed due to the then peaking COVID-19 pandemic.

The Workshop was jointly organized by the Istituto Nazionale Biostrutture e Biosistemi (INBB), Italy, the Department of Pharmacy and Biotechnology and the Rimini Campus of the University of Bologna, Italy (GG), with the support of the German Cancer Research Center, Heidelberg, Germany (DKFZ) (AM).

The decision to organize the meeting as an on-site event allowed us to continue the best tradition of the Parvovirus Workshops, started in 1985 and continuously held every two years, offering the best opportunity to scientists involved in this field of research to meet again, discuss and create networks, in a gratifying venue. About one hundred scientists gathered, contributing to a successful workshop with a total of 64 abstracts.

Following the inaugural session introducing the meeting with three keynote lectures, nine sessions ensued, with communications distributed according to topics, from evolution and structure to receptors, from replication to trafficking, from virus–host interactions to clinical and veterinarian virology, including translational issues related to viral vectors, gene therapy and oncolytic parvoviruses. The oral communications were complemented by a flash poster session, while a poster exhibition remained available for view and discussion during the whole meeting. The abstracts submitted to the conference are reported below as submitted by the authors, in the same order and according to the topics of the actual sessions.

The conference was associated with the Special Issue of *Viruses*, "Advances in Parvovirus Research 2022", and some of the abstracts can be found as contributing articles. The journal sponsored two awards for young scientists, for the best oral presentation and best poster.

Citation: Gallinella, G.; Marchini, A. The XVIII International Parvovirus Workshop Rimini, Italy, 14–17 June 2022. *Viruses* **2023**, *15*, 2129. https://doi.org/10.3390/v15102129

Received: 16 October 2023
Accepted: 18 October 2023
Published: 20 October 2023

The XVIII International Parvovirus Workshop was dedicated to the memory of our dearest colleague Mavis Agbandje-McKenna (1963–2021). At the end of the inaugural session, Arun Srivastava payed her a deeply affectioned tribute on behalf of the whole community.

2. Inaugural Session

In the inaugural session, three keynote speeches were presented. Two of them were reviews on translational aspects in the field. The first, presented by Arun Srivastava, reported on the development of adeno-associated viruses as successful vectors for gene therapy; another, presented by Jürg Nüesch, reported on the potential of a wide portfolio of oncolytic rodent parvoviruses in light of cancer virotherapy. The third speech was presented by Davide Corti, from Humabs BioMed, who offered a wider perspective and reported on the newest techniques and recent applications of human monoclonal antibodies to tackle viral diseases, an issue with the highest relevance to the treatment of severe infections in clinical settings, including parvoviruses.

2.1. Keynote 1: AAV: From Almost a Virus to an Awesome Vector (Or Is It?)

Arun Srivastava

To date, recombinant adeno-associated virus (AAV) vectors, based on a non-pathogenic parvovirus, have been, or are currently in use, in 284 Phase I/II/III clinical trials for a wide variety of human diseases. In some cases, such as Leber's congenital amaurosis, lipoprotein lipase deficiency, hemophilia B, aromatic L-amino acid decarboxylase deficiency, choroideremia, Leber hereditary optic neuropathy, hemophilia A and spinal muscular atrophy, unexpected, remarkable clinical efficacy has also been achieved. Several AAV serotype vectors are available at present, which have shown clinical efficacy in a number of human diseases in animal models. To date, two AAV "drugs"—Luxturna and Zolgensma—have been approved by the Food and Drug Administration (FDA). Despite these remarkable achievements, it has become increasingly clear that the first generation of AAV vectors currently in use are not optimal. For example, despite their efficacy in animal models, these vectors have failed to show clinical efficacy in some cases. In addition, relatively large vector doses are needed to achieve clinical efficacy. The use of high doses has been shown to provoke host immune responses culminating in serious adverse events, and more recently, in the deaths of six patients. Thus, it has become increasingly clear that there is an urgent need for the development of the next generation of AAV vectors that are: (i) safe; (ii) effective; and (iii) human-tropic. Since AAV evolved as a virus, and not as a vector for the purposes of delivery of therapeutic genes, the host immune system cannot distinguish between AAV as a virus versus AAV as a vector. Thus, the use of AAV vectors composed of naturally occurring capsids is likely to induce immune responses, especially at high doses since the host immune response is directly correlated to the AAV vector dose. Similarly, AAV as a virus does not express its own genes effectively since its single-stranded DNA genome is transcriptionally inactive. Most of the ssAAV vectors currently in use are also sub-optimal in expressing therapeutic genes. And finally, the tropisms of AAV vectors in animal models do not necessarily translate well in humans, and hence the need to identify and further develop human-tropic AAV vectors. In this presentation, strategies to overcome each of the limitations of the first generation of AAV vectors will be presented. The next generation of AAV serotype vectors promise to be: (i) efficacious at significant reduced doses; (ii) likely to be less immunogenic, thereby increasing the safety; (iii) obviating the need for the use of immune suppression; (iv) reducing vector production costs; and (v) ensuring translation to the clinic with a higher probability of success, for gene therapy of a wide variety of human diseases.

2.2. Keynote 2: Tackling Viral Infections by Human Monoclonal Antibodies

Davide Corti

Monoclonal antibodies (mAbs) have revolutionized the treatment of several human diseases, including cancer, autoimmunity and inflammatory conditions, and represent a new frontier for the treatment of infectious diseases. In the last twenty years, innovative methods have allowed the rapid isolation of antibodies from convalescent subjects, humanized mice or in vitro libraries, and have proven that the swift isolation of mAbs is a rapid and effective countermeasure to emerging pathogens. During the past two years, an unprecedented wave of monoclonal antibodies has been developed to fight COVID-19. We provide an overview of the preclinical and clinical development of monoclonal antibodies against Ebola virus, SARS-CoV-2, Influenza A virus and hepatitis B virus, including their antiviral and immunological mechanisms of action.

2.3. Keynote 3: Generating a Portfolio of Oncolytic Rodent Parvoviruses

Jürg P.F. Nüesch

Although the initial H-1PV treatment of cancer patients alone, or in combination with approved anticancer agents, provided promising results, there are still significant limitations. In particular, there were patients that did not respond to the therapy and there are cancer entities, which appear to be of limited targets for H-1PV infection. To tackle these drawbacks, we intend to generate a portfolio of oncolytic parvoviruses, based on additional PV strains that were, like H-1PV, originally isolated as an opportunistic infectant of human tumor cell lines. In addition, we intend to improve the propagation and spreading capacity of H-1PV and other isolates through adaptation towards refractory cancer entities. Indeed, the serial adaptation of H-1PV proved to improve the replication and propagation capacity of the original isolate not only for the target human GBM cell lines, but also for a variety of other cancer entities, such as malignant melanoma and PDAC.

In order to enlarge the repertoire of oncolytic PVs, we first assessed viral sequences in the replicative-form DNAs of a number of virus isolates collected mainly in the late 1960s–early 1970s and a few "younger" virus preparations. These sequences founded the basis to generate replication-competent plasmids, essential tools to produce individual virus entities and to characterize them for their propagation capacity in candidate human cancer cell lines. To date, we obtained a number of replication-competent viruses, derived from H-1, KRV, H3, X14, TVX, LuIII and MVM, and generated (specific) monoclonal antibodies enabling us to determine their properties in various target cells. At present, we use these individual viruses to determine their host range and oncosuppressive capacity, targeting human tumor cell lines derived from brain tumors, malignant melanomas, colon cancer and hepato-cell carcinomas.

3. Session 1: Evolution and Structure

3.1. Review Lecture: Evolution of Canine and Feline Parvoviruses, and the Control of Viral Host Range and Antibody Neutralization

Colin R. Parrish, Ian Voorhees, Heather Callaway, Hyunwook Le and *Susan Hafenstein*

Canine parvovirus (CPV) emerged during the mid-1970s, spread globally during 1978 and has maintained a pandemic circulation in dogs. We examined the whole-genome evolution of the virus since it emerged as a variant of a feline-like virus and found that CPV was able to traverse species barriers and rapidly adapt to new hosts, both in nature and in experimental studies. However, only a small number of nucleotide substitutions (fewer than 40 in total) became fixed or widespread throughout the entire evolution of this virus, with parallel evolution and reversion occurring on multiple occasions. Of the substitutions that are fixed or widespread, synonymous changes make up most within the viral non-structural gene (NS1), while most within VP2 are nonsynonymous and many influence host cell receptor binding and infection, mapping within or close to the footprint of the transferrin receptor or antibody binding sites.

We also examined capsid functions and show that the substitutions of residues on the exterior capsid surface altered the binding affinity between the capsid and the transferrin receptor type 1 (TfR). Some altered host range and others allowed uptake into cells without infection, showing that specific interactions between the TfR and the capsid are required for infection. Some of the same mutations also altered antibody binding to the capsid, confirming that they changed the local surface structure. Other changes include a reduction in viral infectivity by 1000-fold or more involved residues inside the capsid structure. These included two cysteine residues and the structures surrounding them. One of these mutations, Cys270Ser, altered capsid stability and influenced a VP2 cleavage that occurs in ~10% of the major capsid proteins. These results confirm the complex nature of the parvovirus capsid and the process of infection of cells.

3.2. Comparative Analysis Reveals the Long-Term Co-Evolutionary History of Parvoviruses and Vertebrates

Matthew A. Campbell, Shannon Loncar, Robert Kotin and *Robert J. Gifford*

Parvoviruses (family *Parvoviridae*) are small DNA viruses that cause numerous diseases of medical, veterinary and agricultural significance and have important applications in gene and anticancer therapy. DNA sequences derived from ancient parvoviruses are common in animal genomes and the analysis of these endogenous parvoviral elements (EPVs) has demonstrated that the family, which includes twelve vertebrate-specific genera, arose in the distant evolutionary past. To date, however, such 'paleovirological' analysis has only provided glimpses into the biology of parvoviruses and their long-term evolutionary interactions with hosts. In this paper, we comprehensively map EPV diversity in 752 published vertebrate genomes, revealing the defining aspects of ecology and evolution within individual parvovirus genera. We identified 364 distinct EPV sequences and show that these represent ~200 unique germline incorporation events, involving at least five distinct parvovirus genera, which took place at points throughout the Cenozoic Era. We used the spatiotemporal and host range calibrations provided by these sequences to infer defining aspects of long-term evolution within individual parvovirus genera, including mammalian vicariance for the genus *Protoparvovirus* and inter-class transmission for the genus *Dependoparvovirus*. Moreover, our findings support a model of virus evolution in which the long-term co-circulation of multiple parvovirus genera in vertebrates reflects the adaptation of each viral genus to fill a distinct ecological niche. Our discovery that parvovirus diversity can be understood in terms of genus-specific adaptations acquired over millions of years has important implications for their development as therapeutic tools—we show that these endeavors can be approached from a rational foundation based on comparative evolutionary analysis. To support this, we published our data in the form of an open, extensible and cross-platform database designed to facilitate the wider utilization of evolution-related domain knowledge in parvovirus research.

3.3. Odegus 4 Is an Endogenous Parvoviral Element with Antiviral Function

Angelica Bravo, Leandro Fernandez, Rodrigo Ibarra-Karmy, Robert J. Gifford and *Gloria Arriagada*

Endogenous viral elements (EVEs) are viral-derived DNA sequences present in the genome of extant species, where an endogenous parvoviral element (EPV) represents an ancestral parvoviral infection in a host germ line. Some of their EVEs possess open reading frames (ORFs) that can express proteins with physiological roles in their host. Furthermore, it has been described that some EVEs exhibit a protective role against exogenous viral infection in their host, but no EPV has been to date associated with this function. Previously, our laboratory demonstrated that an EPV is transcribed in the liver of *Octodon degus* (degu). This EPV, named Odegus4, contains an intact ORF that possess the Rep protein domain of depend-parvovirus. We also demonstrated that, in cell lines transfected with a plasmid that encodes Odegus4, it has nuclear localization. These characteristics lead us to propose that Odegus4 may function as a cellular coopted protein in degu.

We assess whether Odegus4 is protein with an antiviral role against exogenous parvovirus. We cloned the 1527bp sequence of OD4 into bacterial and eukaryotic expression vectors. Using bacterially produced proteins, we obtained polyclonal antibodies that specifically recognize OD4 over other EPVs in Western blot. Using these antibodies, we detected the presence of OD4 protein in degu tissues. To test if Odegus4 could protect against exogenous parvovirus, the minute virus of mice (MVM), a model of autonomous parvovirus, was generated in cells expressing Odegus4 or the control, resulting in a less effective viral infectivity when Odegus4 was present. We also consider if, in cells, the expression of Odegus4 MVM infection was impaired. For this, we transfected cells with Odegus4-encoding plasmids or an empty vector, synchronized them and infected them with MVM. We observed that MVM protein expression, DNA damage induced by replication, viral DNA and cytopathic effect were reduced when Odegus4 was present. Our results show that Odegus4 is expressed as a protein in its host and show, for the first time, that an EPV has a protective role against the extant parvovirus.

3.4. Capsid Structures of Aleutian Mink Disease Virus and Human Parvovirus 4: Adding New Faces to the Family Portrait

Mario Mietzsch, Renuk Lakshmanan, Alberto Jimenez Ybargollin, Paul Chipman, Xiaofeng Fu, Jianming Qiu, Maria Söderlund-Venermo, Robert McKenna and *Mavis Agbandje-McKenna*

Parvoviruses are ssDNA viruses with small, non-enveloped capsids with T = 1 icosahedral symmetry. Determining the capsid structures provides a framework to annotate regions important to the viral life cycle. However, to date, the capsid structures have been determined for only four of the ten *Parvovirinae* genera. Aleutian mink disease virus (AMDV), a pathogen of minks, and human parvovirus 4 (PARV4) infecting humans are parvoviruses belonging to the genera *Amdoparvovirus* and *Tetraparvovirus*, respectively. While Aleutian mink disease caused by AMDV is a major threat to mink farming, resulting in significant economic losses, no clear clinical manifestations have been established following an infection with PARV4 in humans. For both genera *Amdoparvovirus* and *Tetraparvovirus*, no capsid structures have been determined to date. We present the capsid structures of AMDV and PARV4 determined by cryo-electron microscopy and 3D image reconstruction with ~3 Å resolution. Despite the low amino acid sequence identity (10–30%) with parvoviruses of other genera, both viruses share common features previously observed with other parvoviruses, such as depressions at the icosahedral 2-fold axes and surrounding the 5-fold symmetry axes, protrusions surrounding the 3-fold axes and a channel at the 5-fold axes. However, both AMDV and PARV4 display major structural variabilities in the surface loops when the capsid structures are superposed onto other parvoviruses. Of note, AMDV possesses the largest major viral protein (VP) with 647 amino acids compared to known parvovirus capsid structures (including PARV4), in the range of ~530–590 amino acids. These additional amino acids may compensate for AMDV's very short VP1u region, which also lacks a phospholipase A2 (PLA_2) domain and results in large insertions in the majority of the surface loops of the capsid. The capsid structures of AMDV and PARV4 will add to our current knowledge of the structural platform for parvoviruses and permit the future functional annotation of these pathogens, which will help to understand their disease mechanisms at a molecular level towards the development of therapeutics.

4. Session 2: Receptors

4.1. Receptor and Antibody Interactions with AAV by Cryo-EM/ET

Guiqing Hu, Mark Silveria, Edward Large, Nancy Meyer, Grant Zane, Scott Stagg and *Michael S. Chapman*

Most AAV serotypes are dependent on the transmembrane AAV Receptor (AAVR) for endosomal cell entry. Cryo-electron microscopy (cryo-EM) at up to a 2.5 Å resolution reveals interactions of several serotypes with the most strongly bound domain. Intriguingly, AAV5 and the related AAVGo.1 bind PKD1 at a site that is different from that where AAV2 and other viruses interact with PKD2. The epitopes of a dozen monoclonal antibodies have previously been mapped on several serotypes by cryo-EM. The mechanisms of neutralization were sometimes thought to involve interference with glycan attachment or a post-entry step. There is, however, a stronger spatial correlation between neutralizing epitopes and the respective AAVR binding sites than what would be expected if neutralization was conducted by the inhibition of AAVR binding. Upon the re-examination of an exemplary AAV5 antibody, competitive binding inhibition was confirmed in vitro. Although only single domains of AAVR were seen in the high-resolution structures of the complexes, PKD1 has an accessory role (to PKD2) in the interactions of AAV2. The complexes of AAV2 and AAV5 with two-domain fragments of AAVR (PKD12) were examined by cryo-electron tomography (ET) to locate the domains "missing" at a high resolution. Each is in several different configurations extending away without significant interactions at the AAV surface.

Cryo-EM maps of AAV5-PKD12 complexes are low-pass-filtered to reveal a less-ordered structure, including strands of polypeptide adjacent to PKD1 near the AAV5 surface. Side chains are insufficiently ordered for sequence identification, but it is plausible that the peptide is a fragment of either another AAVR subunit or part of the N-terminal region of the AAV capsid protein. The cryo-ET of the AAV2-PKD12 complex shows partially ordered features on the inner surface near the 2-fold axis. Corresponding features have previously been interpreted as the N-terminal region of capsid proteins. The feature is present when βA is weak in high-resolution cryo-EM maps, and this varies among samples of AAV2 complexed with AAVR, but not AAV5. There appears to be a finely balanced conformational equilibrium, perhaps explaining why it has been difficult to rationalize such features in past structures.

4.2. *Characterization of Glycan Binding by AAV44.9, a Member of the New AAV Clade*

G. Di Pasquale, S. Afione, M. Khalaj, C. Zheng, B. Grewe and *J.A. Chiorini*

The recent isolation of novel AAV serotypes has led to significant advances in our understanding of parvovirus biology and vector development for gene therapy by identifying vectors with unique cell tropism and increased efficiency of gene transfer to target cells. AAV44.9 is a natural isolate originally found as a contaminate of the laboratory stock of SV15 adenovirus. Its sequence homology places it between current clades in a small cluster with Rh.8R. Recent studies have suggested that AAV44.9 is a promising candidate for photoreceptor-targeted gene therapies and other tissues. To better understand its activity, we used glycan arrays and competition experiments to define its binding as primarily interacting with glucose or glucosamine on N-linked cell-surface carbohydrates. Mutagenesis experiments were conducted to identified the amino acids responsible for glycan recognition and specificity.

4.3. *Human Parvovirus B19 Infection: A Tale of Two Receptors*

Jan Bieri, Cornelia Bircher, Ruben Assaraf, Remo Leisi and *Carlos Ros*

Parvovirus B19 (B19V) is a human pathogen with a marked tropism for erythroid progenitor cells (EPCs) in the bone marrow. The N-terminal of the VP1 unique region (VP1u) of B19V and related non-human primate erythroparvoviruses contains a receptor-binding domain (RBD). The VP1u RBD mediates virus uptake in EPCs through interaction with an as-yet-unknown receptor, VP1uR. By using a phage-RBD construct, the expression profile of VP1uR was quantitatively analyzed in multiple cell types. The results confirm the exclusive association of VP1uR with cells of erythroid lineage. In contrast to VP1uR, globoside is ubiquitously expressed, and although it is not required for virus uptake, it has an essential role at a post-entry step by facilitating endosomal escape. We found that pH modulates the affinity between the two receptors. At an acidic pH, the affinity for VP1uR decreases and increases for globoside, which allows for the interaction to occur in acidic endosomes. The finding that B19V affinity for VP1uR and globoside is tightly controlled by the pH has major consequences on the overall virus infection. Under the neutral pH conditions of the extracellular milieu, B19V does not interact with globoside. This strategy prevents the redirection of the virus to nonpermissive cells, promoting the selective targeting of the EPCs. However, considering the ubiquitous expression of Gb4, naturally occurring acidic niches become potential targets for the virus.

4.4. Globoside and the Mucosal pH Mediate Parvovirus B19 Entry through the Airway Epithelium

Corinne Suter, *Minela Colakovic*, *Jan Bieri*, *Mitra Gultom*, *Ronald Dijkman* and *Carlos Ros*

The mechanism of entry of parvovirus B19 (B19V) via the respiratory route is unknown. B19V targets the VP1u cognate receptor expressed exclusively on permissive erythroid progenitors in the bone marrow. Following uptake, B19V shifts the receptor in the acidic endosomes and targets globoside, which is required for infectious trafficking. The pH-dependent interaction with globoside may allow virus entry through the naturally acidic nasal mucosa. To test this hypothesis, human airway epithelial cells (hAECs) and polarized monolayers of MDCK II cells were grown on transwell membranes and used as barrier models to study the interaction and transport of viral particles across the airway epithelium. Globoside expression was detected in the ciliated population of hAECs and, under the acidic conditions of the nasal mucosa, B19V was transported to the basolateral side by transcytosis without signs of productive infection. Similarly, MDCK II cells express globoside and support virus transcytosis in a time- and pH-dependent manner. Neither virus attachment nor transcytosis were observed in wild-type cells under neutral pH conditions or in globoside knockout MDCK II cells, demonstrating the direct role of globoside and an acidic pH in the process. Globoside-dependent virus uptake occurred by clathrin-independent, dynamin-, cholesterol- and caveolae-dependent mechanisms and was inhibited by specific antibodies derived from infected individuals. This study provides the first mechanistic insight into the transmission of B19V through the respiratory route and reveals novel vulnerability factors of the airway barrier to viruses.

4.5. Viral Capsid, Antibody and Receptor Interactions: Understanding the Binding, Neutralization, Antibody Escape and Receptor Binding Sites of Canine Parvovirus

Robert A. López-Astacio, *Daniel J. Goetschius*, *Hyunwook Lee*, *Wendy S. Weichert*, *Oluwafemi Adu*, *Brynn K. Alford*, *Ian E.H. Voorhees*, *Sarah Saddoris*, *Laura B. Goodman*, *Edward C. Holmes*, *Susan L. Hafenstein* and *Colin R. Parrish**

Viruses circulating in nature evolve and frequently emerge as new variants due to evolutionary forces that can result from mutation and selection—including key interactions with receptors and antibodies. We study the evolution of canine parvovirus (CPV) incubated with neutralizing antibodies to reveal how they are controlled by the dynamics of binding, neutralization, antibody escape and overlap with the receptor binding site. CPV is a non-enveloped virus with a single-stranded DNA genome, and it causes serious disease in animals worldwide. The original strain (CPV-2) emerged as a new dog pathogen during the late 1970s due to a host jumping event. The subsequent natural evolution of the virus in dogs and other hosts has altered both receptor and antibody binding, with some single changes affecting both functions. Our study reveals that only a small number of mutations arise within the viral capsid (VP2) under the in vitro selection with each of two neutralizing antibodies, which bind distinct sites on the capsid and show the different levels of overlap with the transferrin receptor (TfR) attachment site. Mutations occurred primarily within the antibody footprints, and few changes occurred in the TfR-binding footprint. Remarkably, 54% of the antibody-selected mutations identified were also present in natural circulating variants, showing the connections between our in vitro study and natural infection and also the potential for the emergence of variants in nature due the host humoral immune response. To understand escape mutation dynamics, we also engineered the capsid-binding sites of the two antibodies. The in vitro selection experiments with the engineered antibodies also showed similar mutations to those selected by the wild-type, despite the alternative interactions with the capsid. This study suggests the potential mechanisms by which these variants emerged in nature and provides a better understanding of the coordinated interactions between antibodies and receptors.

5. Session 3: Replication

5.1. Cryo-EM Structure of the Rep68-AAVS1 Complex

R. Jaiswal, V. Santosh and *C.R. Escalante*

Adeno-associated virus (AAV) is the only known eukaryotic virus with the property of establishing latency by integrating site-specifically into the human genome. The integration site known as AAVS1 is located in chromosome 19 and contains multiple GCTC repeats that are recognized by the AAV non-structural Rep proteins. These proteins are multifunctional, with an N-terminal origin-binding domain (OBD) and a helicase domain (HD) joined together by a short linker. In a previous work using analytical ultracentrifugation, we showed that Rep68 binds to AAVS1, forming a heptameric complex. We report the cryo-EM structures of Rep68 bound to a 50 bp AAVS1 fragment in the apo and ATPγS states. The structure shows that, indeed, Rep68 forms a heptameric ring encircling the DNA. In the apo state, most of the contacts are made by the small oligomerization domain. In addition, three of the seven OBDs remain engaged to the RBS sites. Of the remaining four OBDs, we observed three OBDs forming a dimer with each of the DNA-bound OBDs. Upon binding ATPγS, the helicase heptameric ring closes upon the DNA, where three HDs make backbone DNA interactions. We hypothesize that cycles of ATP hydrolysis and the opening and closing of the helicase ring may cause enough distortions to induce the melting of DNA.

5.2. Insights into the ITR Melting Mechanism: Cryo-EM Structure of the Rep68–ITR Complex

R. Jaiswal, V. Santosh, A. Washington, B. Braud and *C.R. Escalante*

The AAV origin of replication consist of three motifs, the Rep binding site (RBS), the terminal resolution site (TRS) and the hairpin Rep binding element (RBE′). During DNA replication, AAV Rep proteins bind to the RBS to perform a site- and strand-specific endonuclease reaction at the TRS that is required to complete the DNA replication of the 3′ hairpin end. A pre-requisite of the nicking reaction is a DNA-melting step using the motor activity of the Rep proteins. To understand the molecular events leading to the melting of DNA, we determined the structure of Rep68 in a complex with AAV-2 ITR. The structure shows that Rep68 forms a heptameric complex in a similar way to the Rep68–AAVS1 complex. The ITR molecule acquires a conformation where two of the arms stacked coaxially and the RBE′ arm protrudes in an antiparallel orientation. The complex shows that one of the OBD molecules interacts with both the RBE′ tip and the RBS at the same time. The structure also shows several residues in the helicase domain that are critical for DNA melting. Taken together, our structure provides insights into how Rep proteins melt the ITRs.

5.3. AAV2 Can Replicate Its DNA by a Rolling Hairpin or Rolling Circle Mechanism, Depending on the Helper Virus

Anouk Lkharrazi, Kurt Tobler, Anita Meie, Bernd Vogt and *Cornel Fraefel*

Adeno-associated virus type 2 (AAV2) is a small, non-pathogenic, helper virus-dependent parvovirus with a single-stranded (ss) DNA genome of approximately 4.7 kb. AAV2 DNA replication requires the presence of a helper virus, such as adenovirus type 5 (AdV5) or herpes simplex virus type 1 (HSV-1), and is generally assumed to occur as a strand-displacement rolling hairpin (RHR) mechanism initiated at the AAV2 3′ inverted terminal repeat (ITR) end. We recently showed that AAV2 replication supported by HSV-1 leads to the formation of double-stranded head-to-tail concatemers, which provides evidence for a rolling circle replication (RCR) mechanism (Meier et al., 2021; doi: 10.1371/journal.ppat.10096389). Using Southern analysis and high-throughput sequencing (Nanopore and PacBio sequencing), we revisit AAV2 DNA replication and specifically compare the formation of AAV2 replication intermediates in the presence of either HSV-1 or AdV5 as the helper virus. The results confirm that the AAV2 DNA replication mechanism is helper-virus-dependent and follows a strand-displacement RHR mechanism, when AdV5 is the helper virus, and primarily an RCR mechanism when HSV-1 is the helper virus. In addition to the monomeric and multimeric products of the AAV2 genome, a considerable fraction of ITR repeats was observed, particularly in the presence of AdV5.

5.4. Consequence and Mechanism of Chk1 Inactivation by MVM during Its Infection

Igor Etingov and David Pintel

We and others have shown that minute virus of mice (MVM) infection causes significant damage to cellular DNA and is accompanied by, and exploits, a DNA damage response (DDR). Viral replication centers are localized in the vicinity of cellular DNA damage sites, which attract numerous factors required for viral expression and replication. The infection-induced DDR is transduced by the ATM kinase, while the ATR kinase is inactivated. During infection, the major cell cycle regulator kinase Chk1, a target of ATR, is not phosphorylated at position S345, which inhibits the activation of its G2/M checkpoint function, despite an ongoing DDR and the presence of RPA-coated viral single-stranded DNA. Chk1 is also involved in additional cellular processes, including the homologous recombination repair (HRR) of DNA, and the phosphorylation of the essential HRR factor RAD51.

We investigate the significance of Chk1 inactivation for MVM replication as well as the mechanism involved in the inhibition of Chk1 phosphorylation upon infection. Using comet assays to assess cellular DNA damage levels and fluorescent reporter constructs to estimate HRR efficiency upon the infection, combined with the overexpression of constitutively active Chk1, we demonstrate that the MVM-induced inactivation of Chk1 significantly reduced the cellular ability to repair its DNA, which facilitates increased levels of viral DNA replication. ATR is known to be recruited to RPA-covered single-stranded DNA fragments in assemblage with its auxiliary factors TopBP1 and the Rad9–Rad1–Hus1 (9-1-1) complex, which are also required for ATR activation and its ability to phosphorylate Chk1. The overexpression of the TopBP1 ATR activation domain (AAD) successfully activated ATR upon infection, demonstrating that MVM incapacitates TopBP1′s ability to support ATR functionality. TopBP1 is known to associate with Rad9, and the phosphorylation of Rad9 at S387 is needed for its capacity to activate ATR. We show that MVM NS1 significantly reduced this phosphorylation, thus identifying a critical role in the prevention of phosphorylation (and thus activation) of Chk1 at S353. The known NS1 association with the casein kinase II α (CKIIα) domain and the possible recruitment of phosphatase PP2C by the NS1–CKIIα complex appeared to be required for the inhibition of Rad9 S387 phosphorylation.

5.5. The Autonomous Parvovirus Minute Virus of Mice Localizes to the Cellular Sites of DNA Damage Using Its Non-Structural Protein NS1

Lauren Bunke, MegAnn Haubold, Clairine Larsen, Rhiannon Abrahams, Sarah Rubin, Isabella Jones, Jessica Pita Aquino and Kinjal Majumder

Minute virus of mice (MVM) is an autonomously replicating parvovirus that is lytic in murine cells and transformed human cells, causing a pre-mitotic cell cycle arrest during which the virus replicates. MVM replicates in nuclear replication centers termed autonomous parvovirus-associated replication (APAR) bodies, rich in factors necessary for virus replication and expression, as well as multiple DNA damage response (DDR) proteins. MVM infection induces ATM-dependent and ATR-independent cellular DDRs. Strikingly, super-resolution imaging and chromatin immunoprecipitation (ChIP) assays revealed that only a subset of cellular DDR proteins, such as MRE11, associates directly with the MVM genome, whereas downstream DDR markers, such as gamma H2AX, surround APAR bodies, likely marking damaged cellular genomic sites. Using chromosome conformation capture assays in trans, we identified the cellular sites of direct interaction between the linear MVM genome and the cellular chromosome, demonstrating that, rather than recruiting DDR proteins to APAR bodies de novo, MVM genomes localize to genomic sites that are abundant in DDR proteins. Some of these cellular DDR sites are fragile sites where oncogenic viruses, such as HPV, localize. These genomic regions are packaged into spatially distinct topologically associating domains (TADs), which also colocalize with accessible Type A chromatin.

Ectopically expressed MVM-NS1 associates with cellular DDR sites at fragile genomic regions. Interestingly, NS1 bound to the MVM genome is essential for the viral genome to localize to cellular genomic DDR sites to jumpstart its replication. NS1 bound to heterologous DNA molecules containing NS1 consensus-binding elements are sufficient to transport DNA molecules to cellular DDR sites, suggesting a novel transport function for MVM-NS1. MVM initiates infection in the early S-phase, inducing additional cellular DNA damage as it amplifies. Using single-molecule DNA fiber assays, we discovered that cellular replication stress is induced prior to the initiation of virus replication. The presence of non-replicating MVM genome in the nucleus is sufficient to induce the shortening of host replication fibers, suggesting the viral genome perturbs cellular DDR pathways prior to the start of replication, implicating the single-stranded viral genome in the induction of cellular replication stress.

5.6. *Carnivore Bocaparvovirus 1 (Minute Virus of Canines) NP1 Modulates Viral Alternative RNA Processing*

Lisa Uhl, Yaming Dong, David J. Pintel and *Olufemi Fasina*

Post-transcriptional mRNA regulation is a critical cellular homeostatic node often hijacked by viruses for a productive life cycle and, at present, is utilized for the design and development of severe acute respiratory coronavirus 2 (SARS-CoV-2) vaccines. Parvoviruses are linear single-stranded DNA viruses and use extensive RNA processing strategies to maximize their coding capacity. This provides an excellent tractable model to elucidate viral RNA processing mechanisms and host interactions geared toward the development of efficient parvovirus gene therapy and oncolytic virotherapy. Carnivore bocaparvovirus 1 (minute virus of canines, MVC) is an autonomous parvovirus in the Bocaparvovirus genus. It has a single promoter that generates a single pre-mRNA that is processed via alternative splicing and alternative polyadenylation to generate at least eight mRNA transcripts. MVC contains two polyadenylation sites, one at the right-hand end (pA)d and another (pA)p that lies within the capsid-coding region. Our previous results showed that the parvovirus non-structural protein NP1 modulates alternative splicing and alternative polyadenylation for efficient capsid production. The mass spectrometry analysis of NP1 interactome revealed a potential interaction with RNA-processing proteins, DNA damage response proteins and chromatin-remodeling proteins. We present the current data addressing the NP1 protein features and potential mechanisms utilized to modulate the alternative processing of MVC RNA. In addition, we address its potential role in nuclear domain reorganization, enabling the formation of nuclear compartments viral RNA processing and viral genome replication. NP1 is the first parvovirus protein implicated in RNA processing, and its discovery provides an excellent model to understand the dynamics and complex regulation of viral RNA processing and viral genome replication in an excellent tractable system.

5.7. *A Functional Minigenome of Parvovirus B19*

Alessandro Reggiani, Erika Fasano, Gloria Bua, Elisabetta Manaresi and *Giorgio Gallinella*

Parvovirus B19 (B19V) is a human pathogenic virus of clinical relevance, characterized by a selective tropism for erythroid progenitor cells in the bone marrow. The study of viral characteristics and lifecycle has always been limited by the availability of just two cellular systems able to support viral replication, the UT7/EpoS1 cell line and PBMC-derived EPCs, and by the difficulties in obtaining high-titer viral replication, hence the need to use patient-derived sera as the viral stock. Relevant information can thus be obtained from experiments involving engineered genetic systems in appropriate in vitro cellular models. Recently, a new model was developed in our laboratory: a genotype 1a consensus sequence was used to generate a genomic clone, named CK, which can replicate in vitro after the nucleofection of UT7/EpoS1 cells and lead to an infectious viral progeny that can be propagated by infecting EPCs, thus reducing the need of clinical samples and improve the manageability of B19V model systems.

In this project, with the dual aim of testing the plasticity of the B19V genome to rearrangements and focusing our attention on the NS1 protein, we design and produce a derived B19V minigenome reduced to a replicon unit. The genome terminal regions were maintained in a form able to sustain viral replication, while the internal region was modified by the deletion of the right-hand half of the internal region and the generation of a new cleavage-polyadenylation site, thus maintaining the coding sequence for the functional NS1 protein. Following transfection in UT7/EpoS1 cells, this minigenome still proved competent for the replication, transcription and production of NS1 protein. Furthermore, the B19V minigenome was able to complement B19-derived, NS1-defective genomes, restoring their ability to express viral capsid proteins. The B19V genome was thus engineered to yield a two-component system with complementing functions, providing a proof of concept of B19V genome-editing possibilities and, at the same time, a useful tool to study the NS1 protein also as an antiviral target.

6. Session 4: Trafficking

6.1. Review Lecture: Nuclear Entry and Egress of Parvoviruses

Maija Vihinen-Ranta

After the endosomal low-pH-induced exposure of the nuclear localization sequence on the capsid surface and escaping into the cytosol, parvovirus capsids are destined to enter the nucleus. Due to the small capsid diameter of 18–26 nm, intact capsids are imported actively to the nucleus through nuclear pore complexes (NPCs). Capsids may also use an alternative NPC-independent nuclear entry pathway that includes the activation of mitosis and the disruption of the nuclear envelope. Once the viral genome is released in the nucleus, viral replication compartments are initiated and the infection proceeds. The viral genome is replicated during the cellular S-phase followed by capsid assembly during virus-induced G2/M cell cycle arrest. The active nuclear egress of progeny capsids through the NPC is mediated by the chromosome region maintenance 1 protein, CRM1, and is enhanced by the phosphorylation of the N-terminal domain of VP2. Alternatively, capsid exit from the nucleus is facilitated by virus-induced transition to mitosis and apoptosis, which leads to an increase in NE permeability.

6.2. A Classical cNLS Is Responsible for the Importin α/β-Dependent Nuclear Transport of Human Parvovirus B19 Non-Structural Protein 1

Gualtiero Alvisi, Elisabetta Manaresi, Emily M. Cross, Nasim Akbari, Gayle F. Petersen, Roberto Garuti, Jade Forwood and *Giorgio Gallinella*

Human parvovirus B19 (B19V) is a major human pathogen that causes a variety of diseases, ranging from fifth disease in children to pure red cell aplasia in immunocompromised individuals, and that is still in need of effective antiviral strategies. In similar fa ashion to all *Parvoviridae* members, the B19V small ssDNA genome is replicated within the nucleus of infected cells through a process that involves both cellular and viral proteins. Among the latter, a crucial role is played by the non-structural protein (NS)1, a multifunctional protein involved in genome replication and transcription, as well as the modulation of host gene expression. Despite the fact that NS1 can be visualized in the host cell nucleus during infection, its nuclear transport pathway and the nuclear localization signal (NLS) have not been characterized to date. In this study, we apply a combination of biochemical and imaging assays to demonstrate that NS1 is actively translocated in the cell nucleus by the importin (IMP) α/β heterodimer in an energy- and Ran-dependent process. Nuclear transport appears to be completely dependent on a short sequence of amino acids 172-GACHAKKPRIT-182, which binds IMPα with nanomolar affinity and confers active nuclear accumulation to GFP and, therefore, represents a classical (c)NLS. Interestingly, the K177T substitution completely abrogated IMPα binding and nuclear import. Furthermore, treatment with Ivermectin, an antiparasitic drug interfering with the IMP α/β-dependent nuclear import pathway, inhibited viral replication in infected UT7 cells. Thus, the NS1 nuclear transport emerges as a potential target of therapeutic intervention against B19V-induced disease.

6.3. Adeno-Associated Virus Type 2 (AAV2) Uncoating Is a Stepwise Process and Is Linked to the Structural Reorganization of the Nucleolus

Sereina O. Sutter, Anouk Lkharrazi, Elisabeth M. Schraner, Anita F. Meier, Kevin Michaelson, Hildegard Büning and *Cornel Fraefel*

Nucleoli are membrane-less nuclear structures formed by liquid–liquid phase separation and are known to be involved in many cellular functions, such as ribosomal RNA (rRNA) synthesis, ribosome biogenesis, stress response and cell cycle regulation. Many viruses can employ the nucleolus or nucleolar proteins to promote different steps of their life cycle, including replication, transcription and assembly. While adeno-associated virus type 2 (AAV2) capsids have previously been reported to enter the host cell nucleus and accumulate in the nucleolus, both the role of the nucleolus in AAV2 infection and the viral uncoating mechanism remain elusive. To elucidate the properties of the nucleolus during AAV2 infection and to assess viral uncoating at a single-cell level, we combined immunofluorescence analysis for the detection of intact AAV2 capsids and capsid proteins with fluorescence in situ hybridization for the detection of AAV2 genomes. The results of our experiments provide evidence that the uncoating of AAV2 particles occurs in a stepwise process that is completed in the nucleolus and supported by the alteration of the nucleolar structure.

6.4. The Phase-Separation Properties of the AAV2 Assembly-Activating Protein

Janine Vetter, Manuel Kley, Catherine Eichwald and *Cornel Fraefel*

Adeno-associated virus 2 (AAV2) is a helper-virus-dependent non-pathogenic Dependoparvovirus studied extensively due to its potential as a gene delivery vector. The 4.7 kb single-stranded DNA genome of AAV2 consists of two coding regions termed *rep* and *cap*, flanked by non-coding inverted terminal repeats. A +1 open reading frame within the *cap* gene encodes a non-structural protein of 204 amino acids named assembly-activating protein (AAP2), which has been attributed a critical role in transporting the viral capsid protein VP3 into the nucleolus for assembly. In the absence of other viral proteins, AAP2 localizes to the nucleolus due to five redundant nuclear and nucleolar localization signals. However, AAP2 remains poorly characterized because of its relatively late discovery and lack of commercial antibodies. Using AAP2 fusions to red or green fluorescent proteins, we assessed the liquid–liquid phase separation (LLPS) properties of AAP2 in transfected cells. Interestingly, AAP2 formed liquid-like condensates in a dose-dependent manner. Similar to other proteins that drive LLPS, fluorescence recovery after photobleaching (FRAP) revealed rapid turnover rates between AAP2-mKO condensates and the nuclear environment. Furthermore, we show that treatment with aliphatic diols, commonly used tools for the characterization of biomolecular condensates, led to the dissolution of AAP2 inclusions. Lastly, we observed AAP2 condensates in cells co-infected with AAV2 and HSV-1. Taken together, these data indicate that AAP2 confers liquid-like properties to viral compartments. However, the role of AAP2 LLPS properties in AAV2 replication remains to be elucidated.

7. Session 5: Virus–Host Interactions

7.1. Identification of Human Monoclonal Antibodies Potently Neutralizing Parvovirus B19

Davide Corti

Infection with Parvovirus B19 is associated with the common childhood disease erythema infectiosum, but also to more severe diseases, including hydrops fetalis, aplastic crises, polyarthralgia and pure red-cell aplasia. The current treatment for patients suffering from persistent B19 virus infection is the administration of high doses of human immunoglobulin preparations (IVIGs). We describe the isolation of a panel of

15 B19-specific monoclonal antibodies directed to multiple antigenic sites on VP1 and VP2. Two antibodies specific for VP1 and VP2 were selected for their neutralizing potency, which was found to be more than 1000-fold higher than IVIGs and mapped to two distinct sites on VP1 and VP2. A cocktail of these two antibodies may represent the basis to develop a novel therapeutic to treat severe B19 infections.

7.2. Enhanced Detection and Production of Parvovirus B19V Depends on the Cell Cycle Status of Erythroid Cells

Zahra Kadri, Amandine Langelé, Bruno You, Céline Ducloux, Olivier Goupille, Emmanuel Payen and *Stany Chrétien*

Human parvovirus B19 (B19V) causes diseases with severities ranging from benign childhood illness to arthropathies, severe anemia or hydrops fetalis, depending on the age, health and hematological status of the patients. Although the propagation of the virus is air-borne or vertical, blood-borne transmission remains possible, especially by the use of labile products. To assess the presence of B19V, the detection of B19V DNA is performed in plasma pools and at each step of the preparation of labile products. However, the detection of B19 nucleic acid does not predict B19V infectivity. Thus, at present, infectious titration systems using animal parvoviruses are used to evaluate the efficacy of inactivation/reduction steps during plasma processing, even though they imperfectly reflect human B19V infectivity. These methods have thus to be revised. Human cell lines permissive to B19V are available (e.g., UT7/Epo-S1), but substantial modifications are required to enable them to detect the presence of viruses and to produce large amounts of infectious viral particles.

We report the improvement of the detection of B19 infectious particles through the quantification of VP1/2 RNA expression and the evaluation of B19 infectious particles' production in selected permissive cells. Of all our tested erythroid cell lines, our UT7/Epo cells (named UT7/Epo-STI) showed the highest sensitivity to B19 infection. We generated stable sub-clones of it and selected those with the highest permissiveness for B19V. Using the FUCCI (fluorescent ubiquitination cell cycle indicator) expression system, we show the direct correlation between infectivity and the cell cycle status of the cells. RNA sequencing showed that new cell lines were significantly different from the previously established UT7/Epo-S1 reference cell clone. The two sub-clones UT7/Epo-B12 and UT7/Epo-E2 had B19V detection and B19 infectious unit production capacities comparable to those obtained with $CD36^+$ primary erythroid progenitor cells, the natural host cells for B19V, and 35-fold higher capacity than the UT7/Epo-S1 cell line. Indeed, 96 h after the inoculation of UT7/Epo-E2 cells by B19V, up to 10^9 genome equivalent/mL of supernatant were obtained and the B19 infectious units' production reached more than 10^4 $TCID_{50}$/mL, a level comparable to that obtained with $CD36^+$ cells.

7.3. Rodent Protoparvoviruses MVMp and H-1PV Are Master Regulators of the Host Antiviral Innate Immune Response

Assia Angelova, Annabel Grewenig, Estelle Santiago, Jürg Nüesch, Jean Rommelaere and *Laurent Daeffler*

Oncolytic rodent protoparvoviruses (PVs) MVMp and H-1PV are considered attractive candidates for cancer therapy since, in addition to exhibiting oncolytic activity, they also drive some anticancer immune responses (AIRs). The production of type-I interferons (IFN) is considered instrumental for the activation of an efficient AIR by immunotherapies. Viruses can achieve IFN production in their host through the detection of viral factors (pathogen-associated molecular patterns, PAMPs) by the cellular receptors (pattern recognition receptors, PRRs) of the antiviral innate machinery. PVs were shown to induce IFN production in normal (mouse embryonic fibroblasts (MEFs) and human peripheral blood mononuclear cells (PBMCs)), but not in transformed/tumor cells, a feature that may therefore limit their immunostimulatory and oncosuppressive potential. The present study shows that the IFN production triggered by MVMp in MEFs requires some level of PV replication. We prove, moreover, that the PV infections of normal but also transformed/tumor cells activate the PRR pathway and that they also produce molecules that have the potential to behave as PRR ligands (PAMPs). Taken together, our data indicate that replicative PV infections are sensed by the innate immune machinery of their hosts, but that a mechanism is triggered by the virus, specifically in neoplastic cells, to prevent IFN production (evasion mechanism). In agreement with this hypothesis, we observed that the pre-infection of transformed/tumor but not normal cells with MVMp or H-1PV prevent a further IFN production triggered by classical PRR ligands, including Poly(I:C) and Newcastle disease virus (NDV). Altogether, we believe that our results will pave the way for the development of second-generation mutant PVs, devoid of this evasion mechanism and endowed, therefore, with an increased immunostimulatory potential through their ability to induce IFN production in infected malignant cells.

7.4. Parvovirus Infection Alters the Nucleolar Structure

Salla Mattola, Simon Leclerc, Satu Hakanen, Vesa Aho, Colin R. Parrish and *Maija Vihinen-Ranta*

The nucleolus is a dynamic nuclear structure that plays important roles in ribosome biogenesis and cellular stress response to stressors, such as viral infections. The nucleolus and nucleolar proteins are essential for the progression of infection by several viruses. Consequently, viral infection often induces alterations in the nucleolar structure and composition. We apply a deep learning algorithm segmentation and nucleolin labeling to analyze the nucleolar changes induced by autonomous parvovirus infection. Our results show that the size of nucleoli decreases and nucleolin is released into the nucleoplasm in late infection. The analysis of ki-67, one of the NS2-associated nucleolar proteins and a key factor in nucleolar organization, showed that the interaction between ki-67 and the DNA increases during infection. The infection initiated by a viral clone lacking an intact NS2 failed to decrease the nucleolar size; however, the orientation of the nucleoli changed. Our results suggest that parvoviruses modify and exploit nucleoli and nucleolar proteins during infection, and NS2 protein might play a role in the regulation of these processes

7.5. Parvovirus Non-Structural Protein 2 Associates with Chromatin-Regulating Proteins

Salla Mattola, Kari Salokas, Vesa Aho, Elina Mäntylä, Sami Salminen, Satu Hakanen, Colin R. Parrish, Markku Varjosalo and *Maija Vihinen-Ranta*

Autonomic parvoviruses encode only a limited number of proteins, making them highly dependent on the functions provided by the host cell. While the non-structural protein 1 is linked to critical nuclear processes required for viral replication, considerably less is known about the role of the non-structural protein 2 (NS2). Specifically, the function of canine parvovirus (CPV) NS2 remains undefined. We used mass spectrometry-based proximity-dependent biotin identification (BioID) to identify the proteins associated with nuclear CPV NS2. Most of the identified proteins were observed in both noninfected and infected cells. However, the location of the interacting proteins shifted from nuclear envelope proteins to chromatin-associated proteins in the infected cells. BioID high-confidence interactions revealed a potential role for NS2 in DNA remodeling and damage response. Further protein–protein interaction analysis by a proximity ligation assay confirmed the nuclear interactions of NS2 with selected key proteins identified by the BioID analysis. Mutations to the NS2 splice donor and acceptor sites affected chromatin organization and DDR-related proteins in infection. Additionally, the mutation of the NS2 splice donor site led to the deficient formation of replication centers. Our findings suggest that CPV NS2 has previously undiscovered roles in the interplay with cellular machinery regulating chromatin functions, replication center formation and DNA damage.

8. Session 6: AAV and Viral Vectors

8.1. Detection of AAV2 in Living Cells

Luisa F. Bustamante-Jaramillo, Josh Fingall and Michael Kann

AAVs are non-pathogenic members of the *Parvovirus* family used in gene therapy. They are mostly applied as self-complementary double-stranded vectors allowing to bypass the wild-type AAVs' requirement of co-infection by a helper virus (herpes or adenovirus). Despite of their use as EMA- and FDA-accredited drugs, their application is hampered by their poor capacity to transduce cells and doses of 10^{13} particles per kg have to be administered. This limitation led us to search for factors restricting scAAV infection with the goal of improving gene therapy, focusing on the poorly understood steps of viral entry and viral genome release. In order to visualize the genomes released from the viral capsid, we used the so-called anchor system, which is based on the accumulation of >400 exogenously expressed fusion proteins, named OR-EGFP, on a double-stranded DNA seed sequence, allowing to detect single DNA sequences by time-lapse microscopy. EGFP-OR binding is dynamic, with a half-life of 52 s, allowing the expression of flanking genes. In our system, we inserted the anchor sequence flanked by m-Cherry ORF under the control of the P_{CMV} promotor into the AAV2 genome. As the dynamic binding of OR-EGFP to the anchor sequence allows the restoration of bleached fluorescent OR-EGFP, we followed the isolated capsid-released scAAV2 genomes and m-Cherry expression for 48 h in real time after the transduction of OR-EGFP-expressing cells. Using this approach, we obtained the kinetics of genome release and protein expression in single cells, also allowing investigations on the cellular factors involved in genome release by using inhibitors, such as e.g., Thapsigargin, that inhibit calcium accumulation in the ER and D-I03, thus blocking Rad52.

8.2. Whole-Genome siRNA and microRNA High-Throughput Screenings to Identify the Molecular Determinants That Govern AAV Vector Transduction

Lorena Zentilin, Edoardo Schneider, Ambra Cappelletto and Mauro Giacca

Adeno-associated viral vectors (AAVs) have emerged as leading gene delivery vectors to treat various inherited, degenerative or acquired conditions. However, despite the patent efficacy of AAV vectors in transducing several tissues in vivo and in vitro, incomplete information is available on the molecular determinants of AAV tissue permissivity.

We previously observed that the host cell DNA damage response machinery and, in particular, the proteins involved in double-stranded DNA break repair (DSB) (including the Mre11–Rad50–Nbs1–MRN complex) interact and negatively regulate incoming AAV genome processing. To systematically identify the host cell factors involved in internalization, intracellular trafficking, the processing of AAV genomes and, eventually, AAV gene expression, either positively or negatively, we previously performed a high-throughput screening using a genome-wide siRNA library (over 18,000 genes were analyzed; Mano et al. PNAS 2015). We also performed a high-throughput screening using a genome-wide library of human microRNA mimics (988 mature sequences, miRBase 13—Dharmacon) in AAV2 Luciferase-transduced HeLa cells. Using this approach, we found that 51 microRNA mimics increased AAV transduction more than 4-fold (up to 23-fold change), while 26 microRNA mimics significantly decreased AAV efficiency.

Hsa-miR-329 and hsa-miR-362-3p, which share the same seed sequence, were identified as the most effective microRNAs when increasing AAV transduction in HeLa cells. However, we also observed that the extent of the effects of the miRNAs on AAV transduction is dependent on the cell line tested, underlining the complexity of the vector–cell interaction. Transcriptomic analysis on the total RNA extracted from HeLa cells transfected with the three miRNAs identified several hundred transcripts that were significantly downregulated. The direct comparison of these results with those obtained from the whole-genome siRNA screening revealed the involvement of proteins that interfere with virus endocytosis or nuclear import or act in intrinsic cellular defense mechanisms. We are confident that a better understanding of the mechanisms of action of the identified genes and RNAs will open the possibility of developing antisense or RNAi-based RNA treatments to improve in vivo AAV vector transduction.

8.3. From AAV Virus to AAV Vectors: Characterization of a Collection of AAV Capsid Variants Isolated from the Human Liver

T. La Bella, B. Bertin, J. Nozi, T. Tedesco, A. Mihaljevic, P. Vidal, S. Imbeaud, N.C. Nault, J. Zucman-Rossi and *G. Ronzitti*

Adeno-associated viral (AAV) vectors represent the leading platform for gene therapy in several genetic diseases. One of the key advantages of AAV vectors is their high versatility: thirteen AAV serotypes and hundreds of naturally occurring variants have been identified, each with varying transduction properties. In 2020, we screened a cohort of 1319 human non-tumor liver tissues to isolate 59 new capsid variants (La Bella T, Imbeaud S et al. 2020). Two distinct AAV subtypes were identified: one similar to AAV2 and the other a hybrid between the AAV2 and AAV13 sequences. The wild-type (wt) AAV2 variants belonged to clade B of AAV classification, whereas the wt AAV2-13 variants were closer to the sequences from clade C. The newly identified capsids were cloned into a plasmid suitable for AAV vector production and the vectors were characterized in terms of manufacturability, in vitro and in vivo transduction efficiency. A total of 70% of the capsids passed the first selection criteria based on manufacturing yields and was infectious in cells. In vivo biodistribution, assessed after intravenous injection in C57BL/6 mice, revealed a marked tropism for muscles for the majority of the capsids, opening the way for a possible muscle-directed AAV gene therapy application. Interestingly, some of the capsids were able to reach the central nervous system (CNS), suggesting a capacity to bypass the blood–brain barrier, a remarkable feature for CNS transduction via systemic administration. In order to understand the impact the amino acid variations on AAV capsid production and transduction efficiency, an analysis of mutations in structural and non-structural proteins was performed, leading to the identification of some indels within the VP sequences, which might be responsible of the destabilization of the VP structure. Moreover, mutations in AAP and protein X genes were identified, suggesting a possible impact on vector production yields.

8.4. Isolation of Novel AAV Serotypes from Pig Tissues for Retinal Gene Therapy

Emanuela Pone, Vivien Temás, Antonella Ferrara, Ferenc Olasz, Anna Furiano, Ivana Trapani, Zadori Zoltán and *Alberto Auricchio*

Due to their excellent efficacy and safety profile, vectors derived from the adeno-associated virus (AAV) are the leading platform for retinal gene therapy. The PCR-based isolation of AAVs from biological samples represents an important source of new AAV variants with unique biological features. In our study, we aim at isolating, from pig tissues, novel AAV variants with potential improved retinal transduction capabilities compared to the existing ones. To this aim, we screened by PCR porcine blood (n = 244) and liver (n = 274) tissues for the presence of AAVs, using primers complementary to conserved and flanking hypervariable regions in the *CAP* gene. We found that about 23% of blood and 28% of liver samples contained AAV sequences. Aminoacidic sequence alignment revealed five novel AAV variants from blood, which have 85–97% homology with the closest porcine AAV5 (AAVpo5) capsid sequence. One of them, AAVpoaa1, transduced pigs' retinal pigmented epithelium and photoreceptors to levels comparable to the gold-standard AAV8 upon subretinal injection. The isolation, cloning and characterization of additional variants of pig origin is ongoing.

8.5. Development of a Synthetic AAV Vector for the Gene Therapy of Hemophilia in Children

Jakob Shoti, Keyun Qing and *Arun Srivastava*

In all previous or currently ongoing clinical trials for the gene therapy of hemophilia, children have not been enrolled since traditional liver-directed AAV gene therapy is unlikely to work for the following reasons: (i) Hepatocytes in the growing liver undergo rapid cell divisions, and with every cell division, the AAV vector genomes would be expected to be diluted due to the episomal nature of the AAV genome; and (ii) Repeat vector dosing is not an option since, following the first administration of the vectors, neutralizing antibodies are generated, making subsequent vector delivery difficult. We previously reported the development of a synthetic AAV vector, named No-End (NE) AAV DNA (*Gene*, 119: 265–272, 1992), which is devoid of AAV capsid proteins and which, upon transfection into human hepatic cells, leads to the sustained expression of a reporter EGFP gene for up to 35 days (*Mol Ther*, 29: 178, 2021). In the present studies, an optimized NE-DNA containing the human Factor IX (hF.IX) gene expression cassette, under the control of a human liver-specific transthyretin (TTR) promoter (optNE-TR75-TTR-hF.IX), was generated. This NE-DNA was transfected into a human hepatocellular carcinoma cell line, HepG2. The same expression cassette as that of a linear DNA was used as an appropriate control. Following transfections, the cells were passaged for up to 28 days. Cell extracts were prepared from replicate cultures and equivalent amounts of total cellular proteins were analyzed on Western blots using a hF.IX-specific monoclonal antibody. These results indicate that ~6-fold higher hF.IX levels were expressed from the optNE-TR75-TTR-hF.IX cassette compared with those from its linear counterpart up to 28 days post-transfection. These data are consistent with our previous studies with NE-DNA containing a reporter gene, suggesting that the observed increased hF.IX gene expression is due to the prolonged stability of the NE-DNA. Studies are currently underway to generate optNE-TTR- DNA containing the human clotting factor VIII (hF.VIII). In future studies, the encapsidation of these optNE-DNAs in liver-targeted synthetic liposomes may provide a viable approach for repeated delivery, and thus, a potential gene therapy of hemophilia in children. (This research was supported by a 2021 Global Hemophilia ASPIRE grant from Pfizer)

9. Session 7: Clinical and Veterinarian Parvovirology

9.1. First Evidence of a New Porcine Parvovirus Species in Italy: A Survey of Reproductive Failure Outbreaks

G. Faustini, C.M. Tucciarone, A. Donneschi, G. Franzo, B. Boniotti, G.L. Alborali and M. Drigo

An epidemiological update on the porcine parvovirus 1 (PPV1) presence and the first evidence of a newly identified species (PPV2-7) circulation in Italy is presented in this paper, filling the current lack of knowledge. Fetuses collected from reproductive failure outbreaks in Northern Italian farms and submitted to the Istituto Zooprofilattico Sperimentale della Lombardia e dell'Emilia Romagna (IZSLER) in the period of 2019–2020 were tested by using four multiplex real-time PCRs, described in previous studies.

PPV1 and new PPV species were respectively detected in 23.8% and 42.5% of the tested farms ($n = 80$), respectively. Considering other pathogens routinely investigated by IZSLER, PPV2-7 co-infections with viral and bacterial agents were observed in 25.0% and 12.5% of the farms, respectively. PCV-2 and at least one PPV2-7 species were the most common co-infections (17.5%). PPV1 and new PPVs were detected in 5% and 15% of the farms, respectively. PPV detection singularly or in co-infection with other pathogens commonly responsible for reproductive failure encourages future studies investigating their biological, clinical and epidemiological roles, for a better preparedness to potential future challenges.

9.2. Phylogenetic and Clinical Relationships among Canine and Feline Parvovirus Strains Collected from Parvovirosis Cases in Italy

Claudia Maria Tucciarone, Giovanni Franzo, Matteo Legnardi, Andrea Zoia, Matteo Petini, Tommaso Furlanello, Marco Caldin, Mattia Cecchinato and *Michele Drigo*

Carnivore protoparvovirus 1 is a relevant species in veterinary medicine that includes canine (CPV) and feline parvovirus (FPV), which can cause severe gastroenteritis and immunosuppression, especially in young animals. CPV heterogeneity has been extensively studied since the discovery of its antigenic variants, to which different virulence levels are occasionally attributed. On the other hand, FPV has been considered less variable and less rapidly evolving than CPV.

Based on these premises, full VP2 sequences were obtained from Italian clinical cases of parvovirosis in dogs and cats. CPV and FPV molecular epidemiology was described by phylogenetic analyses, highlighting the viral heterogeneity and variant exchange within and among countries. Moreover, the relationship between the CPV and FPV strains with the clinicopathological outcome was statistically investigated, revealing that viral phylogeny is associated with host parameters of inflammatory response, even though a statistical significance was proven only for CPV, whose higher heterogeneity likely determined a stronger phylogenetic signal. These results suggest a more complex contribution of viral phylogeny rather than of antigenic features in determining severity.

9.3. Post-Vaccination Polyclonal Antibody Response Mapped by Cryo-EM

Samantha R. Hartmann, Simon Frueh, Robert Lopez-Astacio, Wendy S. Weichart, Nadia Di Nunno, Sung Hung Cho, Carol M. Bato, Colin R. Parrish and *Susan L. Hafenstein*

Canine parvovirus (CPV) is an important pathogen that emerged by cross-species transmission and causes severe disease in dogs, including acute hemorrhagic enteritis, myocarditis and cerebellar disorder. There is overlap on the surface of parvovirus capsids between the A- and B-site antigenic epitopes and the binding site for the host receptor, the transferrin receptor-1 (TfR). Selection pressure by antibodies or TfR has led to closely related variants that differ in antigenicity and host range. Nevertheless, vaccination to canine parvovirus is very effective. To understand the host immune response to vaccination, serum from dogs immunized with live parvovirus were obtained; the polyclonal antibodies were purified and used to obtain the high-resolution cryo-EM structures of the polyclonal Fab-virus complexes. We used a custom software, Icosahedral Subparticle Extraction and Correlated Classification (ISECC), to perform sub-particle analysis and reconstruct polyclonal Fab-virus complexes from two different dogs eight and twelve weeks post-vaccination. In the resulting polyclonal Fab-virus complexes, there were a total of five distinct Fabs identified, directed to the A- and B-sites. Both dogs generated an antibody that recognized the B epitope with identical footprints onto the virus capsid. In both cases, all five antibodies identified would interfere with receptor binding. This polyclonal mapping approach identifies a specific, limited immune response to the live vaccine virus and provides a new method for using cryo-EM to investigate the complex binding of multiple different antibodies or ligands to virus capsids.

9.4. Human Parvovirus Tissue Persistence: Cell Tropism, Activity and Impact

Man Xu, Katarzyna Leskinen, Tommaso Gritti, Valerija Groma, Johanna Arola, Anna Lepistö, Taina Sipponen, Päivi Saavalainen and *Maria Söderlund-Venermo*

Two parvoviruses have been discovered as human pathogens to date, parvovirus B19 and human bocavirus (HBoV) 1. B19V shows extreme tropism to erythroid progenitor cells, resulting in erythema infectiosum, anemia and fetal death. HBoV1 replicates in human airway epithelial cells and causes respiratory tract infections, while HBoV2-4 is enteric. After primary infection, B19V DNA persists in a wide variety of tissues lifelong, whereas HBoVs persist in some. We aim to determine the host cell tropism, virus activity and impact of human parvoviruses in non-permissive host cells. In pediatric tonsillar tissues, we earlier discovered the persistent site of HBoV1 DNA to be lymphoid germinal centers (GCs) and the host cells to be naive, activated and memory B cells and monocytes. In both immortalized and primary tonsillar B-cell cultures, the cellular uptake of HBoV1 occurred through antibody-dependent enhancement (ADE) via the Fc receptor II. HBoV1 did not replicate productively in the tonsils nor in the ADE-mediated cell cultures, despite the detection of spliced mRNAs.

We searched for parvoviral DNA in biopsy specimens of paired diseased and healthy intestinal mucosa of 130 individuals, and detected persistent HBoV1-3 DNA in the intestines of only one individual in each case. Conversely, B19V DNA was detected in the cancerous, inflamed, adenomatous and healthy intestinal biopsy specimens of 50, 47, 31 and 27% of the individuals, respectively. Intra-individually, however, B19V DNA persisted significantly more often in the healthy than in the inflamed paired intestinal segments. By RNAscope-ISH and immunohistochemistry, we located the B19V DNA in the mucosal B cells of lymphoid follicles and vascular endothelial cells. The B19V transcription activity was, however, below the RT-PCR detection level. With RNA-seq analysis, we further identified 272 B19V-modulated, differentially expressed genes in normal ileum specimens, and B19V persistence was shown both to activate cell viability and to inhibit apoptosis. Life-long B19V DNA persistence thus seems to modulate host gene expression, which may lead to clinical outcomes in predisposed individuals.

9.5. *High Prevalence and Activity of Cutavirus in Parapsoriasis Patients*

Ushanandini Mohanraj, Alexander Salava, Liisa Väkevä, Annamari Ranki and *Maria Söderlund-Venermo*

In 2016, metagenomic studies in the diarrheic stool and skin of cutaneous T-cell lymphoma (CTCL) patients revealed a novel human protoparvovirus, cutavirus (CuV). Soon after, we and others detected CuV DNA in CTCL lesions, while all skin biopsy specimens of healthy subjects were CuV-DNA-negative, revealing an association of CuV with CTCL. Most patients with CTCL first present with long-standing reactive inflammatory conditions, such as parapsoriasis en plaques (a form of pre-CTCL). This has led to the hypothesis that chronic antigen stimulation by a pathogen could have a role in CTCL carcinogenesis. Hence, in the present study, we aim to identify the prevalence, activity and cell tropism of CuV in parapsoriasis skin lesions.

We first studied 13 fresh skin biopsy specimens obtained from 12 patients (group A, age: 34–83 years). Of these 12 patients, 7 had CTCL and 5 had parapsoriasis. Next, we studied 24 FFPE (formalin-fixed, paraffin-embedded) skin biopsy samples and 52 skin swabs from 13 parapsoriasis patients (group B, age: 37–86 years). CuV was detected and quantified by qPCR and RT-qPCR. All DNA/mRNA-positive samples were confirmed by cloning and sequencing. By RNAscope in situ hybridization (RISH) and multiplex immunohistochemistry (mIHC), CuV DNA/RNA was visualized in the tissues of CuV DNA-positive individuals. In group A, CuV DNA and spliced mRNA were detected in freshly frozen skin biopsy specimens from 4/12 (33.3%) individuals. Among these four CuV-positive individuals, three had parapsoriasis (3/5, 60%) and one CTCL (1/7, 14.2%). In group B, CuV DNA was detected in swabs from 6/13 (46%) and in FFPE samples from 8/12 (66%) parapsoriasis individuals. Overall, among the 11 CuV-positive parapsoriasis individuals from both groups, 3 progressed to CTCL, while 1 had early stage CTCL. From the ISH + mIHC assays, CuV-specific DNA/RNA signals were observed in both the cytoplasm and nucleus of many cell types, including keratinocytes, T cells and macrophages. We found a very high CuV prevalence in the skin lesions of parapsoriasis en plaques. CuV also actively transcribed mRNA. Hence, it is imperative to clarify if skin-persistent CuV leads to T-cell stimulation and the development of CTCL and if CuV presence could serve as a prognostic marker for CTCL.

10. Session 8: Gene Therapy

10.1. *Dynorphin-Based "Release on Demand" Gene Therapy for Drug-Resistant Temporal Lobe Epilepsy*

Regine Heilbronn, Alexandra S. Agostinho, Mario Mietzsch, Luca Zangrandi, Iwona Kmiec, Anna Mutti, Larissa Kraus, Pawel Fidzinski, Ulf C. Schneider, Martin Holtkamp and *Christoph Schwarzer*

Epilepsy represents one of the most common chronic CNS diseases, with temporal lobe epilepsy as the most frequent clinical presentation. The focus lies in the hippocampus, the site of learning memory and emotional control. The high incidence of drug resistance, devastating comorbidities and insufficient responsiveness to invasive epilepsy surgery are unmet medical challenges. In the quest for novel, disease-modifying treatment strategies, neuropeptides represent promising candidates. We recently provided "proof of concept" that the AAV-vector-based transduction of dynorphin into the epileptogenic focus of clinically well-accepted mouse and rat models for temporal lobe epilepsy leads to the suppression of seizures over months (EMBO Mol Med 2019, e9963). Also, the debilitating long-term decline in learning and memory is prevented. In human hippocampal slice cultures obtained from epilepsy surgery, dynorphins suppressed seizure-like activity, suggestive of their high potential for clinical translation. AAV-delivered neuronal dynorphin expression is focally restricted and its release is dependent on high-frequency stimulation, as it occurs at the onset of seizures. The novel format of the "release on demand" delivery of dynorphin is viewed as a key to prevent habituation and to minimize the risk of adverse effects, leading to the long-term suppression of seizures and of their devastating sequels. Progress on vector validation in the preparation of a clinical trial is presented.

10.2. Structural and Kinetic Characterization of Anti-AAV9 Monoclonal Antibodies Derived from Patients' Post-Zolgensma® Treatment

Jane Hsi, Mario Mietzsch, Austin Nelson, Paul Chipman, Jenny Jackson, Peter Schofield, Daniel Christ, Joanne Reed, Neeta Khandekar, Grant Logan, Ian E. Alexander and *Robert McKenna*

The use of adeno-associated virus (AAV) as a gene transfer vehicle has become increasingly feasible as a clinical option in recent years. Following the FDA approval of Zolgensma® (Novartis), an AAV9-based biologic to treat children under the age of two with spinal muscular atrophy (SMA), there is a growing interest in expanding AAV9 usage due to its ability to transduce cardiac and skeletal muscle, liver, pancreas and eye and its capability to cross the blood–brain barrier to transduce the central nervous system (CNS). However, the presence of pre-existing neutralizing antibodies (NAbs) against AAV9 capsids in a large percentage of the population could reduce the efficacy of AAV9 gene therapy and may lead to the exclusion of patients from treatment. A strategy to circumvent the immune response of a patient for AAV-mediated therapeutic gene delivery is the development of engineered vector capsids by either directed evolution or rational design that are then able to escape antibody recognition. In order to pursue this strategy, the interactions of the NAbs to the capsid binding need to be characterized. Previously, our lab as well as others generated mouse monoclonal antibodies targeting the AAV9 capsids to simulate the immune response against the capsid and map the major antigenic regions. However, this approach has faced criticism as mouse-derived antibodies may not fully mimic the behavior of human-derived antibodies.

We present the structural and kinetic characterization of human monoclonal antibodies that were obtained from patients that received Zolgensma®. Specifically, we determine the binding sites of 13 antibodies obtained from two patients to the AAV9 capsid by cryo-electron microscopy and three-dimensional image reconstruction. Our data show that the 2-fold capsid surface is the antigenically dominant region as ~ three quarters of the antibodies bind there. The binding interactions and kinetics for these antibodies were analyzed using biolayer interferometry and compared to the previously developed murine antibodies. All the antibodies neutralize AAV9 transduction, and some also cross-react and neutralize a range of different AAV serotypes. Structural and kinetic comparisons of human and murine antibodies is presented along with implications for the development of antibody escape variants.

10.3. Development of Optimized (Opt) AAVrh74 Vectors with Increased Transduction Efficiency in Primary Human Skeletal Muscle Cells In Vitro and in Mouse Muscles In Vivo Following Systemic Administration

Keyun Qing, Jakob Shoti, Geoffrey D. Keeler, Barry J. Byrne and *Arun Srivastava*

In a Phase I/II clinical trial sponsored by Solid Biosciences using AAV9 vectors, serious adverse events were reported. In a trial sponsored by Pfizer, also using AAV9 vectors, several serious adverse events and the death of a patient were also reported. Sarepta Therapeutics reported the results of a Phase I/II trial using AAVrh74 vectors with vomiting as the only adverse event, indicating that AAVrh74 vectors are safer, although a high dose of 2×10^{14} vgs/kg was used. We previously reported that capsid-modified next-generation ("NextGen") AAVrh74 vectors (*Mol. Ther.*, 29: 159–160, 2021) and genome-modified generation X ("GenX") AAVrh74 vectors (*Mol. Ther.*, 29: 184–185, 2021) are significantly more efficient than their wild-type (WT) counterpart. In the present study, we combine the two modifications to generate optimized ("Opt") AAVrh74 vectors and evaluate their transduction efficiency in primary human skeletal muscle cells in vitro, which was up to ~5-fold higher than that of the conventional AAVrh74 vectors. The efficacy of the WT and Opt AAVrh74 vectors was also evaluated in mouse muscles in vivo following systemic administration. The transduction efficiency of the Opt AAVrh74 vectors was ~5-fold higher in gastrocnemius (GA) as well as in tibialis anterior (TA) muscles. The total genome copy numbers of either the WT or Opt AAVrh74 vectors in GA, TA, diaphragm and heart muscles were not significantly different, suggesting that the observed increased transduction efficiency of the Opt AAVrh74 vectors was due to improved intracellular trafficking and nuclear transport of these vectors, which is consistent with our previously published studies with other Opt AAV serotype vectors. Taken together, these studies suggest that the use of Opt AAVrh74 vectors may lead to a safe and effective gene therapy of human muscular dystrophies at reduced doses. However, as observed in a recently published study (*Hum. Gene Ther.*, 32: 375–389, 2021), a significant fraction of the AAVrh74 vectors is sequestered in the liver, which is undesirable. Efforts are currently underway to develop liver de-targeted Opt AAVrh74 vectors for their optimal use in the gene therapy of human muscular dystrophies at further reduced doses. (This research was supported by a sponsored research grant from Sarepta Therapeutics).

10.4. Development of Genome-Modified Generation Y (GenY) AAVrh74 Vectors with Improved Transgene Expression in Primary Human Skeletal Muscle Cells In Vitro and in Mouse Muscles In Vivo Following Systemic Administration

Jakob Shoti, *Keyun Qing*, *Geoffrey D. Keeler*, *Barry J. Byrne* and *Arun Srivastava*

Since the naturally occurring AAV contains a single-stranded DNA genome and expresses viral genes poorly because ssDNA is transcriptionally inactive, transgene expression levels from recombinant ssAAV vectors are also negatively impacted. We previously reported that the substitution of the D-sequence in the left inverted terminal repeat (ITR) results in generation X ("GenX") AAV vectors, which mediate up to 8-fold improved transgene expression (*J. Virol.*, 89: 952–961, 2015). More recently, we also reported that the extent of transgene expression from GenX AAVrh74 vectors is ~5-fold higher than that from wild-type (WT) AAVrh74 vectors (*Mol. Ther.*, 29: 184–185, 2021). We previously observed that the distal 10-nucleotides (nts) in the AAV2 D-sequence share a partial homology to the consensus half-site of the glucocorticoid receptor-binding element (GRE), and that the glucocorticoid receptor signaling pathway is activated following AAV2 infection/AAV2 vector transduction (*Mol. Ther.*, 24: S6, 2016). We evaluate whether the substitution of the distal 10 nts in the D-sequence with the authentic GRE leads to increased transgene expression from AAVrh74 vectors, named generation Y ("GenY") vectors. The extent of the transgene expression from GenX and GenY AAVrh74 vectors in primary human skeletal muscle cells was, on average, respectively, ~4-fold and ~6-fold higher compared to that from the WT AAVrh74 vectors. The observed increase in transgene expression was not due to the increased entry of the GenX or the GenY vectors, as documented by approximately similar numbers of vector genome copy numbers quantitated by qPCR analyses of low mol. wt. DNA samples isolated from cells transduced with each of these vectors. The efficacy of the GenY AAVrh74 vectors in skeletal muscles following systemic administration in a murine model was also evaluated in vivo and shown to be higher than that from NextGen AAVrh74 vectors. These studies suggest that the combined use of the capsid-modified NextGen + GenY (Opt^{Y}) AAVrh74 vectors may further reduce the need for the high vector doses currently in use, which has significant implications in the potential use of Opt^{Y} AAVrh74 vectors in the safe and effective gene therapy of muscular dystrophies. (This research was supported by a sponsored research grant from Sarepta Therapeutics)

11. Session 9: Oncolytic Viruses

11.1. *Review Lecture: Characterization of the H-1PV Life Cycle as a Way to Improve Its Anticancer Efficacy*

Amit Kulkarni, Tiago Ferreira, Tiina Marttila, Gayatri Kawishwar, Anna Hartley and *Antonio Marchini*

H-1 parvovirus (H-1PV) is the first member of the Parvoviridae family to be tested as an anticancer agent in early phases clinical studies. The results from these studies in patients with glioblastoma and pancreatic carcinomas showed that H-1PV treatment is safe, well-tolerated and associated with surrogate signs of efficacy. However, the virus alone, in the regimes applied, was unable to eradicate the tumors. The rational design of combination strategies, the development of more effective viruses and the identification of biomarkers that can predict which tumors are most likely to benefit from H-1PV-based therapies are ways to improve H-1PV anticancer efficacy. We review the strategies to improve H-1PV anticancer efficacy, with a special focus on the characterization of the pathways used by H-1PV to infect cancer cells and the identification of the cellular factors involved in virus cell attachment and entry. We propose that the expression levels of these critical modulators may guide the selection of patients whose tumors are more susceptible to H-1PV treatment.

11.2. *Engineering Functional Domains of MVM Capsid with VEGF-Blocking Peptides to Enhance Parvovirus Oncolytic Capacity*

Tania Calvo-López, Esther Grueso, Cristina Sánchez-Martínez and *José M. Almendral*

We attempt to direct the capsid of the prototype strain of the parvovirus minute virus of mice (MVMp) against the tumor vasculature using two strategies: (A) as a platform to induce α-VEGF antibodies and (B) by re-targeting the infection to cells expressing VEGF-R1. For this, peptides from the three functional domains of the MVMp capsid were replaced by peptides that block the binding of VEGF to its receptors (VEbp). (A) In the first approach, although most substitutions caused alterations in the assembly or maturation of the virus, some virus chimeras with VEbp substituting the residues at the 3-fold axis were efficiently propagated in the culture, exposed heterologous peptides on the surface of the capsid and induced native anti-VEGF antibodies in mice. (B) In the re-targeting studies, some virus chimeras bearing VEbp in the 2-fold axis, where the sialic-acid-receptor-binding site localizes, showed greater infectivity than MVMp towards human glioblastoma cells, although they did not infect through VEGF-R1. Instead, the chimeras attached, as MVMp, to distinct types of sialic acid (sia) residues. Our MVM re-targeting study illustrates: (i) the structural constrains to re-target parvoviruses that have evolutionary adopted narrow grooves to allocate small sia receptors; (ii) the critical role that attachment to specific types of sia plays in determining parvovirus; and (iii) the possibility to intervene the tropism of oncolytic parvoviruses by modulating the sia framework on the cancer cell surface.

11.3. *MVM Selectively Infects and Disrupts Glioblastoma-Stem-Cell-Derived Tumors with Patient-Specific p53 Deregulations*

Jon Gil-Ranedo, Carlos Gallego-García and *José M. Almendral*

Glioblastoma multiforme (GBM) remains a major type of cancer with no current effective therapy. Multiple studies support that the efficacy of cancer therapies must be primarily shown against the cancer stem cells driving tumorigenesis. We therefore attempt to develop a GBM therapy using two strains of the minute virus of mice (MVMp and MVMi), a parvovirus that is non-pathogenic for humans. Primary glioblastoma stem cells (GSCs) isolated from GBM patients were challenged with the MVM strains and the system comprehensively studied for cell and virus parameters. GSC neurospheres accumulated assembled capsids, but restrict viral NS1 cytotoxic protein expression by an innate PKR/eIF2α-P response. Inter- and intra-patient GSC heterogeneity was dissected by their diverse innate responses and the ratio between structural and non-structural viral gene expression. Viral infection triggered a comprehensive DNA damage response involving cell cycle arrest, neurosphere disorganization and the bystander disruption of GSC-derived brain tumor architecture in rodent models. Notably, the MVM infection preferably targeted those GSC subpopulations within patients harboring p53 gain-of-function mutants and/or Pp53Ser15 phosphorylation. This study supports MVM as an effective oncolytic agent for personalized parvoviral therapies against devastating glioblastoma and other cancers with deregulated p53 signaling.

11.4. Identification of an Antiviral Drug as a Novel Potentiator of H-1PV-Mediated Oncolysis

Anna Hartley, Valérie Palissot, Tiina Marttila, Toros Tasgin, Céline Jeanty, Gian Mario Dore, Laurent Brino, Anne Maglott-Roth, Richard Harbottle and *Antonio Marchini*

The rat protoparvovirus H-1 (H-1PV) is a small non-enveloped virus with a natural oncolytic capacity. Replication of the virus in human cells is strictly dependent on a transformed phenotype in the host cell, including a dependence on cellular S-phase factors. This has made H-1PV an attractive treatment option for human cancers. The oncolytic activity of H-1PV has been extensively tested in vitro against a wide range of cancer cell lines, including brain cancer, lymphoma and leukemia, pancreatic ductal adenocarcinoma (PDAC) and breast cancer. In the clinics, H-1PV as a monotherapy was shown to be safe and well-tolerated for the treatment of glioblastoma and PDAC, but it was unable to eradicate tumors under the regimes used. Thus, there is a clear need for the improvement of oncolytic H-1PV therapy. We identify a novel combination of H-1PV with an antiviral drug that potentiates the oncolytic capacity of the virus in vitro.

We conducted a high-throughput screening of 1443 FDA-approved drugs in combination with H-1PV in glioma cells to identify drug candidates that are able to potentiate the oncolytic abilities of H-1PV. From this screening, we identified the hepatitis C virus inhibitor ledipasvir as a potentiator of H-1PV-mediated oncolysis and confirmed this in vitro in a variety of cellular backgrounds, including glioblastoma, PDAC, lung cancer and ovarian carcinoma. Importantly, this improved oncolysis was independent of viral replication. The functional kinome profiling (PamGene) in glioma cells co-treated with ledipasvir and H-1PV revealed a number of kinase pathways that are differentially activated in the presence of ledipasvir and H-1PV co-treatment. The causal role of these kinase pathways is under investigation at present. Our data demonstrate, for the first time, that ledipasvir is able to potentiate the oncotoxicity of H-1PV and is a promising candidate for combination therapy in the clinics.

11.5. Oncolytic H-1 Parvovirus in Combination with the Pro-Apoptotic Drug ABT-737 Shows Improved Cytotoxicity and Immune Activation in Prostate Cancer Cells

Gayatri Kavishwar, Alice De Roia, Dirk M. Nettelbeck, Richard Harbottle, Marcelo Ehrlich, Guy Ungerechts and *Antonio Marchini*

In the past decade, novel methodologies have been developed, facilitating the use of immune activation against cancer. This has greatly improved the overall survival and prognosis of various malignancies. However, not all cancer patients benefit from these treatments; therefore, there is an unmet need to find agents that could potentiate the efficacy of immunotherapy. One such field of research is oncolytic-virus-mediated immunotherapy. More than 40 oncolytic viruses (OVs) are presently undergoing clinical testing alone or, increasingly, in combination with other immunotherapeutic agents. OVs specifically target cancer cells, induce tumor cell lysis, tumor antigen release and adjuvant immune response through immunogenic cell death and cytokine release. H-1 parvovirus (H-1PV) is one such "clinically relevant" OV, which has been extensively studied in various cancer models and evaluated in Phase I/II clinical trials for the treatment of patients with glioblastoma and pancreatic ductal adenocarcinoma. It has been shown to be safe, non-toxic and capable of inducing the favorable immune modulation of the tumor microenvironment. However, H-1PV, as a monotherapy, is still not sufficient to completely eradicate the tumors. The development of combination strategies based on H-1PV and other anticancer agents thus seems to be a rational approach to improve efficacy. Previous data from our laboratory showed great promise in using the combination of H-1PV with pro-apoptotic BCL2 inhibitors in different cancer models. In this study, we evaluate whether it is possible to enhance the oncolytic activity of H-1PV by using the pro-apoptotic BH3 mimetic ABT-737 in prostate cancer cells. Our data show that this combination shows an improved killing of prostate cancer cells in a synergistic manner. We also provide first evidence that this cell death is immunogenic, by showing a strong induction of cell surface calreticulin, a classical marker of immunogenic cell death (ICD). To investigate whether the induction of an ICD event also causes the activation of the dendritic cell (DC)/T-cell axis, we established multiple co-culture systems using the prostate cancer cell line PC3 and primary immune cells. Firstly, we observed the maturation and activation of DCs through the upregulation of CD80 and CD86 expression. Furthermore, we observed the peripheral activation of T cells through the upregulation of the early activation marker CD69. The combination also shows an improved activation of natural killer cells through an increase in the degranulation marker CD107a and intracellular IFNγ. Our study thus shows that the combination treatment of H-1PV and ABT-737 shows promise in enhancing direct tumor cell killing as well as anticancer immunity in the context of prostate cancer.

12. Poster Session

A list of the submitted posters is reported below, while the full abstracts are available as Supplemental File S1.

P.01 Variability analysis of Parvovirus B19 sequences obtained through Next-Generation Sequencing
Federica Bichicchi, Niccolò Guglietta, Arthur Daniel Rocha Alves, Gloria Bua, Francesca Bonvicini, Elisabetta Manaresi, Giorgio Gallinella
P.02 In vitro models for the study of B19V interaction with the human placental BeWo monolayer
Francesca Bonvicini, Gloria Bua, Erika Fasano, Elisabetta Manaresi, Giorgio Gallinella
P.03 Mesenchymal stem cells are susceptible but non-permissive to B19V replication
Gloria Bua, Pasquale Marrazzo, Francesco Alviano, Laura Bonsi, Giorgio Gallinella
P.04 The role of Host Cell Factor 1 in the life cycle of AAV
Caroline Dierckx, Zander Claes, Mathieu Bollen, Els Henckaerts
P.05 Analysis of Parvovirus B19 transcriptome in UT7/EpoS1 cells by mRNAseq techniques
Erika Fasano, Gloria Bua, Stefano Amadesi, Alessandro Reggiani, Elisabetta Manaresi, Fabrizio Ferrè, Giorgio Gallinella
P.06 Prevalence of Human Chaphamaparvoviruses
Jingjing Li, and Maria Söderlund-Venermo
P.07 Brain organoids as a platform to study subcellular trafficking of recombinant AAV vectors
Marlies Leysen, Idris Salmon, Sereina O. Sutter, Cornel Fraefel, Adrian Ranga, Benjamien Moeyaert, Els Henckaerts
P.08 Equine Parvovirus Hepatitis qPCR screening of stored equine heparin plasma and serum samples with and without increased liver enzyme activities
Anna Sophie Ramsauer, Ina Mersich, Irina Preining, Jessika-Maximiliane Cavalleri
P.09 FLIM-FRET studies of AAV capsid nuclear disintegration
Visa Ruokolainen, Michael Kann, Maija Vihinen-Ranta
P.10 Enhanced transduction efficiency of AAV vectors mediated by polyvinyl alcohol and human serum albumin is serotype- and cell type-specific
Jakob Shoti, Claire K. Scozzari, Reema Kashif, Hua Yang, Mengqun Tan, Wei Wang, Keyun Qing, Arun Srivastava
P.11 Development of allele-specific dual PCRs to identify members of the 27a cluster of PPV1
Vivien Tamás, Ferenc Olasz, István Mészáros, István Kiss, Zalán G. Homonnay, Preben Mortensen, Zoltán Zádori
P.12 A record of Parvovirus B19 laboratory diagnosis in endemic/epidemic or COVID-19 pandemic
Simona Venturoli; Alessia Bertoldi; Elisabetta Manaresi, Giorgio Gallinella.
P.13 Enhanced muscle transduction by clade F vector AAVhu.32 translates across multiple animal models
Samantha A. Yost, Randolph Qian, April R. Giles, Sungyeon Cho, Chunping Qiao, Olivier Danos, Ye Liu, Andrew C. Mercer

13. Conclusions

The four days of sessions engaged attendees with an intense, but highly rewarding flow of information on the up-to-date and cutting-edge research in the field. Most of the abstracts presented already found their ways into the published literature, promoting research in the ever-fascinating field of Parvoviruses.

The two awards offered by the Journal *Viruses* were conferred to Jan Bieri (presentation 2.3) and Marlies Leysen (poster P.07).

The closing event, a very informal dinner directly on the beach in Rimini (Figure 1), followed by wild dancing until dawn as in the best tradition, provided the link to the next XIX Parvovirus Workshop, which is to be held in Leuven, Belgium, from 3 to 6 September 2024, hosted by Els Henckaerts. Please visit: parvovirusworkshop2024.org.

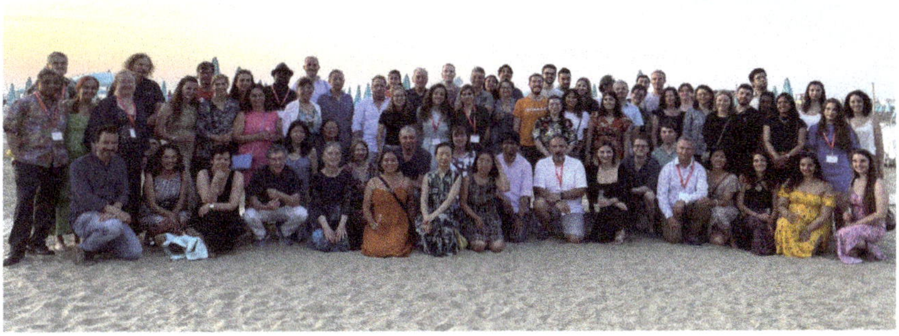

Figure 1. Rimini, 17 June 2022: relax on the beach (courtesy of Maria Söderlund-Venermo).

Supplementary Materials: The following supporting information can be downloaded at: https://www.mdpi.com/article/10.3390/v15102129/s1, Supplemental File S1: Poster Session.

Author Contributions: G.G. and A.M. wrote the introduction and compiled the conference report, based on abstracts submitted by the conference attendees. Abstracts are reported in order of presentation; underlined names are the presenting authors. A list of abstract contributors and related affiliation follows. See also Supplemental File S1 for poster abstracts and authors. All authors have read and agreed to the published version of the manuscript.

Funding: The meeting organization was primarily financed by attendants through a registration fee. The venue was located in an academic building of the University of Bologna, Campus of Rimini. The Journal *Viruses* provided two travel grant awards. Additionally, sponsoring was provided by the following companies: Axion Biosystems (Atlanta, GA, USA); RegenxBio (Rockville, MD, USA); VectorBuilder (Neu-Isenburg, Germany); Vir/Humabs (Bellinzona, Switzerland); Agilent (Santa Clara, CA, USA); Homology Medicine (Bedford, MA, USA); and Lacerta Therapeutics (Alachua, FL, USA).

Data Availability Statement: As a conference report, no new data were created or analyzed in this study. Data sharing is not applicable to this article.

Acknowledgments: The administrative and technical support of Rimini Campus, University of Bologna, and Adria Congrex, Rimini, was crucial to the success of the meetings and is gratefully acknowledged.

Contributor List: A. Srivastava (University of Florida College of Medicine, Gainesville, FA, USA); D. Corti (Humabs BioMed, Bellinzona, Switzerland); J. Nüesch (German Cancer Research Center (DKFZ), Heidelberg, Germany); C.R. Parrish (College of Veterinary Medicine, Cornell University, Ithaca, NY, USA); G. Arriagada (Instituto de Ciencias Biomedicas, Universidad Andres Bello, Chile); M. Mietzsch (University of Florida College of Medicine, Gainesville, FA, USA); M.S. Chapman (Univ. Missouri, Columbia, MO, USA); J.A. Chiorini (National Institutes of Health, Bethesda, MD, USA); J. Bieri (University of Bern, Bern, Switzerland); C. Suter (University of Bern, Bern, Switzerland); R. Lopez-Astacio (College of Veterinary Medicine, Cornell University, Ithaca, NY, USA); C.R. Escalante (Virginia Commonwealth University School of Medicine, Richmond, VA, USA); A. Lkharrazi (University of Zurich, Zurich, Switzerland); D. Pintel (University of Missouri School of Medicine, Columbia, MO, USA); K. Majumder (University of Wisconsin-Madison, Madison, WI, USA); O. Fasina (College of Veterinary Medicine, Iowa State University, Ames, IA, USA); A. Reggiani (University of Bologna,

Bologna, Italy); M. Vihinen-Ranta (University of Jyvaskyla, Jyvaskyla, Finland); G. Alvisi (University of Padova, Padova, Italy); S. Sutter (University of Zurich, Zurich, Switzerland); J. Vetter (University of Zurich, Zurich, Switzerland); Z. Kadri (INSERM and Paris-Saclay University, Fontenay-aux-Roses, France); L. Daeffler (CNRS, Université de Strasbourg, Strasbourg, France); S. Leclerc (University of Jyvaskyla, Jyvaskyla, Finland); S. Mattola (University of Jyvaskyla, Jyvaskyla, Finland); L. Bustamante-Jaramillo (Sahlgrenska Academy, Gothenburg Sweden); L. Zentilin (International Center for Genetic Engineering and Biotechnology (ICGEB), Trieste, Italy); T. La Bella (Genethon, Evry, France); E. Pone (Telethon Institute of Genetics and Medicine (TIGEM), Pozzuoli, Italy); J. Shoti (University of Florida College of Medicine, Gainesville, FA, USA); G. Faustini (University of Padova, Legnaro, Italy); C.M. Tucciarone (University of Padova, Legnaro, Italy); S.L. Hafenstein (Pennsylvania State University, University Park, PA, USA); M. Xu (University of Helsinki, Helsinki, Finland); U. Mohanraj (University of Helsinki, Helsinki, Finland); R. Heilbronn (Charité–Universitätsmedizin, Berlin, Germany); J. His (University of Florida College of Medicine, Gainesville, FA, USA); K. Qing (University of Florida College of Medicine, Gainesville, FA, USA); A. Marchini (German Cancer Research Center (DKFZ), Heidelberg, Germany); T. Calvo-López (Centro de Biología Molecular Severo Ochoa, Madrid, Spain); C. Gallego-García (Centro de Biología Molecular Severo Ochoa, Madrid, Spain); A. Hartley (German Cancer Research Center (DKFZ), Heidelberg, Germany); G. Kavishwar (German Cancer Research Center (DKFZ), Heidelberg, Germany).

Conflicts of Interest: The authors declare no conflict of interest. The sponsors had no direct role in the organization of the meeting nor in the writing of the manuscript.

viruses

MDPI

Article

Antiviral Activity of an Endogenous Parvoviral Element

Angelica Bravo [1,†], Leandro Fernández-García [1,†], Rodrigo Ibarra-Karmy [1], Gonzalo A. Mardones [2], Luis Mercado [3], Fernando J. Bustos [1], Robert J. Gifford [4,*] and Gloria Arriagada [1,*]

1 Instituto de Ciencias Biomedicas, Facultad de Medicina y Facultad de Ciencias de la Vida, Universidad Andres Bello, Santiago 8370071, Chile; ange.bravo@uandresbello.edu (A.B.); leandrofg1990@gmail.com (L.F.-G.); r.ibarrakarmy@gmail.com (R.I.-K.); fernando.bustos@unab.cl (F.J.B.)
2 Facultad de Medicina y Ciencia, Universidad San Sebastián, Valdivia 5110466, Chile; gonzalo.mardonesc@uss.cl
3 Instituto de Biología, Facultad de Ciencias, Pontificia Universidad Católica de Valparaíso, Valparaíso 2373223, Chile; luis.mercado@pucv.cl
4 Centre for Virus Research, MRC-University of Glasgow, 464 Bearsden Rd, Bearsden, Glasgow G61 1QH, UK
* Correspondence: robert.gifford@glasgow.ac.uk (R.J.G.); gloria.arriagada@unab.cl (G.A.)
† These authors equally contributed to this work.

Abstract: Endogenous viral elements (EVEs) are genomic DNA sequences derived from viruses. Some EVEs have open reading frames (ORFs) that can express proteins with physiological roles in their host. Furthermore, some EVEs exhibit a protective role against exogenous viral infection in their host. Endogenous parvoviral elements (EPVs) are highly represented in mammalian genomes, and although some of them contain ORFs, their function is unknown. We have shown that the locus *EPV-Dependo.43-ODegus*, an EPV with an intact ORF, is transcribed in *Octodon degus* (degu). Here we examine the antiviral activity of the protein encoded in this EPV, named DeRep. DeRep was produced in bacteria and used to generate antibodies that recognize DeRep in western blots of degu tissue. To test if DeRep could protect against exogenous parvovirus, we challenged cells with the minute virus of mice (MVM), a model autonomous parvovirus. We observed that MVM protein expression, DNA damage induced by replication, viral DNA, and cytopathic effects are reduced when DeRep is expressed in cells. The results of this study demonstrate that DeRep is expressed in degu and can inhibit parvovirus replication. This is the first time that an EPV has been shown to have antiviral activity against an exogenous virus.

Keywords: parvovirus; immunity; evolution; paleovirology; endogenous viral elements

Citation: Bravo, A.; Fernández-García, L.; Ibarra-Karmy, R.; Mardones, G.A.; Mercado, L.; Bustos, F.J.; Gifford, R.J.; Arriagada, G. Antiviral Activity of an Endogenous Parvoviral Element. *Viruses* **2023**, *15*, 1420. https://doi.org/10.3390/v15071420

Academic Editor: Giorgio Galinella

Received: 7 June 2023
Revised: 19 June 2023
Accepted: 21 June 2023
Published: 23 June 2023

1. Introduction

The genomes of extant species contain numerous DNA sequences derived from viruses. It is proposed that these endogenous viral elements (EVEs) arise when infection of germline cells (i.e., gametes or early embryonic cells) leads to the integration of viral sequences into the chromosomal DNA of ancestral organisms, such that they are subsequently inherited from parent to offspring as novel genes [1]. Most EVEs are derived from viruses that circulated millions of years ago and therefore represent the viral fossil record, providing unique insight into the long-term evolutionary interactions between viruses and cells [2–4]. Because retroviruses integrate into genomic DNA as an obligate step in their replication, most EVE sequences found in mammalian genomes are derived from retroviruses (family *Retroviridae*), compared to a relatively small number of EVE sequences derived from non-retroviral virus families [1,5–7], whose integration is thought to occur only anomalously through non-homologous recombination (DNA viruses) or retrotransposition of viral mRNA (DNA and RNA viruses) [8–10].

Genomic and experimental research has revealed that some of these 'horizontally transferred' viral sequences have been co-opted or exapted to perform physiologically relevant functions. In mammals, EVEs have been shown to be relevant for cell function, embryonic development, and antiviral immunity [11–17]. While most examples involve endogenous retroviruses (ERVs), potentially co-opted/exapted EVEs derived from non-retroviral viruses have also been identified and investigated [16,17]. For example, endogenous bornavirus-like nucleoprotein (EBLN) has been shown to be coopted and expressed as both RNA and proteins in several species. In humans, hsEBLN-1 is expressed in the testis and brain [18]. Although this gene contains an intact ORF, it is proposed to function in gene regulation as a non-coding RNA (ncRNA) [16,18], while hsEBLN-2 encodes the mitochondrial E2 protein that has been shown to interact with apoptosis-related host proteins, affecting cell viability [17]. In the thirteen-lined ground squirrel (*Ictidomys tridecemlineatus*), an EBLN encodes an intact nucleoprotein that co-localizes in the nucleus with viral factories and inhibits in vitro replication of the Borna disease virus (BDV) [15].

Parvoviruses (family *Parvoviridae*) are well represented among the non-retroviral EVEs documented in mammals [1,4,7,19–24]. Parvoviruses are small, non-enveloped viruses of icosahedral symmetry. They have a linear, single-stranded DNA (ssDNA) genome of 4 to 6.3 kilobases (kb) in length [25] and encode at least two major open reading frames (ORFs) that are expressed to produce non-structural (NS or Rep) proteins and structural (VP or Capsid) proteins. Parvovirus replication occurs in the nucleus, and occasionally viral genome integration into host chromosomes can happen through non-homologous recombination, possibly facilitated by single-stranded breaks created by the nickase function of Rep [26]. Thus, incorporation of parvovirus DNA into the germline DNA and the formation of endogenous parvoviruses (EPVs) might be expected to occur at a certain frequency as a natural consequence of the biology of these viruses. However, as is the case for any new allele, the majority of EPVs generated in such events will be rapidly eliminated from the gene pool by genetic drift unless they are selected for some reason. Thus, the presence of several independently acquired, fixed EPV insertions in animal genomes is unexpected and suggests that selective pressures may have favored the retention of EPV genes in animal genomes during their evolution. Intriguingly, several EPV loci containing open reading frames (ORFs) capable of expressing complete or almost complete proteins expressed at least as transcripts have been reported [21,22,27].

We have previously shown that an intact EPV locus (*EPV-Dependo.43-ODegus*), derived from the Rep gene of a dependoparvovirus, is transcribed in the degu (*Octodon degus*) [22]. Degus are small rodents endemic to the Chilean Matorral ecoregion, where they live in colonial burrows. They are intelligent social animals that are responsive to human interaction and are often kept as pets. In the present study, we investigate the protein expression and antiviral activity of the protein encoded in this EPV, named DeRep, which is present in degu.

2. Materials and Methods

2.1. Cell Culture

Human embryonic kidney cells (HEK293T) were used for viral particle production, and mouse fibroblast cells (NIH3T3) were used for infection assays. Both cell lines were maintained at 37 °C with 5% CO_2 in Dulbecco's modified Eagle medium (DMEM) supplemented with 10% fetal bovine serum, 100 IU/mL penicillin, and 100 µg/mL streptomycin.

2.2. Cloning and Plasmids

The infectious parvovirus molecular clones pdBMVp, kindly provided by Peter Tattersall [28], and pcDNA3xFLAG-DeRep [21] have been described previously. To generate pEGFP-DeRep, the DeRep coding sequence was obtained by digestion of pcDNA3xFLAG-DeRep with *BamHI* and *XhoI* and ligated into pEGFP C1 digested with *BglII* and *SalI*. To obtain the lentiviral plasmid pLVX-3xFLAG-DeRep-Puro, the coding sequence of DeRep, including the FLAG epitope was PCR amplified from pcDNA3xFLAG-DeRep using the primers *XhoI*-FLAGstart-F 5′-tatactcgagatggactacaaagaccatga-3′ and DeRep-

*Not*I-R 5′-atatgcggccgcctagagggcgactttttcc-3′, the PCR product was gel purified, digested with *Xho*I and *Not*I and ligated into pLVX-IRES-PURO digested with the same restriction enzymes. The plasmid pcDNA3xFLAG-enRepM9L was previously described [21]. To generate pcDNA3xFLAG-OcenRep, rabbit genomic DNA was amplified using the primers OcRep*BamH*I-F 5′-atggatccatggaagagtatataagggcggct-3′ and OcRep*Xho*I-R 5′-aatctcgagttatcctccgccaagtcttcc-3′. The PCR product was gel purified, digested with *BamH*I and *Xho*I, and ligated into pcDNA3xFLAG digested with the same restriction enzymes. pcDNA3xFLAG-RhTRIM5α was previously described [29].

2.3. Generation of Stable Cell Lines

Lentiviruses for transduction were produced by co-transfection of HEK293T cells with 5 μg of pMD.G (encoding the Vesicular Stomatitis Virus Envelope Glycoprotein), 5 μg of p8.91 (encoding for Gal-Pol of HIV-1), 2.5 μg of pRSVRev (encoding rev from HIV-1), and 10 μg of pLVX-IRES-PURO or pLVX-3xFLAG-DeRep-Puro using polyethyleneimine (PEI) 8 mg/mL in a 3:1 proportion. Viruses were harvested 48 h after transfection, filtered (0.45 μm), and used to transduce NIH3T3 cells in the presence of 8 μg/mL Polybrene. Cells were selected for 1 μg/mL of puromycin.

2.4. Antibody Generation

pcDNA3xFLAG-DeRep was digested with *BamH*I and *Xho*I. The coding sequence of DeRep was purified and ligated into pGEX4T1, digested with the same restriction enzymes. GST-DeRep was purified from bacteria, and DeRep was obtained by digestion with thrombin. DeRep was used to immunize 2 mice, and serum 120 and 121 were obtained. Serums were then affinity purified using GST-DeRep as bait.

2.5. Minute Virus of Mice Production

HEK293T seeded in 150-mm plates were transfected with 10 μg of pdBMVp using PEI 3:1 in fresh media. After 24 h, the media was changed to DMEM with 3% FBS, and cells were cultured until cytopathic effects appeared (days 2–5 post-transfection). Media was collected and filtered to 0.2 μm, and the virus was aliquoted and stored at −80 °C until use.

2.6. Viral DNA Quantification

HEK293T cells (6×10^4 cells/well) were seeded in 6-well plates. Twenty-four hours after plating, cells were co-transfected with 1 μg of pcDNA3xFLAG-DeRep, 1 μg of pcDNA3xFLAG-RhTRIM5α, or with empty vector and 200 ng of pdBMVp using Lipofectamine 2000. Forty-eight hours after transfection, media were recovered and filtered, and the monolayer was recovered in PBS for DNA and protein extraction. DNA was purified by gel and PCR clean-up columns (Machery-Nagel). Recovered DNA was used for qPCR assay with Brilliant II SYBER Green kit and primers directed to MVM NS (NS-F 5′-ACCAGCCAGCACAGGCAAATCTATTAT-3′; NS-R 5′-CATTCTGTCTCTGATTGGTTGAGT-3′) and host 18S (18S-F 5′-GTGGAGCGA TTTGTCTGGTT-3′; 18S-R 5′-CGCTGAGCCAGTCAGTGTAG-3′). Data are expressed as the MVM DNA amount relative to 18S calculated by the ΔΔCt method [30]. Protein overexpression was determined by western blotting using anti-FLAG and anti-tubulin, as described below.

2.7. Western Blot Assays

To analyze the expression of DeRep in fusion with GFP or FLAG, NIH3T3 cells were transfected with 1 μg of either pEGFP, pEGFP-DeRep, pcDNA3xFLAG, pcDNA3xFLAG-DeRep, pcDNA3xFLAG-enRepM9L, or pcDNA3xFLAG-OcenRep using PEI 3:1. Forty-eight hours later, the cells were lysed in Reporter lysis buffer (Promega, Madison, WI, USA). Samples were then boiled in 5× sodium dodecyl sulfate (SDS) loading buffer, and the proteins were resolved by 10% acrylamide SDS-PAGE. After transfer to PVDF membranes, the blots were probed with mouse anti-Flag (Clone M2, Sigma, Kawasaki, Tokyo), mouse anti-GFP B-2 (Santa Cruz Biotechnology, Santa Cruz, CA, USA), mouse anti-DeRep

120, mouse anti-DeRep 121, or mouse anti-α tubulin (Clone DM1A, Sigma). Secondary antibodies conjugated to HRP and ECL reagents were used for development.

To analyze the expression of DeRep in degu, tissues were obtained from a fresh male (3) or female (3) headless *O. degus* cadaver (kindly donated by Dr. Adrian Palacios from the Universidad de Valparaiso, Chile). All experiments were performed according to the protocol approved by the Bioethical Committee of Universidad Andres Bello (Acta 002/2018). Upon obtaining a fresh cadaver, the liver, kidney, heart, lung, muscle, gonad, and adrenal gland were isolated, rinsed with ice-cold phosphate saline buffer (PBS), cut into small pieces, and protein extracts prepared using RIPA buffer (50 mM Tris pH 8.0, 150 mM NaCl, 0.1% SDS, 1% Triton X-100, 0.5% sodium deoxycholate) with protease inhibitors. Samples were homogenized with 20 dounce strokes and maintained for 30 min at 4 °C with rotation. Finally, samples were centrifuged for 20 min at 10,000× *g* at 4 °C. Supernatants were quantified, and 30 μg of protein were used for western blot assays using mouse anti-DeRep 120, mouse anti-DeRep 121, or mouse anti-α tubulin. Samples from *Cavia porcellus* liver and HEK293T cells were prepared as described above. For comparison between degu, HEK293T and guinea pig , 60 μg of protein were used for western blot assays.

To analyze the expression of FLAG-DeRep in HEK293T cells co-transfected with pcDNA3xFLAG-DeRep and pdBMVp or in NIH3T3 cells stably expressing FLAG-DeRep, cells were lysed using RIPA buffer, and 10 μg of each sample were used for western blot assays with anti-FLAG or anti-α tubulin antibodies.

To analyze the expression of viral proteins upon MVM infection, NIH3T3 cells expressing FLAG-DeRep or the control stable cell line were seeded at 5×10^4 cells/well in 6-well plates, and 24 h later they were infected with a $\frac{1}{4}$ MVM dilution and lysed at 0, 12, 16, 20, or 24 h post infection, and western blots were performed using a rabbit anti-NS1/NS2 antibody (kindly donated by Dr. Peter Tattersall), mouse anti-FLAG, or rabbit anti-GAPDH antibody [6C5] (Abcam, Cambridge, UK).

2.8. RNA Extraction and PCR Amplification

Upon obtaining a fresh cadaver, the liver, kidney, heart, lung, muscle, gonad, and adrenal gland were isolated, rinsed with ice-cold phosphate saline buffer (PBS), cut into small pieces, and the RNA extracted with Trizol. One microgram of RNA was used for cDNA synthesis using the iScript gDNA Clear cDNA Synthesis Kit (Bio-Rad, Hercules, CA, USA) according to the manufacturer's instructions. cDNA was PCR amplified and analyzed as described in [22].

2.9. Immunofluorescence Assays

To analyze the DNA damage marker γH2AX upon MVM infection, NIH3T3 cells expressing FLAG-DeRep or the control stable cell line were seeded at 2.5×10^4 cells/well in 12 mm coverslips and infected with a 1/4 MVM dilution for 24 h. Cells were rinsed twice in ice-cold PBS, fixed for 20 min in a freshly prepared solution of 4% paraformaldehyde in PBS, and washed 3 times with PBS; they were permeabilized for 5 min with 0.2% Triton X-100 in PBS, and after 3 rinses in PBS, were incubated in 1% BSA in PBS for 30 min at 37 °C, followed by an overnight incubation at 4 °C with rabbit anti-DYKDDDDK Tag (1:1000; Cell Signalling Cat#14793) and mouse anti-p-Histone H2A.X antibody (Ser 139) (1:1000; Santa Cruz Biotechnology). Cells were washed 3 times with PBS, then incubated with Alexa-conjugated secondary antibodies (ThermoFisher, USA) for 30 min at 37 °C. Cells were washed 3 times with PBS and incubated with NucBlue (ThermoFisher, Waltham, MA, USA) for 15 min. Coverslips were mounted with Fluoromont-G (Electron Microscopy Sciences, Hatfield, PA, USA) and analyzed by confocal laser microscopy (Nikon C2+, Melville, NY, USA). Triple-color immunofluorescent images were captured by multi-tracking imaging of each channel independently to eliminate possible crosstalk between fluorochromes. Images were analyzed using NIH ImageJ software. The quantification of fluorescence was carried out under threshold conditions, measuring signal intensity in a defined ROI.

2.10. MVM Infection Assays

To titrate MVM obtained in HEK293T cells expressing FLAG-DeRep or control cells, NIH3T3 (4×10^3 cells/well) were seeded in 96-well plates. Twenty-four hours later, cells were infected with two-fold serial dilutions of each virus in quadruplicate for 1 h. The media was replaced, and cells were incubated in DMEM with 10% FBS for five days. Cells were fixed with 10% formaldehyde for 1 h at room temperature, washed, and stained with 1% crystal violet for at least 6 h. The stain was dissolved in 1% SDS, and its absorbance was measured at 595 nm.

To challenge cells with MVM, NIH3T3 cells stably expressing FLAG-DeRep or control cells were seeded in 24-well plates (3×10^4 cells/well), and 24 h later, they were infected in triplicate with a two-fold serial dilution of MVM in complete media for 5 h. The media was then changed, and cells were incubated for five days in complete media. Cells were fixed and stained as above.

2.11. Chromatin Immunoprecipitation (ChIP)

NIH3T3 cells were seeded in 150-mm plates with a 3×10^6 cells/mL density. Twenty-four hours later, cells were transfected with 30 µg of pcDNA3xFLAG-DeRep or empty vector, and 24 h after that, they were infected for 2 h with MVM diluted 1/8 in PBS. After changing the media, cells were cultured for 48 h and processed for ChIP according to [31] with modifications. Cells were crosslinked by incubation in DMEM with 1% FBS and 1% formaldehyde for 10 min at 37 °C. Crosslinking was stopped with 0.125 M of glycine. Cells were washed with ice-cold PBS, and Farnham lysis buffer (5 mM PIPES pH 8.0, 85 mM KCl, 0.5% NP-40) was added. Cells were collected, centrifuged at 1000× *g* for 5 min at 4 °C, and the cell pellet was resuspended in 1 mL of Farnham lysis buffer, shred 20 times using a 20-gauge needle, and centrifuged at 1000× *g* for 5 min at 4 °C. The pellet was resuspended in 500 µL of RIPA buffer (1x PBS, 1% NP-40, 0.5% sodium deoxycholate, 0.1% SDS). The suspension was sonicated in Qsonica Q800R3 for 15 min and then centrifuged at 13,000× *g* for 15 min at 4 °C. Four hundred microliters of the supernatant were mixed with 2 µg of anti-FLAG M2 or normal mouse IgG (Santa Cruz) for 1 h at 4 °C, and antibodies were sedimented with a mix of Dynabeads Protein A/G for 2 h at 4 °C. Beads were washed 5 times at 4 °C with 100 mM Tris pH 7.5, 500 mM LiCl, 1% NP-40, and 1% sodium deoxycholate. Crosslinking was reverted over night at 65 °C. The samples were treated with 1 µg/mL proteinase K for 1 h at 37 °C. DNA was purified using gel and PCR clean-up columns (Machery-Nagel) and was used for qPCR assay with the Brilliant II SYBER Green kit and primers directed to MVM NS (NS-F 5′-ACCAGCCAGCACAGGCAAATCTATTAT-3′; NS-R 5′-CATTCTGTCTCTGATTGGTTGAGT-3′) or VP (VP-F 5′-AAATTACTGCACTAGCAAC TAGAC-3′, VP-R 5′-CTTCAGGAAAGGTTGACAGCA-3′).

2.12. Statistical Analysis

Values are presented as the mean ± standard deviation (SD) for 3 or more independent experiments. Statistical analyses with the Student's t test were performed. Values of $p < 0.05$ were considered statistically significant. All statistical analyses were performed using Graphpad Prism (GraphPad Software Inc., San Diego, CA, USA).

3. Results

3.1. Generation of DeRep-Specific Antibodies

EPV-Dependo.43-ODegus is an EPV with an open reading frame of 1527 bp that encodes a protein of 508 amino acids, named DeRep. DeRep has a 62% amino acid identity to AAV2 Rep [22] and a high similarity to other AAV Rep proteins (Figure S1). We have previously shown that *EPV-Dependo.43-ODegus* (Odegus-4 in our previous report) is transcribed in at least 2 organs in degus: the liver and lung [22]. To determine if it is also expressed in vivo, we generated antibodies in mice using a bacterially produced DeRep protein. To test if the antibodies worked on western blot assays, we transfected cell lines with plasmids encoding full-length tagged GFP-DeRep or FLAG-DeRep (Figure 1A). When western blots were performed using anti-GFP antibodies, we detected the presence of GFP when the cells were transfected with the pEGFP vector or the fused protein GFP-DeRep when the cells were transfected with pEGFP-DeRep (Figure 1A, upper panel). Using the anti-FLAG antibody, we detected only one band in cells transfected with pcDNA3xFLAG-DeRep (Figure 1A, second panel). When custom-generated anti-DeRep 120 and anti-DeRep 121 were used, we detected both GFP-DeRep and FLAG-DeRep (Figure 1A, third and fourth panels), showing that both antibodies detect DeRep in western blot assays when it is expressed in cells.

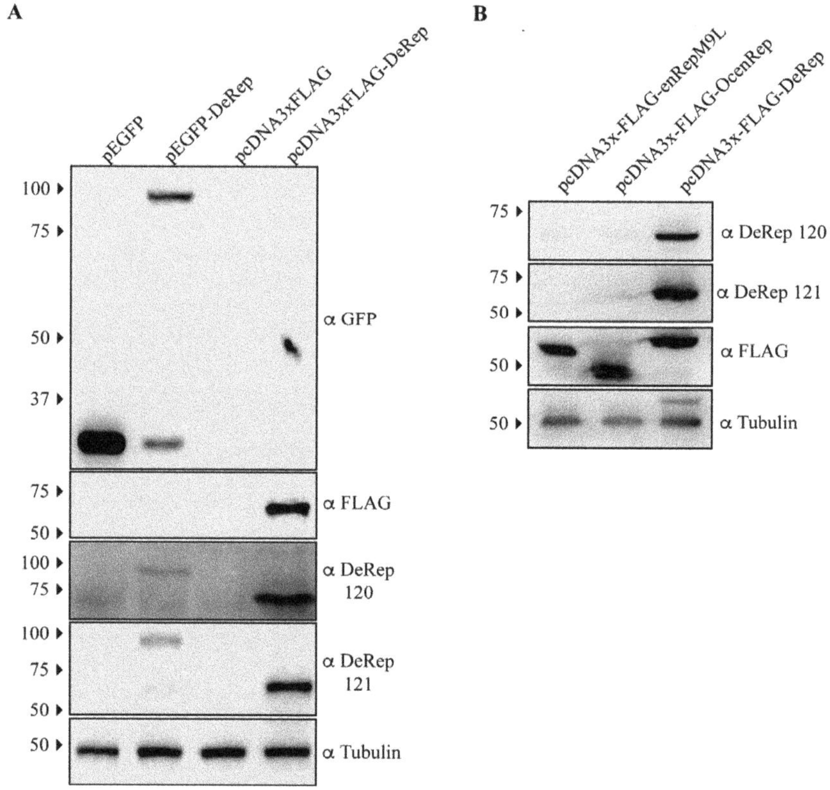

Figure 1. Validation of anti-DeRep antibodies by western blot assays. (**A**) NIH3T3 cells were transfected with plasmids encoding GFP-DeRep, FLAG-DeRep, or empty vectors. Forty-eight hours after transfection, cells were lysed, and western blots were performed using anti-GFP, anti-FLAG, anti-DeRep 120, or anti-DeRep 121. (**B**) NIH3T3 cells were transfected with plasmids encoding FLAG-enRepM9L, FLAG-OcenRep, or FLAG-DeRep. Forty-eight hours after transfection, cells were lysed, and western blots were performed using anti-FLAG, anti-DeRep 120, or anti-DeRep 121. Tubulin was used as a loading control. A representative experiment of at least three independent assays is shown. The migration of the molecular weight marker is indicated on the left-hand side. The antibodies used in each western blot are indicated on the right-hand side.

We also tested if the anti-DeRep antibodies were able to recognize other NS-derived EPVs we have cloned in the same FLAG-expressing vector. We have previously described the transcription and expression in heterologous systems of enRepM9L, an intact EPV found in guinea pigs [21], and include in this analysis an intact EPV cloned from rabbits

(*Oryctolagus cuniculus*) named OcenRep (unpublished data). When a western blot was performed, both anti-DeRep antibodies only recognized DeRep (Figure 1B, first and second panels), while the anti-FLAG antibody recognized the three FLAG-tagged proteins at their expected size. This shows that when expressed in cells, both antibodies specifically detect the expression of DeRep and no other EPV proteins.

3.2. DeRep Expression in Degu

Since both anti-DeRep antibodies can specifically detect DeRep when expressed in cells, we moved on to test if it was possible to detect DeRep in protein extracts obtained from degu tissues. Both antibodies showed similar results: a main band at the expected migration of DeRep (Figure 2A). Unexpectedly, this band was present in all tissue samples analyzed, not only from the liver and lungs. Thus, we revisited the previously analyzed animals and performed RNA extraction in some of the new animals, increasing the starting concentration of RNA for cDNA preparation and finding that the RNA is transcribed in all analyzed tissues (Figure 2B). We also found that both antibodies also detected a second band around 25 kDa, but mainly in liver samples (Figure 2A). To further test the specificity of our antibodies, we performed a second set of western blot assays, comparing one tissue of a different degu from that shown in Figure 2A with lysates from HEK293T cells and *Cavia porcellus* (guinea pig), a relatively closed rodent where we have shown that an intact Rep-derived EPV is transcribed in several tissues [21]. The adrenal sample from degu shows a similar pattern to that observed in Figure 2A with both antibodies; HEK293T shows a non-specific binding with antibody 120 and a weak signal around 25 kDa with antibody 121; more importantly, the liver samples from *C. porcellus* do not show any signal with either antibody (Figure 2C). These results indicate that the DeRep protein is expressed in different tissues of degu, which strongly suggests a functional role for it.

3.3. DeRep Blocks Exogenous Parvovirus Replication

It has not been reported if EPVs have functional roles in their hosts. As a first approach and considering that DeRep has NS/Rep characteristics (Figure S1), it is located in the nucleus when expressed in cell lines [21], and several EVE have a role in immunity [15,32,33], we asked if DeRep could affect parvoviral replication. The virus we decided to use was the 'minute virus of mice' (MVM), a cytolytic autonomous protoparvovirus with 37% homology of the NS1 protein to DeRep.

Our first approach was to analyze the production of MVM in HEK293T cells co-transfected with the MVM molecular clone and the plasmid encoding FLAG-DeRep versus cells co-transfected with the empty vector. We found a significant reduction in viral DNA production in cells expressing FLAG-DeRep (Figure 3A) compared to control cells. When this experiment was performed to co-transfect the retroviral restriction factor TRIM5α [34], we found that viral DNA production has similar levels to that observed in cells co-transfected with the empty vector, while a reduction of around 50% is found in cells co-transfected with FLAG-DeRep (Figure S2). In line with this observation, we performed an infection assay and found that the virus prepared in cells that express FLAG-DeRep was significantly less infective than the virus prepared in cells that do not express it (Figure 3B). This suggested that DeRep could reduce MVM production from the molecular clone. We asked if DeRep could also reduce the replication of MVM upon infection. For this, we generated a stable NIH3T3 cell line that expresses FLAG-DeRep or its control version (Figure 4A) and challenged them with different dilutions of MVM. We found that DeRep can significantly protect cells from the cytopathic effect of MVM replication, even at high doses (Figure 4B). These results strongly suggest that DeRep can inhibit parvoviral replication.

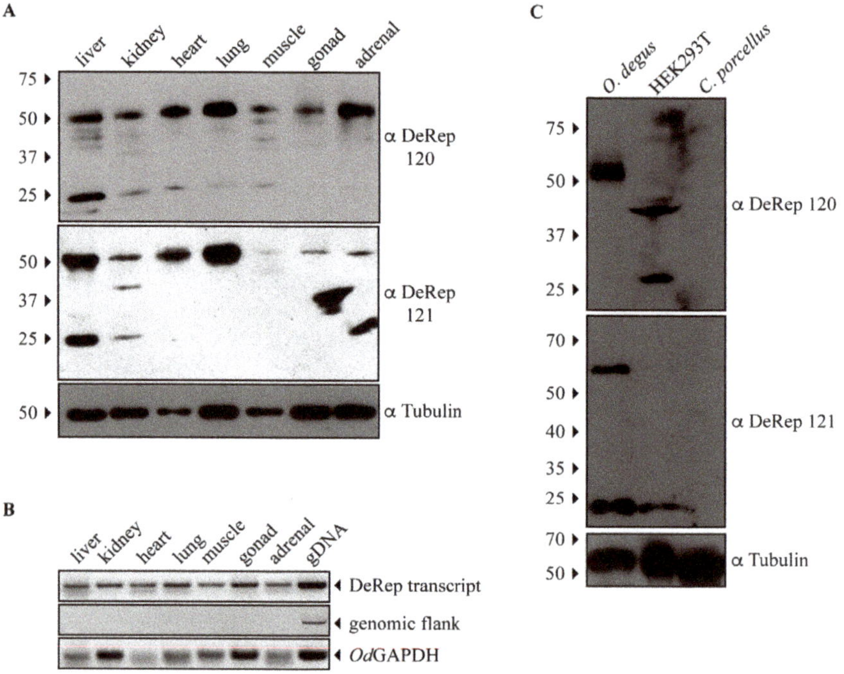

Figure 2. The protein DeRep is expressed in several organs of the degu. (**A**) Different organs of degu were isolated, lysed, and analyzed by western blot using the anti-DeRep 120 (upper panel) or anti-DeRep 121 (middle panel) antibodies. Samples from one representative animal of the six analyzed are shown. Tubulin was used as a loading control. The migration of the molecular weight marker is indicated on the left-hand side. The antibodies used in each western blot are indicated on the right-hand side. (**B**) Different organs of degu were isolated, lysed, and RNA extracted to synthesize cDNA. cDNA was PCR amplified with primers aligning inside the DeRep open reading frame (DeRep transcript), flanking *EPV-Dependo.43-ODegus* (genomic flank), or GAPDH transcript. Amplicons were detected in the agarose gel. One representative animal of the three analyzed is shown. (**C**) Lysates from *O. degus* (adrenal), HEK293T cells, and *C. porcellus* (liver) were analyzed by western blot using the anti-DeRep 120 (upper panel), anti-DeRep 121 (middle panel), and tubulin (lower panel) antibodies. Samples from one representative independent experiment of the three conducted are shown. The migration of the molecular weight marker is indicated on the left-hand side. The antibodies used in each western blot are indicated on the right-hand side.

Since we observed a reduction in viral DNA production in HEK293T cells when they were co-transfected with FLAG-DeRep, we wondered if viral protein production is also affected in FLAG-DeRep-expressing cells when they are infected with MVM. To test this, we performed a western blot assay with samples of cells infected with a single dose of MVM over a time course of 0, 12, 16, 20, and 24 h. We observed that in DeRep-expressing cells there is a delay in NS1 expression; in control cells, it is possible to detect NS1 at 16 h post-infection (hpi), and a clearly defined band is observed at 20 and 24 hpi, while in FLAG-DeRep, we observed a faint band at 20 hpi and a clear band at 24 hpi (Figure 5A). For NS2, we observed a band only at 24 hpi in both cell lines, but much less defined and intense in FLAG-DeRep (Figure 5A). We quantified the western blot signals for NS1 and NS2 at 24 hpi and found a significant reduction in both proteins in cells expressing FLAG-DeRep compared to control cells at the same time point (Figure 5B). In addition, we used immunofluorescence to analyze the presence of the DNA damage marker γH2Ax, which increases with the DNA damage that occurs in cells when MVM replicates [35]. We infected the cells and fixed them at 24 hpi. We then found that in control cells there is a significant increase in the signal of γH2AX upon infection compared to non-infected cells (Figure 5C,D), while in FLAG-DeRep-expressing cells a slight, but non-significant, increase in the γH2Ax signal is observed between non-infected and infected cells. When we compare control and FLAG-DeRep-infected cells, we clearly observe a reduced γH2AX signal in FLAG-DeRep-expressing cells (Figure 5C), which is significantly lower than that in the control cells (Figure 5D). Altogether, these results indicate that although MVM can replicate in cells expressing FLAG-DeRep, its replication is significantly reduced compared to control cells, suggesting a possible antiviral role for DeRep in its host.

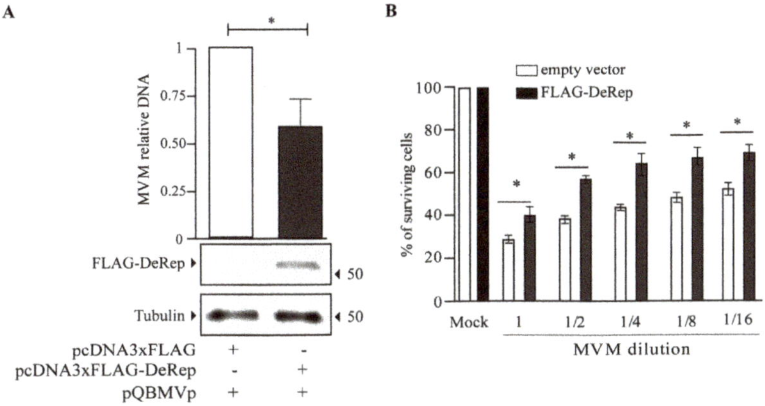

Figure 3. MVM production is reduced in the presence of FLAG-DeRep. (**A**) Quantification of viral DNA in HEK293T cells co-transfected with an empty vector or a FLAG-DeRep coding vector and the MVM molecular clone pQBMVp. The average of three independent experiments is shown. The expression of FLAG-DeRep was confirmed by western blot with an anti-FLAG antibody; tubulin was used as a loading control. The migration of the molecular weight marker is indicated on the right-hand side. The migration of FLAG-DeRep and tubulin is indicated on the left-hand side. (**B**) Infectivity of MVM produced in control (white bars) or FLAG-DeRep (gray bars)-expressing cells. NIH3T3 cells were infected with identical dilutions of each virus, and cell survival was quantified five days post-infection. The average of four independent experiments is shown. * $p < 0.05$.

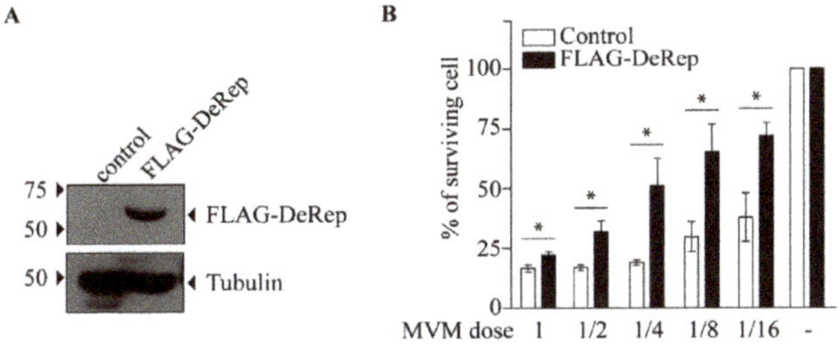

Figure 4. FLAG-DeRep reduces MVM replication in NIH3T3 cells. NIH3T3 cells expressing FLAG-DeRep in a stable manner or stably transfected with an empty vector (control) were generated and then infected with different dilutions of MVM. (**A**) Western blot showing the expression of FLAG-DeRep and its absence in the control cell line using the anti-FLAG antibody. The migration of molecular weight markers is indicated on the left-hand side. The migration of FLAG-DeRep and tubulin is indicated on the right-hand side. (**B**) Infectivity of MVM in control (white bars) or FLAG-DeRep (gray bars)-expressing cells. The average of five independent experiments is shown. The results are expressed as a percent of surviving cells, where 100% are non-infected cells. * $p < 0.05$.

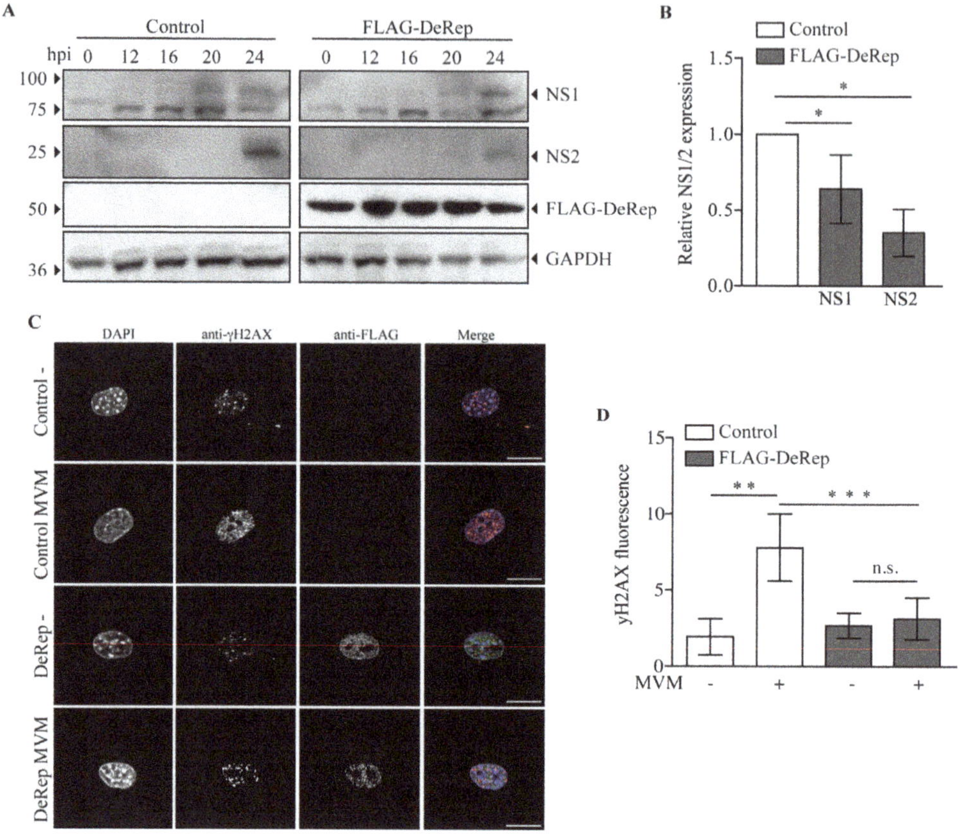

Figure 5. Expression of FLAG-DeRep reduces MVM protein expression and DNA damage induction in MVM-infected cells. (**A**) Control cells or cells stably expressing FLAGDeRep were infected with a $\frac{1}{4}$ MVM dilution and harvested at 0, 12, 16, 20, and 24 h post-infection. Cells were lysed, and western blot assays were performed using anti-NS1/2 serum (first and second panels), anti-FLAG (third panel), and anti-GAPDH (fourth panel). A representative western blot of four independent experiments is shown. (**B**) The NS1 and NS2 protein levels at 24 h post-infection were quantified and expressed relative to the loading control. (**C**) Control cells or cells stably expressing FLAG-DeRep seeded in coverslips were infected or not with a $\frac{1}{4}$ MVM dilution for 24 h. Cells were fixed and stained with mouse anti-γH2AX and rabbit anti-FLAG, followed by anti-mouse Alexa-546, anti-rabbit Alexa-488, and DAPI. A representative cell of 20 quantified cells is shown for each condition. (**D**) Quantification of γH2AX fluorescence labels in control and FLAG-Derep expressing cells the infection status in indicated in the X axis. Scale bar = 20 nm. * $p < 0.05$, ** $p = 0.002$, *** $p < 0.001$, n.s. = not significant.

We observed that the Rep-derived protein DeRep is in the nucleus [21] (Figure 5C), the replication site of MVM. We therefore hypothesize that it could be bound to viral DNA to block its replication and/or transcription. To test whether DeRep is able to bind viral DNA, we performed chromatin immunoprecipitation assays in FLAG-DeRep cells infected with MVM. We found that FLAG-DeRep binds specifically to viral DNA in the NS region but not the VP region (Figure 6). These results are consistent with a role for DeRep as a dominant negative inhibitor of parvovirus replication. Further experiments are needed to determine whether it can form an inactive or partially active complex with the replication machinery or if it is blocking the binding of the replication and/or transcription machinery to viral DNA.

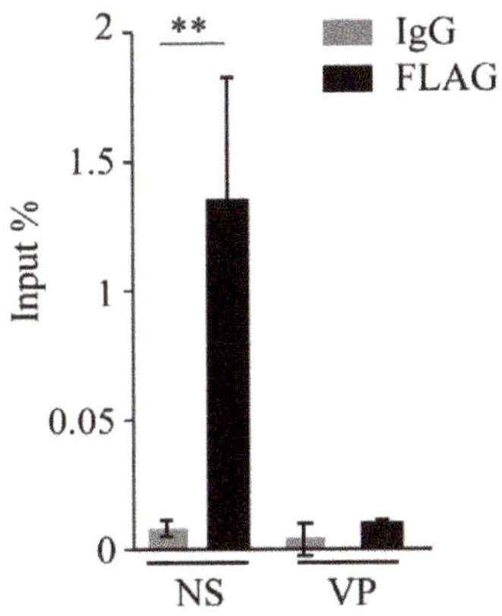

Figure 6. FLAG-DeRep binds to the MVM genome. NIH3T3 cells expressing FLAG-DeRep were infected for 48 h with MVM. Cells were fixed, and chromatin immunoprecipitation was performed with anti-FLAG or non-specific IgG. Immunoprecipitated DNA was recovered and analyzed by qPCR with primers against the NS or VP genes. Results are presented as a percentage of input recovered. ** $p = 0.0094$.

4. Discussion

Intact EPVs have been found at a surprisingly high frequency in mammalian genomes, suggesting that their conservation is associated with a potential physiological role in their host [1,6,21,22]. We and others have found EPVs derived from the Rep genes of dependoparvoviruses that contain intact ORFs and are transcribed in their hosts [21,22,27]. Here we show that one of these EPVs is translated within its host, the degu. Moreover, we have previously reported the expression in vitro of a fusion protein derived in part from an EPV in guinea pigs (*Cavia porcellus*) [21]. Here, however, we demonstrate the expression of a completely EPV-derived protein in vivo; to our knowledge, this is the first such demonstration.

Since our previous study on *EPV-Dependo.43-ODegus* showed transcription in the liver and lung, and the EPV of elephants also showed transcription in the liver [27], we expected a discrete protein expression if it was expressed as protein. To our surprise, we found DeRep protein in all analyzed tissues using either of the two affinity-purified antibodies we developed, although at different expression levels and always more robustly expressed in the liver. We revisited the previously analyzed animals and performed RNA extraction in some of the new animals, increasing the starting concentration of RNA for cDNA preparation and finding that the RNA is transcribed in all tissues (Figure 2B), concomitant with our protein expression patterns. When these antibodies were used in *Cavia porcellus* protein extract, no band was detected with either antibody (Figure 2C). We are therefore confident that the protein detected for both antibodies around 56 kDa is DeRep and not an unspecific binding. We also observed a second band around 25 kDa in some of the degu tissues analyzed with both antibodies. This could be a non-specific band, but it is also possible that Odegus4 mRNA allows the translation of a second protein from an internal AUG codon in Kozak context. Parvoviruses have mainly two genes that can encode several proteins by different mechanisms, such as the use of an internal promoter, splicing, and leaky scanning mechanisms [36], and some of these proteins are in frame with the principal protein that these genes encode. When analyzing the mRNA sequence of DeRep, we identified two putative start codons in a Kozak context that are in frame with the full-length ORF of DeRep. Both can be translated into proteins of 220 or 209 amino acids, respectively, corresponding to the 25 kDa bands we observed. More experiments are required to determine if the smaller protein is also translated from DeRep mRNA by a different transcript from an internal promoter or by a leaky scanning mechanism.

We cloned the coding sequence of the full-length DeRep protein, a 56 kDa protein that localizes in the nucleus [21] (Figure 5C), which is the replication site of parvoviruses. When co-transfecting the DeRep coding sequence along the molecular clone of MVM, we observed a reduction in viral DNA production as well as a lower viral titer when compared to control cells (Figure 3). Similarly, when DeRep-expressing cells are infected with MVM, viral replication is significantly reduced (Figure 4), which correlates with the delay observed in viral protein production (Figure 5A,B). Since DeRep is derived from a Rep parvoviral gene and contains both the Rep (catalytic domain with DNA binding and endonuclease activity) and Parvo_NS1 (DNA helicase and ATPase activity) domains, we tested if it was able to bind viral DNA. We found that DeRep binds to the NS region of the MVM genome (Figure 6), therefore co-localizing with the replication machinery. This has also been observed for itEBLN, which can co-localize with Borna disease virus (BDV) replication factories in the nucleus, reducing BDV replication [15]. Similar to itEBLN, DeRep exhibits antiviral activity against an exogenous virus of the same family. Further experiments are needed to determine its exact mechanism of action, for instance, if DeRep interacts with NS1 and the influence of its localization on its antiviral activity. DeRep's predicted nuclear localization signal (NLS) (Figure S1) must be compared to a real NLS. For now, we can speculate that if an interaction with NS1 is occurring, even in the absence of an NLS in DeRep, we could find DeRep in the nucleus upon infection, still blocking MVM replication. MVM NS1 has been shown to complement nuclear localization-deficient versions of itself [37], and other NS proteins shuttle between cytoplasm and nucleus [38,39], so a putative interaction with DeRep in the cytoplasm could move DeRep to the nucleus. However, if the interaction is only with DNA, blocking NS1 binding to it, an NLS-null DeRep should lose its antiviral activity.

One important limitation of our study is that we have expressed DeRep in mouse cells, and it is in this context that DeRep is able to reduce the replication of a model protoparvovirus, MVM. Since there is no cell line derived from *Octodon degu*, we do not know if the level of expression we achieve in our stable cell line reflects the physiological levels of DeRep in degu cells. If a degu cell line can be established, it would be important to test if they are susceptible and/or permissive to MVM. In this context, DeRep gain and loss of function experiments will show the protein's physiological relevance in the host. So far, no degu parvoviruses have been described, but given the ubiquity of parvovirus infection among mammals, it is likely they exist. We can speculate that if the function of intact EPVs in the host is to act as antivirals, there might exist parvoviruses that have co-evolved with degu. To know this, it will be necessary to understand the diversity of viruses in nature as well as the interaction between native wild animals and domestic animals that can act as vectors of viruses that do not normally circulate in wildlife, such as canine parvovirus.

Other intact, non-retroviral EVEs have been co-opted to perform cellular functions that are not necessarily related to counteracting exogenous viruses. One example is human EBLN, where hsEBLN1 can act as lncRNAs regulating gene expression [18], while hsEBLN2 has acquired a mitochondrial localization signal and is now important to regulate cell survival [17]. If parvoviruses that infect degu in nature are extinct, then we can speculate that the conservation of the *EPV-Dependo.43-ODegus* locus through this rodent evolution is due to domestication to perform a new cellular function as a protein. Its capacity to bind MVM DNA and nuclear localization suggest that it could be participating in DNA metabolism, but unlike hsEBLN1, which functions as RNA, it could be doing it as a protein.

In captivity, degus can live up to 13 years. They are gregarious animals that are models of social behavior [40,41] as well as neurobiology since they are used to study the retina [42,43] and they develop an Alzheimer's-like disease while aging [44–46]. Therefore, they are interesting models that can be genetically manipulated using adeno-associated viruses (AVVs) as delivery vectors. Although we tested replication of a protoparvovirus rather than a dependovirus, our results should be considered when deciding which delivery tools can be used in degu. In favor of using AAVs to manipulate degu, a preliminary assay showed that transduction by a GFP-coding AAV2 vector was not impaired in cells expressing DeRep. More experiments will be needed to demonstrate if there is a saturation phenomenon, as it happened for some retroviral restriction factors such as TRIM5alpha and Fv1 [47], or if AAV infection is indeed not affected by DeRep. It could also be possible that the different levels of DeRep observed in the different tissues analyzed can confer differential protection against parvoviruses or AAV vectors.

5. Conclusions

The endogenous parvovirus (EPV) locus '*EPV-Dependo.43-ODegus*' (Odegus4) is a host gene encoding an intact, Rep-derived protein that is expressed in vivo and named DeRep. This protein, when expressed in cell culture, is able to block parvovirus replication, which suggests an antiviral role.

Supplementary Materials: The following supporting information can be downloaded at: https://www.mdpi.com/article/10.3390/v15071420/s1. Figure S1. Multiple sequence alignment showing homology between DeRep protein and the NS proteins of representative dependoparvoviruses. Figure S2. MVM DNA is reduced in the presence of FLAG-DeRep but not in the presence of FLAG-TRIM5α.

Author Contributions: G.A., A.B. and R.J.G. conceptualize the study; L.M., G.A.M. and F.J.B. generated resources used in this study; A.B., L.F.-G., R.I.-K., F.J.B. and G.A. performed and analyze experiments. G.A. and F.J.B. prepare the figures. G.A. and R.J.G. wrote the paper. All authors have read and agreed to the published version of the manuscript.

Funding: This research was funded by ANID-FONDECYT 1180705 and 1220480 to GA, ANID-FONDECYT 3210343 to LFG, DI-04-19/INI from Universidad Andres Bello to AB.

Institutional Review Board Statement: The animal study protocol was approved by the Institutional Review Board (or Ethics Committee) of Universidad Andres Bello (Acta 002/2018 from 9 May 2019).

Data Availability Statement: All data supporting this work is available upon request.

Acknowledgments: We thank Peter Tattersall for kindly donate the MVM molecular clone and the anti NS antibodies, Adrian Palacios for the degu carcasses used in this study. This article is dedicated to the memory of Andrés Rivera-Dictter who provided technical assistance.

Conflicts of Interest: The authors declare no conflict of interest. The funders had no role in the design of the study; in the collection, analyses, or interpretation of data; in the writing of the manuscript; or in the decision to publish the results.

References

1. Katzourakis, A.; Gifford, R.J. Endogenous viral elements in animal genomes. *PLoS Genet.* **2010**, *6*, e1001191. [CrossRef] [PubMed]
2. Feschotte, C.; Gilbert, C. Endogenous viruses: Insights into viral evolution and impact on host biology. *Nat. Rev. Genet.* **2012**, *13*, 283–296. [CrossRef] [PubMed]
3. Dennis, T.P.W.; Flynn, P.J.; de Souza, W.M.; Singer, J.B.; Moreau, C.S.; Wilson, S.J.; Gifford, R.J. Insights into Circovirus Host Range from the Genomic Fossil Record. *J. Virol.* **2018**, *92*, e00145-18. [CrossRef]
4. Campbell, M.A.; Loncar, S.; Kotin, R.M.; Gifford, R.J. Comparative analysis reveals the long-term coevolutionary history of parvoviruses and vertebrates. *PLoS Biol.* **2022**, *20*, e3001867. [CrossRef] [PubMed]
5. Horie, M.; Tomonaga, K. Non-retroviral fossils in vertebrate genomes. *Viruses* **2011**, *3*, 1836–1848. [CrossRef] [PubMed]
6. Kapoor, A.; Simmonds, P.; Lipkin, W.I. Discovery and characterization of mammalian endogenous parvoviruses. *J. Virol.* **2010**, *84*, 12628–12635. [CrossRef] [PubMed]
7. Belyi, V.A.; Levine, A.J.; Skalka, A.M. Sequences from ancestral single-stranded DNA viruses in vertebrate genomes: The parvoviridae and circoviridae are more than 40 to 50 million years old. *J. Virol.* **2010**, *84*, 12458–12462. [CrossRef]
8. Holmes, E.C. The evolution of endogenous viral elements. *Cell Host Microbe* **2011**, *10*, 368–377. [CrossRef]
9. Horie, M.; Honda, T.; Suzuki, Y.; Kobayashi, Y.; Daito, T.; Oshida, T.; Ikuta, K.; Jern, P.; Gojobori, T.; Coffin, J.M.; et al. Endogenous non-retroviral RNA virus elements in mammalian genomes. *Nature* **2010**, *463*, 84–87. [CrossRef]
10. Shimizu, A.; Nakatani, Y.; Nakamura, T.; Jinno-Oue, A.; Ishikawa, O.; Boeke, J.D.; Takeuchi, Y.; Hoshino, H. Characterisation of cytoplasmic DNA complementary to non-retroviral RNA viruses in human cells. *Sci. Rep.* **2014**, *4*, 5074. [CrossRef]

11. Dewannieux, M.; Heidmann, T. Endogenous retroviruses: Acquisition, amplification and taming of genome invaders. *Curr. Opin. Virol.* **2013**, *3*, 646–656. [CrossRef]
12. Frank, J.A.; Feschotte, C. Co-option of endogenous viral sequences for host cell function. *Curr. Opin. Virol.* **2017**, *25*, 81–89. [CrossRef] [PubMed]
13. Gautam, P.; Yu, T.; Loh, Y.H. Regulation of ERVs in pluripotent stem cells and reprogramming. *Curr. Opin. Genet. Dev.* **2017**, *46*, 194–201. [CrossRef]
14. Horie, M.; Tomonaga, K. Paleovirology of bornaviruses: What can be learned from molecular fossils of bornaviruses. *Virus Res.* **2018**, *262*, 2–9. [CrossRef] [PubMed]
15. Fujino, K.; Horie, M.; Honda, T.; Merriman, D.K.; Tomonaga, K. Inhibition of Borna disease virus replication by an endogenous bornavirus-like element in the ground squirrel genome. *Proc. Natl. Acad. Sci. USA* **2014**, *111*, 13175–13180. [CrossRef] [PubMed]
16. Horie, M. The biological significance of bornavirus-derived genes in mammals. *Curr. Opin. Virol.* **2017**, *25*, 1–6. [CrossRef]
17. Fujino, K.; Horie, M.; Kojima, S.; Shimizu, S.; Nabekura, A.; Kobayashi, H.; Makino, A.; Honda, T.; Tomonaga, K. A Human Endogenous Bornavirus-like Nucleoprotein Encodes a Mitochondrial Protein Associated with Cell Viability. *J. Virol.* **2021**, *95*, e0203020. [CrossRef]
18. Sofuku, K.; Parrish, N.F.; Honda, T.; Tomonaga, K. Transcription Profiling Demonstrates Epigenetic Control of Non-retroviral RNA Virus-Derived Elements in the Human Genome. *Cell Rep.* **2015**, *12*, 1548–1554. [CrossRef]
19. Liu, H.; Fu, Y.; Xie, J.; Cheng, J.; Ghabrial, S.A.; Li, G.; Peng, Y.; Yi, X.; Jiang, D. Widespread endogenization of densoviruses and parvoviruses in animal and human genomes. *J. Virol.* **2011**, *85*, 9863–9876. [CrossRef]
20. Pénzes, J.J.; de Souza, W.M.; Agbandje-McKenna, M.; Gifford, R.J. An ancient lineage of highly divergent parvoviruses infects both vertebrate and invertebrate hosts. *Viruses* **2019**, *11*, 525. [CrossRef]
21. Valencia-Herrera, I.; Faunes, F.; Cena-Ahumada, E.; Ibarra-Karmy, R.; Gifford, R.J.; Arriagada, G. Molecular Properties and Evolutionary Origins of a Parvovirus-Derived Myosin Fusion Gene in Guinea Pigs. *J. Virol.* **2019**, *93*, e00404-19. [CrossRef]
22. Arriagada, G.; Gifford, R.J. Parvovirus-derived endogenous viral elements in two South American rodent genomes. *J. Virol.* **2014**, *88*, 12158–12162. [CrossRef] [PubMed]
23. Smith, R.H.; Hallwirth, C.V.; Westerman, M.; Hetherington, N.A.; Tseng, Y.S.; Cecchini, S.; Virag, T.; Ziegler, M.L.; Rogozin, I.B.; Koonin, E.V.; et al. Germline viral "fossils" guide in silico reconstruction of a mid-Cenozoic era marsupial adeno-associated virus. *Sci. Rep.* **2016**, *6*, 28965. [CrossRef] [PubMed]
24. Hildebrandt, E.; Penzes, J.J.; Gifford, R.J.; Agbandje-Mckenna, M.; Kotin, R.M. Evolution of dependoparvoviruses across geological timescales-implications for design of AAV-based gene therapy vectors. *Virus Evol.* **2020**, *6*, veaa043. [CrossRef]
25. Cotmore, S.F.; Agbandje-McKenna, M.; Chiorini, J.A.; Mukha, D.V.; Pintel, D.J.; Qiu, J.; Soderlund-Venermo, M.; Tattersall, P.; Tijssen, P.; Gatherer, D.; et al. The family Parvoviridae. *Arch. Virol.* **2014**, *159*, 1239–1247. [CrossRef]
26. Berns, K.I. Parvovirus replication. *Microbiol. Rev.* **1990**, *54*, 316–329. [CrossRef] [PubMed]
27. Kobayashi, Y.; Shimazu, T.; Murata, K.; Itou, T.; Suzuki, Y. An endogenous adeno-associated virus element in elephants. *Virus Res.* **2019**, *262*, 10–14. [CrossRef] [PubMed]
28. Kestler, J.; Neeb, B.; Struyf, S.; Van Damme, J.; Cotmore, S.F.; D'Abramo, A.; Tattersall, P.; Rommelaere, J.; Dinsart, C.; Cornelis, J.J. cis requirements for the efficient production of recombinant DNA vectors based on autonomous parvoviruses. *Hum. Gene Ther.* **1999**, *10*, 1619–1632. [CrossRef]
29. Lukic, Z.; Goff, S.P.; Campbell, E.M.; Arriagada, G. Role of SUMO-1 and SUMO interacting motifs in rhesus TRIM5alpha-mediated restriction. *Retrovirology* **2013**, *10*, 10. [CrossRef]
30. Livak, K.J.; Schmittgen, T.D. Analysis of relative gene expression data using real-time quantitative PCR and the 2(-Delta Delta C(T)) Method. *Methods* **2001**, *25*, 402–408. [CrossRef]
31. Johnson, D.S.; Mortazavi, A.; Myers, R.M.; Wold, B. Genome-wide mapping of in vivo protein-DNA interactions. *Science* **2007**, *316*, 1497–1502. [CrossRef] [PubMed]
32. Honda, T.; Tomonaga, K. Endogenous non-retroviral RNA virus elements evidence a novel type of antiviral immunity. *Mob. Genet. Elem.* **2016**, *6*, e1165785. [CrossRef] [PubMed]
33. Parrish, N.F.; Fujino, K.; Shiromoto, Y.; Iwasaki, Y.W.; Ha, H.; Xing, J.; Makino, A.; Kuramochi-Miyagawa, S.; Nakano, T.; Siomi, H.; et al. piRNAs derived from ancient viral processed pseudogenes as transgenerational sequence-specific immune memory in mammals. *RNA* **2015**, *21*, 1691–1703. [CrossRef]
34. Wolf, D.; Goff, S.P. Host restriction factors blocking retroviral replication. *Annu. Rev. Genet.* **2008**, *42*, 143–163. [CrossRef] [PubMed]
35. Adeyemi, R.O.; Landry, S.; Davis, M.E.; Weitzman, M.D.; Pintel, D.J. Parvovirus minute virus of mice induces a DNA damage response that facilitates viral replication. *PLoS Pathog.* **2010**, *6*, e1001141. [CrossRef]
36. Linden, R.M.; Berns, K.I. Molecular biology of adeno-associated viruses. *Contrib. Microbiol.* **2000**, *4*, 68–84. [CrossRef]
37. Nuesch, J.P.; Tattersall, P. Nuclear targeting of the parvoviral replicator molecule NS1: Evidence for self-association prior to nuclear transport. *Virology* **1993**, *196*, 637–651. [CrossRef]
38. Cao, L.; Fu, F.; Chen, J.; Shi, H.; Zhang, X.; Liu, J.; Shi, D.; Huang, Y.; Tong, D.; Feng, L. Nucleocytoplasmic Shuttling of Porcine Parvovirus NS1 Protein Mediated by the CRM1 Nuclear Export Pathway and the Importin alpha/beta Nuclear Import Pathway. *J. Virol.* **2022**, *96*, e0148121. [CrossRef]

39. Alvisi, G.; Manaresi, E.; Cross, E.M.; Hoad, M.; Akbari, N.; Pavan, S.; Ariawan, D.; Bua, G.; Petersen, G.F.; Forwood, J.; et al. Importin alpha/beta-dependent nuclear transport of human parvovirus B19 nonstructural protein 1 is essential for viral replication. *Antivir. Res.* **2023**, *213*, 105588. [CrossRef]
40. Colonnello, V.; Iacobucci, P.; Fuchs, T.; Newberry, R.C.; Panksepp, J. Octodon degus. A useful animal model for social-affective neuroscience research: Basic description of separation distress, social attachments and play. *Neurosci. Biobehav. Rev.* **2011**, *35*, 1854–1863. [CrossRef]
41. Aspillaga-Cid, A.; Vera, D.C.; Ebensperger, L.A.; Correa, L.A. Parental care in male degus (*Octodon degus*) is flexible and contingent upon female care. *Physiol. Behav.* **2021**, *238*, 113487. [CrossRef] [PubMed]
42. Verra, D.M.; Sajdak, B.S.; Merriman, D.K.; Hicks, D. Diurnal rodents as pertinent animal models of human retinal physiology and pathology. *Prog. Retin. Eye Res.* **2020**, *74*, 100776. [CrossRef] [PubMed]
43. Chang, L.Y.; Palanca-Castan, N.; Neira, D.; Palacios, A.G.; Acosta, M.L. Ocular Health of Octodon degus as a Clinical Marker for Age-Related and Age-Independent Neurodegeneration. *Front. Integr. Neurosci.* **2021**, *15*, 665467. [CrossRef] [PubMed]
44. Tarragon, E.; Lopez, D.; Estrada, C.; Ana, G.C.; Schenker, E.; Pifferi, F.; Bordet, R.; Richardson, J.C.; Herrero, M.T. Octodon degus: A model for the cognitive impairment associated with Alzheimer's disease. *CNS Neurosci. Ther.* **2013**, *19*, 643–648. [CrossRef]
45. Rivera, D.S.; Lindsay, C.; Codocedo, J.F.; Morel, I.; Pinto, C.; Cisternas, P.; Bozinovic, F.; Inestrosa, N.C. Andrographolide recovers cognitive impairment in a natural model of Alzheimer's disease (*Octodon degus*). *Neurobiol. Aging* **2016**, *46*, 204–220. [CrossRef]
46. Tan, Z.; Garduño, B.M.; Aburto, P.F.; Chen, L.; Ha, N.; Cogram, P.; Holmes, T.C.; Xu, X. Cognitively impaired aged Octodon degus recapitulate major neuropathological features of sporadic Alzheimer's disease. *Acta Neuropathol. Commun.* **2022**, *10*, 182. [CrossRef]
47. Goff, S.P. Retrovirus restriction factors. *Mol. Cell* **2004**, *16*, 849–859. [CrossRef]

viruses

MDPI

Article

Robust AAV Genotyping Based on Genetic Distances in Rep Gene That Are Maintained by Ubiquitous Recombination

Marina I. Beloukhova [1,*], Alexander N. Lukashev [2], Pavel Y. Volchkov [3,4], Andrey A. Zamyatnin, Jr. [1,5,6,7] and Andrei A. Deviatkin [3,4,8,*]

1 Institute of Molecular Medicine, Sechenov First Moscow State Medical University, 119991 Moscow, Russia; zamyat@belozersky.msu.ru
2 Martsinovsky Institute of Medical Parasitology, Tropical and Vector-Borne Diseases, First Moscow State Medical University (Sechenov University), 119991 Moscow, Russia; alexander_lukashev@hotmail.com
3 Genome Engineering Lab, Moscow Institute of Physics and Technology (National Research University), 141700 Dolgoprudniy, Russia; vpwwww@gmail.com
4 The National Medical Research Center for Endocrinology, 117036 Moscow, Russia
5 Belozersky Institute of Physico-Chemical Biology, Lomonosov Moscow State University, 119992 Moscow, Russia
6 Department of Biotechnology, Sirius University of Science and Technology, 1 Olympic Ave, 354340 Sochi, Russia
7 Department of Immunology, Faculty of Health and Medical Sciences, University of Surrey, Guildford GU2 7XH, UK
8 Laboratory of Postgenomic Technologies, Izmerov Research Institute of Occupational Health, 105275 Moscow, Russia
* Correspondence: beloukhovamarina@gmail.com (M.I.B.); andreideviatkin@gmail.com (A.A.D.)

Abstract: Adeno-associated viruses (AAVs) are a convenient tool for gene therapy delivery. According to the current classification, they are divided into the species AAV A and AAV B within the genus Dependoparvovirus. Historically AAVs were also subdivided on the intraspecies level into 13 serotypes, which differ in tissue tropism and targeted gene delivery capacity. Serotype, however, is not a universal taxonomic category, and their assignment is not always robust. Cross-reactivity has been shown, indicating that classification could not rely on the results of serological tests alone. Moreover, since the isolation of AAV4, all subsequent AAVs were subdivided into serotypes based primarily on genetic differences and phylogenetic reconstructions. An increased interest in the use of AAV as a gene delivery tool justifies the need to improve the existing classification. Here, we suggest genotype-based AAV classification below the species level based on the *rep* gene. A robust threshold was established as 10% nt differences within the 1248 nt genome fragment, with 4 distinct AAV genotypes identified. This distinct sub-species structure is maintained by ubiquitous recombination within, but not between, *rep* genes of the suggested genotypes.

Keywords: adeno-associated virus; AAV; classification; genotype; serotype; intraspecies; pairwise genetic distance; recombination

Citation: Beloukhova, M.I.; Lukashev, A.N.; Volchkov, P.Y.; Zamyatnin, A.A., Jr.; Deviatkin, A.A. Robust AAV Genotyping Based on Genetic Distances in Rep Gene That Are Maintained by Ubiquitous Recombination. *Viruses* **2022**, *14*, 1038. https://doi.org/10.3390/v14051038

Academic Editors: Giorgio Gallinella and Donald Seto

Received: 31 March 2022
Accepted: 9 May 2022
Published: 13 May 2022

1. Introduction

1.1. AAV Biology

Adeno-associated viruses (AAVs) are non-enveloped particles with a size of 18–26 nm. Sixty protein molecules form an icosahedral capsid. The genome is represented by a linear single-stranded DNA of approximately 4.7 thousand bases.

The AAV genome contains two open reading frames (ORFs): (1) *rep*, which encodes four overlapping proteins necessary for the regulation of viral DNA replication: Rep78, Rep68, Rep52, and Rep40 [1,2]; and (2) *cap* encoding viral capsid proteins: VP1, VP2 and VP3 [3,4]. The genome is flanked by inverted terminal repeats (ITRs) [5], which form a

T-shaped self-complementary secondary structure with a free 3′-hydroxyl that acts as a replication primer [6,7].

For effective replication and reproduction in host cells, AAV requires co-infection with an auxiliary virus, e.g., adenovirus (hence the name adeno-associated), although AAV replication is also possible with herpesvirus, cytomegalovirus, and papillomavirus co-infection [8].

The best-known hosts of AAVs are primates and humans [9,10], although these viruses have been found in other animals [11–13]. AAVs do not cause a significant immune response or any notable pathology in the host cells. Consequently, they are not considered pathogenic [4]. Notably, over 90% of the adult population is seropositive to AAVs, i.e., are likely asymptomatic carriers [14]. The prevalence of AAV in distinct tissues varies between 37 and 72% [15].

1.2. AAV Gene Therapy

AAVs are a convenient tool for gene therapy [16,17]. Since wild AAVs persist in the form of episomes (integration into the host genome at AAVS1 19q13.3-qter site is extremely rare [18] and absent in vectors), they are safer compared to retroviruses, which insert into the host genome randomly, leading to oncogenesis [19]. AAVs also have reduced immunogenicity compared to adenoviruses, further supporting their utility as gene therapy vectors [20].

Results of preclinical and clinical studies have demonstrated that AAV vectors are safe and effective tools in gene therapy for a range of diseases including cystic fibrosis, hemophilia B, arthritis, hereditary emphysema, muscular dystrophy, Parkinson's disease, Alzheimer's disease, prostate cancer, malignant melanoma, epilepsy, and others [16,21–23]. To date, three AAV-vector-based products have been approved for use in medical practice: Glybera (familial lipoprotein lipase deficiency) [24], Luxturna (hereditary retinal dystrophy) [25] and Zolgensma (spinal muscular atrophy) [26].

1.3. AAV Classification

Current AAV classification is based on the phenotype (the shape of the virion), replication peculiarities, and the host range [27]. According to these criteria, AAVs are represented by two species—AAV A and AAV B. Besides AAVs, there are eight other species within the genus dependovirus (ICTV: https://talk.ictvonline.org/taxonomy/ accessed 25 June 2021).

Additionally, AAVs are subdivided on the intraspecies level into serotypes. The first reports of serologically distinct AAVs date back to 1966, when the first three serotypes were identified [28].

Further, any newly identified AAV serologically distinct from known types were assigned a new serotype in chronological order. To date, 13 AAV serotypes are known. However, there are significant ambiguities and controversies in the properties and definitions of the AAV serotypes. For instance, AAV4 was identified based on the reaction with antiserum [29], whereas AAV5 was assigned based on the DNA structure differences identified by restriction analysis and blot-hybridization [30,31]. This protocol could correspond to the identification of a new genotype, which is consistent with the later assignment of AAV5 to a separate species within the dependovirus genus by the International Committee on Taxonomy of Viruses [32].

AAV6 was assigned a new serotype based on genetic differences from the complete genomes of AAV2 and AAV3 (82% identity), as well as AAV4 (75–78% identity) [33]. However, its cap genes were 96% similar to AAV1, and most likely AAV6 is a variant of AAV1. Despite this, AAV serotype 6 is still in use.

In 2002, during an investigation of the asymptomatic presence of AAV in primate tissues, Gao et al. identified AAV7 and AAV8 [34]. The authors used signature regions—a fragment of genomic sequence at positions 2886–3143 nt unique to each AAV type (previously identified by Rutledge et al. [33])—to define distinct virus types, and named the newly isolated viruses according to the differences in these regions. The *rep* and *cap* nucleotide sequences and the predicted amino acid sequence comparisons for AAV1-8 (with the exception of AAV5 as obviously incongruent) revealed differences, primarily in the region encoding capsid proteins. AAV7 was shown to have a 63% to 85% similarity to the amino acid sequences and 68% to 84% of the nucleotide sequences of other AAV serotypes; similar results were obtained for AAV8. The serological difference of AAV7, AAV8, and other serotypes was also established based on the absence of neutralization by any antiserum other than their own (anti-AAV7 and anti-AAV8, respectively).

Later, Gao et al. identified 11 phylogenetic groups based on phylogenetic analysis of cap sequences—so-called 'clades'—from A to F, consisting of phylogenetically similar representatives from three or more sources, and five groups of clones (phylogenetically similar representatives from less than three sources) [35].

AAV10 and AAV11 were also identified based on the signature region differences and characterized according to the cap sequence [36]. The serological analysis confirmed that AAV10 and AAV11 were serologically distinct from AAV2.

Similarly, AAV12 was identified based on the *rep* and *cap* sequence differences [37]. Finally, AAV(VR-942) was isolated in 2008 and had a high degree of amino acid sequence similarity of rep with AAV4 (98%) and AAV3 (93%), as well as 93% identity in VP1 as compared to AAV3. Despite this, AAV(VR-942) has a distinct pattern of cellular receptor interaction and was suggested as a new serotype, AAV13 (the name is currently present only in the corresponding GenBank entry); it should be noted that serological studies were not conducted for AAV13 [38].

Thus, since the isolation of AAV4, all subsequent AAVs were subdivided into different serotypes based primarily on genetic differences and phylogenetic reconstructions. In addition to the established 13 serotypes, one of which comprises a separate virus species (AAV5), more than 100 novel genetic variants (so-called serovars [39]) are not assigned to any taxonomic unit below the species level. It is unlikely that they will be all tested serologically, and the genetic boundaries of types are not robust.

Here, we analyzed all available AAV-A sequences to test the possibility of systematically distinguishing AAVs according to genomic sequence data and to suggest a classification based on genotypes with a measurable robust threshold.

2. Materials and Methods

2.1. Sequence Selection for Analysis

All sequences with a length limited to 4000–5100 nt, which approximately corresponds to the full genome, available as of June, 2021, for Dependoparvovirus isolates were retrieved from the GenBank database (artificial sequences were excluded). Since this study aimed to characterize genetic relationships at the intraspecies level, only sequences of the species AAV A were selected. For this purpose, a phylogenetic tree for the retrieved sequences was constructed using neighbor-joining, implemented in MEGA [40].

2.2. Recombination Analysis

The selected sequences were aligned using MAFFT online [41]. Multiple recombination events were analyzed by the RDP4 software [42] (RDP4 output is available at https://github.com/AndreiDeviatkin/repo/blob/main/AAV.rdp, accessed on 11 May 2022). A more comprehensive recombination screening was carried out using pairwise distance deviation matrices (PDDM) and pairwise distance correspondence plots (PDCP) as described earlier [43] with an online Shiny web application (https://v-julia.shinyapps.io/recdplot_app/, accessed on 25 June 2021). Similarity plots for selected sequences were generated using Simplot 3.5.1 [44].

2.3. Nucleotide and Predicted Amino Acid Sequences Analysis

The analysis of nucleotide and inferred amino acid sequence differences was carried out in R software.

3. Results

3.1. The Dataset

A total of 272 Dependoparvovirus sequences (4000–5100 nt length) were retrieved from GenBank. Of them, 105 sequences belonged to the AAV A species based on phylogenetic analysis (Figure S1). The dataset included all previously characterized genotypes, with the exception of AAV9, for which only VP1 coding sequence is available, as well as other unclassified variants available in the database. Two sequences (MK163941.1 and MK163942.1) were significantly different from the others and thus excluded from the dataset.

3.2. Recombination Analysis

Recombination occurs more frequently in some fragments of the virus genome than in others. The root mean square error (RMSE) of all pairwise distances for two genomic regions from the regression line reflects the extent of phylogenetic inconsistency between these fragments of the genome. A high RMSE (indicated by red in Figure 1) indicates more frequent recombination between the corresponding regions of the genome. A pairwise distance deviation matrix (PDDM) was built for all possible pairs of genomic regions using a sliding window (500 nt). Based on the PDDM, a region covering genome positions 200–1700 nt was identified as the region with the lowest relative incidence of recombination, which approximately corresponds to the coding sequence of Rep proteins (Figure 1).

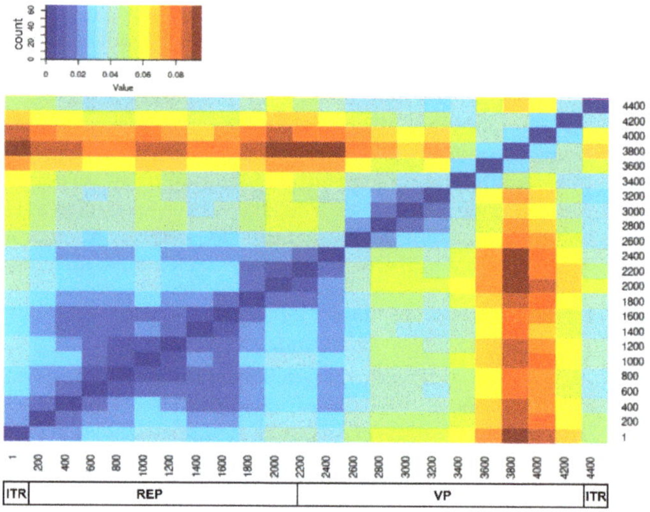

Figure 1. Pairwise distance deviation matrix (PDDM) for AAV A alignment. PDDM summarizes the multitude of pairwise nucleotide distance comparison plots (PDCP) for all possible genome region pairs, visualized as a heatmap. A higher ("red") value of the color key indicates lower overall sequence distance congruence between two genome regions, which is likely caused by recombination.

The PDCP and phylogenetic reconstruction confirmed that recombination in this genome region occurred only between closely related viruses that differed by less than 10% in their nucleotide sequence (Figure 2C, compare to control Figure 2A). Despite ubiquitous recombination within four phylogenetic clades formed by such closely related viruses, there were no signs of recombination between them (Figure 2E). This pattern contrasted with recombination both within and between these four clades when comparing rep and cap genes on the phylogenetic trees (Figure 2E) and signs of recombination between viruses that differed by over 20% nucleotide sequences in cap (Figure 2D). Since complete genomic sequences were not available for all known AAV types (for AAV10-13 only rep + cap complete coding sequences were accessible), alignment positions 453–1700 (genome positions 470–1700 in the reference sequence #NC_001401) were selected for further analysis. Therefore, the region of rep between positions 453 and 1700 was indeed devoid of long-distance recombination and was thus used for further analysis.

3.3. Nucleotide and Amino Acid Pairwise Distance Analysis

Nucleotide or protein sequences may be preferable for distinguishing virus taxa on different levels and in distinct virus groups. A plot of pairwise nucleotide and amino acid distances (Figure 3A) showed that all pairs of viruses formed two clearly distinguishable clouds in the rep gene. Out of a total of 5253 virus pairs, 3558 pairs differed by up to 7.5% nucleotide and up to 8% amino acid sequence, whereas 1695 virus pairs were different in more than 11% nucleotide and 6% amino acid positions. An artificial threshold of 10% nt could be thus suggested for robust AAV subdivision within the species level. At a protein sequence level, there was an overlap between distances within the four phylogenetic groups (below 7.5%) and between them (above 5.5%). Thus, the amino acid sequence is less suitable for the assignment of *rep* genotypes. However, no conclusions could be made according to the plot of pairwise nucleotide and amino acid distances of the cap gene (Figure 3B). The robust separation between AAV4, AAV11, AAV12 and all other serotypes (pairs differing in above 32.5% amino acids in 2250–4400 nt genomic region) was caused by a recombination event that led to the fact that fragments of AAV4, AAV11 and AAV12 capsids have an independent origin from AAV1, AAV2, AAV3, AAV6, AAV7, AAV8, AAV10, AAV13 capsids (Figure 3C).

Analysis of the individual AAV pairs in both plot areas showed that some of them are currently registered as distinct serotypes, but differ by less than 10% of the rep nucleotide sequence and thus may be assigned to the same *rep* genotype (Table 1).

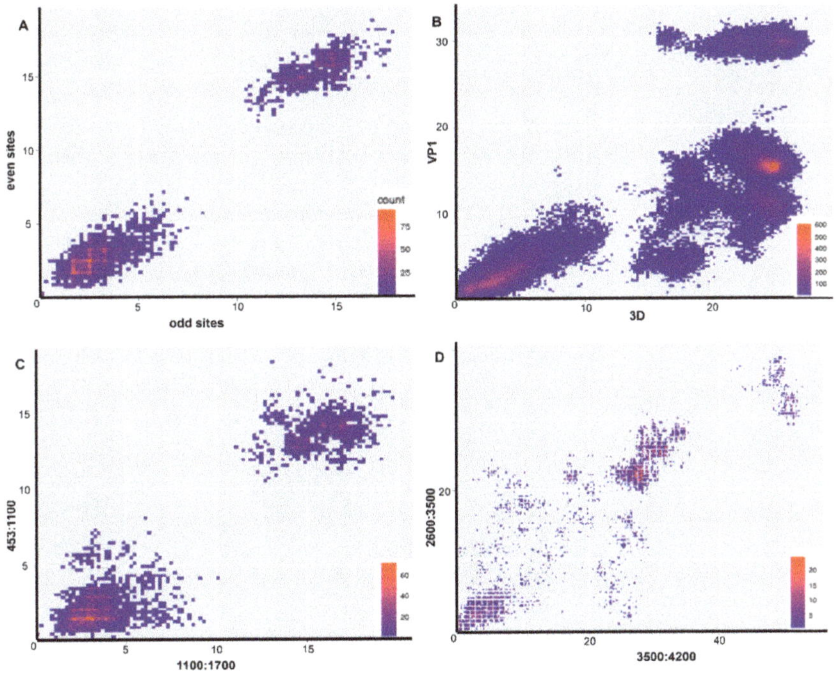

Figure 2. *Cont.*

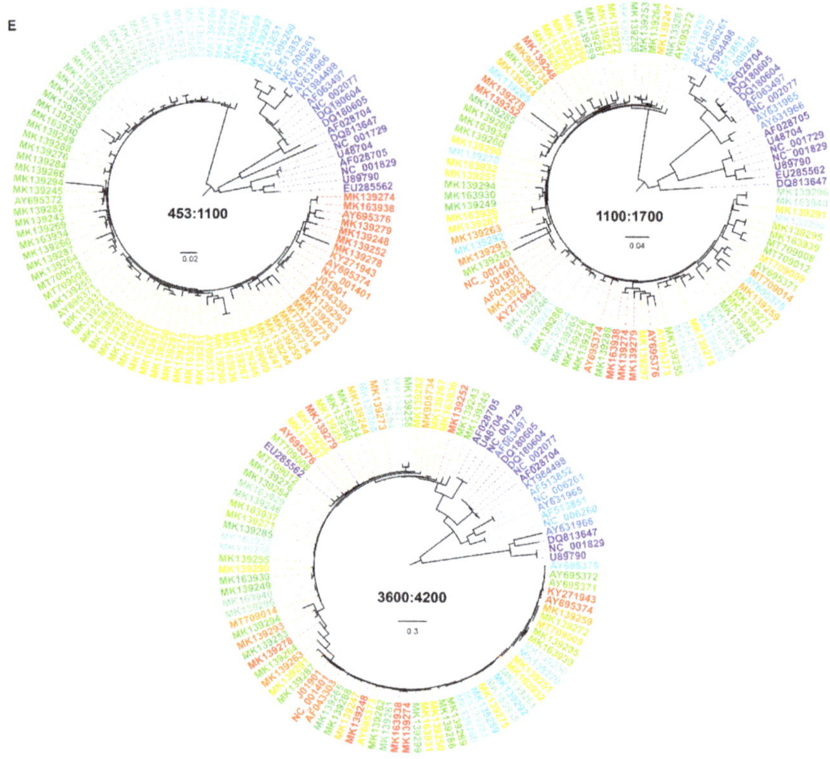

Figure 2. Pairwise nucleotide distance comparison plots (PDCP) indicate recombination between two genetic regions. Each dot corresponds to a pair of nucleotide distances between the same pair of genomes in two genomic regions (axis labels): (**A**) PDCP of even and odd sites in the 453–1700 nt fragment of AAV A alignment (negative control); (**B**) PDCP between VP1 and 3D regions of Enterovirus A species [45], a pattern typical to ubiquitous recombination (positive control); (**C**) PDCP between positions 453 to 1100 nt and 1100 to 1700 of AAV A alignment; (**D**) pairwise distance plot between positions 2600 to 3500 nt and 3500 to 4200 of AAV A alignment. The color indicates the density of overlapping values; (**E**) Phylogenetic trees for three regions in the AAV genome (453–1100; 1100–1700; 3600–4200). The colors of sequences match in trees for each genome region.

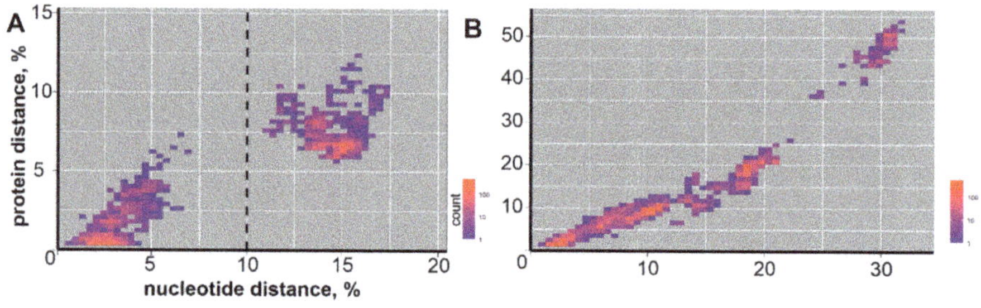

Figure 3. *Cont.*

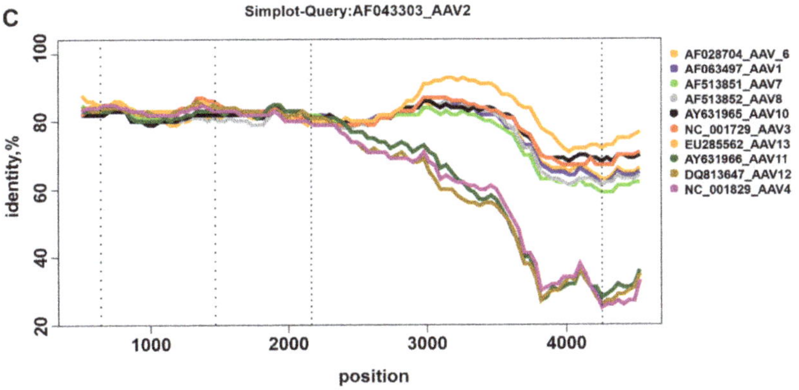

Figure 3. Pairwise amino acid and nucleotide distance plot of AAV A representatives (n = 103): (**A**) for 453–1700 nt region; (**B**) for 2250–4400 nt region. Each dot corresponds to amino acid and nucleotide distances of one virus pair. (**C**) Similarity plot demonstrate mosaic genome patterns in AAV. Similarity scan was conducted using alignments of eleven nucleotide sequences indicated in the legend with window/step size 1000/40 nt. Dotted lines indicate 453–1700 nt and 2250–4400 nt regions.

Table 1. Nucleotide sequence (453–1700 nt positions of full-genome sequence) differences (upper triangle) and inferred amino acid sequence differences (lower triangle) among reference genomes of the currently registered AAV serotypes. Each color indicates a distinct rep genotype based on the nucleotide sequence difference of >10% with representatives of other genotypes and <10% for genomes within a genotype. Nucleotide sequence differences values below 10% (0.10) are highlighted in bold.

	AAV1	AAV2	AAV3	AAV4	AAV6	AAV7	AAV8	AAV10	AAV11	AAV12	AAV13
AAV1	**0**	0.16	0.12	0.11	**0.02**	**0.03**	**0.04**	**0.05**	**0.05**	0.12	0.12
AAV2	0.17	**0**	0.14	0.14	0.15	0.15	0.16	0.16	0.15	0.14	0.14
AAV3	0.16	0.18	**0**	**0.05**	0.13	0.12	0.13	0.12	0.12	0.13	**0.05**
AAV4	0.14	0.19	0.06	**0**	0.12	0.12	0.13	0.12	0.12	0.13	**0.03**
AAV6	0.02	0.18	0.16	0.15	**0**	**0.05**	**0.06**	**0.07**	**0.06**	0.13	0.13
AAV7	0.03	0.16	0.16	0.15	0.04	**0**	**0.03**	**0.05**	**0.04**	0.12	0.12
AAV8	0.05	0.18	0.18	0.16	0.05	0.03	**0**	**0.05**	**0.05**	0.13	0.14
AAV10	0.07	0.17	0.16	0.16	0.08	0.07	0.07	**0**	**0.01**	0.13	0.13
AAV11	0.07	0.16	0.16	0.15	0.07	0.06	0.06	0.02	**0**	0.12	0.13
AAV12	0.15	0.19	0.19	0.17	0.15	0.14	0.16	0.16	0.16	**0**	0.13
AAV13	0.15	0.18	0.06	0.02	0.15	0.15	0.16	0.16	0.15	0.18	**0**

There were no virus pairs in the dataset that were assigned to the same serotype, but differed by more than 10% nucleotide sequence in the rep gene. According to this concept, four distinct rep genotypes could be identified (Table 2, Figure 4).

Table 2. Distinct AAV genotypes identified based on nucleotide sequence differences and the corresponding currently registered serotypes. The table shows the range of the proportions of different nucleotides between the respective genotypes.

	Genotype 1	Genotype 2	Genotype 3	Genotype 4
Genotype 1 (AAV1 + AAV6 + AAV7 + AAV8 + AAV10 + AAV11)	0	0.15–0.16	0.11–0.14	0.12–0.13
Genotype 2 (AAV 2)	-	0	0.14–0.15	0.14
Genotype 3 (AAV3 + AAV4 + AAV13)	-	-	0	0.13
Genotype 4 (AVV12)	-	-	-	0

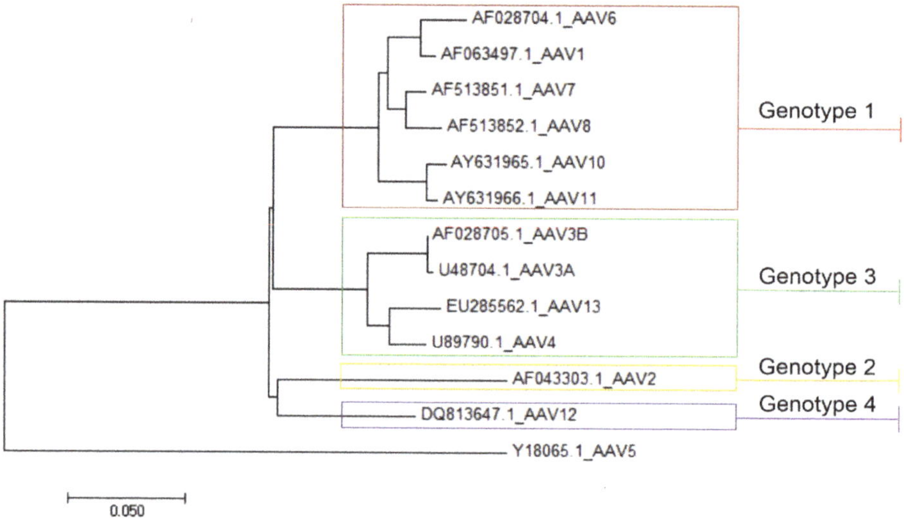

Figure 4. Neighbor-joining phylogenetic tree for the 453–1700 nt region of the AAV A genome. Correlations of currently registered serotypes and four suggested genotypes are presented. AAV B represents an outgroup.

4. Discussion

The lack of an established system for AAV subdivision below the species level results in uncertain classification. There is also no clear, generally accepted definition of such terms as "strain", "variant" and "isolate", and most publications simply reproduce the terminology used previously [46]. The currently used term, "serotype", is not a classical taxonomic category, although such intraspecific division is applicable for practical and scientific purposes [47–49].

According to published studies, the historically established AAV classification based on the serotypes was in some cases not appropriately supported by either serological or genomic data. During early genomic studies, several regions with significant differences between the AAV serotypes were identified within the VP1 sequence, with four domains containing unique sequences for each serotype. These regions were assumed to have a role in serotype-specific functions, such as antigen-antibody or cell receptor binding, which presumably also corresponds to different tissue specificity [33,50,51]. However, the relationship between the serotype and tropism is not clear-cut, because several serotypes efficiently infect similar tissues via both the same and different receptors, implying that capsid proteins may not be the only determinants of tissue tropism.

In subsequent studies, when assigning new AAVs into distinct serotypes, genetic differences (primarily in the capsid proteins) were used. However, conflicts and incongruences in AAV serotype assignment have been accumulating (see above). They were further complicated by serological cross-reactivity [14,50]. Uncertain serological distinction was reported not just for AAV1 and AAV6 [34,36,52], but also for AAV1 and AAV5 [35]. Cross-neutralization between AAV11 and AAV4 was also noted [36]. Many inconsistencies in AAV classification that historically relied on a mix of phenotypic and genetic data could be explained by natural recombination.

Recombination is a physical interaction of viral genomes that leads to gene combinations not existing in any parent. Natural recombination has been described in all known viruses. In the case of some, it may be relatively rare, but in many viruses, it is a regular occurrence that shapes the genetics of taxa. Recombination is commonly seen as a typical feature of RNA viruses, and distinct genome regions of a virus often have different recombination profiles [51,53]; however, small DNA viruses [52,54–57] and adenoviruses [58] also commonly recombine, which may complicate their taxonomic assignment. For instance, recombination within the VP1 sequences was shown for another ssDNA virus—human parvovirus B19 [59]. Genetic analysis of canine parvovirus (CPV) VP1 indicated that recombinants emerged from CPV-2 and CPV-2a or CPV-2b viruses [60]. It was also found that human bocavirus HBoV3 is a recombinant of HBoV and HBoV4 with a recombination breakpoint located near the VP1 start codon [61], and a recombinant of HBoV3 and HBoV4 was further revealed [62]. Apparently, this was also true in the case of AAVs.

Analysis of the genetic sequences of several AAV clones isolated from various primates showed recombination signs in cap genes [57]. The recombination events were also observed in some clones associated with AAV2 and AAV3 [35]. Genetic mosaicism of VP genes of AAVs was shown to be a result of recombination events [62]. Furthermore, the AAV6 genome was shown to be the result of AAV2 and AAV1 recombination [63].

Our analysis confirmed that natural recombination in AAV is ubiquitous and needs to be considered for any taxonomic implications. The effect of recombination on taxonomy may both be negative, when it shuffles genomes and precludes a definitive phylogeny and sequence distance criteria, and positive, when it mixes genes within, but not between, taxa, as seen in enteroviruses [53] or adenoviruses [58], for example. It is likely that the same phenomenon, the shuffling of rep genes within the suggested genotypes, but not between them, explains a very robust separation of within- and between-genotype genetic distances. This hypothesis is supported by phylogenetic analysis (Figure 2E) and many incongruent pairwise genetic distances within genotypes (under 10%, Figure 2C). When it comes to recombination (frequently within the rep genotypes, but never between them), the AAV genotype acts similar to enterovirus [64] and adenovirus species [60].

The difference between the suggested AAV *rep* genotypes is objective, measurable, robust, and unambiguous. To assign viruses to a particular genotype, their genome needs to be sequenced and the sequence has to be analyzed with phylogenetic methods. The same strategy has been suggested and successfully implemented previously for adenovirus classification [65].

Genetic analysis allowed for robust segregation of AAV into *rep* genotypes. However, the biological implications of such a classification remain largely unknown, as most AAV properties have been associated with the capsid. Thus, the suggested classification is not intended to replace the classical VP1-based one, but to supplement it, and further studies are required to assay its phenotypic implications. In other viruses, it is not uncommon to have different classifications for distinct genome regions. One example is rotaviruses that have a segmented genome and feature ubiquitous reassortment [66]. However, there are also examples in viruses with non-segmented genomes, when distinct recombination profiles in different genome regions shape taxonomic units linked with structural proteins and with non-structural (replication-associated) ones. Examples include both RNA viruses, such as picornaviruses [66], and DNA viruses, such as adenoviruses [58]. In these examples, there is a fixed set of capsids (corresponding to types) that are compatible with a variety of non-structural genes within a species. Each species has a defined set of types, and structural genes from different species are not compatible. In AAVs, however, we did not observe obvious limitations on recombination between various rep and cap genes. This is concordant with the possibility of the so-called pseudotyped recombinant AAV vectors, i.e., a genome of one serotype used as a cassette for a therapeutic gene of interest, while the other serotype genome is used to supply *rep* and *cap*. Satisfactory transfection and expression were shown for AAV2/4, AAV2/5, AAV2/6, AAV2/8 and AAV2/9 constructs [17].

Knowledge about AAV genetic diversity remains fragmentary. For instance, the complete genome or rep gene of AAV9 has not been sequenced yet (the only record available in GenBank refers to the VP1 complete coding sequence). Thus, our dataset lacks this serotype for analysis (conducted based on Rep coding sequence) and we could not assign AAV9 to any of the determined genotypes. It is likely that the robust rep genotype criteria suggested here would need to be refined in the future. Additionally, although the suggested classification is robust and is explained by an obvious biological phenomenon (recombination), its practical implications require further study.

5. Conclusions

Based on genome analysis, we have identified four distinct *rep* genotypes, which are proposed as an auxiliary classification within the AAV A species: AAV A genotype 1 (including serotypes AAV1, AAV6, AAV7, AAV8, AAV10, AAV11); AAV A genotype 2 (including AAV2 and other unclassified AAVs that differ genetically between each other by less than 10%—the majority of the currently known sequences); AAV A genotype 3 (including AAV3, AAV4, AAV13 and other unclassified AAVs that differ genetically by less than 10%); and AAV A genotype 4 (represented by AAV12).

Supplementary Materials: The following are available online at https://www.mdpi.com/article/10.3390/v14051038/s1, Figure S1: Neighbor-joining phylogenetic tree for Dependoparvovirus genomic sequences (4000–5100 nt length, n = 272) retrieved from GenBank. AAV-A (n = 105) sequences were indicated by red color.

Author Contributions: Conceptualization, A.A.D., A.N.L., P.Y.V. and A.A.Z.J.; bioinformatic analysis, M.I.B. and A.A.D.; data curation, M.I.B.; writing—original draft preparation, M.I.B.; writing—review and editing, M.I.B., A.A.D., A.N.L., P.Y.V. and A.A.Z.J.; visualization, M.I.B. and A.A.D.; supervision, A.A.D. All authors have read and agreed to the published version of the manuscript.

Funding: The study was supported by the Ministry of Science and Higher Education of the Russian Federation (agreement No. 075-15-2020-899).

Institutional Review Board Statement: Not applicable.

Informed Consent Statement: Not applicable.

Data Availability Statement: The data and source code presented in this study are openly available in the GitHub repository https://github.com/MarinaBeloukhova/AAVgenotypes (accessed on 21 April 2022).

Conflicts of Interest: The authors declare no conflict of interest. The funders had no role in the design of the study; in the collection, analyses, or interpretation of data; in the writing of the manuscript, or in the decision to publish the results.

References

1. Im, D.S.; Muzyczka, N. Partial purification of adeno-associated virus Rep78, Rep52, and Rep40 and their biochemical characterization. *J. Virol.* **1992**, *66*, 1119–1128. [CrossRef] [PubMed]
2. Kyöstiö, S.R.; Owens, R.A.; Weitzman, M.D.; Antoni, B.A.; Chejanovsky, N.; Carter, B.J. Analysis of adeno-associated virus (AAV) wild-type and mutant Rep proteins for their abilities to negatively regulate AAV p5 and p19 mRNA levels. *J. Virol.* **1994**, *68*, 2947–2957. [CrossRef] [PubMed]

3. Trempe, J.P.; Carter, B.J. Alternate mRNA splicing is required for synthesis of adeno-associated virus VP1 capsid protein. *J. Virol.* **1988**, *62*, 3356–3363. [CrossRef] [PubMed]
4. Carter, P.J.; Samulski, R.J. Adeno-associated viral vectors as gene delivery vehicles. *Int. J. Mol. Med.* **2000**, *6*, 17–27. [CrossRef] [PubMed]
5. Gonçalves, M.A.F.V. Adeno-associated virus: From defective virus to effective vector. *Virol. J.* **2005**, *2*, 43. [CrossRef]
6. Bohenzky, R.A.; Lefebvre, R.B.; Berns, K.I. Sequence and symmetry requirements within the internal palindromic sequences of the adeno-associated virus terminal repeat. *Virology* **1988**, *166*, 316–327. [CrossRef]
7. Wang, X.-S.; Ponnazhagan, S.; Srivastava, A. Rescue and Replication Signals of the Adeno-associated Virus 2 Genome. *J. Mol. Biol.* **1995**, *250*, 573–580. [CrossRef]
8. Meier, A.F.; Fraefel, C.; Seyffert, M. The Interplay between Adeno-Associated Virus and Its Helper Viruses. *Viruses* **2020**, *12*, 662. [CrossRef]
9. Parks, W.P.; Boucher, D.W.; Melnick, J.L.; Taber, L.H.; Yow, M.D. Seroepidemiological and Ecological Studies of the Adenovirus-Associated Satellite Viruses. *Infect. Immun.* **1970**, *2*, 716–722. [CrossRef]
10. Gao, G.; Vandenberghe, L.; Wilson, J. New Recombinant Serotypes of AAV Vectors. *Curr. Gene Ther.* **2005**, *5*, 285–297. [CrossRef]
11. Bossis, I.; Chiorini, J.A. Cloning of an Avian Adeno-Associated Virus (AAAV) and Generation of Recombinant AAAV Particles. *J. Virol.* **2003**, *77*, 6799–6810. [CrossRef] [PubMed]
12. Schmidt, M.; Katano, H.; Bossis, I.; Chiorini, J.A. Cloning and Characterization of a Bovine Adeno-Associated Virus. *J. Virol.* **2004**, *78*, 6509–6516. [CrossRef] [PubMed]
13. Arbetman, A.E.; Lochrie, M.; Zhou, S.; Wellman, J.; Scallan, C.; Doroudchi, M.M.; Randlev, B.; Patarroyo-White, S.; Liu, T.; Smith, P.; et al. Novel Caprine Adeno-Associated Virus (AAV) Capsid (AAV-Go.1) Is Closely Related to the Primate AAV-5 and Has Unique Tropism and Neutralization Properties. *J. Virol.* **2005**, *79*, 15238–15245. [CrossRef] [PubMed]
14. Louis Jeune, V.; Joergensen, J.A.; Hajjar, R.J.; Weber, T. Pre-existing anti-adeno-associated virus antibodies as a challenge in AAV gene therapy. *Hum. Gene Ther. Methods* **2013**, *24*, 59–67. [CrossRef] [PubMed]
15. Wright, J.F. Transient transfection methods for clinical adeno-associated viral vector production. *Hum. Gene Ther.* **2009**, *20*, 698–706. [CrossRef]
16. Kotterman, M.A.; Schaffer, D.V. Engineering adeno-associated viruses for clinical gene therapy. *Nat. Rev. Genet.* **2014**, *15*, 445–451. [CrossRef]
17. Naso, M.F.; Tomkowicz, B.; Perry, W.L.; Strohl, W.R. Adeno-Associated Virus (AAV) as a Vector for Gene Therapy. *BioDrugs* **2017**, *31*, 317–334. [CrossRef]
18. Surosky, R.T.; Urabe, M.; Godwin, S.G.; McQuiston, S.A.; Kurtzman, G.J.; Ozawa, K.; Natsoulis, G. Adeno-associated virus Rep proteins target DNA sequences to a unique locus in the human genome. *J. Virol.* **1997**, *71*, 7951–7959. [CrossRef]
19. Lukashev, A.N.; Zamyatnin, A.A. Viral vectors for gene therapy: Current state and clinical perspectives. *Biochem.* **2016**, *81*, 700–708. [CrossRef]
20. Thomas, C.E.; Ehrhardt, A.; Kay, M.A. Progress and problems with the use of viral vectors for gene therapy. *Nat. Rev. Genet.* **2003**, *4*, 346–358. [CrossRef]
21. Daya, S.; Berns, K.I. Gene Therapy Using Adeno-Associated Virus Vectors. *Clin. Microbiol. Rev.* **2008**, *21*, 583–593. [CrossRef] [PubMed]
22. Santiago-Ortiz, J.L.; Schaffer, D.V. Adeno-associated virus (AAV) vectors in cancer gene therapy. *J. Control. Release* **2016**, *240*, 287–301. [CrossRef] [PubMed]
23. Nienhuis, A.W.; Nathwani, A.C.; Davidoff, A.M. Gene Therapy for Hemophilia. *Mol. Ther.* **2017**, *25*, 1163–1167. [CrossRef] [PubMed]
24. Ylä-Herttuala, S. Endgame: Glybera finally recommended for approval as the first gene therapy drug in the European union. *Mol. Ther.* **2012**, *20*, 1831–1832. [CrossRef] [PubMed]
25. Spark Therapeutics LUXTURNA (voretigene neparvovec-rzyl) [Package Insert]. Available online: https://www.fda.gov/media/109906/download (accessed on 25 June 2021).
26. Zhu, H.; Wang, T.; John Lye, R.; French, B.A.; Annex, B.H. Neuraminidase-mediated desialylation augments AAV9-mediated gene expression in skeletal muscle. *J. Gene Med.* **2018**, *20*, e3049. [CrossRef] [PubMed]
27. Simmonds, P.; Adams, M.J.; Benk, M.; Breitbart, M.; Brister, J.R.; Carstens, E.B.; Davison, A.J.; Delwart, E.; Gorbalenya, A.E.; Harrach, B.; et al. Consensus statement: Virus taxonomy in the age of metagenomics. *Nat. Rev. Microbiol.* **2017**, *15*, 161–168. [CrossRef]
28. Hoggan, M.D.; Blacklow, N.R.; Rowe, W.P. Studies of small DNA viruses found in various adenovirus preparations: Physical, biological, and immunological characteristics. *Proc. Natl. Acad. Sci. USA* **1966**, *55*, 1467–1474. [CrossRef]
29. Parks, W.P.; Melnick, J.L.; Rongey, R.; Mayor, H.D. Physical Assay and Growth Cycle Studies of a Defective Adeno-Satellite Virus. *J. Virol.* **1967**, *1*, 171–180. [CrossRef]
30. Bantel-Schaal, U.; Zur Hausen, H. Characterization of the DNA of a defective human parvovirus isolated from a genital site. *Virology* **1984**, *134*, 52–63. [CrossRef]
31. Bantel-Schaal, U.; Delius, H.; Schmidt, R.; zur Hausen, H. Human Adeno-Associated Virus Type 5 Is Only Distantly Related to Other Known Primate Helper-Dependent Parvoviruses. *J. Virol.* **1999**, *73*, 939–947. [CrossRef]

32. Murphy, F.A.; Fauquet, C.M.; Bishop, D.H.L.; Ghabrial, S.A.; Jarvis, S.A.; Martelli, G.; Mayo, P.M.A.; Summers, M.D. Virus Taxonomy. Sixth report of the International Committee on Taxonomy of Viruses. *Arch. Virol. Suppl.* **1995**, *10*, 175.
33. Rutledge, E.A.; Halbert, C.L.; Russell, D.W. Infectious Clones and Vectors Derived from Adeno-Associated Virus (AAV) Serotypes Other Than AAV Type 2. *J. Virol.* **1998**, *72*, 309–319. [CrossRef] [PubMed]
34. Gao, G.-P.; Alvira, M.R.; Wang, L.; Calcedo, R.; Johnston, J.; Wilson, J.M. Novel adeno-associated viruses from rhesus monkeys. *Proc. Natl. Acad. Sci. USA* **2002**, *99*, 11854–11859. [CrossRef] [PubMed]
35. Gao, G.; Vandenberghe, L.H.; Alvira, M.R.; Lu, Y.; Calcedo, R.; Zhou, X.; Wilson, J.M. Clades of Adeno-Associated Viruses Are Widely Disseminated in Human Tissues. *J. Virol.* **2004**, *78*, 6381–6388. [CrossRef]
36. Mori, S.; Wang, L.; Takeuchi, T.; Kanda, T. Two novel adeno-associated viruses from cynomolgus monkey: Pseudotyping characterization of capsid protein. *Virology* **2004**, *330*, 375–383. [CrossRef]
37. Schmidt, M.; Voutetakis, A.; Afione, S.; Zheng, C.; Mandikian, D.; Chiorini, J.A. Adeno-Associated Virus Type 12 (AAV12): A Novel AAV Serotype with Sialic Acid- and Heparan Sulfate Proteoglycan-Independent Transduction Activity. *J. Virol.* **2008**, *82*, 1399–1406. [CrossRef]
38. Schmidt, M.; Govindasamy, L.; Afione, S.; Kaludov, N.; Agbandje-McKenna, M.; Chiorini, J.A. Molecular Characterization of the Heparin-Dependent Transduction Domain on the Capsid of a Novel Adeno-Associated Virus Isolate, AAV(VR-942). *J. Virol.* **2008**, *82*, 8911–8916. [CrossRef]
39. Ronzitti, G.; Gross, D.A.; Mingozzi, F. Human Immune Responses to Adeno-Associated Virus (AAV) Vectors. *Front. Immunol.* **2020**, *11*, 670. [CrossRef]
40. Kumar, S.; Stecher, G.; Tamura, K. MEGA7: Molecular Evolutionary Genetics Analysis Version 7.0 for Bigger Datasets. *Mol. Biol. Evol.* **2016**, *33*, 1870–1874. [CrossRef]
41. Katoh, K.; Rozewicki, J.; Yamada, K.D. MAFFT online service: Multiple sequence alignment, interactive sequence choice and visualization. *Brief. Bioinform.* **2018**, *20*, 1160–1166. [CrossRef]
42. Martin, D.P.; Murrell, B.; Golden, M.; Khoosal, A.; Muhire, B. RDP4: Detection and analysis of recombination patterns in virus genomes. *Virus Evol.* **2015**, *1*, 1–5. [CrossRef] [PubMed]
43. Vakulenko, Y.; Deviatkin, A.; Drexler, J.F.; Lukashev, A. Modular evolution of coronavirus genomes. *Viruses* **2021**, *13*, 1270. [CrossRef] [PubMed]
44. Lole, K.S.; Bollinger, R.C.; Paranjape, R.S.; Gadkari, D.; Kulkarni, S.S.; Novak, N.G.; Ingersoll, R.; Sheppard, H.W.; Ray, S.C. Full-Length Human Immunodeficiency Virus Type 1 Genomes from Subtype C-Infected Seroconverters in India, with Evidence of Intersubtype Recombination. *J. Virol.* **1999**, *73*, 152–160. [CrossRef] [PubMed]
45. Lukashev, A.N.; Elena, Y.; Belalov, I.S.; Ivanova, O.E.; Eremeeva, T.P.; Reznik, V.I.; Trotsenko, O.E.; Drexler, J.F.; Drosten, C. Recombination strategies and evolutionary dynamics of the Human enterovirus A global gene pool. *J. Gen. Virol.* **2014**, *95*, 868–873. [CrossRef] [PubMed]
46. Kuhn, J.H.; Bao, Y.; Bavari, S.; Becker, S.; Bradfute, S.; Brister, J.R.; Bukreyev, A.A.; Chandran, K.; Davey, R.A.; Dolnik, O.; et al. Virus nomenclature below the species level: A standardized nomenclature for natural variants of viruses assigned to the family Filoviridae. *Arch. Virol.* **2013**, *158*, 301–311. [CrossRef] [PubMed]
47. Ellis, B.L.; Hirsch, M.L.; Barker, J.C.; Connelly, J.P.; Steininger, R.J.; Porteus, M.H. A survey of ex vivo/in vitro transduction efficiency of mammalian primary cells and cell lines with Nine natural adeno-associated virus (AAV1-9) and one engineered adeno-associated virus serotype. *Virol. J.* **2013**, *10*, 74. [CrossRef]
48. Srivastava, A. In vivo tissue-tropism of adeno-associated viral vectors. *Curr. Opin. Virol.* **2016**, *21*, 75–80. [CrossRef]
49. Korneyenkov, M.A.; Zamyatnin, A.A. Next step in gene delivery: Modern approaches and further perspectives of aav tropism modification. *Pharmaceutics* **2021**, *13*, 750. [CrossRef]
50. Boutin, S.; Monteilhet, V.; Veron, P.; Leborgne, C.; Benveniste, O.; Montus, M.F.; Masurier, C. Prevalence of serum IgG and neutralizing factors against adeno-associated virus (AAV) types 1, 2, 5, 6, 8, and 9 in the healthy population: Implications for gene therapy using AAV vectors. *Hum. Gene Ther.* **2010**, *21*, 704–712. [CrossRef]
51. Simmonds, P. Recombination and selection in the evolution of picornaviruses and other Mammalian positive-stranded RNA viruses. *J. Virol.* **2006**, *80*, 11124–11140. [CrossRef]
52. Lukashov, V.V.; Goudsmit, J. Evolutionary Relationships among Parvoviruses: Virus-Host Coevolution among Autonomous Primate Parvoviruses and Links between Adeno-Associated and Avian Parvoviruses. *J. Virol.* **2001**, *75*, 2729–2740. [CrossRef] [PubMed]
53. Lukashev, A.N. Recombination among picornaviruses. *Rev. Med. Virol.* **2010**, *20*, 327–337. [CrossRef] [PubMed]
54. Shackelton, L.A.; Hoelzer, K.; Parrish, C.R.; Holmes, E.C. Comparative analysis reveals frequent recombination in the parvoviruses. *J. Gen. Virol.* **2007**, *88*, 3294–3301. [CrossRef] [PubMed]
55. Hoelzer, K.; Parrish, C.R. *Evolution and Variation of the Parvoviruses*, 2nd ed.; Elsevier: Amsterdam, The Netherlands, 2008; ISBN 9780123741530.
56. Martin, D.P.; Biagini, P.; Lefeuvre, P.; Golden, M.; Roumagnac, P.; Varsani, A. Recombination in eukaryotic single stranded DNA viruses. *Viruses* **2011**, *3*, 1699–1738. [CrossRef]
57. Gao, G.; Alvira, M.R.; Somanathan, S.; Lu, Y.; Vandenberghe, L.H.; Rux, J.J.; Calcedo, R.; Sanmiguel, J.; Abbas, Z.; Wilson, J.M. Adeno-associated viruses undergo substantial evolution in primates during natural infections. *Proc. Natl. Acad. Sci. USA* **2003**, *100*, 6081–6086. [CrossRef]

58. Lukashev, A.N.; Ivanova, O.E.; Eremeeva, T.P.; Iggo, R.D. Evidence of frequent recombination among human adenoviruses. *J. Gen. Virol.* **2008**, *89*, 380–388. [CrossRef]
59. Shackelton, L.A.; Holmes, E.C. Phylogenetic Evidence for the Rapid Evolution of Human B19 Erythrovirus. *J. Virol.* **2006**, *80*, 3666–3669. [CrossRef]
60. Mochizuki, M.; Ohshima, T.; Une, Y.; Yachi, A. Recombination between vaccine and field strains of canine parvovirus is revealed by isolation of virus in canine and feline cell cultures. *J. Vet. Med. Sci.* **2008**, *70*, 1305–1314. [CrossRef]
61. Cheng, W.; Chen, J.; Xu, Z.; Yu, J.; Huang, C.; Jin, M.; Li, H.; Zhang, M.; Jin, Y.; Duan, Z. jun Phylogenetic and recombination analysis of human bocavirus 2. *BMC Infect. Dis.* **2011**, *11*, 50. [CrossRef]
62. Tyumentsev, A.I.; Tikunova, N.V.; Tikunov, A.Y.; Babkin, I.V. Recombination in the evolution of human bocavirus. *Infect. Genet. Evol.* **2014**, *28*, 11–14. [CrossRef]
63. Xiao, W.; Chirmule, N.; Berta, S.C.; Gao, G.; Wilson, J.M.; Cullough, B.M.C. Gene Therapy Vectors Based on Adeno-Associated Virus Type 1 Gene Therapy Vectors Based on Adeno-Associated Virus Type 1. *J. Virol. Methods* **1999**, *73*, 3994. [CrossRef] [PubMed]
64. Lukashev, A.N. Role of recombination in evolution of enteroviruses. *Rev. Med. Virol.* **2005**, *15*, 157–167. [CrossRef] [PubMed]
65. Seto, D.; Chodosh, J.; Brister, J.R.; Jones, M.S. Using the Whole-Genome Sequence To Characterize and Name Human Adenoviruses. *J. Virol.* **2011**, *85*, 5701–5702. [CrossRef]
66. Simsek, C.; Corman, V.M.; Everling, H.U.; Lukashev, A.N.; Rasche, A.; Maganga, G.D.; Binger, T.; Jansen, D.; Beller, L.; Deboutte, W.; et al. At Least Seven Distinct Rotavirus Genotype Constellations in Bats with Evidence of Reassortment and Zoonotic Transmissions. *mBio* **2021**, *12*, 1–17. [CrossRef] [PubMed]

viruses

MDPI

Communication

Carnivore protoparvovirus 1 (CPV-2 and FPV) Circulating in Wild Carnivores and in Puppies Illegally Imported into North-Eastern Italy

Stefania Leopardi [1], Adelaide Milani [1], Monia Cocchi [2], Marco Bregoli [2], Alessia Schivo [1], Sofia Leardini [1], Francesca Festa [1], Ambra Pastori [1], Gabrita de Zan [2], Federica Gobbo [1], Maria Serena Beato [1,†], Manlio Palei [3], Alessandro Bremini [3,4], Marie-Christin Rossmann [4,5], Paolo Zucca [3,4], Isabella Monne [1] and Paola De Benedictis [1,*]

1 National Reference Centre/WOAH Collaborating Centre for Diseases at the Animal-Human Interface, Istituto Zooprofilattico Sperimentale Delle Venezie, 35020 Legnaro, Italy
2 Istituto Zooprofilattico Sperimentale Delle Venezie, Sezione Territoriale di Udine, 33030 Basaldella di Campoformido, Italy
3 Central Directorate for Health, Social Policies and Disabilities, Friuli Venezia Giulia Region, 34123 Trieste, Italy
4 Biocrime Veterinary Medical Intelligence Centre, c/o International Police and Custom Cooperation Centre, Thörl-Maglern, 9602 Arnoldstein, Austria
5 Agiculture, Forestry, Rural Areas Veterinary Department, Land Carinthia, 9020 Klagenfurt, Austria
* Correspondence: pdebenedictis@izsvenezie.it
† Current address: Istituto Zooprofilattico Sperimentale dell'Umbria e delle Marche "Togo Rosati", Via G. Salvemini 1, 06126 Perugia, Italy.

Abstract: The illegal trade of animals poses several health issues to the global community, among which are the underestimated risk for spillover infection and the potential for an epizootic in both wildlife and domestic naïve populations. We herein describe the genetic and antigenic characterization of viruses of the specie *Carnivore protoparvovirus 1* detected at high prevalence in puppies illegally introduced in North Eastern Italy and compared them with those circulating in wild carnivores from the same area. We found evidence of a wide diversity of canine parvoviruses (CPV-2) belonging to different antigenic types in illegally imported pups. In wildlife, we found a high circulation of feline parvovirus (FPV) in golden jackals and badgers, whereas CPV-2 was observed in one wolf only. Although supporting a possible spillover event, the low representation of wolf samples in the present study prevented us from inferring the origin, prevalence and viral diversity of the viruses circulating in this species. Therefore, we suggest performing more thorough investigations before excluding endemic CPV-2 circulation in this species.

Keywords: CPV-2; FPV; illegal trade; companion animals; wildlife; spillover

Citation: Leopardi, S.; Milani, A.; Cocchi, M.; Bregoli, M.; Schivo, A.; Leardini, S.; Festa, F.; Pastori, A.; de Zan, G.; Gobbo, F.; et al. *Carnivore protoparvovirus 1* (CPV-2 and FPV) Circulating in Wild Carnivores and in Puppies Illegally Imported into North-Eastern Italy. *Viruses* **2022**, *14*, 2612. https://doi.org/10.3390/v14122612

Academic Editor: Giorgio Gallinella

Received: 19 October 2022
Accepted: 22 November 2022
Published: 23 November 2022

1. Introduction

Parvoviruses are non-enveloped viruses with a short genome of non-segmented single-stranded DNA encoding for two open reading frames (ORFs), among which ORF1 encodes for non-structural proteins NS1 and NS2 and ORF2 encodes for the capsid proteins VP1 and VP2 [1]. Parvoviruses of companion animals belong to the species *Carnivore protoparvovirus 1*, genus *Protoparvovirus*, and family *Parvoviridae*. Canine parvovirus type-2 (CPV-2) arose in the mid-1970s as a variant of a virus similar to but distinct from FPV [2]. Historically, typing of CPV-2 was based on the antigenic variability of strains assessed using monoclonal antibodies or amino acid (aa) substitutions (at aa residues 297 and 426) within the gene coding for the major capsid protein VP2 [3], although phylogenetic analyses based on either the VP2 or the whole genome do not completely reflect the antigenic properties [1]. Since its first emergence, CPV-2 was selected in dogs giving rise to several antigenic and genetic variants: CPV-2a, CPV-b, and the most recent subtypes new CPV-2a, new CPV-2b and CPV-2c, that gradually replaced the original type [3,4].

Nowadays, CPV-2 is occasionally detected worldwide likely due to its use as attenuated live vaccine [5,6]. Compared to the original CPV-2, the new variants recovered the ability to infect felids and showed increased pathogenicity [2,7].

Regardless of the classification used and based on the sequences publicly available, parvoviruses fail to show any significant geographical clustering in dogs, thus suggesting high admixing between populations due to the extensive movement of persons and their pets and, very likely, to the ever-growing commercialization, legal and not, of pups [1]. In this context, it hast been suggested that the black market of puppies might contribute to the spread and evolution of CPV-2 in European count ries with high vaccination coverage, such as Italy [6].

The European Commission considers the illegal trade of pets an emerging risk for Member States. Indeed, considering the sanitary impacts, the illegal distribution not only poses risks to the pet itself due to the possible bad practices in keeping, breeding and transporting, but also represents a risk for the introduction of epizootic and zoonotic diseases into free areas [8,9]. Within this frame, the important sanitary impacts driven by the illegal transport of puppies through Northeastern Italy has been underlined. Indeed, a three-year survey demonstrated that illegally imported puppies displayed poor vaccine immunity—with canine parvovirus and giardia recognized as the infections most frequently associated to fatal gastroenteritis and, most importantly, identified *Salmonella* and *Microsporum canis* as major zoonotic pathogens [10]. In 2015, the cat and dog trade involved 61 million dogs and 67 million cats in twelve EU Member States, representing € 1.3 billion and generating a direct employment of about 300,000 workers [8]. The illegal trade of puppies also represents a source of illegal market, thus an unfair competition for complaint breeders and sellers [11].

Both CPV-2 and FPV have been detected in wild carnivores of different genera across the world, with cross-species transmission at the domestic-wildlife interface still evident in some countries, such as South America, making virus dynamics and evolution rather complex [1]. In other areas, including most European countries investigated so far, CPV-2 and FPV strains have mostly become endemic in wild reservoirs, even if sporadic spillover events are still detected [12]. As for dogs and cats, the pathogenicity of parvoviruses in wildlife is variable, spanning from asymptomatic infection to severe diarrhea in pups, possibly affecting the health of fragile populations [12–14].

In the present study, we characterized viruses of the specie *Carnivore protoparvovirus 1* (FPV and CPV-2) circulating in wild carnivores from Friuli Venezia-Giulia (North Eastern Italy) and compared them to the strains that have been introduced in the same area through the illegal trade of puppies [10].

2. Materials and Methods

The sample set included (i) n = 256 feces samples collected from puppies admitted in quarantine facilities in Friuli Venezia-Giulia between 2018 and 2021 after their illegal introduction from Central and Eastern Europe and (ii) n = 79 intestines collected post-mortem in case of the animal death during the observation period [10]. In addition, we analyzed intestinal samples of wild carnivores collected since 2021 in the framework of passive surveillance for rabies from the same region. These include n = 55 from Eurasian badgers (*Meles meles*), n = 21 from red foxes (*Vulpes vulpes*), n = 12 from golden jackals (*Canis aureus*), n = 5 from gray wolves (*Canis lupus lupus*), and n = 4 from beech martens (*Martes foina*). Samples were homogenized and nucleic acids were extracted using QIAsymphony DSP Virus/Pathogen Midi kit on the QIAsymphony SP instrument (QIAGEN, Hilden, Germany) or MagMAX Viral/Pathogen II on KingFisher Magnetic Particle Processors (Thermo Fisher Scientific, Waltham, Massachusetts) for dog and wildlife samples, respectively. All samples were screened using molecular testing for canine parvovirus and feline panleukopenia virus [6] using the QuantiFast® Pathoghen PCR+IC (QIAGEN, Hilden, Germany) as amplification kit and CFX 96 BIO-RAD (BIO-RAD, Hercules, CA, USA) as platform.

We characterized the near complete genome of all wildlife strains and of strains from selected samples of seventy-four positive dogs. More specifically, samples from dogs were selected using a random stratified sampling, according to the year of detection and the type of sample. In order to do this, we used a target PCR approach and Next Generation Sequencing (NGS). Primers were modified from Perez et al. (2014) [15] or designed de novo to obtain two or three overlapping amplicons using alternative protocols (Tables 1 and 2).

Table 1. Primers used within the study.

Primer	Sequence 5′→3′	Nucleotide Positions	Direction	Reference
NS-Rext	GAAGGGTTAGTTGGTTCTCC	2441–2460	reverse	[15]
F194short	ATAAAAGACAAACCATAGACCGT	194–223	forward	Modified from [15]
NS-Fext	GACCGTTACTGACATTCGCTTC	206–227	forward	
2161For	TTGGCGTTACTCACAAAGACGTGC	2161–2184	forward	
4823Rev	ACCAACCACCCACACCATAACAAC	4800–4823	reverse	
3475R	GTTGGTGTGCCACTAGTTCCAGTA	3452–3475	reverse	
CPV2-2776midF	ATCTTGCMCCAATGAGTGATG	2776–2797	forward	This study
CPV2-4928R	TGGTAAGGTTAGTTCACCTTATA	4905–4928	reverse	

Table 2. Protocols used for sequencing the complete genome of *Carnivore protoparvovirus 1*.

Protocol	Primer Combination for 5′ Fragment	Amplicon Size	Primer Combination for 3′ Fragment	Amplicon Size
1	F194short forward + NS-Rext reverse → In case of PCR failure use protocol 2	2400	2161 For forward + 4823 Rev reverse → In case of PCR failure use protocol 3	2700
2	NS-Fext forward + NS-Rext reverse	2200		
3			2161For forward + 3475 R reverse CPV2-2776midF forward + CPV2-4928R reverse	1314 2150

All PCR protocols were run in a final volume of 25 μL, using 1 to 5 ng of sample DNA, 0.7 μM of each primer, 1X PCR buffer, 0.8 M $MgCl_2$ and 1 U of Platinum Taq polymerase (Invitrogen). The amplification included 5 min at 94 °C, followed by 40 cycles at 94 °C for 30 s, 58 °C for 30 s and 72 °C for 3 min and by a final extension of 10 min at 72 °C. For sequencing, we pooled amplicons belonging to the same sample in equimolar ratio, prepared libraries using the Nextera XT DNA sample preparation kit (Illumina, San Diego, CA, USA) and processed them on an Illumina MiSeq platform with the MiSeq reagent kit V3 (2 × 300) or V2 (2 × 250) (paired-end [PE] mode; Illumina, San Diego, CA, USA) following the company's instructions.

After assessing the quality of raw reads with FastQC v0.11.7 (https://www.bioinformatics.babraham.ac.uk/projects/fastqc/, accessed on 23 September 2022), we used scythe v0.991 (https://github.com/vsbuffalo/scythe, accessed on 23 September 2022) to clip them from Illumina Nextera XT adaptors sequences (Illumina, San Diego, CA, USA) and cutadapt v2.10 to trim the adaptors and filter raw reads with length below 80 nucleotides and Q score below 30. We then generated complete genomes through a reference-based approach using BWA v0.7.12 (https://github.com/lh3/bwa, accessed on 23 September 2022) [16]. Finally, we used Picard-tools v2.1.0 (http://picard.sourceforge.net (accessed on 23 September 2022)) and GATK v3.5 (https://github.com/moka-guys/gatk_v3.5, accessed on 23 September 2022) to process alignments, loFreq v2.1.2 (https://github.com/CSB5/lofreq, accessed on 23 September 2022) to call Single Nucleotide Polymorphisms (SNPs) and an in-house script to obtain consensus sequences, setting 50% of allele frequency as threshold for base calling and 10X as the minimum coverage.

In order to investigate the diversity of parvovirus strains circulating in the area, we performed genetic and phylogenetic analyses for the whole genome and the complete VP2 gene, which is more widely used across the literature. Datasets included positive original samples and the first three non-identical best matches for each sequence, as determined using BLAST reference strains that were previously associated either with dogs in the study area [6] or with wildlife across the world. The selection from the public database included sequences from Italy or wild species tested positive in our study. Sequences were aligned using the G-INS-1 parameters implemented in Mafft [17] and Maximum likelihood (ML) nucleotide phylogenetic trees were inferred using PhyML (version 3.0), employing the GTR+Γ4 substitution model, a heuristic SPR branch-swapping algorithm and 1000 bootstrap replicates [18]; the obtained trees were then graphically edited using iTOL [19]. In order to achieve the typing of the CPV-2/FPV strains, we derived amino acidic sequences using MEGA6 and considered VP2 amino acid residues at positions 87, 297, 300, 305, 426 and 555, as described elsewhere [1].

3. Results

Overall, we screened n = 387 fecal samples and intestines from dogs and different wildlife species, achieving a total of n = 298 positive samples among dogs (n = 290/343, 84.5%), Eurasian badgers (n = 4/55, 7.2%), golden jackals (n = 3/12, 25%), and grey wolves (n = 1/5, 20%). All samples from red foxes (n = 21) and beech martens (n = 4) tested negative (Table 3). Pathological findings in positive dogs were in accordance with a moderate to severe hemorrhagic/necrotic-hemorrhagic enteritis. Similarly, the positive wolf was an adult male presenting a severe hemorrhagic enteritis, whereas the golden jackals were all young individuals and did not show any gut lesion. On the other hand, we could not evaluate the association between virus positivity and clinical or pathological conditions of badgers, which were submitted for rabies surveillance as carcasses at various degrees of putrification, or after severe car accidents, both conditions preventing reliable necropsies.

Table 3. Details of samples including the genetic and antigenic characterization of positive samples.

Host	N of Positive/Tested Samples	% of Positivity	Viral Type/Variant (% Out of Positive Samples)
Dog	290/343	84.5	CPV-2 (12.2), new CPV-2a (74.3), CPV-2b (8.1), new CPV-2b (2.7), CPV-2c (2.7)
Eurasian badger	4/55	7.2	FPV (100)
Red fox	0/21	0	-
Golden jackal	3/12	25	FPV (100)
Grey wolf	1/5	20	CPV-2c (100)
Beech marten	0/4	0	-

Seventy-four positive samples from dogs and all positive samples from wildlife were further characterized throughout whole genome sequencing. The majority of CPV-2 detected and characterized in dogs were new CPV-2a (Table 3) followed by CPV-2, new CPV-2b, CPV-2b, and CPV-2c. Whereas viral strains from wildlife were characterized as FPV (from Eurasian badgers and golden jackals) and CPV-2c (from one grey wolf) (Table 3; Figure 1).

All positive samples were sequenced using one of the three molecular approaches described, obtaining consensus sequences of a total length of 4000–4300 nucleotides that mostly excluded only non-coding terminal regions (160–400 bp on 5′ and 140 bp on 3′). However, we failed to amplify around 2000 bp on 5′ in nine samples, including four dogs, the wolf, one jackal and three badgers, and on 3′ in three badger samples. In addition, another jackal's sample did not provide an interpretable sequence across 1000 bp towards the 5′ end. The obtained sequences have all been deposited under the GenBank accession numbers OP587964 to OP588036 and OP595737 to OP595745. Alignments used for phylogenetic analyses accounted for 130 and 230 sequences for the whole genome and the VP2 region, respectively. Of these, 73 and nine, respectively, have been obtained in the present Investigation. The topology of the phylogenetic trees based on the whole genome sequences and on the VP2 gene sequences were comparable, showing that sequences of viral strains from wildlife were included in a separate branch, along with the sequences of other FPV strains, except for the one from the grey wolf, included in a cluster within the sequences of CPV-2 strains. Sequences related to illegally imported puppies displayed a high differentiation of canine parvoviruses included in several clusters across the whole phylogenetic tree (Figures 1 and 2).

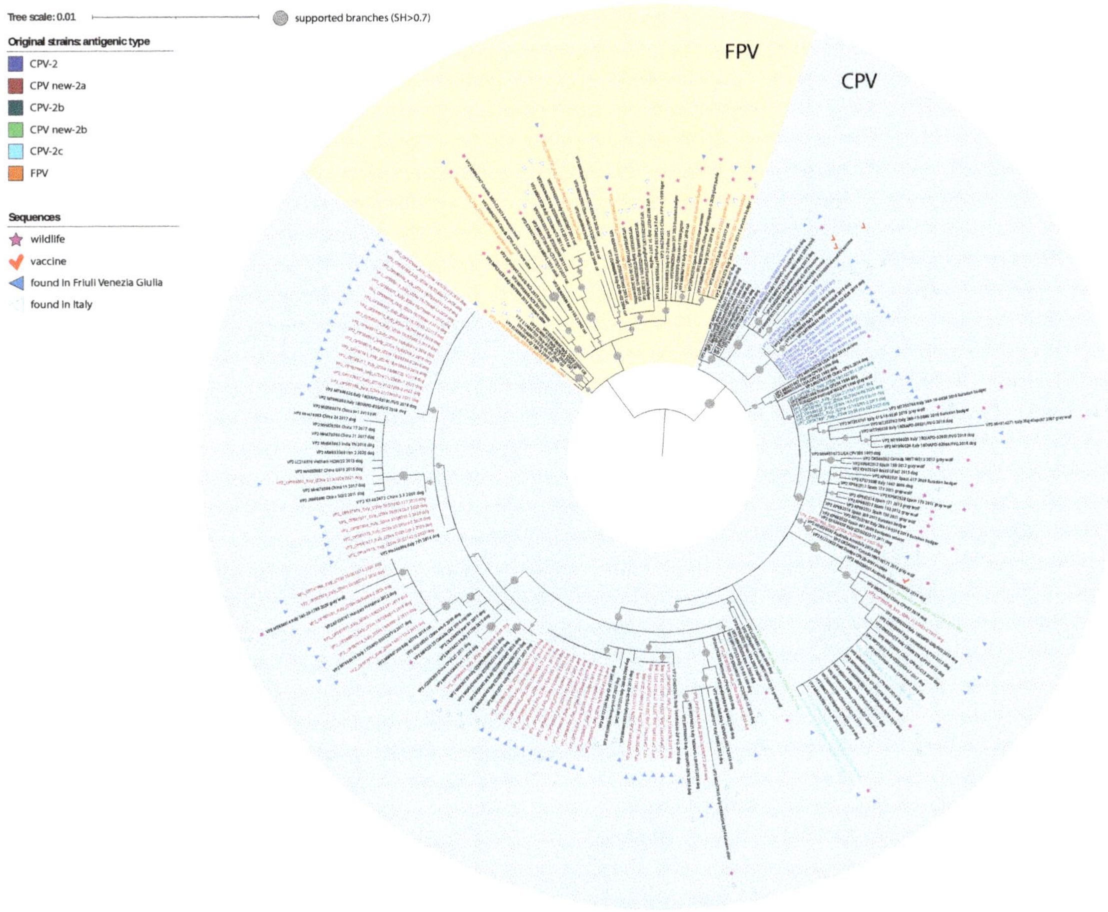

Figure 1. ML phylogenetic tree of *Carnivore Protoparvovirus 1* analyzed in this study, based on the complete VP2 gene sequences, divided in canine (blue) and feline (yellow) parvoviruses. Branches supported with SH value higher than 0.7 are marked with grey circles, with size proportional to the SH value. Original strains sequenced for this work are shown with colored labels based on their antigenic classification as CPV-2 (blue), new CPV-2a (red), CPV-2b (petrol), new CPV-2b (green), CPV-2c (light blue). Sequences (original and reference) associated with wildlife and found in the study area are indicated with pink stars and blue circles, respectively (full for the region of Friuli Venezia-Giulia and empty for some other areas in Italy), while vaccine strains are marked with a red checkmark.

Almost all published available CPV-2/FPV sequences detected in the Italian domestic dogs and cats, as well as in European wildlife, accounted for partial genomes. In this framework, phylogeny based on the VP2 gene sequences provided better reference to interpret phylogenetic trees. Indeed, FPV sequences from Eurasian badgers generated in this study formed a stand-alone cluster within FPV considering the whole genome (Figure 2). Conversely, considering the VP2 only, the FPV strains sequenced from wildlife appeared scattered in the phylogenetic tree, showing high correlation with strains described in Italian cats but also in Eurasian badgers and stone martens from Spain and the UK

(Figure 1). Interestingly, two of these sequences (OP595737 and OP595738) were identical to Italian FPVs associated with cats at the VP2 level (KX434461 and KX434462, respectively).

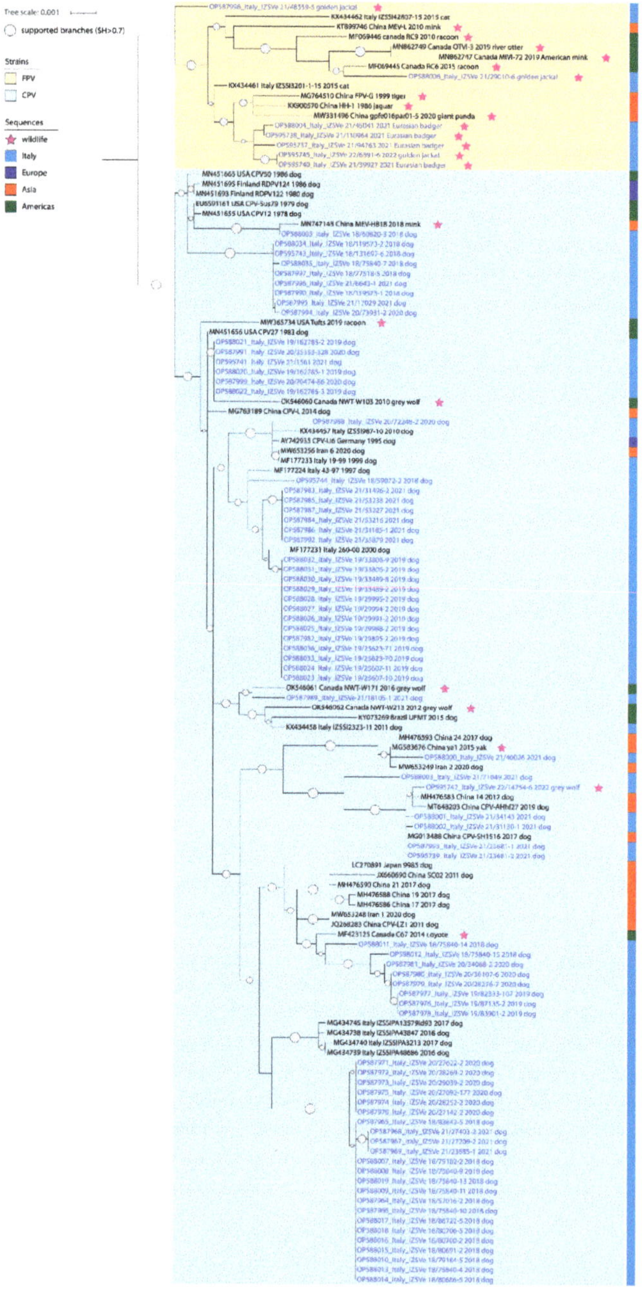

Figure 2. ML phylogenetic tree of *Protoparvovirus 1* analyzed in this study, based on the complete genome, divided in canine (blue) and feline (yellow) parvoviruses. Branches supported with SH value higher than 0.7 are marked with grey circles, with size proportional to the SH value. Original strains sequenced for this work are shown with blue labels. Sequences (original and reference) associated with wildlife and found in the study area are indicated with pink stars.

FPV sequences generated from golden jackals (n = 3) were not related to each other (Figure 1). One (OP595745) clustered with the FPV sequence (OP595740) from Eurasian badger characterized in this study and with the FPV sequences from Italian cats and wildlife, a second one (OP588006) with the FPV sequence from Canadian wildlife, and the last one (OP587998) with the FPV sequences from Italian domestic cats. As for FPV strains from Eurasian badgers, this last sequence (OP587998) was highly related with sequences obtained from cats only at the level of VP2, while it occupied a basal branch with no evident clustering upon analyses using the complete genomes (Figure 2).

Similarly, the analysis of the VP2 sequences allowed us to show that most clusters identified in dogs in our study were highly related with strains already described in Friuli Venezia-Giulia or, more generally, in Italy (Figure 1). Interestingly and similarly to what previously noticed by [6], in the present study the VP2 phylogenetic tree showed that the CPV-2 strains sequenced from illegally imported dogs are grouped according to the antigenic type (Figure 1). Considering the antigenic characterization, 55 sequences classified as new CPV-2a, six as CPV-2b, two as new CPV-2b, and two as CPV-2c (Figure 1). The high prevalence of the new CPV-2a variant in illegally imported dogs is similar to the one recently observed in dogs in the same Italian geographical area [6]. Of note, nine sequences obtained from puppies clustered within CPV-2 strains actively circulating in dogs in the 1980s and were included in widely used attenuated vaccines (Figures 1 and 2). By analyzing their amino acid sequence, we were able to confirm their antigenic classification as CPV-2 strains (Figure 1). Eight out of nine sequences, clustering with previously characterized CPV-2 in Italy, showed mutations I219V and Q386K typical of one of the live-attenuated vaccines available in the market (MG264079) [20]. Interestingly, four of the identified CPV-2 strains were associated with severe clinical signs and mortality in puppies, three of them (including two sequences displaying the two vaccine signatures as of MG264079) in absence of other pathogens detected (data not shown).

Finally, the VP2 phylogenetic tree evidenced that CPV new-2a strains identified in the present study from illegally imported dogs make up distinct groups reflecting the detection year to a certain extent (Figure 1). Interestingly, the 2018 new CPV-2a cluster groups together with two new CPV-2a strains of the same year and same region (Friuli Venezia Giulia) that were reported to be suspected of illegal importation from East Europe most probably [6].

The strain detected in the grey wolf was the only CPV-2 we found in the screened widlife (OP595742). This sequence was antigenically classified as CPV-2c and phylogenetically closely related with Asian-origin CPV-2c circulating in dogs, showing a maximum nucleotide identity with dog strains of 99.9% across the whole genome and in the VP2 region (Figures 1 and 2). Analyses of the VP2 highlighted that a related sequence (MT454909) had already been associated with wolves in Southern Italy in 2020 (Figure 1) [13]. The analysis of aa residues showed that both the OP595742 sequence identified in the present study and the MT454909 sequence [13] retained tyrosine and threonine at positions 324 and 440 of VP2, respectively, contrasting with the puppies' sequences retaining only threonine at position 440, out of the three signatures likely caused from vaccine immune pressure (F267Y/Y324I/T440A) [21].

4. Discussion

This study provides a snapshot of parvoviruses circulating in wild carnivores from Friuli Venezia-Giulia, in comparison with strains imported in the region from Central and Eastern Europe through the illegal market of pups. Despite the vaccination of puppies against canine parvovirus is widely implemented in North Eastern Italy, this practice likely represents a major evolutionary source of old and new strains [6]. The high prevalence of CPV-2 in the tested puppies highlights the risk for domestic dogs posed by the illegal introduction. Indeed, genetic and phylogenetic evaluations of the samples sequenced from illegally traded dogs confirmed that the CPV-2 strains introduced in the area of study belong to several groups across the phylogenetic tree of CPV-2, with eight to twelve clusters identified using the complete VP2 and the whole genome, respectively. Among these, most samples were included in three clusters identified almost exclusively in Italy, with the exception of a single sequence found in Hungary in 2008. Nine sequences clustered with original strains CPV-2 circulating in the 1980s [1], even if most of them formed a sister clade that was exclusive of this work. Similar sequences were reported from neighboring areas in Italy, in particular in the Veneto region and were classified as being likely vaccine strains [6]. Indeed, viruses included in several live attenuated vaccines (shown with red checkmarks in Figure 1) cluster within the original clade of CPV-2. These vaccines are still widely used worldwide, because they induce a strong long-lasting immunity without inducing severe clinical signs [22]. However, the virus replicates within the host so that shedding is frequent after inoculation [23,24]. Because CPV-2 strains do not seem to be actively circulating in European dogs, it is likely that our findings also relate to post-vaccination shedding, as elsewhere already assumed [6]. In this context, it is noteworthy that eight out of nine typed sequences presented two mutations that are included in the patent of a widely used CPV-2 vaccine (MG264079) [20], strongly supporting our hypothesis. Of note, although vaccine replication and shedding are considered non-pathogenic for puppies, we found three cases indicating severe signs of gastroenteritis and mortality linked with vaccine virus. This finding is only partially in line with previous field detections, linking the shedding of vaccine strains with mild diarrhea in pups [25]. In this context, we might not exclude that clinical signs in our study were exacerbated by the poor health of pups under investigation, mostly younger than the recommended vaccination age and transported illegally in poor conditions and not in compliance with animal welfare and sanitary requirements [10].

Despite the whole genome provided a much better resolution of the phylogenetic relationship between viruses identified in the area, the phylogenetic tree based on the VP2 allowed a clearer interpretation thanks to the presence of a greater number of sequences from other areas, especially Italian and European from both dogs and wildlife. Indeed, there are still few studies that provide the complete genome of *Carnivore protoparvovirus 1*, despite they are progressively increasing. In this context, our sequencing protocols allowed us to characterize successfully most strains and were able to provide a cost-effective tool for future studies as well.

The analyzed CPV-2 strains were associated with most antigenic types currently circulating worldwide (CPV-2, new CPV-2a, CPV-2b, new CPV-2b and CPV-2c), among which new CPV-2a was the most widespread in the area, as previously reported in the same geographic area (North East Italy) [6].

In addition, our data support that this subtype completely replaced CPV-2a in the area, while CPV-2b still co-circulates with the recently emerged subtype new CPV-2b. The differentiation of antigenic types mirrored only partially the topology of the phylogenetic tree [1]. In particular, all CPV-2 strains clustered with the "original" clade and all sequences classified as CPV-2c were included within a single cluster diverging from the others. CPV2-b also clustered together, with strains of the new diverging subtype also in the phylogenetic tree. In 2008, CPV-2b reappeared in Italy after ten years, and since then it has maintained a low prevalence [6,26], raising several doubts on the origin of such a renewed circulation. Indeed, CPV-2b has been introduced as vaccine component, due to its notable capability of inducing a broad-spectrum immunity against both CPV-2a and CPV-2c strains [27]. The origin of the CPV-2b sequences identified in the illegally imported puppies in the present study could therefore be due to vaccine strain occurrence rather than to an active circulation of the "old" CPV-2b variant. Of note, all dogs carrying CPV-2b sequences displayed no signs of acute gastroenteritis. Finally, clusters of sequences typed as CPV-2a were sparse across the phylogenetic tree, although clustering together according to the detection year (Figure 1).

Overall, our phylogenetic and genetic data support the assumption that strains detected and sequenced in imported dogs are highly related to what previously observed in the local canine population, suggesting that either the illegal pet trade accounts for most of the variability in parvoviruses in the area, or else that similar strains are circulating in

Central and Eastern Europe. However, more recent data from these areas are needed to corroborate one of the two hypotheses.

In order to test the assumption that parvoviruses introduced in the area with the trade of puppies might pose a risk for local wildlife, we analyzed a large repository of intestinal samples collected from diverse carnivore species widespread in the region. We found only one sample positive for CPV-2 in a grey wolf out of five analyzed in 2022, belonging to the antigenic type CPV-2c. Despite this type was the least represented in dogs from our investigation, this strain was correlated with sequences detected in Asia and also reported in Italian domestic dogs. Similarly to what found elsewhere in Southern Italy, the CPV-2c detected in the wolf retained two aa residues out of the three that had probably emerged from vaccine immune pressure, and may represent current circulation in wildlife following an ancestral spillover event [13,21]. However, investigating the ecopathology of this virus in the grey wolf and its relationship with the domestic dogs deserves a wider investigation.

No other species was found positive for the presence of CPV-2, differently to that described elsewhere [13,14]. On the other hand, we found that FPV circulates among carnivores in the study area, with percentage of positivity of 7.2 detected in Eurasian badgers, consistently with what reported in Spain [14]. Similarly, a higher circulation of FPV compared to CPV has been described in Portugal, together with a high frequency in Eurasian badgers [28]. To the best of our knowledge, this is the first report of golden jackals resulted positive for FPV in Europe, with the highest percentage of positivity corresponding to 25% (3/12), compared to the other tested carnivores. The high diversity of FPV found in jackals could be explained either by the repopulation of the areas with individuals from different populations or by multiple cross-species transmission. Remarkably, several evidences suggest interactions between jackals and domestic animals, including cats. In addition, the scavenger-like feeding behavior performed by golden jackals in anthropogenic territory may provide the opportunity for spillover from domestic animals to wild carnivores and vice versa. Of note, all foxes tested negative in our study despite the number of individuals tested, thus excluding a prevalence of at least 15% considering the estimated fox population in Friuli Venezia Giulia. This result was expected based on previous findings estimating 2.8% prevalence of FPV in red foxes in other areas of Italy [13] and might be due to the fox susceptibility to *Carnivore protoparvovirus 4* species, of which the prototype virus has been identified in a red fox [29]. Nevertheless, enhanced surveillance in the red fox should be implemented in light of its susceptibility to both FPV and CPV-2 viruses [14,28] and its well-known proximity with human settlements.

Interestingly, FPV sequences detected in this study did not all cluster together based on the widely used VP2, but were correlated with viruses found in both wildlife and domestic cats in Italy and abroad (Figure 1). Similarly, no sequences shared 100% ID based on the whole genome, which suggests a considerable mixing of strains within wildlife populations, including possible cross-species transmissions in the wild and across the interface with domestic cats, as already suggested [14]. Finally, all FPV shared the classical antigenic signature described in domestic animals across all the amino acid residues analyzed.

5. Conclusions

In this study, we showed that puppies illegally imported in North-Eastern Italy introduce a wide diversity of canine parvoviruses, belonging to different antigenic types, among which the new CPV-2a is the most represented. However, this diversity matches the one reported elsewhere in Italy, preventing us further speculations.

In wildlife, we found evidence for the infection with CPV-2 only in one wolf, showing a high correlation with a cluster already described in the same species in Southern Italy. Severe clinical signs and mortality associated with original and vaccine strains might be explained by the young age and poor health conditions of the illegally traded pups. Negative findings in foxes and Eurasian badgers suggested that no CPV is circulating at high prevalence in these species in Friuli Venezia Giulia. On the other hand, we found a significant circulation of FPV in golden jackals and, to a lesser extent, in badgers. As for CPV-2, FPV found in wildlife clustered with sequences from wild as well as domestic carnivores, thus describing a complex ecology of *Carnivore protoparvovirus 1*. This ecological complexity is further enhanced by the rapid viral spatial movement associated with the illegal trafficking of puppies from Eastern to Western Europe.

Author Contributions: Conceptualization, P.Z., I.M. and P.D.B.; methodology, S.L. (Stefania Leopardi), A.M., I.M. and P.D.B.; software, S.L. (Stefania Leopardi), A.M. and A.P.; validation, A.M., A.P. and A.S.; formal analysis, S.L. (Stefania Leopardi), A.M., A.S., S.L. (Sofia Leardini), F.F. and A.P.; investigation, M.C., M.B., G.d.Z. and F.G.; resources, M.C., I.M. and P.D.B.; data curation, A.M.; writing—original draft preparation, S.L. (Stefania Leopardi); writing—review and editing, S.L. (Stefania Leopardi), A.M., M.C., M.B., A.S., S.L. (Sofia Leardini), F.F., A.P., G.d.Z., F.G., M.S.B., M.P., A.B., M.-C.R., P.Z., I.M. and P.D.B.; visualization, S.L. (Stefania Leopardi) and P.D.B.; supervision, P.D.B.; project administration, A.B. and P.D.B.; funding acquisition, M.P., M.-C.R., P.Z. and P.D.B. All authors have read and agreed to the published version of the manuscript.

Funding: This study was supported by the European Regional Development Fund—Interreg V-A Italia-Österreich, Biocrime Project, project Code ITAT3002.

Institutional Review Board Statement: The present study was performed on samples either collected from live animals by Public Health Authorities for official sanitary surveillance or from dead animals. All samples were collected under a legal framework and submitted to the reference laboratory for the Friuli Venezia-Giulia Region. In Europe, such procedures do not require any specific ethical approval and the sampling procedures were performed in compliance with the country's own legislation and the recommendations of international institutions. According to the national legislation regulating animal experimentation, no ethical approval or permit was required for collecting and processing the type of samples examined for this study.

Informed Consent Statement: Not applicable.

Data Availability Statement: Sequences have been deposited in GenBank public database under accession numbers OP587964 to OP588036 and OP595737 to OP595745.

Acknowledgments: The authors wish to thank the technical laboratory staff members at the Istituto Zooprofilattico Sperimentale delle Venezie.

Conflicts of Interest: The authors declare no conflict of interest. The funders had no role in the design of the study; in the collection, analyses, or interpretation of data; in the writing of the manuscript, or in the decision to publish the results.

References

1. De Oliveira Santana, W.; Silveira, V.P.; Wolf, J.M.; Kipper, D.; Echeverrigaray, S.; Canal, C.W.; Truyen, U.; Lunge, V.R.; Streck, A.F. Molecular phylogenetic assessment of the canine parvovirus 2 worldwide and analysis of the genetic diversity and temporal spreading in Brazil. *Infect. Genet. Evol.* **2022**, *98*, 105225. [CrossRef] [PubMed]
2. Callaway, H.; Welsch, K.; Weichert, W.; Allison, A.; Hafenstein, S.; Huang, K.; Iketani, S.; Parrish, C. Complex and Dynamic Interactions between Parvovirus Capsids, Transferrin Receptors, and Antibodies Control Cell Infection and Host Range. *J. Virol.* **2018**, *92*, e00460-18. [CrossRef] [PubMed]
3. Chung, H.C.; Kim, S.J.; Nguyen, V.G.; Shin, S.; Kim, J.Y.; Lim, S.K.; Park, Y.H.; Park, B.K. New genotype classification and molecular characterization of canine and feline parvoviruses. *J. Vet. Sci.* **2020**, *21*, e43. [CrossRef]
4. Shackelton, L.A.; Parrish, C.R.; Truyen, U.; Holmes, E.C. High rate of viral evolution associated with the emergence of carnivore parvovirus. *Proc. Natl. Acad. Sci. USA* **2005**, *102*, 379–384. [CrossRef] [PubMed]
5. Giraldo-Ramirez, S.; Rendon-Marin, S.; Ruiz-Saenz, J. Phylogenetic, evolutionary and structural analysis of canine parvovirus (CPV-2) antigenic variants circulating in Colombia. *Viruses* **2020**, *12*, 500. [CrossRef] [PubMed]
6. Carrino, M.; Tassoni, L.; Campalto, M.; Cavicchio, L.; Mion, M.; Corrò, M.; Natale, A.; Beato, M.S. Molecular Investigation of Recent Canine Parvovirus-2 (CPV-2) in Italy Revealed Distinct Clustering. *Viruses* **2022**, *14*, 917. [CrossRef]
7. Sacristán, I.; Esperón, F.; Pérez, R.; Acuña, F.; Aguilar, E.; García, S.; José, M.; Elena, L.; Cabello, J.; Karen, E.H.; et al. Epidemiology and molecular characterization of Carnivore protoparvovirus-1 infection in the wild felid Leopardus guigna in Chile. *Transbound. Emerg. Dis.* **2021**, *2*, 3335–3348. [CrossRef] [PubMed]
8. Zucca, P.; Rossmann, M.C.; Osorio, J.E.; Karem, K.; De Benedictis, P.; Haißl, J.; De Franceschi, P.; Calligaris, E.; Kohlweiß, M.; Meddi, G.; et al. The "Bio-Crime Model" of Cross-Border Cooperation Among Veterinary Public Health, Justice, Law Enforcements, and Customs to Tackle the Illegal Animal Trade/Bio-Terrorism and to Prevent the Spread of Zoonotic Diseases Among Human Population. *Front. Vet. Sci.* **2020**, *7*, 593683. [CrossRef] [PubMed]

9. Schrijver, R.; Sikkema, R.; de Vries, H.; Dewar, D.; Bergevoet, R.; Messori, S.; D'Albenzio, S.; Barnard, S. Study on the Welfare of Dogs and Cats Involved in Commercial Practices (Specific Contract SANCO 2013/12364). 2015. Available online: https://www.un.org/en/development/desa/population/migration/generalassembly/docs/globalcompact/A_RES_66_288.pdf (accessed on 23 September 2022).
10. Cocchi, M.; Danesi, P.; De Zan, G.; Leati, M.; Gagliazzo, L.; Ruggeri, M.; Palei, M.; Bremini, A.; Rossmann, M.C.; Lippert-Petscharnig, M.; et al. A three-year biocrime sanitary surveillance on illegally imported companion animals. *Pathogens* **2021**, *10*, 1047. [CrossRef]
11. Eurogroup for Animals. *The Illegal Pet Trade: Game Over*; Eurogroup for Animals: Brussels, Belgium, 2020.
12. Canuti, M.; Fry, K.; Cluff, H.D.; Mira, F.; Fenton, H.; Lang, A.S. Co-circulation of five species of dog parvoviruses and canine adenovirus type 1 among gray wolves (*Canis lupus*) in northern Canada. *Transbound. Emerg. Dis.* **2022**, *69*, e1417–e1433. [CrossRef]
13. Ndiana, L.A.; Lanave, G.; Desario, C.; Berjaoui, S.; Alfano, F.; Puglia, I.; Fusco, G.; Loredana, M.; Vincifori, G.; Camarda, A.; et al. Circulation of diverse protoparvoviruses in wild carnivores, Italy. *Transbound. Emerg. Dis.* **2021**, *68*, 2489–2502. [CrossRef]
14. Calatayud, O.; Esperón, F.; Velarde, R.; Oleaga, Á.; Llaneza, L.; Ribas, A.; Negre, N.; de la Torre, A.; Rodríguez, A.; Millán, J. Genetic characterization of Carnivore Parvoviruses in Spanish wildlife reveals domestic dog and cat-related sequences. *Transbound. Emerg. Dis.* **2020**, *67*, 626–634. [CrossRef]
15. Pérez, R.; Calleros, L.; Marandino, A.; Sarute, N.; Iraola, G.; Grecco, S.; Blanc, H.; Vignuzzi, M.; Isakov, O.; Shomron, N.; et al. Phylogenetic and genome-wide deep-sequencing analyses of Canine parvovirus reveal co-infection with field variants and emergence of a recent recombinant strain. *PLoS ONE* **2014**, *9*, e111779. [CrossRef] [PubMed]
16. Van der Auwera, G.A.; Carneiro, M.O.; Hartl, C.; Poplin, R.; del Angel, G.; Levy-Moonshine, A.; Jordan, T.; Shakir, K.; Roazen, D.; Thibault, J.; et al. From FastQ Data to High-Confidence Variant Calls: The Genome Analysis Toolkit Best Practices Pipeline. *Curr. Protoc. Bioinforma.* **2013**, *43*, 11.10.1–11.10.33. [CrossRef]
17. Katoh, K.; Misawa, K.; Kuma, K.; Miyata, T. MAFFT: A novel method for rapid multiple sequence alignment based on fast Fourier transform. *Nucleic Acids Res.* **2002**, *30*, 3059–3066. [CrossRef]
18. Dereeper, A.; Guignon, V.; Blanc, G.; Audic, S.; Buffet, S.; Chevenet, F.; Dufayard, J.F.; Guindon, S.; Lefort, V.; Lescot, M.; et al. Phylogeny.fr: Robust phylogenetic analysis for the non-specialist. *Nucleic Acids Res.* **2008**, *36*, 465–469. [CrossRef]
19. Letunic, I.; Bork, P. Interactive tree of life (iTOL) v3: An online tool for the display and annotation of phylogenetic and other trees. *Nucleic Acids Res.* **2016**, *44*, W242–W245. [CrossRef]
20. Calatayud, O.; Esperón, F.; Cleaveland, S.; Biek, R.; Keyyu, J.; Eblate, E.; Neves, E.; Lembo, T.; Lankester, F. Carnivore Parvovirus Ecology in the Serengeti Ecosystem: Vaccine Strains Circulating and New Host Species Identified. *J. Virol.* **2019**, *93*, e02220-18. [CrossRef] [PubMed]
21. Zhou, P.; Zeng, W.; Zhang, X.; Li, S. The genetic evolution of canine parvovirus-A new perspective. *PLoS ONE* **2017**, *12*, e0175035. [CrossRef]
22. Decaro, N.; Buonavoglia, C.; Barrs, V.R. Canine parvovirus vaccination and immunisation failures: Are we far from disease eradication? *Vet. Microbiol.* **2020**, *247*, 108760. [CrossRef] [PubMed]
23. Martella, V.; Decaro, N.; Elia, G.; Buonavoglia, C. Surveillance activity for canine parvovirus in Italy. *J. Vet. Med. Ser. B* **2005**, *52*, 312–315. [CrossRef]
24. Decaro, N.; Crescenzo, G.; Desario, C.; Cavalli, A.; Losurdo, M.; Colaianni, M.L.; Ventrella, G.; Rizzi, S.; Aulicino, S.; Lucente, M.S.; et al. Long-term viremia and fecal shedding in pups after modified-live canine parvovirus vaccination. *Vaccine* **2014**, *32*, 3850–3853. [CrossRef] [PubMed]
25. Decaro, N.; Desario, C.; Elia, G.; Campolo, M.; Lorusso, A.; Mari, V.; Martella, V.; Buonavoglia, C. Occurrence of severe gastroenteritis in pups after canine parvovirus vaccine administration: A clinical and laboratory diagnostic dilemma. *Vaccine* **2007**, *25*, 1161–1166. [CrossRef]
26. Battilani, M.; Modugno, F.; Mira, F.; Purpari, G.; Di Bella, S.; Guercio, A.; Balboni, A. Molecular epidemiology of canine parvovirus type 2 in Italy from 1994 to 2017: Recurrence of the CPV-2b variant. *BMC Vet. Res.* **2019**, *15*, 393. [CrossRef] [PubMed]
27. Wilson, S.; Illambas, J.; Siedek, E.; Stirling, C.; Thomas, A.; Plevová, E.; Sture, G.; Salt, J. Vaccination of dogs with canine parvovirus type 2b (CPV-2b) induces neutralising antibody responses to CPV-2a and CPV-2c. *Vaccine* **2014**, *32*, 5420–5424. [CrossRef] [PubMed]
28. Duarte, M.D.; Henriques, A.M.; Barros, S.C.; Fagulha, T.; Mendonça, P.; Carvalho, P.; Monteiro, M.; Fevereiro, M.; Basto, M.P.; Rosalino, L.M.; et al. Snapshot of Viral Infections in Wild Carnivores Reveals Ubiquity of Parvovirus and Susceptibility of Egyptian Mongoose to Feline Panleukopenia Virus. *PLoS ONE* **2013**, *8*, e59399. [CrossRef] [PubMed]
29. Bodewes, R.; van der Giessen, J.; Haagmans, B.L.; Osterhaus, A.D.M.E.; Smits, S.L. Identification of multiple novel viruses, including a parvovirus and a hepevirus, in feces of red foxes. *J. Virol.* **2013**, *87*, 7758–7764. [CrossRef] [PubMed]

viruses

MDPI

Article

Not Asian Anymore: Reconstruction of the History, Evolution, and Dispersal of the "Asian" Lineage of CPV-2c

Giovanni Franzo [1,*], Francesco Mira [2,3], Giorgia Schirò [2,3] and Marta Canuti [4,5,6,*]

1 Department of Animal Medicine, Production and Health (MAPS), Padua University, 35020 Legnaro, Italy
2 Istituto Zooprofilattico Sperimentale della Sicilia "A. Mirri", 90129 Palermo, Italy; francesco.mira@izssicilia.it (F.M.); giorgia.schiro91@gmail.com (G.S.)
3 Department of Veterinary Science, University of Messina, Polo Universitario dell'Annunziata, 98168 Messina, Italy
4 Department of Pathophysiology and Transplantation, Università degli Studi di Milano, 20122 Milan, Italy
5 Coordinate Research Centre EpiSoMI (Epidemiology and Molecular Surveillance of Infections), Università degli Studi di Milano, 20122 Milan, Italy
6 Centre for Multidisciplinary Research in Health Science (MACH), Università degli Studi di Milano, 20122 Milan, Italy
* Correspondence: giovanni.franzo@unipd.it (G.F.); marta.canuti@gmail.com (M.C.)

Abstract: Variability has been one of the hallmarks of canine parvovirus type 2 (CPV-2) since its discovery, and several lineages and antigenic variants have emerged. Among these, a group of viruses commonly called Asian CPV-2c has recently been reported with increasing frequency in different regions. Currently, its global epidemiology and evolution are essentially unknown. The present work deals with this information gap by evaluating, via sequence, phylodynamic, and phylogeographic analyses, all the complete coding sequences of strains classified as Asian CPV-2c based on a combination of amino acid markers and phylogenetic analysis. After its estimated origin around 2008, this lineage circulated undetected in Asia until approximately 2012, when an expansion in viral population size and geographical distribution occurred, involving Africa, Europe, and North America. Asia was predicted to be the main nucleus of viral dispersal, leading to multiple introduction events in other continents/countries, where infection establishment, persistence, and rapid evolution occurred. Although the dog is the main host, other non-canine species were also involved, demonstrating the host plasticity of this lineage. Finally, although most of the strains showed an amino acid motif considered characteristic of this lineage, several exceptions were observed, potentially due to convergent evolution or reversion phenomena.

Keywords: canine parvovirus type 2; CPV-2; molecular epidemiology; *Protoparvovirus carnivoran1*; parvovirus; virus evolution

Citation: Franzo, G.; Mira, F.; Schirò, G.; Canuti, M. Not Asian Anymore: Reconstruction of the History, Evolution, and Dispersal of the "Asian" Lineage of CPV-2c. *Viruses* **2023**, *15*, 1962. https://doi.org/10.3390/v15091962

Academic Editor: Giorgio Gallinella

Received: 24 August 2023
Revised: 14 September 2023
Accepted: 18 September 2023
Published: 20 September 2023

1. Introduction

In the 1970s, a novel parvovirus capable of infecting canines emerged as a dog pathogen, quickly becoming a major health threat for pets and wild canine populations globally. This virus was named canine parvovirus type 2 (CPV-2) to distinguish it from the only other parvovirus known at that time to infect dogs, the minute virus of canines [1,2]. CPV-2 causes severe enteric disease in affected dogs, which can lead to acute hemorrhagic diarrhea and death, sometimes complicated by myocarditis and lymphopenia-associated immunodepression with consequent super-infections. While the infection can be acquired at any age, the disease is more severe in younger individuals [2–4]. CPV-2 infection in cats is similar in its course to what is observed in dogs, but panleukopenia is usually predominant [2,4,5]. Not much is known about the clinical manifestations among wild animals.

CPV-2 belongs to the species *Protoparvovirus carnivoran1* (family *Parvoviridae*, subfamily *Parvovirinae*), together with another virus that circulates among terrestrial felids and mustelids, feline panleukopenia virus (FPV or FPLV) [6,7]. However, before genetic studies clarified that only these two main genetic lineages existed within the species, CPV-2 and FPV were named differently when found in other hosts, such as mink enteritis virus (MEV), raccoon parvovirus (RPV), or blue fox parvovirus (BFPV) [2,8–10]. Like all other parvoviruses, viruses within this species are characterized by ~25 nm naked T = 1 icosahedral capsids composed of two viral proteins, VP1 and VP2, which contain a single-stranded DNA molecule of approximately 5 Kb, covalently linked to the main viral non-structural protein, NS1 [6]. The genome includes two gene cassettes—one for the non-structural (NS) and one for the structural (VP) proteins—which, thanks to the alternative splicing of host-transcribed messenger RNAs, produce all open reading frames (ORF) coding for viral proteins. These cassettes are flanked by terminal non-coding regions that fold into hairpin-like structures that are important for viral DNA replication [6].

CPV-2 emerged from an FPV-like virus after acquiring specific mutations that allowed its capsid to bind the transferrin receptor of canine cells, extending its tropism to canines and enabling its fast pandemic spread [1,2,11]. The original CPV-2 strain, which now no longer circulates among dogs, did not possess the ability to infect felines, but the variant that replaced it in the 1980s, known as CPV-2a, (re)gained this ability [1,2]. Since then, CPV-2a and its descendants have been found in several carnivoran hosts, predominantly canids, felids, and mustelids, and even in non-carnivoran mammals [5,8,9,12–17]. Despite this difference in host ranges, the genomes of CPV-2 and FPV are approximately 98% identical to each other, and only six amino acid (AA) mutations distinguish their VP2s, while only three amino acid mutations distinguish CPV-2 from CPV-2a. Additionally, mutations at amino acid 300 of VP2 can alter the virus–host tropism, and several different residues have been detected at this position in various members of *Protoparvovirus carnivoran1* infecting different hosts [8,18].

After the emergence of CPV-2a, several new mutations were reported for this virus, seemingly, without shifts in host tropism. The classification of this virus into three antigenic variants depending on the amino acid, featuring position 426 of VP2 (N in CPV-2a, D in CPV-2b, and E in CPV-2c), gained significant consensus [2,19,20]. However, there are contradictory opinions about these mutations' antigenic and biological relevance, as vaccines remain cross-protective, and the virulence of the three variants seems similar [4,21]. Nonetheless, these and other mutations continuously emerge, and several studies have shown variation in their frequency over the years [2,4,22,23]. Some amino acid mutations, including the one at AA 426, arose in different lineages at various times and places, likely as a result of convergent evolution due to positive selection pressure [24,25]. In fact, the groups of viruses belonging to the same variant are paraphyletic [24].

Given these convergences, the presence of one specific phenotypic mutation cannot be used for virus classification. However, the presence of a pattern of mutations, combined with phylogenetic analyses, allows us to more specifically define evolutionary-related strains and monitor their circulation [24–26]. This is the case for the so-called "Asian CPV-2c" lineage, a monophyletic group of viruses characterized by a specific set of mutations in both structural and non-structural proteins [25]. This clade was recorded for the first time in Asian countries, where it became more and more prevalent as years passed by, and it was recently introduced to several other countries worldwide, where it is now spreading and locally evolving [12,27–32]. However, the understanding of the real success, population dynamics, and spreading patterns of this clade are hindered by sparse and biased diagnostic and sequencing activity. As the success of this clade is intriguing from an evolutionary and epidemiological perspective, in this study, we investigated the origin and evolution of Asian CPV-2c-like viruses, using dedicated statistical and bioinformatic approaches that are less susceptible to sampling structure to gain a deeper understanding of CPV-2 global transmission and evolutionary dynamics.

2. Materials and Methods

2.1. Datasets

All sequences of members of the species *Protoparvovirus carnivoran1*, available in GenBank as of 2 April 2023, were downloaded and combined with additional sequences deposited later (accession numbers OR463583–OR463704) [32], resulting in a set of 8804 sequences. Three subsets were then created, including full coding (from NS1 start codon plus, at most, 3 AAs to VP2 stop codon minus, at most, 3 AAs), full NS1 (minus, at most, 3 AAs), and full VP2 (minus, at most, 3 AAs) sequences. From the three sets, sequences with ambiguities, frameshift mutations, and premature stop codons were removed. This resulted in three datasets of 733 complete, 901 NS1, and 4765 VP2 coding sequences. For each sequence, the collection host, country, and date were recorded if available, and the sequence name was edited to include this information.

2.2. Asian CPV-2c Lineage Definition

Sequence alignments (NS1, VP2, complete genome) were performed with MAFFT [33]. For coding regions, an alignment was initially performed at the amino acid level, and then sequences were back-translated as nucleotides using TranslatorX [34].

Since different methods can lead to slightly different results, especially in the case of high genetic identity and convergent mutations, for each dataset, three phylogenetic trees were reconstructed, and the results were compared. Trees were built using IQ-Tree [35], RAxML [36], and Fasttree2 [37], and using the substitution model with the lowest Bayesian information criterion (BIC) as calculated by JModelTest2 [38]. The Asian CPV-2 lineage was defined based on three expert opinions according to the following:

(1) The presence of the amino acid motif 5A/G, 267Y, 297A, 324I, 370R, 426E, and 440T in VP2 and 630P in NS1. Motif identification was automatically performed using specifically designed R scripts.
(2) Being part of a monophyletic clade, including the majority of strains featured in the above-mentioned markers. This choice was necessary to classify as part of the "Asian CPV-2c" clade some strains that, although originating from an Asian ancestor, lost, because of amino acid toggling and reversion, the peculiar phenotypic pattern.
(3) The strains were identified based on different trees and expert opinions were compared to classify them based on a majority consensus rule: strains fulfilling the second rule in at least two out of three trees built with at least one of the three alignments were classified as "Asian CPV-2c".

2.3. Phylodynamic Analyses

The selected datasets (VP2, NS1, and complete genome) were analyzed to reconstruct several population parameters, including the time to the most recent common ancestor (tMRCA), the evolutionary rate, and viral population dynamics using the Bayesian serial coalescent approach implemented in BEAST 1.10 [39]. The nucleotide substitution model was selected based on a BIC score calculated using JmodelTest [38]. The molecular clock method was selected to calculate the marginal likelihood estimation through path-sampling and stepping-stone methods, as suggested by Baele et al. [40]. A non-parametric Bayesian skygrid [39] was implemented to reconstruct the viral population (relative genetic diversity: effective population size x generation time; Ne x τ) over time.

Based on the higher sequence number and more representative geographic origin compared with other genomic regions, a discrete-state phylogeographic analysis was also performed as described by Lemey et al., 2009 [41], on the VP2 dataset only. An asymmetric migration model with Bayesian stochastic search variable selection (BSSVS) was implemented, allowing us to identify the most parsimonious description of the spreading process and calculate a BF indicative of the statistical significance of the inferred migration path between areas. Since sampling and sequencing biases are likely, this phenomenon and its impact on analysis results were assessed via subsampling without replacing the available sequences and allowing for a maximum of 8 sequences for each country–date pair. Moreover, this allowed us to create more balanced sequence datasets.

The history and evolution over time of marker amino acids featuring the Asian CPV-2c lineage were also reconstructed using discrete trait analysis (DTA) in BEAST 1.10. For each analysis, an independent run of 200 million generations was performed. The results were analyzed using Tracer 1.7 [42] after the removal of a burn-in of 20% and accepted only if the estimated sample size (ESS) was greater than 200 and the convergence and mixing were adequate. Parameter estimation was summarized in terms of mean and the 95% highest posterior density (95HPD). Maximum clade credibility (MCC) trees were constructed and annotated using TreeAnnotator (BEAST package). SpreaD3 [43] was used to calculate the BF associated with each migration route. All non-zero transition rates among countries were considered significant when the BF was greater than 10. Additional summary statistics and graphical outputs were generated using homemade R scripts (Team, 2014).

The presence of sites under episodic diversifying selection was assessed using MEME [44], implemented in HyPhy [45], while the positive pervasive selection was evaluated using FEL [46] and FUBAR [47], implemented in the same program. The statistical significance was set at $p < 0.05$ and the posterior probability at >0.9.

3. Results

3.1. Details of the Sequences Identified as Belonging to the Asian CPV-2c Lineage

After searching the NCBI sequence database, a total of 917 sequences belonging to the Asian CPV-2c lineage were identified. The earliest sequences (2013) originated from Asian (Vietnamese and Indonesian) dogs, but since 2017, viruses belonging to this clade started to be detected on other continents as well (Figure 1), having been recorded in dogs but also cats (*Felis silvestris catus*), raccoon dogs (*Nyctereutes procyonoides*) (Republic of Korea), and pangolins (*Manis pentadactyla*) (Taiwan and China). In total, 872 of these strains could be classified as CPV-2c, 7 as CPV-2b, and 3 as CPV-2a, depending on the amino acid present at residue 426 of VP2. Supplementary Table S1 details how many sequences were identified for each year, country, host, and antigenic type, while the Supplementary File provides the accession numbers and a description of each identified sequence.

By analyzing the amino acid residues that were used in the literature to determine whether a strain belonged to this clade (60V, 544F, 545V, and 630P in NS1 and 5G, 267Y, 297A, 324I, 370R, 426E, and 440T in VP2) [25], we observed that, while none of these mutations are unique to this clade, and not all sequences in this clade possess all of these mutations, specific combinations of mutations were significantly associated with this clade and not other clades (Figure 2). Specifically, NS1-630P was found in all sequences belonging to the Asian CPV-2c lineage, and VP2 324I, 297A, 267Y, 370R, 426E, and 440T were simultaneously present in 94.3% of sequences in this clade. Interestingly, the monophyletic Asian lineage also included a few CPV-2b (426D) and CPV-2a (426N) strains (see Section 3.4). A summary of amino acid residues present in all other strains is available in Supplementary Figure S1.

3.2. Phylodynamic Analyses

The VP2-based analyses led to concordant results regardless of the randomly generated dataset. The average evolutionary rate was 4.62×10^{-4} subs/site/year (95HPD: 2.21×10^{-4}–7.78×10^{-4}), and the tMRCA was estimated in 2006.43 (95HPD: 1972.41–2009). The reconstruction of the population dynamics allowed us to identify three main phases: the first one, right after the origin of the lineage, featured a substantially stable population size; this was followed by a rapid increase in diversity approximately in the period 2012–2017 and, finally, after the population peak, by a slow decline (Figure 3).

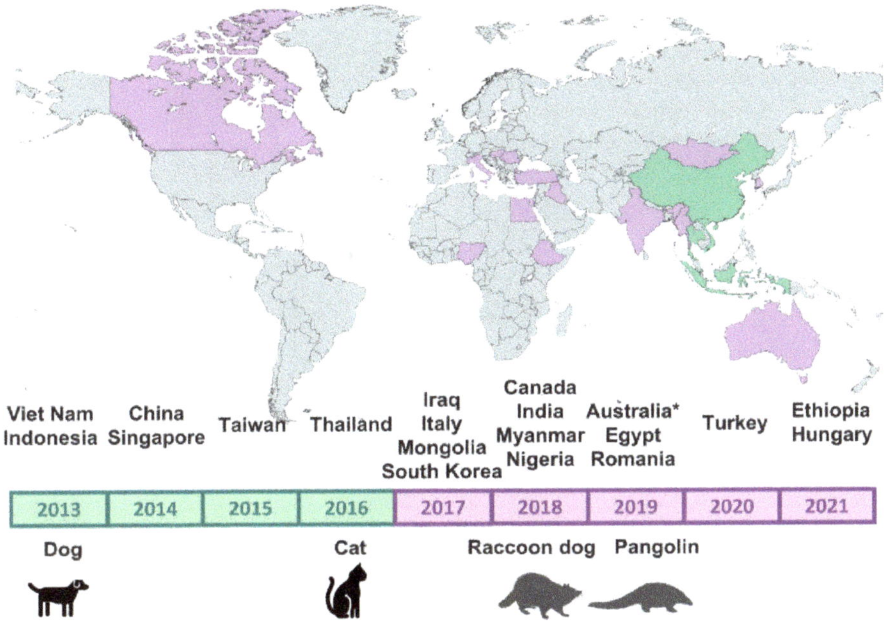

Figure 1. Temporal, host, and country distribution of sequences belonging to the Asian CPV-2c lineage annotated in GenBank. In the map at the top, the countries where the earliest sequences (2013–2016) were identified are indicated in green, while those where the viruses were found later (2017–2021) are in purple. The gray on the map indicates no sequences reported as of yet. In the lower part, countries (top) and hosts (bottom: in black, domestic animals, and in gray, other animals) are indicated in correspondence to the years when they were detected for the first time. The map was created with Mapchart.net ©. * Classified based on NS1.

VP2

								Asian		Non-Asian	
	5	267	297	324	370	426	440	N	%	N	%
CPV-2c	G	Y	A	I	R	E	T	**573**	**64.5**	0	0.0
	A	Y	A	I	R	E	T	**262**	**29.8**	0	0.0
	A	Y	A	I	Q	E	T	10	1.1	1	0.0
	A	Y	A	I	R	E	A	9	1.0	0	0.0
	G	Y	A	I	Q	E	T	7	0.8	0	0.0
	A	Y	A	I	Q	E	A	5	0.6	0	0.0
	G	Y	A	I	R	E	A	2	0.2	0	0.0
	G	F	A	I	R	E	T	2	0.2	0	0.0
	G	Y	A	L	R	E	T	1	0.1	0	0.0
CPV-2b	G	Y	A	I	R	D	T	3	0.3	0	0.0
	G	Y	A	I	Q	D	T	2	0.2	48	1.6
	A	Y	A	I	R	D	T	1	0.1	0	0.0
CPV-2a	G	Y	A	I	R	N	A	1	0.1	0	0.0
	A	Y	A	I	R	N	T	1	0.1	0	0.0
	G	Y	A	I	Q	N	T	1	0.1	0	0.0

NS1

				Asian		Non-Asian	
60	544	545	630	N	%	N	%
V	F	V	P	**233**	**98.3**	0	0.0
I	F	V	P	3	1.3	0	0.0
V	Y	E	P	1	0.4	0	0.0

Figure 2. Key amino acids at specific residues in VP2 (**left**) and NS1 (**right**), defining Asian CPV-2c strains. In each panel, the amino acid position is indicated at the top, while the number (N) of times and percentages (%) that these sequences were found in the CPV-2c Asian (Asian) clade and in all other CPV-2 strains (non-Asian) are indicated on the right.

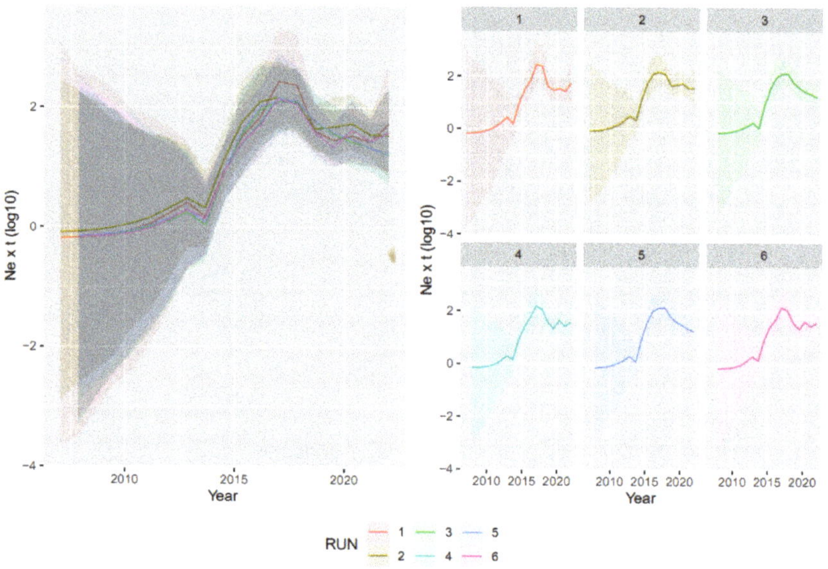

Figure 3. Relative genetic diversity (Ne x t) of the Asian CPV-2c lineage over the years. The results of the six independent runs have been color-coded. Mean, median, and upper and lower 95HPD values are reported for each run on the right and superimposed on the left.

Comparable results were obtained for the NS1 dataset, whose evolutionary rate was estimated to be 4.87×10^{-4} subs/site/year (95HPD: 2.26×10^{-4}–6.94×10^{-4}), and the tMRCA was 2008.97 (95HPD: 1969.26–2013). Although it had a relatively broad uncertainness, a stabler population size was inferred using NS1, with minor fluctuations occurring over the last decade (Supplementary Figure S2).

Finally, the estimated evolutionary rate of the complete genome was 6.64×10^{-4} subs/site/year (95HPD: 4.22×10^{-4}–1.24×10^{-3}), and the tMRCA was 2010.19 (95HPD: 2006.4–2012.56) (Supplementary Figure S3). A relatively constant population size, with minor fluctuations, was also reconstructed.

3.3. *Phylogeographic Analyses*

The phylogeographic analyses performed on randomly and independently generated datasets, despite minor variations due to the differences in strains included, highlighted an essentially common pattern (Figure 4). Almost all statistically supported migration rates pointed to centrifugal spreading and multiple, independent introductions from Asia (China) to other Asian, African, and European countries (Figure 4).

Specifically, after an Asian origin, potentially in Indonesia or China, the "Asian CPV-2c" lineage persisted in the region until approximately 2012, when new continents started to be involved, including European and, essentially in the same period, African countries. Multiple independent introductions occurred from Asian countries to both Europe and Africa. These events were followed by local persistence and evolution (Figure 5). In addition to within-continent clustering, the tendency of strains collected in the same country to cluster together was apparent. Nevertheless, the clustering of strains sampled in different countries of the same continent and the circulation of highly divergent strains in the same country were observed (Figures 5 and S4).

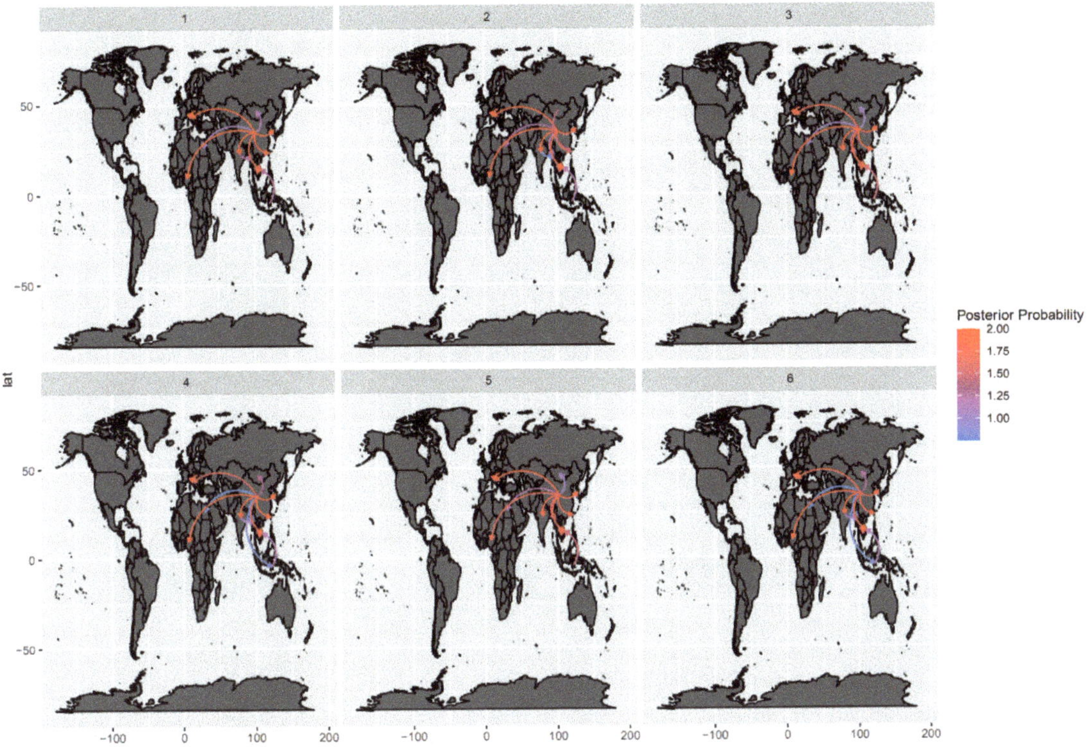

Figure 4. Well-supported migration paths (i.e., BF > 10) of strains belonging to the Asian CPV-2c lineage among countries are depicted as edges whose colors are proportional to the base-10 logarithm of the migration rate. The location of each country is matched with its centroid. The results of the 6 independent analyses are reported in different panels.

3.4. Marker Amino Acid Evolution

Although the Asian CPV-2c lineage has been traditionally defined based on the presence of amino acid markers in specific VP2 positions, a certain variability was observed among its strains. To understand whether this feature was ascribable to basal branches (i.e., ancestral strains not fully displaying the final phenotype) or to reversion/toggling phenomena, the evolution of variable marker positions was reconstructed through a DTA. In all instances, the variability affected recent, terminal branches, providing evidence for the second hypothesis. Although single-terminal branches were mainly affected, some clades with 370Q persisted for a certain period. A minor recent clade with European (Italy and Hungary) sequences showing 426D was also present (Figure 6).

MEME analysis detected amino acids 5, 119, 354, 426, and 542 (including two Asian CPV-2c markers) under episodic diversifying selection at the set significance level ($p < 0.05$). FEL and FUBAR detected amino acids 5 and 440 (both Asian CPV-2c markers) and 5, 13, 440, and 426 (three of which are Asian CPV-2c markers) under diversifying selection, respectively. In NS1, AAs 492 and 665 were detected under diversifying selection with FUBAR, while AAs 647, 664, and 665 were detected with MEME.

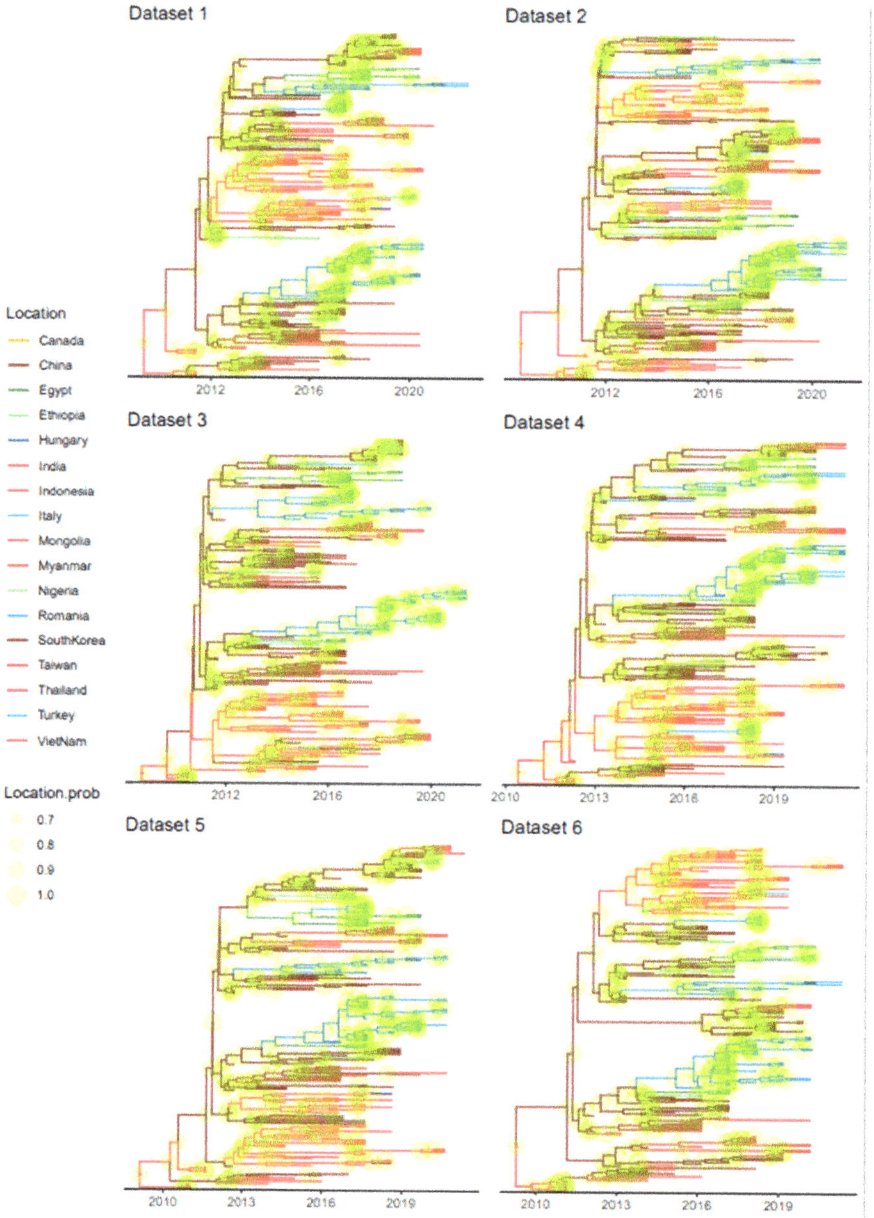

Figure 5. Maximum clade credibility trees based on the Asian CPV-2c lineage VP2 dataset. The results of the phylogeographic analyses are reported with different colors. Tips and branches are color-coded according to the collection country or the one estimated with the higher posterior probability, respectively. Countries are reported in different shades of color featuring the same continent. Node size is proportional to the posterior probability of the inferred locations. The results of different datasets are reported in different panels. A comparable figure with reported tip names is provided in Supplementary Figure S4.

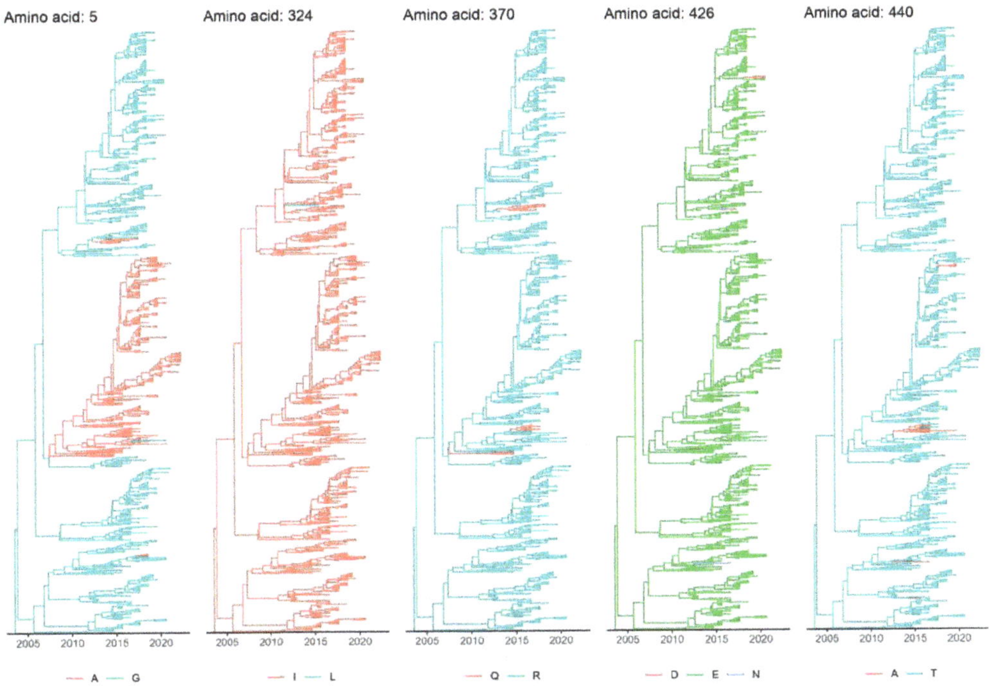

Figure 6. Maximum clade credibility trees based on the Asian CPV-2c lineage VP2 dataset. The results of the DTA analysis—reconstructing the evolution, over time, of the amino acids traditionally used as markers to define Asian CPV-2c strains—are reported in different panels. Tips and branches are color-coded according to the detected amino acid or the one estimated with the higher posterior probability, respectively.

4. Discussion

Since it emerged as a devastating dog pathogen, CPV-2 has demonstrated a high evolutionary rate, which has led to the emergence of remarkable genetic and phenotypic variability [10]. For a long time, the primary research interest was the description and characterization of phenotypic/antigenic variants, which are defined based on the presence of peculiar combinations of amino acidic markers in specific positions of the VP2 protein [1,2]. CPV-2a, -2b, and -2c are the most widely recognized variants, whose definition is largely shared by most research groups [2,19,20]. Over time, different studies have reported a plethora of other potential genetic variants, which have shown inconsistent epidemiological success. Most recently, an increase in the detection frequency of the so-called "Asian CPV-2c" lineage was observed [27–30,32,48]. However, no systematic study has been performed to evaluate its molecular epidemiology and evolution on a broader scale. The present work deals with this knowledge gap.

According to our models, the origin of the Asian CPV-2c lineage was estimated to be approximately in 2008 in Asian countries. Thereafter, it likely circulated in the area, undetected or unreported for years, progressively but slowly increasing in population size in accordance with what was previously reported [49]. Comparably to what was previously reported for other CPV-2 variants, the Asian lineage featured an overall high evolutionary rate [10,48–50]. A major change in this pattern was observed after 2012 when an abrupt expansion occurred. This period coincided with the first official description of Asian CPV-2c strains, whose detection was facilitated by an increase in infection (and likely disease) prevalence. The first available sequences were, in fact, from samples collected in 2013 (dogs from Vietnam and Indonesia), 2014 (dogs from China and Singapore), and 2015 (dogs from Taiwan and China). However, from 2016 onward, an increase in the number of the sequences submitted yearly to GenBank was observed, likely corresponding to more sustained viral circulation. This finding confirms the huge spreading potential that has characterized the history of CPV-2 and, thus, the need for more effective and systematic monitoring activities to promptly detect and effectively react to emerging viruses. In fact, the increase in population size also mirrored the viral introduction to new areas of the world, and strains belonging to this lineage have been reported particularly in Asia [30,51,52], Europe [25,27,29,53], and Africa [31,54,55], although there is also a report from North America [12]. Furthermore, in recent years, an increasing number of studies from Asia have highlighted not only the progressive spread of the Asian CPV-2c lineage but also the progressive replacement of the circulating CPV-2 strains by this lineage, as if it had potentially greater viral fitness [56–59]. Similarly, a strong expansion of this lineage, which replaced other locally circulating CPV-2c variants soon after its first occurrence, was also recently observed in Italy [32]. Although a biological advantage of the CPV-2c Asian lineage over other CPV-2 variants could be speculated, no definitive proof is present, opening interesting new research fields regarding this topic.

The higher infection rates in Asian countries, likely also favored by lower vaccination coverage, could have increased the likelihood of strain exportations. Epidemiological links mediated by both human and animal movement between Asia and Europe have been proven for several companion animal infections, including CPV-2 [28,60–63]. Similarly, the rising political, economic, and cultural interactions occurring between Asian (especially China) and African countries might have favored the introduction of this lineage, as previously suggested [48,55].

Alternatively, the increase in the viral population size could have followed the introduction into new areas, allowing this lineage to benefit from a broader host population. Vaccination is especially rare in African dog populations [48], which may have favored viral expansion. Although vaccination rates are much higher in Europe, understanding whether immunity induced by other strains confers less protection against this new lineage is intriguing and requires further investigation. The final stabilization and slow decline of the viral population size modeled in the present study could support this hypothesis, reflecting the progressive establishment of lineage-specific immunity. A combination of the two phenomena should also not be excluded.

The spreading dispersal pattern analysis suggests Asia is the central nucleus of viral spread, mediating multiple independent introductions to other continents, followed by successful infection establishment, persistence, and local evolution. Although a tendency toward country-based clustering was present, evidence of within-continent dispersal was also observed, although with higher among-dataset variability. Accordingly, none of those connections were statistically significant. Overall, local persistence and spreading were the dominant phenomena, as we also observed elsewhere [32], while transboundary dispersal was more sporadic. This pattern, featuring multiple independent introduction events as a consequence of inter- and intracontinental migrations, followed by local differentiation and competition between populations, is a hallmark of CPV-2 epidemiology [64–66] and reveals the remarkable evolutionary consequences of poorly constrained viral circulation.

Besides dogs, infections with this lineage have also been reported multiple times in cats (Thailand and China), although FPV is still the dominant virus in felids [67–69]. Additionally, Asian CPV-2c strains have also been observed in wild canids, such as in one raccoon dog (Republic of Korea), and even in non-carnivoran hosts, including two pangolins (China and Taiwan) that likely died because of the infection [15,17]. This indicates that these viruses are capable of cross-species transmission, even to non-carnivorans, and should be monitored because they pose a potential danger to wildlife. Whether this lineage emerged in wild animals and then spilled over to dogs, as happened with CPV-2a strains [70], or originated in dogs and then spilled over to other animals remains to be established.

The above-mentioned pattern could be at least partially explained by the biased and unbalanced number of sequences (especially complete genome sequences) among countries, which might have led to an overestimation of the contribution of more represented countries. For example, while several investigations of the molecular epidemiology of CPV-2 have been performed in Europe and Asia, almost no studies have investigated viral diversity in North America, and very few studies have assessed viral presence among wild animals. Nonetheless, the substantial agreement between the randomly generated datasets seems to contradict this proposition and supports the robustness of the obtained findings. However, the absence of a proper sampling design necessitates caution in results interpretation. While the overall patterns can be considered reliable, specific county pair connections must not be overstated. The long branch length separating several clades likely conceals additional spatial movements between multiple locations, and intermediate links between country pairs might have been lost because of limited diagnostic and sequencing activity.

While marker positions are still often used to classify CPV-2 strains, the incongruence between genetic- and phenotypic-based clustering has also been demonstrated by other authors [24,66]. Strains with a separate evolutionary history can share the same amino acid because of convergent evolution, while reversion phenomena can cause closely related strains to show different phenotypic features. Such phenomena feature in the Asian CPV-2c lineage too. Although not common since >94% of the sequences from this lineage present the same amino acids at key residues (namely, 630P in NS1 and 324I, 297A, 267Y, 370R, 426E, and 440T in VP2), some of the strains classified in this lineage revealed a different phenotypic pattern. In all instances, the amino acid mutations affected terminal branches rather than basal ones, demonstrating episodes of reversion. Establishing whether such mutations can provide an evolutive advantage or are an incidental finding is challenging. Since mostly single branches were involved, low-fitness, epidemiological dead ends are likely. However, some long-lasting clades harboring 5A, 370Q, and 440A were observed. Of note, a phenotypically CPV-2b (AA 426D) clade was observed, including Italian strains from 2022 and a Hungarian one sampled in 2021 [25,32,71]. A similar mutation also independently affected three strains from China sampled since 2016. Two strains sampled in 2017 and 2018 from China and one from India independently acquired 426N. Since positions 5, 426, and 440 were detected under diversifying selection, a potential beneficial effect and fitness advantage induced by phenotypic variability might be speculated. Whether this is ascribable to immune pressures or other forces remains to be established. Biological meaning aside, our results again stress the unreliability of marker-based classification and the importance of integrating sequence and phylogenetic analyses when studying the molecular epidemiology of this virus, as we highlighted in previous studies [25,26,66,72].

5. Conclusions

The present study reconstructs the history, evolution, and spread of the Asian CPV-2c lineage from its origin to the present day. After likely relatively long and undetected circulation in Asia, it was able to spread worldwide, increasing its prevalence and relative genetic diversity. Asia was estimated to be the central nucleus of viral dispersal, mediating multiple independent introductions to other continents, followed by successful infection establishment, local persistence, and evolution. A certain phenotypic variability was observed within this clade, resulting from a combination of high mutation rates and selective pressure action. Our results stress one more time the need for systematic epidemiological studies, monitoring, and reporting for CPV-2 activity and diversity to promptly detect new CPV-2 variants and lineages, whose behavior is currently hardly predictable, creating the best conditions for their control.

Supplementary Materials: The following supporting information can be downloaded at https://www.mdpi.com/article/10.3390/v15091962/s1: Table S1: Number of sequences within the Asian CPV-2c lineage identified in each country, year, and host and for each variant. Figure S1: Key amino acids at specific residues in VP2 and NS1, defining Asian CPV-2c viruses in strains that do not belong to the Asian CPV-2 lineage. Figure S2: Relative genetic diversity (Ne x t) of the Asian CPV-2c lineage over the years, estimated using the NS1 gene. Figure S3: Relative genetic diversity

(Ne x t) of the Asian CPV-2c lineage over the years, estimated using the complete genome. Figure S4: Maximum clade credibility trees based on the Asian CPV-2c lineage VP2 dataset.

Author Contributions: Conceptualization, G.F., F.M. and M.C.; methodology, G.F. and M.C.; validation, G.F., F.M. and M.C.; formal analysis, G.F. and M.C.; investigation, G.F., F.M., G.S. and M.C.; data curation, G.F. and M.C.; writing—original draft preparation, G.F., F.M., G.S. and M.C.; writing—review and editing, G.F., F.M. and M.C.; visualization, G.F. and M.C.; supervision, G.F., F.M. and M.C.; project administration, G.F., F.M. and M.C. All authors have read and agreed to the published version of the manuscript.

Funding: This research received no external funding.

Institutional Review Board Statement: Not applicable.

Informed Consent Statement: Not applicable.

Data Availability Statement: The sequences used in this study are all available in GenBank under the accession numbers listed in the Supplementary File.

Conflicts of Interest: The authors declare no conflict of interest.

References

1. Parrish, C.R.; Have, P.; Foreyt, W.J.; Evermann, J.F.; Senda, M.; Carmichael, L.E. The Global Spread and Replacement of Canine Parvovirus Strains. *J. Gen. Virol.* **1988**, *69*, 1111–1116. [CrossRef] [PubMed]
2. Miranda, C.; Thompson, G. Canine Parvovirus: The Worldwide Occurrence of Antigenic Variants. *J. Gen. Virol.* **2016**, *97*, 2043–2057. [CrossRef]
3. Parrish, C.R. Pathogenesis of Feline Panleukopenia Virus and Canine Parvovirus. *Baillière's Clin. Haematol.* **1995**, *8*, 57–71. [CrossRef] [PubMed]
4. Decaro, N.; Buonavoglia, C. Canine Parvovirus—A Review of Epidemiological and Diagnostic Aspects, with Emphasis on Type 2c. *Vet. Microbiol.* **2012**, *155*, 1–12. [CrossRef]
5. Miranda, C.; Parrish, C.R.; Thompson, G. Canine Parvovirus 2c Infection in a Cat with Severe Clinical Disease. *J. Vet. Diagn. Investig.* **2014**, *26*, 462–464. [CrossRef]
6. Cotmore, S.F.; Agbandje-McKenna, M.; Canuti, M.; Chiorini, J.A.; Eis-Hubinger, A.-M.; Hughes, J.; Mietzsch, M.; Modha, S.; Ogliastro, M.; Pénzes, J.J.; et al. ICTV Virus Taxonomy Profile: *Parvoviridae*. *J. Gen. Virol.* **2019**, *100*, 367–368. [CrossRef]
7. Pénzes, J.J.; Söderlund-Venermo, M.; Canuti, M.; Eis-Hübinger, A.M.; Hughes, J.; Cotmore, S.F.; Harrach, B. Reorganizing the Family *Parvoviridae*: A Revised Taxonomy Independent of the Canonical Approach Based on Host Association. *Arch. Virol.* **2020**, *165*, 2133–2146. [CrossRef]
8. Allison, A.B.; Kohler, D.J.; Ortega, A.; Hoover, E.A.; Grove, D.M.; Holmes, E.C.; Parrish, C.R. Host-Specific Parvovirus Evolution in Nature Is Recapitulated by in Vitro Adaptation to Different Carnivore Species. *PLOS Pathog.* **2014**, *10*, e1004475. [CrossRef] [PubMed]
9. Canuti, M.; Todd, M.; Monteiro, P.; Van Osch, K.; Weir, R.; Schwantje, H.; Britton, A.P.; Lang, A.S. Ecology and Infection Dynamics of Multi-Host Amdoparvoviral and Protoparvoviral Carnivore Pathogens. *Pathogens* **2020**, *9*, 124. [CrossRef]
10. Shackelton, L.A.; Parrish, C.R.; Truyen, U.; Holmes, E.C. High Rate of Viral Evolution Associated with the Emergence of Carnivore Parvovirus. *Proc. Natl. Acad. Sci. USA* **2005**, *102*, 379–384. [CrossRef]
11. Hueffer, K.; Parker, J.S.L.; Weichert, W.S.; Geisel, R.E.; Sgro, J.-Y.; Parrish, C.R. The Natural Host Range Shift and Subsequent Evolution of Canine Parvovirus Resulted from Virus-Specific Binding to the Canine Transferrin Receptor. *J. Virol.* **2003**, *77*, 1718–1726. [CrossRef] [PubMed]
12. Canuti, M.; Mira, F.; Sorensen, R.G.; Rodrigues, B.; Bouchard, É.; Walzthoni, N.; Hopson, M.; Gilroy, C.; Whitney, H.G.; Lang, A.S. Distribution and Diversity of Dog Parvoviruses in Wild, Free-Roaming and Domestic Canids of Newfoundland and Labrador, Canada. *Transbound. Emerg. Dis.* **2022**, *69*, e2694–e2705. [CrossRef] [PubMed]
13. Nur-Farahiyah, A.N.; Kumar, K.; Yasmin, A.R.; Omar, A.R.; Camalxaman, S.N. Isolation and Genetic Characterization of Canine Parvovirus in a Malayan Tiger. *Front. Vet. Sci.* **2021**, *8*, 660046. [CrossRef] [PubMed]
14. Canuti, M.; Fry, K.; Cluff, H.D.; Mira, F.; Fenton, H.; Lang, A.S. Co-Circulation of Five Species of Dog Parvoviruses and Canine Adenovirus Type 1 among Gray Wolves (*Canis lupus*) in Northern Canada. *Transbound. Emerg. Dis.* **2022**, *69*, e1417–e1433. [CrossRef]
15. Wang, S.-L.; Tu, Y.-C.; Lee, M.-S.; Wu, L.-H.; Chen, T.-Y.; Wu, C.-H.; Tsao, E.H.-S.; Chin, S.-C.; Li, W.-T. Fatal Canine Parvovirus-2 (CPV-2) Infection in a Rescued Free-Ranging Taiwanese Pangolin (*Manis pentadactyla pentadactyla*). *Transbound. Emerg. Dis.* **2020**, *67*, 1074–1081. [CrossRef]
16. Kurucay, H.N.; Tamer, C.; Muftuoglu, B.; Elhag, A.E.; Gozel, S.; Cicek-Yildiz, Y.; Demirtas, S.; Ozan, E.; Albayrak, H.; Okur-Gumusova, S.; et al. First Isolation and Molecular Characterization of Canine Parvovirus-Type 2b (CPV-2b) from Red Foxes (*Vulpes vulpes*) Living in the Wild Habitat of Turkey. *Virol. J.* **2023**, *20*, 27. [CrossRef]

17. Lina, Z.; Kai, W.; Fuyu, A.; Dongliang, Z.; Hailing, Z.; Xuelin, X.; Ce, G.; Hongmei, Y.; Yingjie, K.; Zhidong, Z.; et al. Fatal Canine Parvovirus Type 2a and 2c Infections in Wild Chinese Pangolins (*Manis pentadactyla*) in Southern China. *Transbound. Emerg. Dis.* **2022**, *69*, 4002–4008. [CrossRef]
18. Allison, A.B.; Organtini, L.J.; Zhang, S.; Hafenstein, S.L.; Holmes, E.C.; Parrish, C.R. Single Mutations in the VP2 300 Loop Region of the Three-Fold Spike of the Carnivore Parvovirus Capsid Can Determine Host Range. *J. Virol.* **2016**, *90*, 753–767. [CrossRef]
19. Parrish, C.R.; Aquadro, C.F.; Strassheim, M.L.; Evermann, J.F.; Sgro, J.Y.; Mohammed, H.O. Rapid Antigenic-Type Replacement and DNA Sequence Evolution of Canine Parvovirus. *J. Virol.* **1991**, *65*, 6544–6552. [CrossRef]
20. Buonavoglia, C.; Martella, V.; Pratelli, A.; Tempesta, M.; Cavalli, A.; Buonavoglia, D.; Bozzo, G.; Elia, G.; Decaro, N.; Carmichael, L. Evidence for Evolution of Canine Parvovirus Type 2 in Italy. *J. Gen. Virol.* **2001**, *82*, 3021–3025. [CrossRef]
21. Wilson, S.; Illambas, J.; Siedek, E.; Stirling, C.; Thomas, A.; Plevová, E.; Sture, G.; Salt, J. Vaccination of Dogs with Canine Parvovirus Type 2b (CPV-2b) Induces Neutralising Antibody Responses to CPV-2a and CPV-2c. *Vaccine* **2014**, *32*, 5420–5424. [CrossRef] [PubMed]
22. Zhou, P.; Zeng, W.; Zhang, X.; Li, S. The Genetic Evolution of Canine Parvovirus—A New Perspective. *PLoS ONE* **2017**, *12*, e0175035. [CrossRef] [PubMed]
23. Hao, X.; He, Y.; Wang, C.; Xiao, W.; Liu, R.; Xiao, X.; Zhou, P.; Li, S. The Increasing Prevalence of CPV-2c in Domestic Dogs in China. *PeerJ* **2020**, *8*, e9869. [CrossRef]
24. Voorhees, I.E.H.; Lee, H.; Allison, A.B.; Lopez-Astacio, R.; Goodman, L.B.; Oyesola, O.O.; Omobowale, O.; Fagbohun, O.; Dubovi, E.J.; Hafenstein, S.L.; et al. Limited Intrahost Diversity and Background Evolution Accompany 40 Years of Canine Parvovirus Host Adaptation and Spread. *J. Virol.* **2019**, *94*, e01162-19. [CrossRef] [PubMed]
25. Schirò, G.; Mira, F.; Canuti, M.; Vullo, S.; Purpari, G.; Chiaramonte, G.; Di Bella, S.; Cannella, V.; Randazzo, V.; Castronovo, C.; et al. Identification and Molecular Characterization of a Divergent Asian-like Canine Parvovirus Type 2b (CPV-2b) Strain in Southern Italy. *Int. J. Mol. Sci.* **2022**, *23*, 11240. [CrossRef] [PubMed]
26. Mira, F.; Canuti, M.; Purpari, G.; Cannella, V.; Di Bella, S.; Occhiogrosso, L.; Schirò, G.; Chiaramonte, G.; Barreca, S.; Pisano, P.; et al. Molecular Characterization and Evolutionary Analyses of *Carnivore protoparvovirus 1* NS1 Gene. *Viruses* **2019**, *11*, 308. [CrossRef]
27. Mira, F.; Purpari, G.; Lorusso, E.; Di Bella, S.; Gucciardi, F.; Desario, C.; Macaluso, G.; Decaro, N.; Guercio, A. Introduction of Asian Canine Parvovirus in Europe through Dog Importation. *Transbound. Emerg. Dis.* **2018**, *65*, 16–21. [CrossRef]
28. Mira, F.; Purpari, G.; Bella, S.D.; Colaianni, M.L.; Schirò, G.; Chiaramonte, G.; Gucciardi, F.; Pisano, P.; Lastra, A.; Decaro, N.; et al. Spreading of Canine Parvovirus Type 2c Mutants of Asian Origin in Southern Italy. *Transbound. Emerg. Dis.* **2019**, *66*, 2297. [CrossRef]
29. Balboni, A.; Niculae, M.; Di Vito, S.; Urbani, L.; Terrusi, A.; Muresan, C.; Battilani, M. The Detection of Canine Parvovirus Type 2c of Asian Origin in Dogs in Romania Evidenced Its Progressive Worldwide Diffusion. *BMC Vet. Res.* **2021**, *17*, 206. [CrossRef]
30. Mon, P.P.; Thurain, K.; Charoenkul, K.; Nasamran, C.; Wynn, M.; Tun, T.N.; Amonsin, A. Emergence of Canine Parvovirus Type 2c (CPV-2c) of Asian Origin in Domestic Dogs in Myanmar. *Comp. Immunol. Microbiol. Infect. Dis.* **2022**, *90–91*, 101901. [CrossRef]
31. Ogbu, K.I.; Mira, F.; Purpari, G.; Nwosuh, C.; Loria, G.R.; Schirò, G.; Chiaramonte, G.; Tion, M.T.; Bella, S.D.; Ventriglia, G.; et al. Nearly Full-length Genome Characterization of Canine Parvovirus Strains Circulating in Nigeria. *Transbound. Emerg. Dis.* **2020**, *67*, 635. [CrossRef] [PubMed]
32. Mira, F.; Schirò, G.; Franzo, G.; Canuti, M.; Purpari, G.; Giudice, E.; Decaro, N.; Vicari, D.; Antoci, F.; Guercio, A. Evaluation of Canine Parvovirus Type 2 (CPV-2) Molecular Epidemiology in Sicily, Southern Italy: A Geographical Island, an Epidemiological Continuum. *Heliyon* **2023**. *submitted*.
33. Katoh, K.; Standley, D.M. MAFFT Multiple Sequence Alignment Software Version 7: Improvements in Performance and Usability. *Mol. Biol. Evol.* **2013**, *30*, 772–780. [CrossRef] [PubMed]
34. Abascal, F.; Zardoya, R.; Telford, M.J. TranslatorX: Multiple Alignment of Nucleotide Sequences Guided by Amino Acid Translations. *Nucleic. Acids Res.* **2010**, *38*, W7–W13. [CrossRef] [PubMed]
35. IQ-TREE: A Fast and Effective Stochastic Algorithm for Estimating Maximum-Likelihood Phylogenies | Molecular Biology and Evolution | Oxford Academic. Available online: https://academic.oup.com/mbe/article/32/1/268/2925592 (accessed on 25 July 2023).
36. RAxML Version 8: A Tool for Phylogenetic Analysis and Post-Analysis of Large Phylogenies | Bioinformatics | Oxford Academic. Available online: https://academic.oup.com/bioinformatics/article/30/9/1312/238053 (accessed on 25 July 2023).
37. Price, M.N.; Dehal, P.S.; Arkin, A.P. FastTree 2—Approximately Maximum-Likelihood Trees for Large Alignments. *PLoS ONE* **2010**, *5*, e9490. [CrossRef]
38. Darriba, D.; Taboada, G.L.; Doallo, R.; Posada, D. jModelTest 2: More Models, New Heuristics and Parallel Computing. *Nat. Methods* **2012**, *9*, 772. [CrossRef]
39. Hill, V.; Baele, G. Bayesian Estimation of Past Population Dynamics in BEAST 1.10 Using the Skygrid Coalescent Model. *Mol. Biol. Evol.* **2019**, *36*, 2620–2628. [CrossRef]
40. Baele, G.; Lemey, P.; Bedford, T.; Rambaut, A.; Suchard, M.A.; Alekseyenko, A.V. Improving the Accuracy of Demographic and Molecular Clock Model Comparison While Accommodating Phylogenetic Uncertainty. *Mol. Biol. Evol.* **2012**, *29*, 2157–2167. [CrossRef]
41. Lemey, P.; Rambaut, A.; Drummond, A.J.; Suchard, M.A. Bayesian Phylogeography Finds Its Roots. *PLoS Comput. Biol.* **2009**, *5*, e1000520. [CrossRef]

42. Rambaut, A.; Drummond, A.J.; Xie, D.; Baele, G.; Suchard, M.A. Posterior Summarization in Bayesian Phylogenetics Using Tracer 1.7. *Syst. Biol.* **2018**, *67*, 901–904. [CrossRef]
43. Bielejec, F.; Baele, G.; Vrancken, B.; Suchard, M.A.; Rambaut, A.; Lemey, P. SpreaD3: Interactive Visualization of Spatiotemporal History and Trait Evolutionary Processes. *Mol. Biol. Evol.* **2016**, *33*, 2167–2169. [CrossRef] [PubMed]
44. Murrell, B.; Wertheim, J.O.; Moola, S.; Weighill, T.; Scheffler, K.; Kosakovsky Pond, S.L. Detecting Individual Sites Subject to Episodic Diversifying Selection. *PLoS Genet.* **2012**, *8*, e1002764. [CrossRef] [PubMed]
45. Pond, S.L.K.; Frost, S.D.W.; Muse, S.V. HyPhy: Hypothesis Testing Using Phylogenies. *Bioinformatics* **2005**, *21*, 676–679. [CrossRef] [PubMed]
46. Pond, S.L.K.; Frost, S.D.W. Not so Different after All: A Comparison of Methods for Detecting Amino Acid Sites under Selection. *Mol. Biol. Evol.* **2005**, *22*, 1208–1222. [CrossRef]
47. Murrell, B.; Moola, S.; Mabona, A.; Weighill, T.; Sheward, D.; Kosakovsky Pond, S.L.; Scheffler, K. FUBAR: A Fast, Unconstrained Bayesian Approximation for Inferring Selection. *Mol. Biol. Evol.* **2013**, *30*, 1196–1205. [CrossRef]
48. Franzo, G.; De Villiers, L.; De Villiers, M.; Ravandi, A.; Gyani, K.; Van Zyl, L.; Coetzee, L.M.; Khaiseb, S.; Molini, U. Molecular Epidemiology of Canine Parvovirus in Namibia: Introduction Pathways and Local Persistence. *Prev. Vet. Med.* **2022**, *209*, 105780. [CrossRef]
49. Lin, Y.-C.; Chiang, S.-Y.; Wu, H.-Y.; Lin, J.-H.; Chiou, M.-T.; Liu, H.-F.; Lin, C.-N. Phylodynamic and Genetic Diversity of Canine Parvovirus Type 2c in Taiwan. *Int. J. Mol. Sci.* **2017**, *18*, 2703. [CrossRef]
50. Nguyen Manh, T.; Piewbang, C.; Rungsipipat, A.; Techangamsuwan, S. Molecular and Phylogenetic Analysis of Vietnamese Canine Parvovirus 2C Originated from Dogs Reveals a New Asia-IV Clade. *Transbound. Emerg. Dis.* **2021**, *68*, 1445–1453. [CrossRef]
51. Wardhani, S.W.; Wongsakul, B.; Kasantikul, T.; Piewbang, C.; Techangamsuwan, S. Molecular and Pathological Investigations of Selected Viral Neuropathogens in Rabies-Negative Brains of Cats and Dogs Revealed Neurotropism of Carnivore Protoparvovirus-1. *Front. Vet. Sci.* **2021**, *8*, 710701. [CrossRef]
52. Temuujin, U.; Tserendorj, A.; Fujiki, J.; Sakoda, Y.; Tseren-Ochir, E.-O.; Okamatsu, M.; Matsuno, K.; Sharav, T.; Horiuchi, M.; Umemura, T.; et al. The First Isolation and Identification of Canine Parvovirus (CPV) Type 2c Variants during 2016–2018 Genetic Surveillance of Dogs in Mongolia. *Infect. Genet. Evol.* **2019**, *73*, 269–275. [CrossRef]
53. Carrino, M.; Tassoni, L.; Campalto, M.; Cavicchio, L.; Mion, M.; Corrò, M.; Natale, A.; Beato, M.S. Molecular Investigation of Recent Canine Parvovirus-2 (CPV-2) in Italy Revealed Distinct Clustering. *Viruses* **2022**, *14*, 917. [CrossRef] [PubMed]
54. Ndiana, L.A.; Lanave, G.; Zarea, A.A.K.; Desario, C.; Odigie, E.A.; Ehab, F.A.; Capozza, P.; Greco, G.; Buonavoglia, C.; Decaro, N. Molecular Characterization of *Carnivore protoparvovirus 1* Circulating in Domestic Carnivores in Egypt. *Front. Vet. Sci.* **2022**, *9*, 932247. [CrossRef] [PubMed]
55. Tegegne, D.; Tsegaye, G.; Faustini, G.; Franzo, G. First Genetic Detection and Characterization of Canine Parvovirus Type 2 (*Carnivore protoparvovirus 1*) in Southwestern Ethiopia. *Vet. Res. Commun.* **2023**, *47*, 975–980. [CrossRef] [PubMed]
56. Nguyen Van, D.; Le, T.D.H.; Maeda, K. Transition of Dominant Canine Parvovirus Genotype from 2b to 2c in Vietnamese Dogs. *Vet. Ital.* **2022**, *58*, 199–206. [CrossRef]
57. Hao, X.; Li, Y.; Xiao, X.; Chen, B.; Zhou, P.; Li, S. The Changes in Canine Parvovirus Variants over the Years. *Int. J. Mol. Sci.* **2022**, *23*, 11540. [CrossRef] [PubMed]
58. Chen, Y.; Wang, J.; Bi, Z.; Tan, Y.; Lv, L.; Zhao, H.; Xia, X.; Zhu, Y.; Wang, Y.; Qian, J. Molecular Epidemiology and Genetic Evolution of Canine Parvovirus in East China, during 2018–2020. *Infect. Genet. Evol.* **2021**, *90*, 104780. [CrossRef]
59. Chen, B.; Zhang, X.; Zhu, J.; Liao, L.; Bao, E. Molecular Epidemiological Survey of Canine Parvovirus Circulating in China from 2014 to 2019. *Pathogens* **2021**, *10*, 588. [CrossRef]
60. Decaro, N.; Campolo, M.; Elia, G.; Buonavoglia, D.; Colaianni, M.L.; Lorusso, A.; Mari, V.; Buonavoglia, C. Infectious Canine Hepatitis: An "Old" Disease Reemerging in Italy. *Res. Vet. Sci.* **2007**, *83*, 269–273. [CrossRef]
61. Martella, V.; Cirone, F.; Elia, G.; Lorusso, E.; Decaro, N.; Campolo, M.; Desario, C.; Lucente, M.S.; Bellacicco, A.L.; Blixenkrone-Møller, M.; et al. Heterogeneity within the Hemagglutinin Genes of Canine Distemper Virus (CDV) Strains Detected in Italy. *Vet. Microbiol.* **2006**, *116*, 301–309. [CrossRef]
62. Alfano, F.; Lanave, G.; Lucibelli, M.G.; Miletti, G.; D'Alessio, N.; Gallo, A.; Auriemma, C.; Amoroso, M.G.; Lucente, M.S.; De Carlo, E.; et al. Canine Distemper Virus in Autochtonous and Imported Dogs, Southern Italy (2014–2021). *Animals* **2022**, *12*, 2852. [CrossRef]
63. Willi, B.; Spiri, A.M.; Meli, M.L.; Grimm, F.; Beatrice, L.; Riond, B.; Bley, T.; Jordi, R.; Dennler, M.; Hofmann-Lehmann, R. Clinical and Molecular Investigation of a Canine Distemper Outbreak and Vector-Borne Infections in a Group of Rescue Dogs Imported from Hungary to Switzerland. *BMC Vet. Res.* **2015**, *11*, 154. [CrossRef]
64. Maya, L.; Calleros, L.; Francia, L.; Hernández, M.; Iraola, G.; Panzera, Y.; Sosa, K.; Pérez, R. Phylodynamics Analysis of Canine Parvovirus in Uruguay: Evidence of Two Successive Invasions by Different Variants. *Arch. Virol.* **2013**, *158*, 1133–1141. [CrossRef] [PubMed]
65. Grecco, S.; Iraola, G.; Decaro, N.; Alfieri, A.; Alfieri, A.; Gallo Calderón, M.; da Silva, A.P.; Name, D.; Aldaz, J.; Calleros, L.; et al. Inter- and Intracontinental Migrations and Local Differentiation Have Shaped the Contemporary Epidemiological Landscape of Canine Parvovirus in South America. *Virus Evol.* **2018**, *4*, vey011. [CrossRef]

66. Tucciarone, C.M.; Franzo, G.; Mazzetto, E.; Legnardi, M.; Caldin, M.; Furlanello, T.; Cecchinato, M.; Drigo, M. Molecular Insight into Italian Canine Parvovirus Heterogeneity and Comparison with the Worldwide Scenario. *Infect. Genet. Evol.* **2018**, *66*, 171–179. [CrossRef] [PubMed]
67. Tang, Y.; Tang, N.; Zhu, J.; Wang, M.; Liu, Y.; Lyu, Y. Molecular Characteristics and Genetic Evolutionary Analyses of Circulating Parvoviruses Derived from Cats in Beijing. *BMC Vet. Res.* **2022**, *18*, 195. [CrossRef] [PubMed]
68. Charoenkul, K.; Tangwangvivat, R.; Janetanakit, T.; Boonyapisitsopa, S.; Bunpapong, N.; Chaiyawong, S.; Amonsin, A. Emergence of Canine Parvovirus Type 2c in Domestic Dogs and Cats from Thailand. *Transbound. Emerg. Dis.* **2019**, *66*, 1518–1528. [CrossRef] [PubMed]
69. Tucciarone, C.M.; Franzo, G.; Legnardi, M.; Lazzaro, E.; Zoia, A.; Petini, M.; Furlanello, T.; Caldin, M.; Cecchinato, M.; Drigo, M. Genetic Insights into Feline Parvovirus: Evaluation of Viral Evolutionary Patterns and Association between Phylogeny and Clinical Variables. *Viruses* **2021**, *13*, 1033. [CrossRef]
70. Allison, A.B.; Harbison, C.E.; Pagan, I.; Stucker, K.M.; Kaelber, J.T.; Brown, J.D.; Ruder, M.G.; Keel, M.K.; Dubovi, E.J.; Holmes, E.C.; et al. Role of Multiple Hosts in the Cross-Species Transmission and Emergence of a Pandemic Parvovirus. *J. Virol.* **2012**, *86*, 865–872. [CrossRef]
71. Boros, Á.; Albert, M.; Urbán, P.; Herczeg, R.; Gáspár, G.; Balázs, B.; Cságola, A.; Pankovics, P.; Gyenesei, A.; Reuter, G. Unusual "Asian-Origin" 2c to 2b Point Mutant Canine Parvovirus (*Parvoviridae*) and Canine Astrovirus (*Astroviridae*) Co-Infection Detected in Vaccinated Dogs with an Outbreak of Severe Haemorrhagic Gastroenteritis with High Mortality Rate in Hungary. *Vet. Res. Commun.* **2022**, *46*, 1355–1361. [CrossRef]
72. Franzo, G.; Tucciarone, C.M.; Casagrande, S.; Caldin, M.; Cortey, M.; Furlanello, T.; Legnardi, M.; Cecchinato, M.; Drigo, M. Canine Parvovirus (CPV) Phylogeny Is Associated with Disease Severity. *Sci. Rep.* **2019**, *9*, 11266. [CrossRef]

viruses

MDPI

Article

A Phylogeographic Analysis of Porcine Parvovirus 1 in Africa

Giovanni Franzo [1,*], Habibata Lamouni Zerbo [2], Bruno Lalidia Ouoba [2], Adama Drabo Dji-Tombo [2], Marietou Guitti Kindo [2], Rasablaga Sawadogo [2], Jelly Chang'a [3], Stella Bitanyi [3], Aloyce Kamigwe [3], Charles Mayenga [3], Modou Moustapha Lo [4], Mbengué Ndiaye [4], Aminata Ba [4], Gaye Laye Diop [4], Iolanda Vieira Anahory [5], Lourenço P. Mapaco [5], Sara J. Achá [5], Valere Kouame Kouakou [6], Emmanuel Couacy-Hymann [6], Stephen G. Gacheru [7], Jacqueline K. Lichoti [7], Justus K. Kasivalu [7], Obadiah N. Njagi [7], Tirumala B. K. Settypalli [8], Giovanni Cattoli [8], Charles E. Lamien [8], Umberto Molini [9,10] and William G. Dundon [8]

1 Department of Animal Medicine, Production and Health, University of Padova, viale dell'Università 16, 35020 Legnaro, Italy
2 Laboratoire National d'Elevage (LNE), Ouagadougou 03 BP 907, Burkina Faso
3 Centre for Infectious Diseases and Biotechnology, Tanzania Veterinary Laboratory Agency, Dar es Salaam P.O. Box 9254, Tanzania
4 Laboratoire National de l'Elevage et de Recherches Vétérinaires, Institut Sénégalais de Recherches Agricoles (ISRA), Dakar BP 3120, Senegal
5 Central Veterinary Laboratory, Agricultural Research Institute of Mozambique, Directorate of Animal Science, Maputo 1922, Mozambique
6 Centre National de Recherche Agronomique (CNRA), Abidjan 1740, Côte d'Ivoire
7 Central Veterinary Laboratory, Directorate of Veterinary Services, Kabete P.O. Box 00100-34188, Kenya
8 Animal Production and Health Laboratory, Animal Production and Health Section, Joint FAO/IAEA Division, Department of Nuclear Sciences and Applications, International Atomic Energy Agency, P.O. Box 100, 1400 Vienna, Austria
9 School of Veterinary Medicine, Faculty of Health Sciences and Veterinary Medicine, University of Namibia, Neudamm Campus, Windhoek Private Bag 13301, Namibia
10 Central Veterinary Laboratory (CVL), 24 Goethe Street, Windhoek Private Bag 18137, Namibia
* Correspondence: giovanni.franzo@unipd.it; Tel.: +39-0498272968

Abstract: Porcine parvovirus 1 (PPV1) is recognized as a major cause of reproductive failure in pigs, leading to several clinical outcomes globally known as SMEDI. Despite being known since the late 1960s its circulation is still of relevance to swine producers. Additionally, the emergence of variants such as the virulent 27a strain, for which lower protection induced by vaccines has been demonstrated, is of increasing concern. Even though constant monitoring of PPV1 using molecular epidemiological approaches is of pivotal importance, viral sequence data are scarce especially in low-income countries. To fill this gap, a collection of 71 partial VP2 sequences originating from eight African countries (Burkina Faso, Côte d'Ivoire, Kenya, Mozambique, Namibia, Nigeria, Senegal, and Tanzania) during the period 2011–2021 were analyzed within the context of global PPV1 variability. The observed pattern largely reflected what has been observed in high-income regions, i.e., 27a-like strains were more frequently detected than less virulent NADL-8-like strains. A phylogeographic analysis supported this observation, highlighting that the African scenario has been largely shaped by multiple PPV1 importation events from other continents, especially Europe and Asia. The existence of such an international movement coupled with the circulation of potential vaccine-escape variants requires the careful evaluation of the control strategies to prevent new strain introduction and persistence.

Keywords: porcine parvovirus 1; Africa; epidemiology; phylogeography; phylogeny; VP2

Citation: Franzo, G.; Zerbo, H.L.; Ouoba, B.L.; Dji-Tombo, A.D.; Kindo, M.G.; Sawadogo, R.; Chang'a, J.; Bitanyi, S.; Kamigwe, A.; Mayenga, C.; et al. A Phylogeographic Analysis of Porcine Parvovirus 1 in Africa. *Viruses* **2023**, *15*, 207. https://doi.org/10.3390/v15010207

Academic Editor: Giorgio Gallinella

Received: 21 November 2022
Revised: 5 January 2023
Accepted: 8 January 2023
Published: 11 January 2023

1. Introduction

Porcine parvovirus 1 (PPV1) is a virus classified in the species *Ungulate protoparvovirus 1* of the genus *Protoparvovirus* in the virus family *Parvoviridae* (https://ictv.global/taxonomy, accessed 10 January 2023). It is a non-enveloped virus with a single-stranded DNA genome of about 5 kb including two main coding regions that encode non-structural (NS1, NS2, and NS3) and structural (VP1, VP2, and VP3) proteins [1,2]. PPV1 has been recognized as the etiological agent of reproductive disorders in swine for a long time, globally known as SMEDI (i.e., stillbirth, mummification, embryonic death, and infertility), causing significant economic losses worldwide [1–3]. Similar to other ssDNA viruses, PPV1 is characterized by a relatively high evolutionary rate, ranging from 10^{-6} to 10^{-4} substitutions·site^{-1}·year^{-1}, depending on the cited study and the genomic region [1,4,5]. This rapid evolution has generated significant genotypic and phenotypic variability over time that has been classified according to different systems proposed by different authors [6–8] (sub-species classification has not yet been well standardized).

Such heterogenicity has been associated with variation in tropism and virulence, whose determinants are most likely confined to the structural proteins. For example, among the VP2 amino acids, three of them, and their relative heterogeneity (i.e., D378G, H383Q, and S436P), have been considered to be responsible for different tissue tropism [9,10]. Similarly, viral variability could negatively impact neutralizing antibodies' pivotal role in host protection. Cross-protection among strains has been assessed in experimental studies, revealing higher protection against homologous compared to heterologous challenge [11]. The lower affinity to neutralizing antibodies has been linked to amino acid substitution in the 3-fold spike region.

Vaccines against PPV1 have been used since the early 80s and have largely been administered in the last 30 years [5]. However, despite broad application, an increase in SMEDI cases has been reported in the last few years in Europe [5]. This increase is often associated with the new variant 27a or 27a-like strains that have become predominant in Europe [5,6]. It has been suggested that the appearance of 27a over the last decades is the result of viral adaptation to vaccine pressure on a viral population circulating in a partially immune population [4,5,8]. Overall, a reduction in viral diversity in favor of viruses more able to deal with vaccine-induced pressure has been postulated. In silico and in vitro analyses, plus the evidence that strains detected in wild boars showed a higher variability compared to their domestic counterparts, seem to confirm such a hypothesis [8].

Although the consequences in terms of clinical protection are far more debated [12], the implications that potential differential cross-protection has on PPV1 epidemiology justifies a constant updating of the molecular epidemiology of the virus. Nevertheless, this information is still limited and biased according to temporal and spatial distribution. Data from Africa are especially scarce even though such knowledge is of particular relevance for several reasons: the impact of the productive losses on society with already limited resources; the growing economic and commercial relationship of many African countries with more developed regions; the characteristics of the African farming system, its heterogeneity and the frequent contact opportunities with wild species, which could enhance the persistence, circulation, and evolution of strains with unusual features, as demonstrated for other swine pathogens [13]. Unfortunately, limited resources and capacity often prevent significant diagnostic and sequencing efforts in many African countries.

The present study aimed to provide, despite these limitations, an as extensive as possible characterization of PPV1 strains in Africa and evaluate the potential introduction sources thereby providing important data for local and regional veterinary authorities involved in porcine disease management.

2. Materials and Methods

2.1. Swine Samples

Archived DNA purified from samples (i.e., spleen, lung, liver, blood, serum) collected from pigs as part of routine diagnostic activities in Burkina Faso (*n* = 52), Ivory Coast (*n* = 54), Kenya (*n* = 9), Mozambique (*n* = 96), Senegal (*n* = 17), and Tanzania (n = 123) between 2011 and 2021 (Table S1) were screened by PCR for the presence of PPV1 as previously described [14]. Positive amplicons of a 739 bp region of the VP2 were purified and sequenced commercially by LGC Genomics (Berlin, Germany)

2.2. Sequence Analysis

PPV1 nucleotide sequences spanning the same VP2 region obtained in the present study and originating from Europe, North and South America, and Asia were downloaded from GenBank (when the sampling country and date were available). In addition, sequences (n = 40) from two African countries Namibia and Nigeria were included [14–16]. All the sequences were merged with the ones generated in the present study and aligned using MAFFT [17] and their quality was evaluated. Partial or poorly aligned sequences, those displaying unknown bases, premature stop codons, or frameshift mutations were excluded from further analysis. Recombination analysis was performed using GARD [18] and RDP4 [19] to identify and remove recombinant strains from the dataset. RDP4 analysis settings were selected based on the dataset features according to the recommendations of the RDP manual. A recombination event was accepted as significant if detected by more than two methods with a significance level of 0.05 after Bonferroni correction. The presence of adequate phylogenetic and temporal signals was tested using the likelihood mapping approach implemented in IQ-Tree [20] and the TempEst [21] programs, respectively. A phylogenetic tree was reconstructed using IQ-Tree selecting the substitution model with the lowest Akaike information criterion (AIC) score calculated using the same software and assessing the robustness of detected clades performing 1000 bootstrap replicates.

2.3. Viral Population Dynamics and Phylogeography

Considering that the sequence selection was biased for collection country and date, more balanced datasets were obtained by randomly subsampling a maximum of three sequences per country-year. To assess the effect of sampling, five random datasets were generated and independently analyzed. PPV1 population parameters, including time to the most recent common ancestor (tMRCA), evolutionary rate, and population size variation over time were estimated using the Bayesian serial coalescent approach implemented in BEAST 1.10.4 [22]. The nucleotide substitution model was selected based on the Bayesian information criterion (BIC) calculated using JModelTest2 [23] while the best-fitting molecular clock model was selected by calculating the Bayesian factor (BF) estimating the marginal likelihood of the evaluated models using the path sampling (PS) and stepping stones (SS) methods [24]. The non-parametric Skygrid [25] model was selected to reconstruct the trend of the relative genetic diversity (i.e., effective population size $\times$ generation time; Ne $\times$ t) over time. Strain migration among countries was estimated using the discrete state phylogeographic approach [26]. The Bayesian stochastic search variable selection (BSSVS) was also implemented to allow for the identification of the most parsimonious description of the phylogeographic diffusion process and to construct a BF test assessing the statistical significance of such links. All parameters were jointly estimated using a 100 million generation Markov chain Monte Carlo (MCMC) chain, sampling the population parameters and trees every 10 thousand generations. Run performances were summarized and evaluated using Tracer 1.7 after removing the first 20% as burn-in. Run results were accepted if the estimated sample size (ESS) was higher than 200 and the mixing and convergence, evaluated by visual inspection of the run's trace, were adequate. A maximum clade credibility tree (MCC) was obtained using the Treeannotator suite of the BEAST package. SPREAD3 [27] was used to identify the statistically supported migration rates between country pairs. The significance level was set to BF > 10 for all considered analyses. Additional summary statistics and graphics were generated using R [28] and specific libraries [29,30].

3. Results

Of the 351 samples screened by PCR in this study, 31 (8.8%) were positive for PPV1 [i.e., Burkina Faso (n = 2; positivity ratio = 3.85%), Ivory Coast (n = 7; positivity ratio = 12.96%), Kenya (n = 1; positivity ratio = 11.11%), Mozambique (n = 17; positivity ratio = 17.71%),

Senegal (n = 2; positivity ratio = 11.76%), Tanzania (n = 2; positivity ratio = 1.63%)]. Additionally, 40 sequences previously obtained from Namibia (positivity ratio = 36.35%) and Nigeria (positivity ratio = 20.6%) were included in the study [14–16].

In total, 71 sequences originating from eight African countries (Burkina Faso, Ivory Coast, Kenya, Mozambique, Namibia, Nigeria, Senegal, Tanzania) in the period 2011–2021 were analyzed in the present study (Table S1). The obtained sequences covered a region from position 3035 to 3608 of the U44978 reference genome. After merging all of the African sequences with the other sequences available in GenBank, 312 sequences from 24 countries sampled between 1963 and 2021 were included in the final dataset (Table S2). Phylogenetic and temporal signals were adequate for further analysis. The average distance among the strains was 1.00% (interval: 0–4.2%) while it ranged between 0 and 3% (average = 0.7%) when considering the African strains only (Table S3). No significant recombination event was detected in the region considered using the selected analysis settings.

Overall, 47 African strains were related to the 27a strain (Cluster PPV1b, according to the Vereecke et al., classification), 21 to the NADL-8 (Cluster PPV1d), and three to the Cluster PPV1a (Figure S1).

The analysis of the five independent datasets provided highly concordant results. The tMRCA was estimated in 1918.08 [95HPD: 1872.06–1952.65] (average of the five datasets) and the evolutionary rate was 1.735×10^{-4} [95HPD: 7.944×10^{-5}–3.12×10^{-4}]. The viral population size demonstrated a constant increase from the tMRCA until approximately 2010 when a progressive decrease was observed (Figure 1).

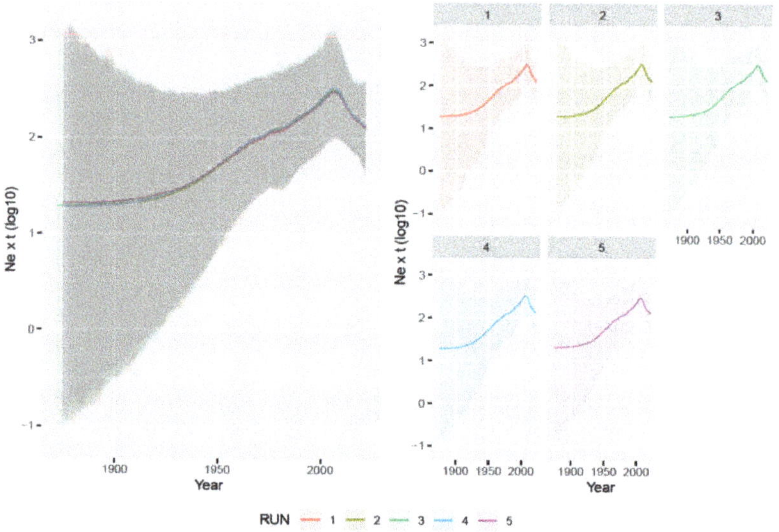

Figure 1. Left figure: mean relative genetic diversity (Ne × t) of the worldwide PPV1 population over time. The results of the five independent runs have been color-coded. Right figure: mean and upper and lower 95HPD values are reported for each run.

The phylogeographic analysis highlighted several well-supported migration rates connecting African countries with others, especially from Asia and Europe (Figure S2). More specifically, although with minor differences among datasets, significant connections linked Denmark with Mozambique, Ivory Coast, and Tanzania. Mozambique had also significant connections with China and other African counties such as Namibia and Tanzania. Finally, a connection between Senegal and South Korea and the USA was detected. Other links involving African counties were also present, although they did not reach the fixed significance level. Phylogenetic tree analysis highlighted a close relationship between Namibian and Mozambican strains and between strains from Nigeria, Ivory Coast, and Mozambique

(Figure S1). More specifically, based on the ML phylogenetic tree, it was possible to identify different clades to which African strains belonged (herein named Clade A-H; see Figure S1). Clade A included two strains from Ivory Coast and one from Tanzania, in addition to European (mostly from Denmark but also Germany, Ireland, and Romania) and Asian (China) strains. Clade B, including one strain from Tanzania, was composed essentially of strains from Asia, i.e., China and South Korea). Clade C comprised strains from Namibia and Mozambique plus three strains from Romania. Clade D included Nigerian strains only, although a certain relationship with European strains was observed. Clade E included strains from Mozambique, Denmark, and the Netherlands. Clade F included Namibian and Denmark strains only. Clade G included European sequences plus one from Burkina Faso. Finally, Clade H, although genetically homogenous, was highly heterogenous in terms of the countries from which the strains were collected, since it included viruses from Ivory Coast, Kenya, Nigeria, and Mozambique, in addition to European (i.e., Denmark, Romania, the Netherlands, France, Belgium, Germany, and Spain) and Asian (i.e., China, India, and South Korea) countries. One strain from Mozambique, Ivory Coast, Kenia, Burkina Faso, and two from Senegal were not part of a well-defined clade, although they were closely related to Asian and European strains.

Therefore, several countries harbored strains belonging to different clades, highly suggestive of multiple introduction events: Burkina Faso (2 clades), Ivory Coast (4 clades), Mozambique (3 clades), Namibia (2 clades), Nigeria (2 clades), and Tanzania (2 clades).

Viral dispersal over time suggested a probable European origin of the virus (Figures 2 and S3), where it persisted until the 1960s and thereafter migrated to Asia and North America in the following twenty years. Since the beginning of the new millennium, Asia and Europe emerged as the main sources of viral dispersal and introduction into African countries. Within Africa spreading was also observed, although with higher uncertainty and variability among datasets.

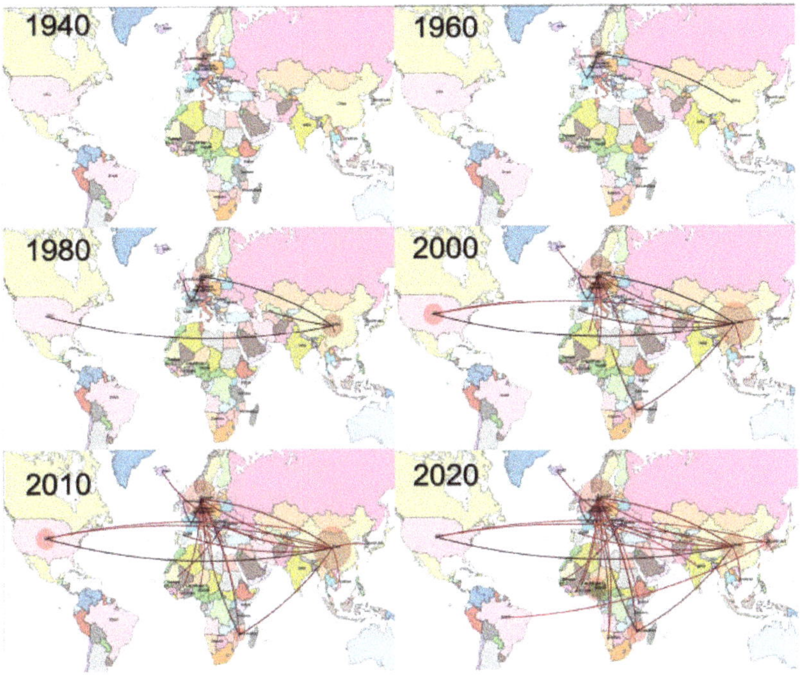

Figure 2. Phylogeographic reconstruction of PPV1 migration among countries over time. Each picture represents a different decade. The edges connecting the countries have been color-coded from black to red based on the estimated age.

4. Discussion

This study represents the first attempt to investigate PPV1 molecular epidemiology in Africa and contextualize it within a worldwide scenario. The obtained results describing the evolutionary dynamics of PPV1 are in complete agreement with those of previous studies. Similarly, the high repeatability of output data using the independently generated datasets testifies that sampling bias does not significantly affect the present inferences, supporting the reliability of our results. The estimated substitution rate was approximately 10^{-5} substitutions·site^{-1}·year^{-1}, which reflects other authors' work [4,5] and highlights the high evolutionary potential of PPV1, as observed for several other ssDNA viruses. As reported by Vereecke et al., using VP2 sequences, PPV1(tMRCA) was predicted at the beginning of the previous century and, similarly to what transpired for other pig pathogens, a constant increase in the population size occurred [5]. This highlights a prolonged, undetected viral circulation in the European swine population which initially likely caused limited damage. The progressive intensification of farming systems sustained the increase in viral circulation and prevalence and thereafter its global spread [31,32]. Modern farming conditions likely contributed, together with the emergence of other co-infections and predisposing factors, to the emergence of PPV1 as an economically relevant, clinically overt disease. A successive decrease in the viral population size was predicted from the mid-2010s, in agreement with Vereecke et al. [5]. Such evidence is of particular interest since the first vaccines were introduced in the early 1980s, although adequate vaccination coverage was reached only years later and with high variability among countries. The long latent period between vaccine introduction and its effect on viral circulation, although also most probably confounded by the parallel increase in swine populations that sustained an increase in the viral population, testify to the need for extensive immunization campaigns and high population coverage to achieve successful results. Additional improvements in biosecurity measures and the better control of other co-infections (e.g., PCV-2, PRRSV) that occurred in those years probably also had a direct impact on PPV1 dynamics.

Viral circulation in a partially immune environment has also been proposed to be involved in the evolution of PPV1 and the emergence of vaccine escape variants [5]. Particular attention has been paid to the 27a strain that has become predominant in Europe and for which lower protection from infection with currently available vaccines has been demonstrated [1]. Most of the African strains were closely related to this variant and, to a lesser extent, to NADL-8. The phylogeographic analysis confirms these findings since several links were estimated between African countries and Europe or Asia. Therefore, the evolution of the epidemiological scenario in these regions directly affected the African one. Overall, several clades that included strains collected in Africa were identified. Some of these clades consisted of strains identified in Asian and European countries, strengthening the evidence for intense worldwide circulation of PPV1 and the role of these regions in strain importation in Africa. Of note, strains collected in the African countries were often part of different, poorly related clades, which is highly suggestive of multiple introduction events. Denmark, and to a lesser extent China, emerged as the most common origins of viral dispersal. However, the limitations in data availability and the close genetic relationship among strains circulating in Europe and Asia make it difficult to identify specific links and to establish specific sources of virus since other countries seemed to be involved both directly or as part of more extensive, undetected, transmission chains. Therefore, it is often challenging to understand if the clustering of African strains with specific countries is due to real epidemiological links or sequence paucity. Caution should therefore be exercised when interpreting connections between countries in this context. Nevertheless, the overall pattern can be assumed with a certain degree of confidence, being also supported by epidemiological evidence. Live swine or semen importation in Africa, although not common, occurred (https://www.fao.org/faostat/) especially in periods when internal sources such as South Africa were excluded from trade due to African Swine Fever (2005 and 2016) and Foot and Mouth disease outbreaks (2019 and 2022). Moreover, significant numbers of pork products were also imported by South Africa which, in turn, was the main source of exportation to other African countries [33]. Unfortunately, the lack of data from this region prevents definitive conclusions and so, more intensive sampling and sequencing are recommended. Interestingly, several introduction events were predicted in the early 2000s, which is compatible with the above-mentioned hypothesis. Similarly, Asia and China in particular, have played an increasing role in African countries' economies [34], including the agricultural sector, thus increasing the risk of direct or indirect contact between animals and their by-products. Similar connections have been reported for several infections affecting both companion animals and livestock [35,36]. The high environmental resistance of PPV1 could also point to more obscure, indirect, and long-distance transmission pathways. Moreover, pig by-products are still commonly used for animal nutrition in several African farms and could thus represent an important source of virus importation from foreign countries. Once introduced, some African strains were detected more than once, testifying to the establishment of successful and persistent infections. Although some links between African countries were also present, they were rare and involved mostly neighboring countries, which suggests that PPV1 epidemiology in Africa is mainly shaped by strain introduction (even through multiple events) from non-African countries followed by local evolution, rather than intra-continental spread. However, the low number of African countries for which sequences were available for this study could conceal a more complex scenario.

The present study has several limitations. The first is ascribable to the overall scarcity and biased nature of global PPV1 molecular epidemiology data. The good concordance among the randomly generated datasets and with other studies allows for confidence in the obtained results, at least when interpreted in terms of overall trends and patterns. On the other hand, we discourage any overstatement of fine-level interaction and connection between country pairs since other links could be concealed by undersampling.

The other main limitation is that only partial VP2 sequences were obtained from a limited number of African countries, which prevented an in-depth investigation of phenotypic features and association with viral clinical/biological features. While we recognize that complete VP2 sequences from a higher number of regions would have been preferable to allow a better characterization of African PPV1 molecular epidemiology and evaluate the potential determinants of virulence, tropism, and cross-protection [9], we also need to stress the challenges of undertaking a standardized research project involving several countries with different priorities and limited resources. Therefore, this study was mainly based on the samples collected during non-specific animal disease diagnostic activities. We hope that these results, although preliminary and improvable, will prompt new efforts to refine such investigations.

Despite these shortcomings, it was possible to imply the circulation of several PPV1 strains characterized by significant genetic variability, largely originating from multiple introductions from Europe and Asia. Most of the strains were closely related to virulent strains, including the 27a, for which a sub-optimal cross-protection conferred by the currently available vaccine has been proven. Currently, PPV1 vaccination is extremely rare in Africa, even in intensive farms due to economical constraints. Although current vaccines still appear to be beneficial in the control of clinical disease, their introduction should be carefully considered in light of their limitations and the peculiarities of the African scenario. Therefore, significant efforts should be made to decrease the risk of the introduction of new strains, evaluate the efficacy of vaccination, assess the economic impact of PPV1 in the African context, and estimate the cost–benefits of different control strategies to allow a proper prioritization of limited resources.

Supplementary Materials: The following supporting information can be downloaded at: https://www.mdpi.com/article/10.3390/v15010207/s1, Figure S1: Maximum likelihood phylogenetic tree based on the partial VP2 gene. The collection continents have been color-coded. Figure S2: Well-supported viral migration rates among countries estimated using different runs. The Bayesian Factor (BF) featuring each connection has been color-coded. Figure S3: Time-scaled maximum clade credibility trees obtained based on different datasets. The tree branches have been color-coded according to the most likely estimated country while the country posterior probability is displayed as a circle whose size is proportional to the probability value. Table S1: Dataset reporting the African strains used in the present study and the relative metadata. The Accession numbers of the strains obtained in the present study are also reported. Table S2: Dataset reporting the sequences used in the present study and the relative metadata. Table S3. Pairwise genetic distance calculated for both worldwide and African strains.

Author Contributions: Conceptualization, W.G.D., G.F. and U.M.; methodology, T.B.K.S.; software, G.F.; formal analysis, G.F. and W.G.D.; investigation, H.L.Z., J.C., S.B., C.M., M.M.L., S.J.A., E.C.-H. and J.K.L.; resources, B.L.O., A.D.D.-T., M.G.K., R.S., A.K., M.N., A.B., G.L.D., I.V.A., L.P.M., V.K.K., S.G.G., O.N.N. and J.K.K.; data curation, W.G.D. and G.F.; writing—original draft preparation, G.F., W.G.D. and U.M.; supervision, C.E.L. and G.C. funding acquisition, C.E.L. and G.C. All authors have read and agreed to the published version of the manuscript.

Funding: This study was supported by funds from the IAEA Peaceful Uses Initiative (PUI) VETLAB Network (US and Japan).

Institutional Review Board Statement: Ethical review and approval were waived for this study since all samples were obtained during the routine veterinary activity. No additional experimental procedures were performed.

Informed Consent Statement: Not applicable.

Data Availability Statement: Sequence accession numbers and datasets are reported in Supplementary material.

Acknowledgments: The sequences were generated through the Sequencing Services of the Animal Production and Health sub-programme of the Joint Food and Agricultural Organization of the United Nations/International Atomic Energy Agency (IAEA) Division.

Conflicts of Interest: The authors declare no conflict of interest.

References

1. Streck, A.F.; Truyen, U. Porcine Parvovirus. *Curr. Issues Mol. Biol.* **2020**, *37*, 33–45. [CrossRef] [PubMed]
2. Mészáros, I.; Olasz, F.; Cságola, A.; Tijssen, P.; Zádori, Z. Biology of Porcine Parvovirus (Ungulate Parvovirus 1). *Viruses* **2017**, *9*, 393. [CrossRef] [PubMed]
3. Parke, C.R.; Burgess, G.W. An Economic Assessment of Porcine Parvovirus Vaccination. *Aust. Vet. J.* **1993**, *70*, 177–180. [CrossRef] [PubMed]
4. Oh, W.T.; Kim, R.Y.; Nguyen, V.G.; Chung, H.C.; Park, B.K. Perspectives on the Evolution of Porcine Parvovirus. *Viruses* **2017**, *9*, 196. [CrossRef]
5. Vereecke, N.; Kvisgaard, L.K.; Baele, G.; Boone, C.; Kunze, M.; Larsen, L.E.; Theuns, S.; Nauwynck, H. Molecular Epidemiology of Porcine Parvovirus Type 1 (PPV1) and the Reactivity of Vaccine-Induced Antisera against Historical and Current PPV1 Strains. *Virus Evol.* **2022**, *8*, veac053. [CrossRef]
6. Zimmermann, P.; Ritzmann, M.; Selbitz, H.J.; Heinritzi, K.; Truyen, U. VP1 Sequences of German Porcine Parvovirus Isolates Define Two Genetic Lineages. *J. Gen. Virol.* **2006**, *87*, 295–301. [CrossRef] [PubMed]
7. Cadar, D.; Dán, Á.; Tombácz, K.; Lorincz, M.; Kiss, T.; Becskei, Z.; Spînu, M.; Tuboly, T.; Cságola, A. Phylogeny and Evolutionary Genetics of Porcine Parvovirus in Wild Boars. *Infect. Genet. Evol.* **2012**, *12*, 1163–1171. [CrossRef]
8. Streck, A.F.; Canal, C.W.; Truyen, U. Molecular Epidemiology Evolution of Porcine Parvoviruses. *Infect. Genet. Evol.* **2015**, *36*, 300–306. [CrossRef]
9. Streck, A.; Bonatto, S.L.; Homeier, T.; Souza, C.K.; Gonçalves, K.R.; Gava, D.; Canal, C.W.; Truyen, U. High Rate of Viral Evolution in the Capsid Protein of Porcine Parvovirus. *J. Gen. Virol.* **2011**, *92*, 2628–2636. [CrossRef]
10. Bergeron, J.; Hébert, B.; Tijssen, P. Genome Organization of the Kresse Strain of Porcine Parvovirus: Identification of the Allotropic Determinant and Comparison with Those of NADL-2 and Field Isolates. *J. Virol.* **1996**, *70*, 2508–2515. [CrossRef]
11. Zeeuw, E.J.L.; Leinecker, N.; Herwig, V.; Selbitz, H.J.; Truyen, U. Study of the Virulence and Cross-Neutralization Capability of Recent Porcine Parvovirus Field Isolates and Vaccine Viruses in Experimentally Infected Pregnant Gilts. *J. Gen. Virol.* **2007**, *88*, 420–427. [CrossRef] [PubMed]
12. Jóźwik, A.; Manteutel, J.; Selbitz, H.J.; Truyen, U. Vaccination against Porcine Parvovirus Protects against Disease, but Does Not Prevent Infection and Virus Shedding after Challenge Infection with a Heterologous Virus Strain. *J. Gen. Virol.* **2009**, *90*, 2437–2441. [CrossRef] [PubMed]
13. Molini, U.; Franzo, G.; Gous, L.; Moller, S.; Hemberger, Y.M.; Chiwome, B.; Marruchella, G.; Khaiseb, S.; Cattoli, G.; Dundon, W.G. Three Different Genotypes of Porcine Circovirus 2 (PCV-2) Identified in Pigs and Warthogs in Namibia. *Arch. Virol.* **2021**, *166*, 1723–1728. [CrossRef] [PubMed]

14. Luka, P.D.; Adedeji, A.J.; Jambol, A.R.; Ifende, I.V.; Luka, H.G.; Choji, N.D.; Weka, R.; Settypalli, T.B.K.; Achenbach, J.E.; Cattoli, G.; et al. Coinfections of African Swine Fever Virus, Porcine Circovirus 2 and 3, and Porcine Parvovirus 1 in Swine in Nigeria. *Arch. Virol.* **2022**, *167*, 2715–2722. [CrossRef]
15. Molini, U.; Franzo, G.; Settypalli, T.B.K.; Hemberger, M.Y.; Khaiseb, S.; Cattoli, G.; Dundon, W.G.; Lamien, C.E. Viral Co-Infections of Warthogs in Namibia with African Swine Fever Virus and Porcine Parvovirus 1. *Animals* **2022**, *12*, 1697. [CrossRef]
16. Molini, U.; Coetzee, L.M.; Hemberger, M.Y.; Khaiseb, S.; Cattoli, G.; Dundon, W.G. Evidence Indicating Transmission of Porcine Parvovirus 1 between Warthogs and Domestic Pigs in Namibia. *Vet. Res. Commun.* **2022**. [CrossRef]
17. Standley, K. MAFFT Multiple Sequence Alignment Software Version 7: Improvements in Performance and Usability. (Outlines Version 7). *Mol. Biol. Evol.* **2013**, *30*, 772–780. [CrossRef]
18. Kosakovsky Pond, S.L.; Posada, D.; Gravenor, M.B.; Woelk, C.H.; Frost, S.D.W. GARD: A Genetic Algorithm for Recombination Detection. *Bioinformatics* **2006**, *22*, 3096–3098. [CrossRef]
19. Martin, D.P.; Murrell, B.; Golden, M.; Khoosal, A.; Muhire, B. RDP4: Detection and Analysis of Recombination Patterns in Virus Genomes. *Virus Evol.* **2015**, *1*, vev003. [CrossRef]
20. Nguyen, L.T.; Schmidt, H.A.; von Haeseler, A.; Minh, B.Q. IQ-TREE: A Fast and Effective Stochastic Algorithm for Estimating Maximum-Likelihood Phylogenies. *Mol. Biol. Evol.* **2015**, *32*, 268–274. [CrossRef]
21. Rambaut, A.; Lam, T.T.; Max Carvalho, L.; Pybus, O.G. Exploring the Temporal Structure of Heterochronous Sequences Using TempEst (Formerly Path-O-Gen). *Virus Evol.* **2016**, *2*, vew007. [CrossRef] [PubMed]
22. Suchard, M.A.; Lemey, P.; Baele, G.; Ayres, D.L.; Drummond, A.J.; Rambaut, A. Bayesian Phylogenetic and Phylodynamic Data Integration Using BEAST 1.10. *Virus Evol.* **2018**, *4*, vey016. [CrossRef] [PubMed]
23. Darriba, D.; Taboada, G.L.; Doallo, R.; Posada, D. JModelTest 2: More Models, New Heuristics and Parallel Computing. *Nat. Methods* **2012**, *9*, 772. [CrossRef]
24. Baele, G.; Lemey, P.; Bedford, T.; Rambaut, A.; Suchard, M.A.; Alekseyenko, A.V. Improving the Accuracy of Demographic and Molecular Clock Model Comparison While Accommodating Phylogenetic Uncertainty. *Mol. Biol. Evol.* **2012**, *29*, 2157–2167. [CrossRef] [PubMed]
25. Hill, V.; Baele, G. Bayesian Estimation of Past Population Dynamics in BEAST 1.10 Using the Skygrid Coalescent Model. *Mol. Biol. Evol.* **2019**, *36*, 2620–2628. [CrossRef] [PubMed]
26. Lemey, P.; Rambaut, A.; Drummond, A.J.; Suchard, M.A. Bayesian Phylogeography Finds Its Roots. *PLoS Comput. Biol.* **2009**, *5*, e1000520. [CrossRef] [PubMed]
27. Bielejec, F.; Baele, G.; Vrancken, B.; Suchard, M.A.; Rambaut, A.; Lemey, P. SpreaD3: Interactive Visualization of Spatiotemporal History and Trait Evolutionary Processes. *Mol. Biol. Evol.* **2016**, *33*, 2167–2169. [CrossRef]
28. Team, R.C. *R: A Language and Environment for Statistical Computing*; R Foundation for Statistical Computing: Vienna, Austria, 2013.
29. Ginestet, C. Ggplot2: Elegant Graphics for Data Analysis. *J. R. Stat. Soc. Ser. A Stat. Soc.* **2011**, *174*, 245–246. [CrossRef]
30. Yu, G.; Smith, D.K.; Zhu, H.; Guan, Y.; Lam, T.T.Y. Ggtree: An R Package for Visualization and Annotation of Phylogenetic Trees With Their Covariates and Other Associated Data. *Methods Ecol. Evol.* **2017**, *8*, 28–36. [CrossRef]
31. Segalés, J.; Kekarainen, T.; Cortey, M. The Natural History of Porcine Circovirus Type 2: From an Inoffensive Virus to a Devastating Swine Disease? *Vet. Microbiol.* **2013**, *165*, 13–20. [CrossRef]
32. Franzo, G.; Faustini, G.; Legnardi, M.; Cecchinato, M.; Drigo, M.; Tucciarone, C.M. Phylodynamic and Phylogeographic Reconstruction of Porcine Reproductive and Respiratory Syndrome Virus (PRRSV) in Europe: Patterns and Determinants. *Transbound. Emerg. Dis.* **2022**, *69*, e2175–e2184. [CrossRef]
33. A Profile of the South African Pork Market Value Chain 2020. Available online: https://dalrrd.gov.za (accessed on 10 January 2023).
34. Stein, P.; Uddhammar, E. China in Africa: The Role of Trade, Investments, and Loans Amidst Shifting Geopolitical Ambitions. *ORF Occasional Paper* **2021**. Available online: https://policycommons.net/artifacts/1808834/china-in-africa/2543755/ (accessed on 10 January 2023).
35. Franzo, G.; Settypalli, T.B.K.; Agusi, E.R.; Meseko, C.; Minoungou, G.; Ouoba, B.L.; Habibata, Z.L.; Wade, A.; de Barros, J.L.; Tshilenge, C.G.; et al. Porcine Circovirus-2 in Africa: Identification of Continent-Specific Clusters and Evidence of Independent Viral Introductions from Europe, North America and Asia. *Transbound. Emerg. Dis.* **2021**, *69*, e1142–e1152. [CrossRef] [PubMed]
36. Tegegne, D.; Tsegaye, G.; Aman, S.; Faustini, G.; Franzo, G. Molecular Epidemiology and Genetic Characterization of PCV2 Circulating in Wild Boars in Southwestern Ethiopia. *J. Trop. Med.* **2022**, *2022*, 5185247. [CrossRef] [PubMed]

viruses MDPI

Article

Next Generation Sequencing for the Analysis of Parvovirus B19 Genomic Diversity

Federica Bichicchi [1], Niccolò Guglietta [1], Arthur Daniel Rocha Alves [2], Erika Fasano [1], Elisabetta Manaresi [1], Gloria Bua [1,*] and Giorgio Gallinella [1,3]

1 Department of Pharmacy and Biotechnology, University of Bologna, 40138 Bologna, Italy
2 Laboratory of Technological Development in Virology, Oswaldo Cruz Foundation/FIOCRUZ, Brasil Avenue 4365, Manguinhos, Rio de Janeiro 21040-900, Brazil
3 Microbiology Section, IRCCS Sant'Orsola Hospital, 40138 Bologna, Italy
* Correspondence: gloria.bua2@unibo.it

Abstract: Parvovirus B19 (B19V) is a ssDNA human virus, responsible for an ample range of clinical manifestations. Sequencing of B19V DNA from clinical samples is frequently reported in the literature to assign genotype (genotypes 1–3) and for finer molecular epidemiological tracing. The increasing availability of Next Generation Sequencing (NGS) with its depth of coverage potentially yields information on intrinsic sequence heterogeneity; however, integration of this information in analysis of sequence variation is not routinely obtained. The present work investigated genomic sequence heterogeneity within and between B19V isolates by application of NGS techniques, and by the development of a novel dedicated bioinformatic tool and analysis pipeline, yielding information on two newly defined parameters. The first, α-diversity, is a measure of the amount and distribution of position-specific, normalised Shannon Entropy, as a measure of intra-sample sequence heterogeneity. The second, σ-diversity, is a measure of the amount of inter-sample sequence heterogeneity, also incorporating information on α-diversity. Based on these indexes, further cluster analysis can be performed. A set of 24 high-titre viraemic samples was investigated. Of these, 23 samples were genotype 1 and one sample was genotype 2. Genotype 1 isolates showed low α-diversity values, with only a few samples showing distinct position-specific polymorphisms; a few genetically related clusters emerged when analysing inter-sample distances, correlated to the year of isolation; the single genotype 2 isolate showed the highest α-diversity, even if not presenting polymorphisms, and was an evident outlier when analysing inter-sample distance. In conclusion, NGS analysis and the bioinformatic tool and pipeline developed and used in the present work can be considered effective tools for investigating sequence diversity, an observable parameter that can be incorporated into the quasispecies theory framework to yield a better insight into viral evolution dynamics.

Keywords: Parvovirus B19; genetic diversity; viral quasispecies; Next Generation Sequencing; Shannon Entropy; cluster analysis

Citation: Bichicchi, F.; Guglietta, N.; Rocha Alves, A.D.; Fasano, E.; Manaresi, E.; Bua, G.; Gallinella, G. Next Generation Sequencing for the Analysis of Parvovirus B19 Genomic Diversity. *Viruses* **2023**, *15*, 217. https://doi.org/10.3390/v15010217

Academic Editor: Jianming Qiu

Received: 21 December 2022
Revised: 2 January 2023
Accepted: 7 January 2023
Published: 12 January 2023

1. Introduction

Within the family *Parvoviridae*, Parvovirus B19 (B19V) is a widespread human virus, responsible for an ample range of clinical manifestations [1]. B19V is mostly transmitted through the respiratory route, while the major tropism is towards erythroid progenitor cells in bone marrow (EPCs) that are susceptible and permissive to viral replication, dependent on their differentiation state and replicative rate [2]. Infected cells allow a sustained viral replication that leads to the release of virus into the bloodstream that can be in excess of 10^{12} genome copies/mL, and undergo apoptosis, with the consequence of a temporary block in erythropoiesis that can be clinically relevant [3,4]. The viraemic phase is followed by systemic distribution of the virus to other non-erythroid cell types, including endothelial, stromal, or synovial cells, that are also susceptible but mainly non-permissive [5]. In these cells, infection can trigger inflammatory responses and consequent tissue damage, leading for example to the common clinical presentations of erythema infectiosum and arthritis/arthralgia, and generally resulting in long-term persistence of viral DNA within tissues [6]. The development of a neutralising immune response is functional to the clearance of the virus from the blood and termination of infection, but may also contribute to pathogenesis in peripheral tissues [7].

The genome of B19V is a ssDNA molecule, of either polarity, 5596 nt long, composed of two terminal regions, 383 nt, that provide the origins of replication, flanking a unique internal region, 4830 nt, containing all open reading frames. Three genotypes (1–3) have been recognised for B19V [8,9]. Genotype 1 is prevalent worldwide [10], apparently having replaced, in the last fifty years, genotype 2 [11], which is now found sporadically [12], while genotype 3 can be found at lower frequency in restricted geographic areas [10]. Genetic distance between the three different genotypes is in the order of 10%, while intragenotype distance values are different—higher for genotypes 2 and 3 (3–8%), lower for genotype 1 (1–3%)—possibly reflecting a shorter evolutionary history for the latter [9,13]. As of present, research did not reveal differences in the biological [14], immunological or pathogenetic characteristics among the different genotypes [15], except for the closer association of genotype 2 with tissue persistence in elder people [11,16]. Experimentally, sequence determination of B19V DNA from clinical samples is frequently reported in literature to assign genotype and for finer molecular epidemiological tracing. Quite predictably, isolate clusters can be distinguished mainly based on sample population composition, but due to limited investigation, a comprehensive picture of genetic diversity within B19V is still lacking. Based on the available data, a relatively high mutation/substitution rate has been predicted for B19V, in the order of 10^{-4} and similar to other ssDNA viruses, implying high intrinsic genetic diversity and evolutionary potential [17,18]. However, such prediction is in some contrast to experimental data showing a more conserved evolutionary pathway over longer time periods [19,20]. Moreover, high rates would also predict a high heterogeneity and dynamicity of viral populations as a result of the replicative process, therefore implying a quasispecies structure [21], a hypothesis that can be tested.

Technically, until now, genome sequencing has been mainly carried out by a standard Sanger sequencing technique, though the increasing availability and use of Next Generation Sequencing (NGS) with its depth of coverage incorporates additional relevant information on intrinsic sequence heterogeneity [22,23]. However, integration of this information in analysis of sequence variation is not routinely obtained. The present work has been carried out as a first exploratory study to investigate genomic sequence heterogeneity within and between B19V isolates, by application of NGS techniques, and by the development of a novel dedicated bioinformatic tool and analysis pipeline. As a result, experimental output yielded the following: (i) for each isolate, representation of NGS sequence data via a position-specific probability matrix, and an assessment of genomic heterogeneity using Shannon entropy as an index of intra-sample diversity; (ii) for the set of isolates, evaluation of diversity among the position-specific probability matrices, and an assessment of genetic distances by indexes combining both intra- and inter-sample diversity. This information can yield a finer insight into the genetics of B19V, and in perspective can be incorporated into a theoretical approach conforming to quasispecies theory.

2. Materials and Methods

Samples. Reference samples, deriving from the consensus B19V EC genotype 1 sequence (GenBank KY940273.1) and the related synthetic genetic system previously developed [24], included: (i) cloned DNA, excised from plasmid CJ0, as an in-process control; ii) a B19V laboratory strain stock sample, EC1622, propagated in vitro in differentiated erythroid progenitor cells as described. A panel of high-titre B19V viraemic serum samples (>10^6 genome copies/mL) was collected in the course of institutional diagnostic service at the Microbiology Unit, S. Orsola Hospital, Bologna, in the period 2012–2020. Samples were available for virologic investigation according to institutional guidelines and compliance with Italian Privacy law, for the sole purpose of viral DNA sequencing, waiving patient informed consent.

Sample processing. For each sample, a 100 μL volume was processed by Maxwell Viral Total Nucleic Acid Kit (Promega) on a Maxwell MDX platform, to obtain a purified total nucleic acid fraction. For sequencing, a target genomic region spanning positions 2210–3342 was selected, corresponding to the region between A1.2 splice acceptor and pAp2 cleavage-polyadenylation signals. Target DNA was amplified by high-fidelity PCR, using primers R2210 (forward) and R3342 (reverse) [25,26]. Amplification was carried out by using the High Fidelity PCR System (Roche), according to manufacturer's instructions, with a thermal profile consisting of initial denaturation 94 °C, 2′; 10 cycles of denaturation 94 °C, 15″, annealing 50 °C, 30″, extension 72 °C, 2′30″; 20 cycles of denaturation 94 °C, 15″, annealing 50 °C, 30″, extension 72 °C, 2′30″ incremented by 5″/cycle; final extension 72 °C, 7′. Following agarose gel electrophoresis analysis, the amplification product was purified from the reaction volume by using a Wizard® SV Gel and PCR Clean-Up System kit (Promega), and finally quantified by the Qubit 2.0 Fluorometer (Promega). For each sample, a minimal amount of 0.2 μg DNA was processed for sequencing.

Next Generation Sequencing. Library preparations and NGS were carried out by an external service (IGA Technology, Udine, Italy). Following DNA fragmentation, library preparation was made with Celero DNA-Seq kit (Tecan). Both input and final libraries were quantified by Qubit 2.0 Fluorometer, and quality tested by the Agilent 2100 Bioanalyzer Sensitivity DNA assay. Libraries were then sequenced on Illumina NovaSeq 6000 in paired-end mode, with reads of 120 bps. The preliminary analyses performed were base calling and demultiplexing, by the Bcl2Fasq 2.20 version of the Illumina pipeline, followed by adapters masking using Cutadapt v1.11 from raw fastq data. As an output, IGA returned fastq reads files for further data processing conducted in our laboratory.

Sequence Data Processing. Received fastq reads files were examined for Quality control by FastQC; then, high-quality reads were processed by trimming (Trim Galore!), whereas duplicate removal (Prinseq v0.20.4) was not necessary. Alignment of high-quality reads and genome indexing was performed using BowTie2 v2.5.0. The reference sequence used for these operations is the consensus B19V EC, genotype 1, previously developed by the research group (GenBank KY940273.1). After alignment, the SAM files generated by BowTie2 were converted into BAM files via SAMTools, to allow visualisation of the alignment on Integrative Genomics Viewer (IGV) [27]. For a preliminary analysis on genome variability, individual consensus sequences were obtained starting from the multiple alignment files by a dedicated pipeline, using different functions from SAMtools v1.16.1, BCFtools v1.15, and setqk v1.2-r94. The resulting fasta files with individual consensus sequences could be imported into MEGA11 software [28] for alignment and further analysis.

Sequence Data Analysis. NGS data were analysed by an in-house developed tool, QSA (Quasi-Species Analyser). QSA, still in its beta version (https://github.com/ovaltriangle/qsa, accessed on 2 January 2023), was specifically developed within this project to carry out analyses on sequence variability data embedded in BAM files. QSA is a unique tool, whose functions allow: (i) processing of aligned reads from BAM files to create a position frequency and a position probability matrix; (ii) calculation of position-specific normalised Shannon entropy values (called α-diversity) and obtainment of a graphical display; (iii) calculation of aggregate, inter-sample entropy values (called 'δ-diversity); (iv) calculation of inter-sample genetic distance based on inter-sample entropy values (called 'σ-diversity'). Further analysis and graphical elaboration were carried out using Python on IDLE Spyder (packages numpy, pandas, matplotlib for boxplot analysis) [29] and R Studio (packages stringr, pvclust for hierarchical clustering, cluster for K-means analysis) (https://posit.co/, accessed on 2 January 2023).

Data availability. NGS raw fastq reads have been submitted to the European Nucleotide Archive, Study ID PRJEB58863 (ERP143941).

3. Results

3.1. Samples and NGS Output

A total of 26 samples were included in the study (Table 1). Reference samples, deriving from the consensus B19V EC genotype 1 sequence and the related synthetic genetic system previously developed, included: (i) cloned DNA, excised from plasmid CJ0, as an in-process control; (ii) a B19V laboratory strain stock sample, EC1622, propagated in vitro in differentiated erythroid progenitor cells as described. Tested clinical samples consisted of a panel of 24 high-titre B19V viraemic serum samples (>10^6 genome copies/mL), collected in the course of an institutional diagnostic service at the Microbiology Unit, S.Orsola Hospital, Bologna, in the period 2012–2020. For investigation, a target genomic region spanning positions 2210–3342 was selected, corresponding to the region between A1.2 splice acceptor and pAp2 cleavage-polyadenylation signals, encompassing the VP1 N-terminal unique region (Figure 1). Target was amplified by high-fidelity PCR, the resulting amplification products were purified and then processed for NGS, first by DNA fragmentation and library preparation, then by sequencing on Illumina NovaSeq 6000 in paired-end mode, with reads of 120 bps length. As output for each sample, reads received were in the range 0.82–6.0 × 10^6, yielding a depth of coverage in the range 0.87–6.3 × 10^5 counts per position. Quality control on reads reported a high overall score, excluding systematic sequencing errors, so all of the obtained reads were used for further analysis.

Table 1. Sample set in the study and derived distance and diversity values.

Sample [1]	Date	Viral Load	Variations [2]	Distance to CJ0 [3]	Mean Distance [3,5]	α-Diversity [4]	δ-Diversity [4,5]
CJ0	—	1.00 × 10^6	0	0.0000	0.0067	0.0403	0.9376
EC1622	—	1.00 × 10^6	0	0.0000	0.0067	0.0595	1.0601
S08	04/09/2019	8.26 × 10^6	14	0.0127	0.0105	0.0735	0.4695
S26	21/03/2012	1.00 × 10^{10}	8	0.0072	0.0063	0.0663	0.4555
S27	14/04/2012	1.20 × 10^8	6	0.0054	0.0047	0.0699	0.3891
S29	11/06/2012	5.40 × 10^6	6	0.0053	0.0099	0.0635	0.6682
S30	14/06/2012	5.00 × 10^9	6	0.0053	0.0099	0.0674	0.4018
S31	15/06/2012	6.00 × 10^9	5	0.0045	0.0052	0.0737	0.4735
S32	27/06/2012	2.00 × 10^6	2	0.0018	0.0084	0.0744	0.5090
S33	06/11/2012	2.00 × 10^{10}	10	0.0063	0.0050	0.0647	0.5663
S35	06/06/2013	1.00 × 10^{10}	7	0.0081	0.0070	0.0759	0.6108
S36	25/06/2013	1.00 × 10^{10}	11	0.0090	0.0079	0.0654	0.5164
S37	12/09/2013	1.00 × 10^9	6	0.0053	0.0099	0.0677	0.3932
S38	26/09/2013	1.00 × 10^7	4	0.0036	0.0056	0.0742	0.5011
S42	07/05/2015	3.00 × 10^6	11	0.0099	0.0098	0.0681	0.3863
S43	27/06/2015	1.00 × 10^6	7	0.0062	0.0050	0.0787	0.8703
S48	27/01/2016	1.50 × 10^7	8	0.0072	0.0074	0.0670	0.4206
S49	03/03/2016	2.00 × 10^6	7	0.0062	0.0046	0.0716	0.4116
S50	23/08/2016	3.00 × 10^6	7	0.0072	0.0054	0.0680	0.3872
S51	23/03/2017	1.00 × 10^{10}	7	0.0062	0.0046	0.0669	0.4247
S52	01/06/2017	2.00 × 10^8	7	0.0062	0.0046	0.0717	0.4125
S53	29/07/2017	5.00 × 10^7	8	0.0081	0.0081	0.0620	0.8029
S54	28/11/2018	1.86 × 10^6	6	0.0054	0.0042	0.0687	0.3837
S56	26/06/2019	2.69 × 10^6	6	0.0054	0.0042	0.0763	0.6484
S57	23/07/2019	2.96 × 10^6	13	0.0117	0.0100	0.0754	0.5745
Mean for Genotype 1			7	0.0067	0.0069	0.0700	0.5077
S20	02/05/2020	7.65 × 10^6	53	0.0509	0.0547	0.0828	3.0858

[1] CJ0 is the reference plasmid DNA, EC1622 is a reference virus stock. All samples (S08–S57) are genotype 1 with the exception of sample S20, which is genotype 2. [2] For all samples, variations are nucleotide differences with respect to the reference sequence (KY940273.1). [3] Distance to CJ0 and mean distance calculated under MCL substitution model by using MEGA 11 software. [4] α-diversity and δ-diversity values calculated as described in the text. [5] Mean distance and δ-diversity values for CJ0, EC1622 and S20 are calculated with respect to genotype 1 samples; genotype 1 sample values are calculated excluding CJ0, EC1622. and S20.

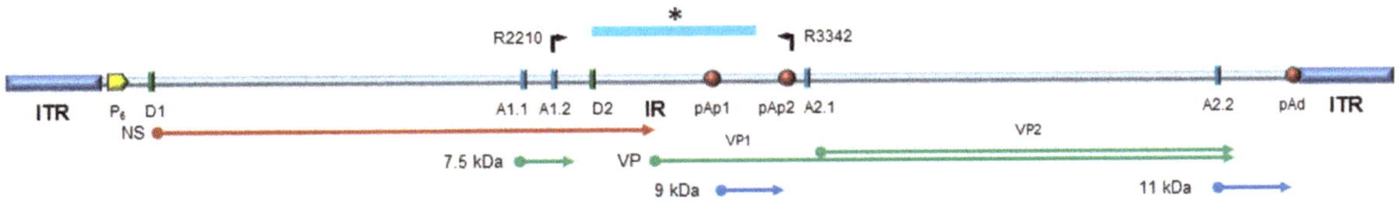

Figure 1. Schematic diagram of B19V genome. ITR, inverted terminal regions; IR, internal region; cis-acting functional sites: P6, promoter; pAp1, pAp2, proximal cleavage-polyadenylation sites; pAd, distal cleavage-polyadenylation site; D1, D2, splice donor sites; A1.1, A1.2, A2.1, A2.2, splice acceptor sites. Top: primer location and genome segment included in NGS analysis (*). Bottom: open reading frames and coding sequences for the viral proteins. NS, non-structural protein NS1; VP, structural proteins, colinear VP1 and VP2, assembled in a T1 icosahedral capsid; 7.5 kDa, 9.0 kDa, 11 kDa: minor non-structural proteins. Modified from [30].

3.2. Sequence Alignment

Reads obtained from each individual sample were aligned to the B19V EC genotype 1 reference sequence. B19V EC is a genotype 1 consensus, obtained from alignment of a set of 50 genomic-length sequences, of representative isolates collected in different areas ante year 2010, and coincident with a possible ancestral state as determined from an ML phylogenetic tree [24]. Alignment generated individual consensus sequences that were imported into MEGA11 software for visualisation, further alignment, and investigation of the presence of sequence variants with respect to the reference sequence, calculation of pairwise genetic distances and graphical representation of distances. For the purpose of our work, results provided a comparison term to further analysis aimed at incorporating depth of sequencing as obtained from NGS.

At first, analysis of NGS-derived consensus sequences confirmed the perfect identity of the reference CJ0 and EC1622 samples to the B19V EC genotype 1 reference sequence from which they were derived. Then, all of the clinical samples, except sample S20, could be aligned to this same genotype 1 reference sequence. For each genotype 1 sample, a range of 2–14 individual base differences were found, dispersed over 47 base positions, 6 of which were common to more than 12 samples. Sample S20 was a notable exception, showing 53 base differences to consensus, with only 9 being in common with other samples, and unexpectedly turning out to align with a genotype 2 consensus sequence (Table 1) (Supplemental Table S1).

3.3. Sequence Variability Analysis

In the analysis of the individual consensus sequences only, all information on sequence diversity embedded in reads obtained from NGS techniques is lost. IGV allows for visual inspection of diversity at individual positions for each obtained read, but cannot allow for further aggregate analysis. For the purpose of incorporating NGS information in the analysis of intra-sample sequence variability, a novel algorithm was carried out by using a specific, in-house developed bioinformatic tool, QSA, and a related analysis pipeline.

For the scope of this work, to ensure homogenous coverage and avoid background noise linked to reads misalignment, an effect observed at the extremes of the sequenced products, all samples were analysed to a restricted sequence—spanning position 2390 to 3242, for a total of 852 base positions. For each single sample, aligned reads in BAM files were processed by QSA to create first a position frequency matrix (PFM), and then a position probability matrix (PPM). PPM gives information on the normalised probability of occupation at each position by each one of the bases. On the PPM matrix, for each position i, and j $\in \{T, C, G, A\}$, $[j] = 4$, a normalised Shannon entropy was calculated as:

$$\eta(\mathrm{i}) = \frac{-\sum_j p_{ij}\log_2 p_{ij}}{\log_2[j]}$$

The quantity η_i, termed as efficiency, is a normalisation of Shannon's entropy to assess position-specific variability in a set of aligned sequences, in this case obtained from the totality of NGS reads. First, Shannon's entropy values are calculated at each position in the sequence. Afterwards, values are divided by the maximum value of Shannon's entropy (in binary notation, 2 bits) to find the efficiency at each position. Efficiency values at each position can be represented as a line graph over the sequence length (Figure 2), while values distribution can be calculated and represented in a box-plot graph (Figure 3).

The overall sum of the entropy values at each position in the sequence (total efficiency), normalised by the sequence's length, yields an averaged quantity that can be named an 'α-diversity' index (Table 1). Considering the reference samples, CJ0 is a plasmid-derived insert, while EC1622 is representative of an actual replicating viral population, where some variation is expected to occur. Thus, α-diversity of CJ0 was at the lowest, while the higher value in EC1622 likely reflects this fact. Only for the genotype 1 samples, the mean α-diversity was 0.070 (range 0.062–0.079); the genotype 2 sample showed indeed the highest value of 0.083 (Table 1). The α-diversity index is a unique value related to overall genomic variability, while the distribution of efficiency values yields indication on sequence homogeneity. Low or high outlier values indicate more conserved or variable positions on the sequence that can be identified on the line graph representation. It should be remarked how these quantities only refer to position specific variability as detectable from the totality of aligned NGS reads, not taking into consideration any possible linkage into whole-length genomic sequences as a means of reconstruction of individual sequences' identity and abundance.

3.4. Sequence Distances Analysis

For the purpose of inter-sample diversity analysis, NGS-derived consensus sequences were first analysed by using the functions available in MEGA11 software. A pairwise distance plot was constructed under an MCL (Maximum Composite Likelihood, gamma-distributed) substitution model. The mean normalised distance of genotype 1 samples to CJ0/EC1622 reference sequences was 0.007 (range 0.005–0.012), similar to the mean of normalised distances within samples that was 0.007 (range 0.004–0.011). The genotype 2 sample was an evident outlier with a distance to reference sequence of 0.051, and a mean distance to genotype 1 samples of 0.055 (range 0.052–0.058) (Table 1) (Figure 4) (Supplemental Table S2).

For the same purpose of inter-sample diversity analysis, to exploit the information embedded in reads obtained from NGS techniques, a measure analogous to a genetic distance was calculated on the basis of the position probability matrices previously obtained, thus incorporating both intra- and inter-sequence variability. Comparison between any two samples was carried out by calculating the Manhattan Distance, that is, the difference matrix between each of the samples' PPMs, as a measure of sequence diversity over each single position. Then, for each difference matrix, a total normalised efficiency value was obtained as a measure of pairwise genetic distance, a quantity that could be termed 'δ-diversity'. Repeating the procedure for all pairs, a cumulative distance matrix was obtained, analogous to a standard genetic distance matrix, but critically incorporating all position-specific information as derived from the NGS output. Such a distance matrix, implying both intra- and inter-sample diversity, yields information on what can be named 'σ-diversity' in a set of sequences. The σ-diversity in a set of sequences can be calculated as the normalised amount of δ-diversity, or diversity between α-diversity values.

The mean δ-diversity values, normalised to 100 nt positions, of genotype 1 samples to CJ0/EC1622 reference sequences were 0.94–1.06, higher than the mean of normalised distances within samples that was 0.51 (range 0.38–0.87). The genotype 2 sample had a mean diversity to reference sequences of 4.08, and a mean diversity to genotype 1 samples of 3.09 (range 2.22–3.89) (Table 1) (Figure 4) (Supplemental Table S2).

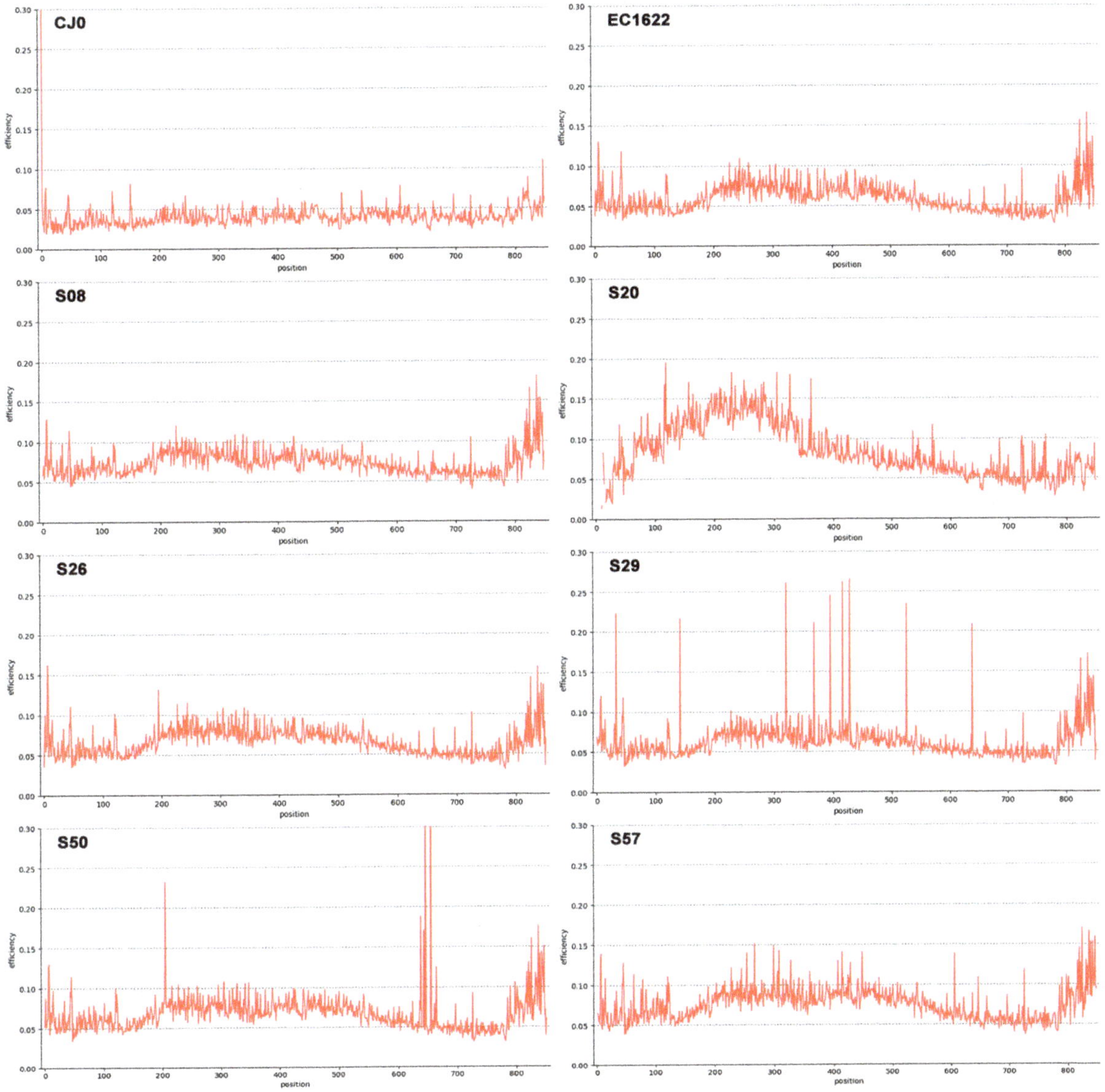

Figure 2. Line graph representation of Shannon Entropy Efficiency values in the genome segment from nt. 2390 to nt. 3242. A selection of representative samples is shown (see also Figure 3 for the complete set). CJ0 is the reference, control plasmid DNA. EC1622 is a reference B19V laboratory strain stock sample. S08, S20, S26, S29, S50 and S57 are clinical isolates. Low efficiency values and low dispersion are typical for control CJ0, virus stock EC1622 and also evident in samples S08 and S26. Higher efficiency and dispersed values can be observed for samples S20, S29, S50 and S57. In particular, sample S20 is a genotype 2 isolate showing higher variability in the first 400 nts; samples S29 and S50 show relatively low efficiency values, but distinct position-specific peaks that can be interpreted as polymorphisms; sample S57 shows a relatively higher efficiency value along with higher, more distributed dispersion.

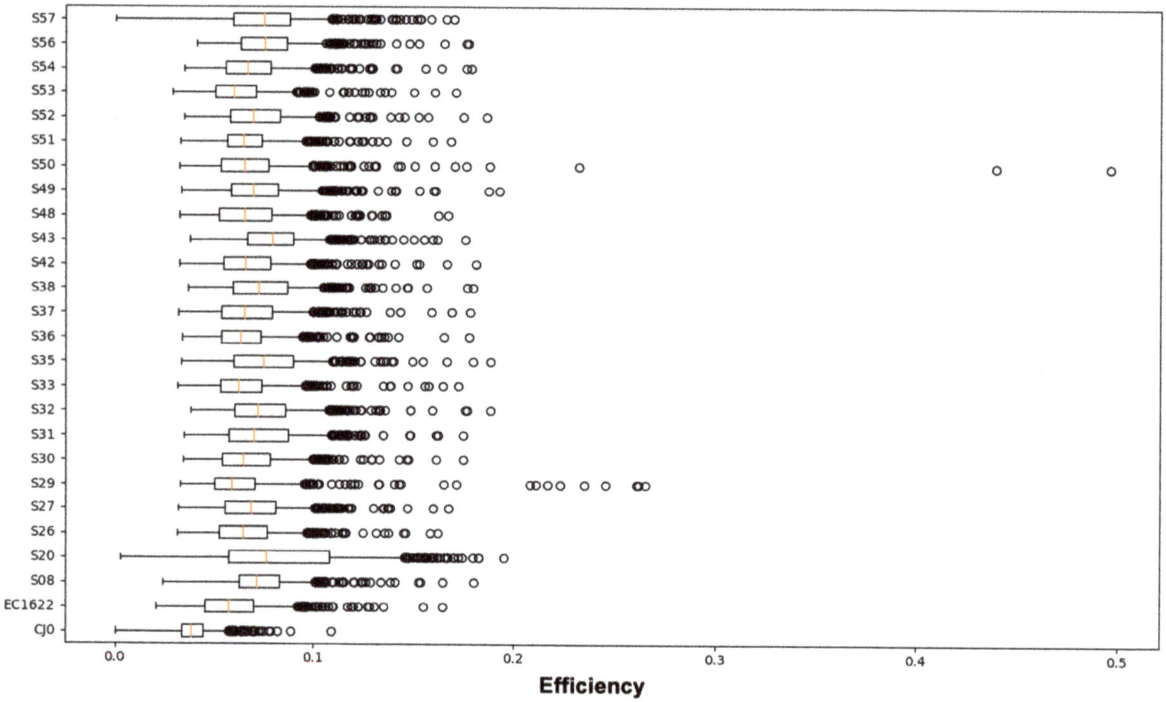

Figure 3. Boxplot representation of the distribution of Shannon Entropy Efficiency values in the genome segment from nt. 2390 to nt. 3242, each position individually contributing. For each sample, the average, 25–75% interquartile range, SD interval and single high-range outlier values are shown. Average value is termed as 'α-diversity' index. For interpretation of data, see also Figure 2.

A dendrogram representation of distances was built based on both the consensus distance and δ-diversity matrices of values, by Hierarchical Clustering (Figure 5A,B). Since the source matrices are different, the resulting tree topology is not equivalent. However, in the case of the distance based dendrogram (5A), the resulting topology is not supported by bootstrap analysis, while the δ-diversity based dendrogram (5B) has supporting unbiased bootstrap p values for nodes > 0.96.

To further investigate any possible correlation within the sample set, K-means analysis was carried out on both datasets. While average distance and δ-diversity did not yield separate clusters, discrete clustering was obtained when considering the year of isolation and either average distance or δ-diversity. When analysing genotype 1 samples only, the best separation was achieved by partitioning the sample set in seven subsets (Figure 6A,B). Given the lack of direct correlation between the two variables, the distribution of subgroups was not identical for the two datasets, but in both cases, analysis suggests the occurrence of a series of epidemiologically related isolate clusters in a distinct temporal replacement pattern (Figure 6C,D).

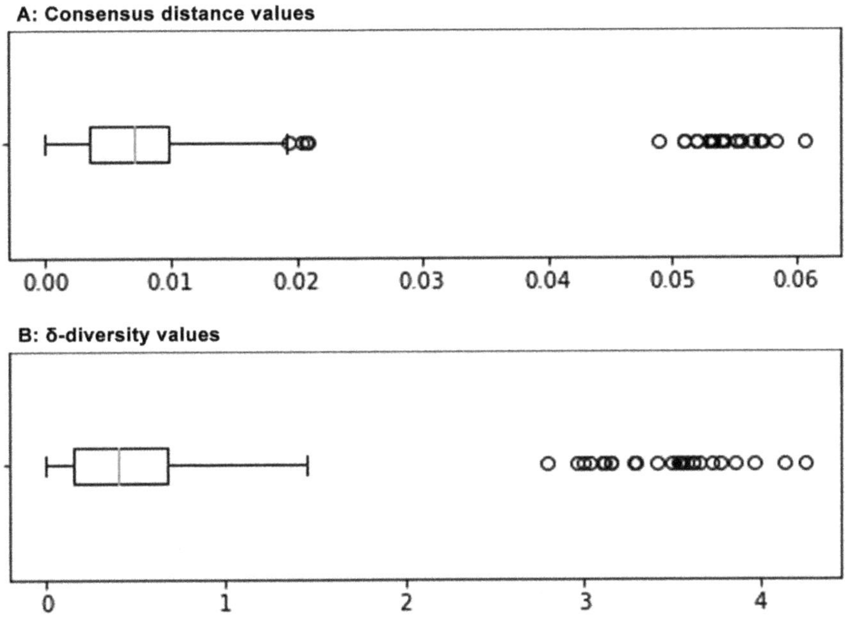

Figure 4. Boxplot graph of the distribution of consensus distance values (**A**) and of δ-diversity values (**B**) in the sample set. For both, average, 25–75% interquartile range, SD interval and single high-range outlier values are shown. Average δ-diversity value is termed as 'σ-diversity' index.

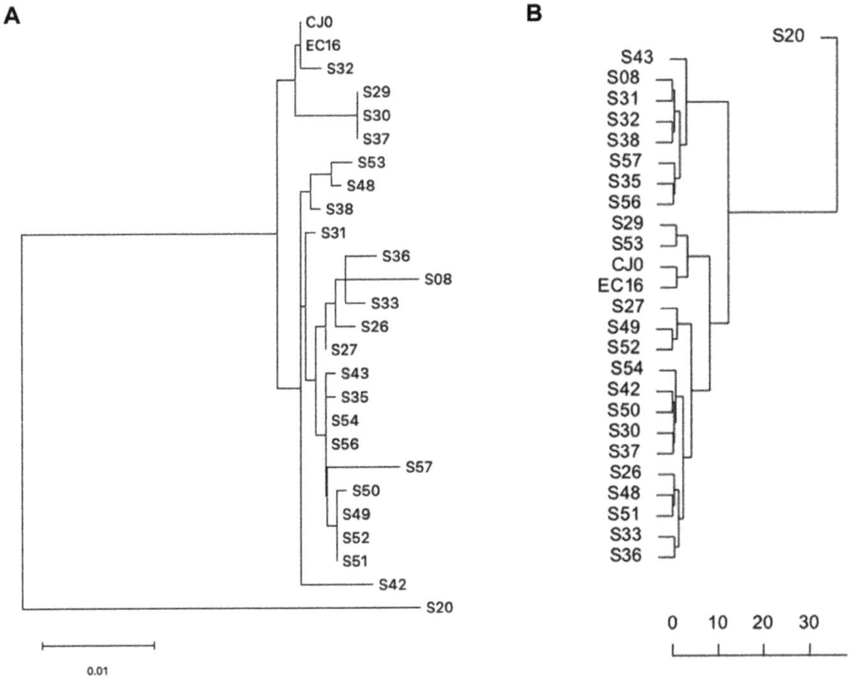

Figure 5. Dendrogram representation of consensus distances and δ-diversity values, hierarchical clustering. (**A**) Distance based dendrogram (MEGA 11); (**B**) δ-diversity based dendrogram (PVClust).

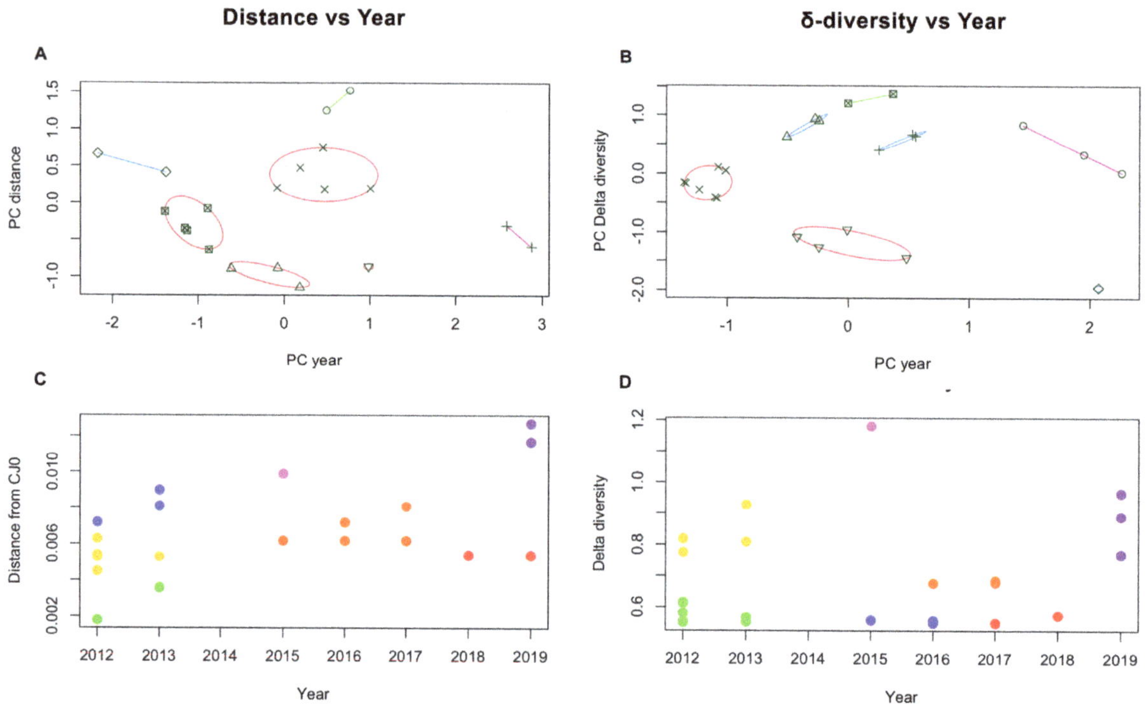

Figure 6. K-means analysis of sample clustering, based on either consensus distances (**A**,**C**) or δ-diversity values (**B**,**D**). Principal Component (PC) analysis indicates clustering according to year of isolation, and best separation was achieved when K = 7 for both datasets. Groups are separated on the PC graphs (**A**,**B**), and identified by colour code in the year vs. distance graphs (**C**,**D**). While the distribution of each isolate among groups is not equivalent for the two datasets, a similar dependence on year of isolation suggests a temporal replacement pattern of different isolate groups.

4. Discussion

NGS techniques are increasingly replacing Sanger sequencing techniques in virologic applications: from sequencing of individual isolates to detection of variants of interest; from diagnostics in clinical settings to virus discovery and comprehensive virome analysis; and last but not least, for wide epidemiological surveillance and preparedness for novel pandemic threats [31]. The enormously increased amount of information obtained from NGS, compared to Sanger sequencing, provides an opportunity for expanded knowledge and insights into system biology and reconstruction of virus evolution.

In addition to the opportunity of whole genome sequencing and identification, high-coverage NGS can provide information on the amount of sequence heterogeneity that can be found within a viral population, one of the key parameters directing viral adaption and evolution, including evolving relationships with hosts [32]. Although NGS can be carried out directly on clinical samples in a 'metagenomic' approach, this may not be suitable to detect sequence heterogeneity within a viral population representing a low-fraction of the accessible targets. For this purpose, a higher depth of coverage is needed; thus an amplification step of the target of interest is required, with the necessary assumption that the original sequence diversity is represented in the amplification product [31].

Although the high output content is a key asset of NGS techniques, information on sequence heterogeneity is not easily incorporated into downstream analysis. In most cases, NGS reads are aligned against a reference sequence and a novel consensus is obtained, which can highlight majority variants with respect to the reference. However, the presence and distribution of minority variants, whose information is embedded into NGS output, is not easily extrapolated and available as information for deeper analysis [33]. Further, several bioinformatic tools are available that can attempt at reconstructing viral genomes by progressive assembly of reads; in this case, the output is a predicted partition of the total set of different viral sequences into subsets of more homogenous sequences [34]. However, short reads, as obtained from Illumina sequencing, cannot be definitely assigned to the same template on the basis of variation patterns; on the other hand, longer reads, as can be obtained for example by Nanopore techniques, often have a higher error rate, being thus unsuitable for the analysis of minority variants. Given these limits, a compromise in the informative potential of NGS must be sought [35].

In the frame of the quasispecies theory, a viral population needs to be considered as a set of variant sequences [21]. The complexity of a viral population is determined by the number and relative abundance of the different subsets of variant sequences, as well by the degree of sequence diversity among variants [36]. In a quantitative approach, complexity indexes usually refer to quasispecies composition, given the number and relative frequency of variant sequences. This approach requires a reliable reconstruction of variant genomes, which by themselves are not experimentally determined data. On the other hand, converting an alignment of reads into a position-specific frequency matrix, an index of sequence complexity can also be obtained by evaluating the degree of heterogeneity at single positions within the viral population; such analysis would bring the advantage of being accurately descriptive and not relying on inferential algorithms, usually with a low predictive value when compared. A generally accepted index such as Shannon entropy can be successfully adapted and exploited for this purpose.

Given such considerations, and in the pursuit of a more informative approach exploiting NGS data, we developed a novel bioinformatic tool, named QSA. It is unique in its functions, and has established a dedicated analysis pipeline for investigation of viral sequence heterogeneity. The challenge was in the exploration of sequence diversity embedded within NGS reads, as compared to information obtained from standard, consensus-based analysis. Starting from aligned NGS reads, via the construction of position-specific probability matrixes, the experimental pipeline yielded information on two inherent basic parameters. The first, which we defined as α-diversity, is a measure of intra-sample sequence heterogeneity, derived from the amount and distribution of position-specific, normalised Shannon Entropy. The second, which we defined as σ-diversity, is a combined measure of intra- and inter-sample sequence heterogeneity, derived from the amount of inter-sample sequence heterogeneity, defined as δ-diversity, also incorporating the amount and distribution of samples' α-diversity. While α-diversity is a parameter that characterises each viral population and can be considered in addition to the definition of a unique, individual consensus sequence, the δ-diversity and σ-diversity parameters incorporate both intra- and inter-sample diversity, and can be considered in comparison to other measures of genetic distances, normally derived from unique consensus sequences. In this way, information from NGS data becomes incorporated into genomic information.

Concerning the specific aim of investigating sequence heterogeneity within B19V, by using this conceptual approach and bioinformatic tools, results yielded the following information: (i) the reference strain stock yielded the expected consensus sequence, without any mutation; its α-diversity was in the lowest range of observed experimental values, 0.060, thus confirming stability of the genome in the experimental system; (ii) clinical isolates, genotype 1, also showed low α-diversity values, in the range 0.062–0.079, while a few samples showed distinct position-specific polymorphisms; polymorphisms at specific positions are suggestive of the emergence of minority variants, although the presence of a coinfecting cell population cannot be formally excluded by NGS analysis; (iii) distance values of genotype 1 samples within the sample set and with respect to reference samples are comparable, thus confirming the characteristics of the consensus-derived reference strain; however, diversity values are lower within the sample set than to reference samples, thus suggesting different evolutionary dynamics; (iv) a few genetically related clusters emerged when analysing inter-sample distances, correlated to the year of isolation; (v) the single genotype 2 isolate showed the highest efficiency value, 0.083, even if not presenting polymorphisms, and was an evident outlier when analysing inter-sample distance and diversity.

Implications of the results are that the accumulation of diversity in B19V occurs at a low pace. Intra-sample diversity is low; the data can be anticipated because of the dependence of the virus on cellular DNA polymerase for its replication. Inter-sample diversity is also low considering the distance between the reference samples, which are based on a consensus, possibly 'ancestral' sequence, and the clinical isolates collected in the past ten years over a defined geographical setting. Higher substitution rates, as reported in the literature, are probably an overestimate, possibly due to a confounding effect of temporal and spatial heterogeneity in sampling [37]. However, statistical analysis suggests that more closely related isolate clusters can circulate in defined temporal patterns, an observation favoured by the close geographical area of sample isolation. Interestingly, the genotype 2 isolate has a higher intrinsic heterogeneity, a phenomenon possibly linked to an association in the host, in a long-term persistent/latent state, followed by reactivation and high-titre viraemia as detected in the collected sample (since a de novo, exogenous infection can be deemed most unlikely in our case, although not formally excluded). Extension of the investigation to the whole genome, rather than to a limited genome segment, and inclusion of more numerous and diverse samples is required in future research to validate the model, extend validity of α- and σ-diversity parameters and derive a clearer picture of B19V sequence diversity and evolution.

In conclusion, NGS analysis is an effective tool for investigating sequence diversity, itself an observable that can be incorporated into the quasispecies theory framework to yield a better insight into viral evolution dynamics. The bioinformatic tool and pipeline that we developed and used in the present work can be considered functional to this aim.

Supplementary Materials: The following supporting information can be downloaded at: https://www.mdpi.com/article/10.3390/v15010217/s1, Table S1: consensus sequence nt and aa variations; Table S2: MEGA11 genetic distance and NGS δ-diversity values matrices.

Author Contributions: Conceptualisation, G.G.; data curation, F.B., A.D.R.A., E.F. and G.G.; funding acquisition, G.G.; investigation, F.B., A.D.R.A., E.F., E.M. and G.B.; methodology, F.B., N.G., A.D.R.A., E.F. and E.M.; software, F.B. and N.G.; validation, N.G.; writing—original draft, E.M., G.B. and G.G.; writing—review and editing, G.B. and G.G. All authors have read and agreed to the published version of the manuscript.

Funding: This research was funded by the Italian Ministry of University and Research, grant PRIN 2017 9JHAMZ_007 to G.G. ADRA was supported by the Coordenação de Aperfeiçoamento de Pessoal de Nível Superior-Brasil (CAPES)-Finance Code 001.

Institutional Review Board Statement: Samples were available for virologic investigation according to institutional guidelines and in compliance with Italian Privacy law, for the sole purpose of viral DNA sequencing.

Informed Consent Statement: Patient consent was waived according to institutional guidelines and in compliance with Italian Privacy law.

Data Availability Statement: NGS raw fastq reads have been submitted to the European Nucleotide Archive, Study ID PRJEB58863 (ERP143941).

Conflicts of Interest: The authors declare no conflict of interest. The funders had no role in the design of the study; in the collection, analyses, or interpretation of data; in the writing of the manuscript; or in the decision to publish the results.

References

1. Gallinella, G. Parvoviridae. In *Encyclopedia of Infection and Immunity*; Rezaei, N., Ed.; Elsevier: Oxford, UK, 2022; pp. 259–277. [CrossRef]
2. Bua, G.; Manaresi, E.; Bonvicini, F.; Gallinella, G. Parvovirus B19 Replication and Expression in Differentiating Erythroid Progenitor Cells. *PLoS ONE* **2016**, *11*, e0148547. [CrossRef] [PubMed]

3. Brown, K.E. Haematological consequences of parvovirus B19 infection. *Baillieres Clin. Haematol.* **2000**, *13*, 245–259. [CrossRef] [PubMed]
4. Kerr, J.R. A review of blood diseases and cytopenias associated with human parvovirus B19 infection. *Rev. Med. Virol.* **2015**, *25*, 224–240. [CrossRef] [PubMed]
5. Bua, G.; Gallinella, G. How does parvovirus B19 DNA achieve lifelong persistence in human cells? *Futur. Virol.* **2017**, *12*, 549–553. [CrossRef]
6. Adamson-Small, L.A.; Ignatovich, I.V.; Laemmerhirt, M.G.; Hobbs, J.A. Persistent parvovirus B19 infection in non-erythroid tissues: Possible role in the inflammatory and disease process. *Virus Res.* **2014**, *190*, 8–16. [CrossRef]
7. Young, N.S.; Brown, K.E. Parvovirus B19. *N. Engl. J. Med.* **2004**, *350*, 586–597. [CrossRef]
8. Servant, A.; Laperche, S.; Lallemand, F.; Marinho, V.; De Saint Maur, G.; Meritet, J.F.; Garbarg-Chenon, A. Genetic diversity within human erythroviruses: Identification of three genotypes. *J. Virol.* **2002**, *76*, 9124–9134. [CrossRef]
9. Gallinella, G.; Venturoli, S.; Manaresi, E.; Musiani, M.; Zerbini, M. B19 virus genome diversity: Epidemiological and clinical correlations. *J. Clin. Virol.* **2003**, *28*, 1–13. [CrossRef]
10. Hübschen, J.M.; Mihneva, Z.; Mentis, A.F.; Schneider, F.; Aboudy, Y.; Grossman, Z.; Rudich, H.; Kasymbekova, K.; Sarv, I.; Nedeljkovic, J.; et al. Phylogenetic analysis of human parvovirus B19 sequences from eleven different countries confirms the predominance of genotype 1 and suggests the spread of genotype 3b. *J. Clin. Microbiol.* **2009**, *47*, 3735–3738. [CrossRef]
11. Norja, P.; Hokynar, K.; Aaltonen, L.-M.; Chen, R.; Ranki, A.; Partio, E.K.; Kiviluoto, O.; Davidkin, I.; Leivo, T.; Eis-Hübinger, A.M.; et al. Bioportfolio: Lifelong persistence of variant and prototypic erythrovirus DNA genomes in human tissue. *Proc. Natl. Acad. Sci. USA* **2006**, *103*, 7450–7453. [CrossRef]
12. Eis-Hübinger, A.M.; Reber, U.; Edelmann, A.; Kalus, U.; Hofmann, J. Parvovirus B19 genotype 2 in blood donations. *Transfusion* **2014**, *54*, 1682–1684. [CrossRef]
13. Bonvicini, F.; Manaresi, E.; Bua, G.; Venturoli, S.; Gallinella, G. Keeping pace with parvovirus B19 genetic variability: A multiplex genotype-specific quantitative PCR assay. *J. Clin. Microbiol.* **2013**, *51*, 3753–3759. [CrossRef] [PubMed]
14. Chen, Z.; Guan, W.; Cheng, F.; Chen, A.Y.; Qiu, J. Molecular characterization of human parvovirus B19 genotypes 2 and 3. *Virology* **2009**, *394*, 276–285. [CrossRef] [PubMed]
15. Ekman, A.; Hokynar, K.; Kakkola, L.; Kantola, K.; Hedman, L.; Bondén, H.; Gessner, M.; Aberham, C.; Norja, P.; Miettinen, S.; et al. Biological and immunological relations among human parvovirus B19 genotypes 1 to 3. *J. Virol.* **2007**, *81*, 6927–6935. [CrossRef] [PubMed]
16. Pyöriä, L.; Toppinen, M.; Mäntylä, E.; Hedman, L.; Aaltonen, L.M.; Vihinen-Ranta, M.; Ilmarinen, T.; Söderlund-Venermo, M.; Hedman, K.; Perdomo, M.F. Extinct type of human parvovirus B19 persists in tonsillar B cells. *Nat. Commun.* **2017**, *8*, 14930. [CrossRef]
17. Norja, P.; Eis-Hübinger, A.M.; Söderlund-Venermo, M.; Hedman, K.; Simmonds, P. Rapid sequence change and geographical spread of human parvovirus B19: Comparison of B19 virus evolution in acute and persistent infections. *J. Virol.* **2008**, *82*, 6427–6433. [CrossRef]
18. Stamenković, G.G.; Cirkovic, V.; Siljic, M.; Blagojevic, J.; Knezevic, A.; Joksić, I.D.; Stanojević, M.P. Substitution rate and natural selection in parvovirus B19. *Sci. Rep.* **2016**, *6*, 35759. [CrossRef]
19. Mühlemann, B.; Margaryan, A.; Damgaard, P.D.B.; Allentoft, M.E.; Vinner, L.; Hansen, A.J.; Weber, A.; Bazaliiskii, V.I.; Molak, M.; Arneborg, J.; et al. Ancient human parvovirus B19 in Eurasia reveals its long-term association with humans. *Proc. Natl. Acad. Sci. USA* **2018**, *115*, 7557–7562. [CrossRef]
20. Guzmán-Solís, A.A.; Villa-Islas, V.; Bravo-López, M.J.; Sandoval-Velasco, M.; Wesp, J.K.; Gómez-Valdés, J.A.; Moreno-Cabrera, M.D.L.L.; Meraz, A.; Solís-Pichardo, G.; Schaaf, P.; et al. Ancient viral genomes reveal introduction of human pathogenic viruses into Mexico during the transatlantic slave trade. *elife* **2021**, *10*. [CrossRef]
21. Domingo, E.; Perales, C. Viral quasispecies. *PLoS Genet.* **2019**, *15*, e1008271. [CrossRef]
22. Beerenwinkel, N.; Zagordi, O. Ultra-deep sequencing for the analysis of viral populations. *Curr. Opin. Virol.* **2011**, *1*, 413–418. [CrossRef] [PubMed]
23. Posada-Cespedes, S.; Seifert, D.; Beerenwinkel, N. Recent advances in inferring viral diversity from high-throughput sequencing data. *Virus Res.* **2016**, *239*, 17–32. [CrossRef] [PubMed]
24. Manaresi, E.; Conti, I.; Bua, G.; Bonvicini, F.; Gallinella, G. A Parvovirus B19 synthetic genome: Sequence features and functional competence. *Virology* **2017**, *508*, 54–62. [CrossRef] [PubMed]
25. Bonvicini, F.; Filippone, C.; Delbarba, S.; Manaresi, E.; Zerbini, M.; Musiani, M.; Gallinella, G. Parvovirus B19 genome as a single, two-state replicative and transcriptional unit. *Virology* **2006**, *347*, 447–454. [CrossRef] [PubMed]
26. Bonvicini, F.; Filippone, C.; Manaresi, E.; Zerbini, M.; Musiani, M.; Gallinella, G. Functional analysis and quantitative determination of the expression profile of human parvovirus B19. *Virology* **2008**, *381*, 168–177. [CrossRef]
27. Robinson, J.T.; Thorvaldsdóttir, H.; Winckler, W.; Guttman, M.; Lander, E.S.; Getz, G.; Mesirov, J.P. Integrative genomics viewer. *Nat. Biotechnol.* **2011**, *29*, 24–26. [CrossRef]
28. Tamura, K.; Stecher, G.; Kumar, S. MEGA11: Molecular Evolutionary Genetics Analysis Version 11. *Mol. Biol. Evol.* **2021**, *38*, 3022–3027. [CrossRef]
29. Harris, C.R.; Millman, K.J.; van der Walt, S.J.; Gommers, R.; Virtanen, P.; Cournapeau, D.; Wieser, E.; Taylor, J.; Berg, S.; Smith, N.J.; et al. Array programming with NumPy. *Nature* **2020**, *585*, 357–362. [CrossRef]

30. Manaresi, E.; Gallinella, G. Advances in the Development of Antiviral Strategies against Parvovirus B19. *Viruses* **2019**, *11*, 659. [CrossRef]
31. Houldcroft, C.J.; Beale, M.A.; Breuer, J. Clinical and biological insights from viral genome sequencing. *Nat. Rev. Microbiol.* **2017**, *15*, 183–192. [CrossRef]
32. Pérez-Losada, M.; Arenas, M.; Galán, J.C.; Bracho, M.A.; Hillung, J.; García-González, N.; González-Candelas, F. High-throughput sequencing (HTS) for the analysis of viral populations. *Infect. Genet. Evol.* **2020**, *80*, 104208. [CrossRef] [PubMed]
33. King, D.; Freimanis, G.; Lasecka-Dykes, L.; Asfor, A.; Ribeca, P.; Waters, R.; King, D.; Laing, E. A Systematic Evaluation of High-Throughput Sequencing Approaches to Identify Low-Frequency Single Nucleotide Variants in Viral Populations. *Viruses* **2020**, *12*, 1187. [CrossRef] [PubMed]
34. Prosperi, M.C.F.; Yin, L.; Nolan, D.J.; Lowe, A.D.; Goodenow, M.M.; Salemi, M. Empirical validation of viral quasispecies assembly algorithms: State-of-the-art and challenges. *Sci. Rep.* **2013**, *3*, 2837. [CrossRef] [PubMed]
35. Lu, I.N.; Muller, C.P.; He, F.Q. Applying next-generation sequencing to unravel the mutational landscape in viral quasispecies. *Virus Res.* **2020**, *283*, 197963. [CrossRef] [PubMed]
36. Gregori, J.; Perales, C.; Rodriguez-Frias, F.; Esteban, J.I.; Quer, J.; Domingo, E. Viral quasispecies complexity measures. *Virology* **2016**, *493*, 227–237. [CrossRef]
37. Simmonds, P.; Aiewsakun, P.; Katzourakis, A. Prisoners of war—Host adaptation and its constraints on virus evolution. *Nat. Rev. Microbiol.* **2019**, *17*, 321–328. [CrossRef]

viruses

MDPI

Article

Capsid Structure of Aleutian Mink Disease Virus and Human Parvovirus 4: New Faces in the Parvovirus Family Portrait

Renuk Lakshmanan [1,†], Mario Mietzsch [1,*,†], Alberto Jimenez Ybargollin [1], Paul Chipman [1], Xiaofeng Fu [2], Jianming Qiu [3], Maria Söderlund-Venermo [4] and Robert McKenna [1,*]

1 Department of Biochemistry and Molecular Biology, Center for Structural Biology, McKnight Brain Institute, College of Medicine, University of Florida, Gainesville, FL 32603, USA
2 Biological Science Imaging Resource, Department of Biological Sciences, Florida State University, Tallahassee, FL 32306, USA
3 Department of Microbiology, Molecular Genetics and Immunology, University of Kansas Medical Center, Kansas City, KS 66160, USA
4 Department of Virology, University of Helsinki, 00014 Helsinki, Finland
* Correspondence: mario.mietzsch@ufl.edu (M.M.); rmckenna@ufl.edu (R.M.)
† These authors contributed equally to this work.

Abstract: Parvoviruses are small, single-stranded DNA viruses with non-enveloped capsids. Determining the capsid structures provides a framework for annotating regions important to the viral life cycle. Aleutian mink disease virus (AMDV), a pathogen in minks, and human parvovirus 4 (PARV4), infecting humans, are parvoviruses belonging to the genera *Amdoparvovirus* and *Tetraparvovirus*, respectively. While Aleutian mink disease caused by AMDV is a major threat to mink farming, no clear clinical manifestations have been established following infection with PARV4 in humans. Here, the capsid structures of AMDV and PARV4 were determined via cryo-electron microscopy at 2.37 and 3.12 Å resolutions, respectively. Despite low amino acid sequence identities (10–30%) both viruses share the icosahedral nature of parvovirus capsids, with 60 viral proteins (VPs) assembling the capsid via two-, three-, and five-fold symmetry VP-related interactions, but display major structural variabilities in the surface loops when the capsid structures are superposed onto other parvoviruses. The capsid structures of AMDV and PARV4 will add to current knowledge of the structural platform for parvoviruses and permit future functional annotation of these viruses, which will help in understanding their infection mechanisms at a molecular level for the development of diagnostics and therapeutics.

Keywords: parvovirus; capsid; AMDV; PARV4; cryo-EM; *Amdoparvovirus*; *Tetraparvovirus*; pathogen; VP1u

Citation: Lakshmanan, R.; Mietzsch, M.; Jimenez Ybargollin, A.; Chipman, P.; Fu, X.; Qiu, J.; Söderlund-Venermo, M.; McKenna, R. Capsid Structure of Aleutian Mink Disease Virus and Human Parvovirus 4: New Faces in the Parvovirus Family Portrait. *Viruses* **2022**, *14*, 2219. https://doi.org/10.3390/v14102219

Academic Editor: Giorgio Gallinella

Received: 22 September 2022
Accepted: 7 October 2022
Published: 9 October 2022

1. Introduction

The *Parvoviridae* is a family of small, non-enveloped, single-stranded DNA viruses [1]. This virus family is divided into three subfamilies: *Parvovirinae*, *Densovirinae*, and *Hamaparvovirinae* [2]. Members of the *Parvovirinae* are further split into ten genera: *Amdo-*, *Arti-*, *Ave-*, *Boca-*, *Copi-*, *Dependo-*, *Erythro-*, *Lori-*, *Proto-*, and *Tetraparvovirus*. The capsids of the *Parvovirinae* are ~260 Å in diameter and their proteins are encoded in the right-hand open reading frame of the viral genomes [3]. Different members of this subfamily either express two or three viral proteins (VPs) that overlap at their C-termini. The larger VPs are extended at their N-termini and have different important functions, including a phospholipase A_2 (PLA_2) domain, nuclear localization signals, and/or receptor-binding domains [4–6]. These N-terminal-extended VPs are expressed at about a 10-fold lower ratio relative to their shortest (major) VP, in the case of viruses expressing two VPs, 1:10 (VP1:VP2), and in the case of the viruses expressing three VPs, 1:1:10 (VP1:VP2:VP3) [7]. Their icosahedral capsids are composed of 60 VPs that assemble via two-, three-, and five-fold symmetry-related VP interactions. The viral capsids are critical components of the viral infectious life cycle: they protect the viral genome, are the determinants of the tissue type and host that is targeted (tropism), and remain intact while the virus escapes the endo-/lysosomal pathway and trafficks to the nucleus where the genome is released [8], leading to viral genome replication.

The capsid structures of several members of the *Parvovirinae* have been determined by X-ray crystallography and/or cryo-electron microscopy (cryo-EM) [3,9–11]. However, to date, these capsid structures originate from only four of the ten genera (*Boca-*, *Dependo-*, *Erythro-*, and *Protoparvovirus*). In all these structures, the N-terminal extended regions of the larger VPs, as well as the N-terminal 20–40 amino acids (aa) of the smaller VPs, have not been resolved [3]. They are believed to be highly flexible, likely due to a glycine-rich region near the N-terminus of the major VP, and are located in the interior of the capsid. Upon receptor-mediated endocytosis and subsequent acidification of the endosome, the VP1 unique (VP1u) with its PLA_2 enzymatic domain is externalized [12]. One described exception is parvovirus B19 (B19), of the *Erythroparvovirus* genus, which possesses a receptor-binding domain in its VP1u which needs to be located on the exterior side of the capsid for attachment to its target cells [6]. The structurally ordered regions of the VPs, which comprise most of the major VPs, display significant similarities among the members of the different genera, despite low sequence identities (10–30%) [13]. All VP monomers of members in the *Parvovirinae* consist of a core, eight-stranded (βB to βI), anti-parallel β-barrel motif, also known as a jelly-roll motif, with a BIDG sheet that forms the inner surface of the capsid. Additionally, a βA strand that runs anti-parallel to the βB strand and a helix αA that is located between the strands βC and βD are also conserved [3]. Between the β-strands of the VPs, connecting loops are inserted, which form the surface of the capsid. These loops are named after the connecting β-strands; for example, the HI loop connects the βH and βI strands. These surface loops exhibit the greatest amino acid sequence and structural diversity among members of the same genus and between the different genera. Differences at the apexes of these loops are termed variable regions (VRs), defined as two or more amino acids with Cα positions greater than 2 Å apart when their VPs are superposed. Despite these structural differences on the capsid surface, members of the *Parvovirinae* share the same overall characteristic features, including channels at the icosahedral five-fold symmetry axes, protrusions at or around the three-fold symmetry axes, and depressions at the two-fold symmetry axes and surrounding the five-fold channels, which depressions are separated by a raised region termed the two/five-fold wall [3].

Members of the *Parvovirinae* infect a wide range of vertebrate hosts, including humans [1,14]. Parvovirus 4 (PARV4) is a human parvovirus, first reported in 2005 in the serum of an intravenous drug user infected with hepatitis B virus [15]. The virus has been detected worldwide in plasma and different tissues, and it seems to be transmitted parenterally to hemophiliacs and injection-drug users, but with no clear clinical manifestations (reviewed in [14]). However, a recent study reported a strong association between PARV4 and individuals showing severe respiratory illness, and its DNA was found in cerebrospinal fluid from two children with encephalitis [16,17]. PARV4 has been assigned to the genus *Tetraparvovirus*, along with other members infecting pigs, sheep, cattle, yaks, and bats [18].

Aleutian mink disease virus (AMDV) is a member of the genus *Amdoparvovirus*. Viruses of this genus primarily infect carnivores, as well as some rodents and bats [19]. AMDV is known to cause Aleutian disease, which results in the enlargement of the kidneys, the spleen, and the lymph nodes and manifests in deadly plasmacytosis and hyperglobulinemia [20]. Outbreaks of this virus are a significant threat to mink farms. Currently, there are no vaccines available against AMDV [20].

To date, for PARV4, AMDV, and other viruses in their genera, no capsid structures have been determined. This study reports the capsid structures of PARV4 and AMDV determined by cryo-EM at 3.12 and 2.37 Å resolutions, respectively. These capsid structures of members of the genera *Tetraparvovirus* and *Amdoparvovirus* have been compared with capsid structures of viruses of the known genera—the *Boca-*, *Dependo-*, *Erythro-*, and *Protoparvovirus* capsids. Despite low sequence identities, these viruses share common capsid features with the viruses in the *Parvovirinae* subfamily but display major differences in the surface loops, with several large insertions and/or deletions. In particular, the capsid of AMDV possesses the largest major VP, with ~60 to 115 additional aa compared to other *Parvovirinae* members for which capsid structures have been determined. In contrast, AMDV's VP1u is very short and does not contain a PLA_2 domain. On the other hand, PARV4 possesses a VP1u that is much longer than those of other members of the *Parvovirinae*. It contains a PLA_2 domain and likely also a receptor-binding domain.

These studies provide a structural platform for functional annotation of these viruses that will help to understand their disease mechanisms at a molecular level. This information could be applicable in the development of therapeutics.

2. Materials and Methods

2.1. Production of Virus-like Particles (VLPs)

The open reading frames expressing VP2 for PARV4 (nt: 3464–5122; accession no.: AY622943) and AMDV (nt: 2406–4349; accession no.: M20036) were cloned into the pFastBac1 plasmid vector. For the AMDV construct expressing VP1 and VP2, nt 2204–4349 were cloned into pFastBac1, excluding the intron sequences (nt 2214–2286), and the VP1 start codon was changed to ACG. These constructs were used to generate the recombinant baculoviruses by following the standard Bac-to-Bac Baculovirus Expression System protocol (Invitrogen, Waltham, MA, USA). The recombinant baculoviral stocks were used to infect Sf9 cells in the mid-logarithmic phase at a multiplicity of infection (MOI) of 5 plaque-forming units (PFUs). The Sf9 cells were harvested after 72 h by centrifugation at 1000× *g* for 20 min at 4 °C. Following centrifugation, the supernatants were separated from the cell pellets. The Sf9 cell pellets were resuspended in TNTM buffer (25 mM Tris-HCl, 100 mM NaCl, 0.2% Triton X-100, 2 mM $MgCl_2$, pH 8.0), and the supernatants were subjected to polyethylene glycol (PEG) treatment with the addition of 10% (*w*/*v*) PEG 8000 and overnight stirring at 4 °C. The PEG-treated samples were centrifuged at 14,300× *g* for 90 min at 4 °C, followed by resuspension of the PEG pellets in TNTM buffer. Furthermore, the resuspended PEG and cell pellets were combined and lysed using the LM10 Microfluidizer (Microfluidics, Westwood, MA, USA) at 5000 psi. The lysates were benzonase-treated and clarified by centrifugation at 12,000× *g* for 30 min to remove cell debris. The supernatants were loaded onto a 20% sucrose cushion (*w*/*v* sucrose in TNTM buffer) and centrifuged at 45,000 rpm, using a Ti70 rotor for 3 h at 4 °C. The sucrose cushion pellet was resuspended in TNTM buffer, loaded onto a 10–40% sucrose step gradient (*w*/*v* sucrose in TNTM buffer), and centrifuged using a SW41 rotor for 3 h at 4 °C. The sample fractions were then recovered by fractionation, analyzed by SDS-PAGE, dialyzed in phosphate-buffered saline (PBS), concentrated to ~1 mg/mL using Apollo concentrators (Orbital Biosciences, Topsfield, MA, USA), and stored at −20 °C.

2.2. Cryo-EM Data Collection

Purified VLPs were loaded onto a glow-discharged holey carbon-coated grid (Quantifoil, Großlöbichau, Germany) and incubated at 4 °C at 95% humidity for 30 s in a Vitrobot Mark IV (Thermo Fisher Scientific, Waltham, MA, USA). Following this, excess sample was blotted by the machine and the grids were vitrified by plunging into liquid ethane. The ice quality of the vitrified grids as well as sample distribution were probed by imaging on a 200 kV FEI Tecnai G2 F20-TWIN transmission electron microscope (FEI, Hillsboro, OR, USA) at ~20 $e^-/Å^2$. After confirming the quality of the grid, high-resolution data collections were performed at the Biological Science Imaging Resource (BSIR) at Florida State University. Data were collected on a Titan Krios electron microscope operating at 300 kV and equipped with the DE64 or DE-Apollo direct electron detector (Direct Electron, San Diego, CA, USA), with 52 or 102 movie frames collected per micrograph at a total electron dose of ~60 $e^-/Å^2$. Furthermore, motion-corrected micrographs were obtained by aligning the movie frames, using MotionCor2 (version 1.5.0) with dose weighting [21].

2.3. 3D Image Reconstruction

The motion-corrected micrographs were imported into the cisTEM software package, which was used for 3D image reconstruction of the PARV4 and AMDV capsids [22]. CTF estimation was used to exclude micrographs of poor quality, as well as micrographs with overlapping or damaged particles. Particles were picked automatically and subjected to 2D classification by imposing icosahedral symmetry. The 2D classes containing clear virus features were used for generation of an ab initio model by 3D reconstruction. The 3D model was then auto-refined using default settings, and the final density map was sharpened with a pre-cutoff B-factor value of −90 Å^2 and a post-cutoff B-factor value of 20 Å^2. The resolution of the density map was calculated based on a Fourier shell correlation of 0.143 (Table 1).

Table 1. Summary of cryo-EM data collection and refinement statistics for PARV4 and AMDV.

Cryo-EM Data and Refinement Parameters	PARV4	AMDV
Total number of micrographs	1324	2254
Defocus range (µm)	0.5–2.0	0.5–2.0
Electron dose (e$^-$/Å^2)	60	59
Frames/micrograph	52	102
Pixel size (Å/pixel)	0.91	0.95
Capsids used for final map	5248	93,393
Resolution of final map (Å)	3.12	2.37
PHENIX model refinement statistics		
Residue range	15–552	19–565
Map CC	0.846	0.889
RMSD bonds (Å)	0.02	0.01
RMSD angles (°)	1.05	0.92
All-atom clash score	17.6	9.12
Ramachandran plot		
Favored (%)	98.0	95.1
Allowed (%)	2.0	4.6
Outliers (%)	0	0.3
Rotamer outliers (%)	0	0.2
C-β deviations	0	0

2.4. Model Building

In silico models of PARV4 and AMDV were generated using the SWISS-MODEL homology-modeling server [23]. Furthermore, VIPERdb was used to generate a T = 1 icosahedral capsid from the in silico model [24]. The newly generated capsid 60-mer was then docked into the EM density map using the 'fit in map' feature of UCSF Chimera [25]. The fit of the 60-mer with respect to the EM density map was then improved by adjusting the voxel size, which maximizes the correlation coefficient. The voxel-size-adjusted EM density map was then imported into Coot, where manual model building and real-space refinement tools were used to improve the 60-mer model [26]. Finally, the 60-mer was automatically refined using the real-space-refine subroutine in PHENIX, which also provided refinement statistics [27]. Based on their primary amino acid sequences, in silico models of VP1u and AMDV VR-VII were generated using AlphaFold v2.0 run on HiPerGator (UF research computing).

3. Results and Discussion

3.1. Determination of the Human Parvovirus 4 Capsid Structure

Following the production and purification of PARV4-virus-like particles (VLPs), the purified fraction, analyzed by SDS-PAGE, contained a band consistent with PARV4 VP2, migrating at ~60 kDa (Figure 1a). Cryo-EM micrographs showed intact particles ~250 Å in diameter (Figure 1b). Thus, the PARV4 sample was deemed suitable for structural determination by cryo-EM. Three-dimensional-image reconstruction of the PARV4 capsids, utilizing a total of 5248 individual particles, resulted in a resolution of 3.12 Å, based on an FSC threshold of 0.143 (Table 1). The reconstructed capsid of PARV4, the first structure of the genus *Tetraparvovirus*, displayed familiar surface features, similar to those observed in the capsids of other genera in the *Parvovirinae* subfamily, with channels at the icosahedral five-fold axes, protrusions near the three-fold axes, and depressions at the two-fold axes and surrounding the five-fold axes (Figure 1c) [3]. Despite these common features, the specific shapes of the protrusions and depressions were found to be unique when compared to other parvoviruses. Overall, the PARV4 capsid has a "flatter" appearance, similar to some densoviruses [3], since the three-fold protrusions do not project radially outwards and instead are positioned towards the two-fold, three-fold, and five-fold symmetry axes. This results in very small depressions at the two-fold axes and more segmented depressions surrounding the five-fold channel. While most viruses of the *Parvovirinae* subfamily possess three separated protrusions surrounding the three-fold symmetry axis [3], in PARV4, density near the three-fold axis fuses the three-fold protrusions in the shape of a concaved triangle. Additionally, fused three-fold protrusions have been previously observed for various animal protoparvoviruses [13], though with a differently shaped three-fold region compared to PARV4. Structural order in the density map of the PARV4 VP started at lysine 15 (VP2 numbering). The amino acids in the VP monomer were generally well-ordered (Figure 1d) to the C-terminal leucine 552, with the exception of aa 380–401, located near the three-fold symmetry axis, where only diffuse electron density was observed at a sigma (σ) threshold of ~1, preventing reliable placement of the amino acid chain.

3.2. Determination of the Aleutian Mink Disease Virus Capsid Structure

Similar to PARV4, AMDV VLPs were produced using the Bac-to-Bac system. However, in contrast to PARV4 VLPs, the AMDV VLPs composed of VP1 and VP2 were generated by modifying the VP1 start codon to ACG (Figure 2a). The same strategy was not possible for PARV4, as its VP1u region is very long and contains multiple ATGs prior to the VP2 start codon. For AMDV, the VP1u region is very short (43 aa) compared to those of other members of the *Parvovirinae* and does not possess a PLA_2 domain. In addition, AMDV capsid proteins were shown to be cleaved by caspases in Crandell feline kidney (CrFK) cells [28]. This cleavage event was also observed following the production and purification of AMDV VLPs in insect Sf9 cells (Figure 2b). Nonetheless, this cleavage event did not affect the integrity of the capsids, as homogenous, intact particles ~250 Å in diameter were visible by cryo-EM (Figure 2c). Previously, pan-caspase inhibitors were shown to be effective in preventing this cleavage in CrFK cells [28] however, this inhibitor was not functional in Sf9 cells.

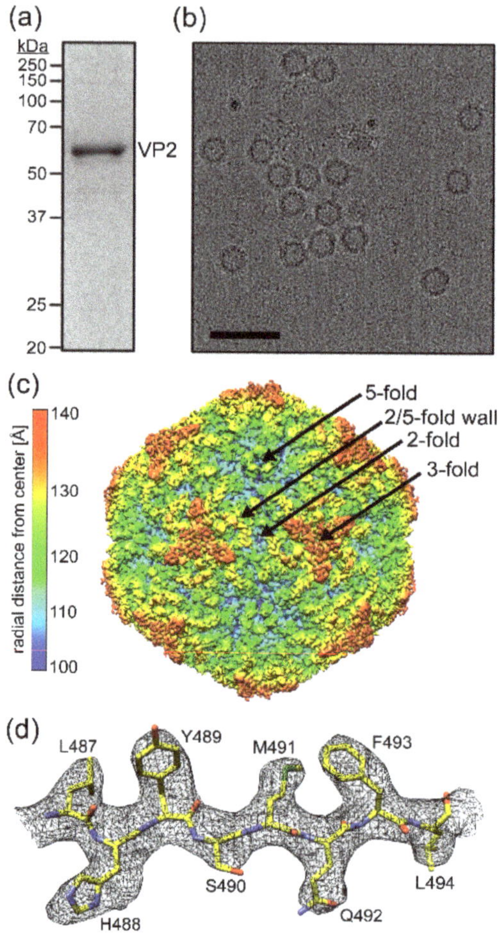

Figure 1. Determination of the PARV4 capsid structure. (**a**) SDS-PAGE of purified PARV4 VLPs, with a band at ~60 kDa equivalent to the size of VP2. (**b**) Example cryo-electron micrograph of PARV4. Scale bar: 500 Å. (**c**) The capsid surface density map contoured at a sigma (σ) threshold level of 1.0. The map is radially colored (blue to red) according to distance to the capsid center, as indicated by the scale bar on the left. The approximate icosahedral two-, three-, and five-fold axes are indicated. (**d**) Amino acid residues modeled for the βI strand are shown inside their density maps (in black). The amino acid residues are as labeled and shown as stick representations and colored according to atom type: C = yellow, O = red, N = blue, S = green. Panels (**c**,**d**) were generated using UCSF-Chimera [25].

As the capsids appeared uniform, the AMDV sample was deemed suitable for high-resolution structural determination. Three-dimensional-image reconstruction of a total of 93,393 individual AMDV capsids resulted in a resolution of 2.37 Å, based on an FSC threshold of 0.143 (Table 1). The reconstructed capsid of AMDV, the first determined structure of the genus *Amdoparvovirus*, also displayed familiar surface features, as described above, with channels at the icosahedral five-fold axes, protrusions near the three-fold axes, and depressions at the two-fold axes and surrounding the five-fold axes (Figure 2d) [3]. Previously, the capsid structure of AMDV was determined by cryo-EM at ~22 Å resolution and showed the same overall capsid surface features [29].

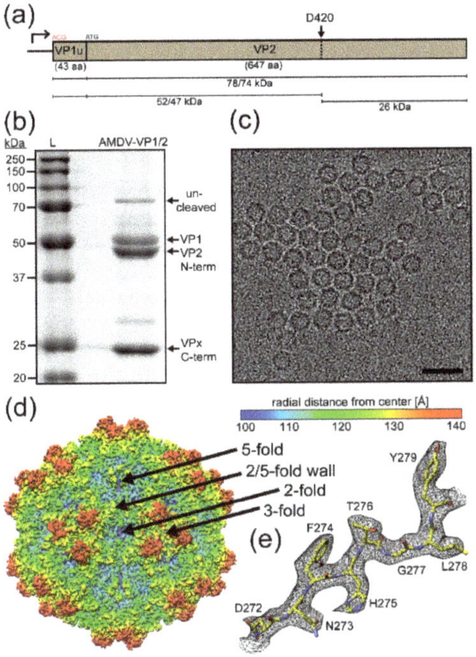

Figure 2. Determination of the AMDV capsid structure. (**a**) Depiction of the AMDV-VP1/2 expression construct. A cleavage of the AMDV VPs at D420 has been described previously [28]; the results for the VP1 and VP2 fragments as shown below. (**b**) SDS-PAGE of purified AMDV VLPs with bands at ~75, 52, 47, and 25 kDa equivalent to the size of uncleaved VP2, the N-terminal VP1 and VP2 fragments, and the C-terminal VPx fragment, respectively. (**c**) Example cryo-electron micrograph of AMDV. Scale bar: 500 Å. (**d**) The capsid surface density map contoured at a sigma (σ) threshold level of 2.0. The map is radially colored (blue to red) according to distance to the capsid center, as indicated by the scale bar on the right. The approximate icosahedral two-, three-, and five-fold axes are indicated. (**e**) Amino acid residues modeled for the βG strand are shown inside their density maps (in black). The amino acid residues are as labeled and shown as stick representations and colored according to atom type: C = yellow, O = red, N = blue. Panels (**d**,**e**) were generated using UCSF-Chimera [25].

Unlike PARV4, the three-fold protrusions were separated and radiated further outwards (the maximum capsid diameter of AMDV being ~300 Å compared to ~270 Å for PARV4). Overall, the AMDV capsid looks similar to bufavirus capsids [13]. Structural ordering in the density map was observed, starting at threonine 42 (VP2 numbering). The amino acids, including their side chains in the VP monomers, were generally very well-ordered (Figure 2e) to the C-terminal tyrosine 647, with the exception of the apexes of the loops at the three-fold protrusion, involving aa 93–94 and 238–239, which showed only weak density at a sigma (σ) threshold of ~1, preventing reliable placement of the amino acid side chains. In addition, no density was observed for aa 420–449. This stretch of amino acids is located at the caspase cleavage site (Figure 2a).

In addition to the AMDVs containing VP1 and VP2, the capsid structure of AMDV VLPs only containing VP2 was also determined by cryo-EM at 3.1 Å resolution (data deposited in EMDB). However, the capsid structure was indistinguishable from the VP1/VP2 capsids and similar to other parvovirus capsid structures, due to the low copy numbers of the minor VPs and the flexibility of their N termini [3].

3.3. The Three-Fold Protrusions Are Formed by Different Loops in PARV4 and AMDV

The VP monomers of PARV4 and AMDV (Figure 3a,b) conserve the β-barrel core motif (βB–βI) with the additional βA strand and the α-helix A (αA) observed in other parvoviruses. The structurally ordered N-terminus is situated in both viruses in approximately the same location underneath the βBIDG sheet. However, for most capsid structures of the *Parvovirinae*, the N-terminus is located directly below the five-fold channel, except for parvovirus B19 [3]. This is mediated by a conserved hydrophobic valine to leucine interaction of the N-terminus and the DE loop (canine parvovirus (CPV): V38-L169, human bocavirus 1 (HBoV1): V36-L151, adeno-associated virus serotype 2 (AAV2): V221-L336) [30,31]. Neither parvovirus B19 nor PARV4 conserves these residues, which might explain their differently structured VP N-termini. In contrast, AMDV conserves both residues, V38 and L175, but valine 38 is embedded in a 17 aa-long glycine-rich sequence element (aa 22–39) which introduces a lot of flexibility and might prevent interaction with the DE loop.

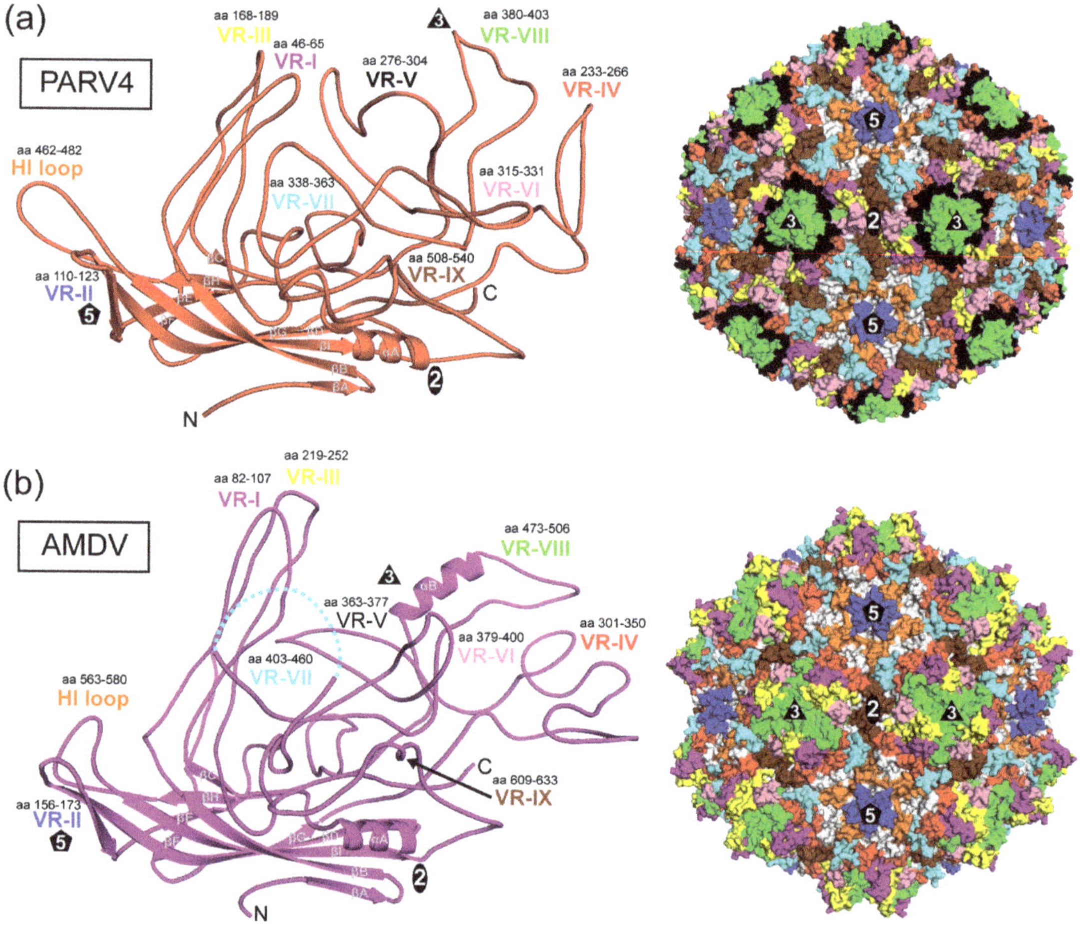

Figure 3. The PARV4 and AMDV VP structures. (**a**) Ribbon diagram (left) of PARV4 VP. The conserved β-barrel core motif (βB–βI), βA, the αA helix, the N- and C-termini are indicated. The VRs (VR-I to -IX) are labeled and the approximate icosahedral two-, three-, and five-fold axes are represented by ovals, triangles, and pentagons, respectively. Right: The location of the VRs, colored as in the ribbon diagram, on the capsid surface of PARV4. (**b**) Ribbon diagram (left) and capsid surface map of AMDV VP, as in (**a**).

Large loops are inserted between the β-strands that form the surface of the capsid (Figure 3). The largest loop is the GH loop with multiple subloops comparable to other capsid structures of members in the *Parvovirinae*. Despite the significant structural variability of these surface loops, the base of each loop originates from approximately the same location in the capsid core as for all viruses of this subfamily. Thus, the previously described variable-region (VR) terminology for other genera can also be applied to PARV4 and AMDV to describe these loops.

The PARV4 capsid utilizes VR-II to form the five-fold channel; VR-I, VR-III, and VR-IX for the two-/five-fold wall; and VR-IV, VR-V, and VR-VIII for the three-fold protrusions (Figure 3a). The fused three-fold protrusions are caused by VR-VIII with its subloop leading towards the three-fold symmetry axis. Interestingly, the fused three-fold protrusions of the animal protoparvoviruses (e.g., CPV) are generated by the equivalent loop, though without any sequence similarity [10]. The small depression at the two-fold symmetry axis is the result of VR-VI covering most of the depression from both sides (Figure 3a, right panel). Around the five-fold channel, the depression is interrupted by VR-VII interacting with the HI loop.

The AMDV capsid also utilizes VR-II to form the five-fold channel (Figure 3b). However, in contrast to PARV4, the elongated VR-I and VR-III (15 and 18 aa longer, respectively) are responsible for the three-fold protrusions in AMDV. The region at the three-fold symmetry axis between the protrusions is primarily formed by VR-VIII, while VR-V is not surface-exposed. The VR-VIII loop possesses an additional α-helix B (Figure 3b). To date, only the viruses of the *Bocaparvovirus* genus have been described as possessing a long α-helix at the capsid surface [11,32]. However, in contrast to AMDV, the surface helix of the bocaviruses is located in VR-III at the two/five-fold wall. The α-helix B in AMDV is located very close to the three-fold symmetry axis. In fact, three helices from three symmetry-related VPs are positioned around the three-fold symmetry axis, creating a small pore with a diameter of ~3.5 Å (Figure 4a). Interestingly, leucine 506 is located at the center and represents the narrowest point of the three-fold pore. In the five-fold pore with a larger diameter (~7.6 Å), leucines (L175) are also located at its narrowest point. It remains to be seen whether the three-fold pore fulfills specific functions in the viral life cycle. Possible amino acid substitutions of leucine 506 may help to characterize the pore, as in experiments performed on the five-fold channel [30,33].

The two/five-fold wall of the AMDV capsid is formed by VR-IV, VR-VII, and VR-IX (Figure 3b). However, due to the cleavage of the AMDV VPs at D420, no density was observed for aa 420 to 449, but both ends of VR-VII, leucine 419 and proline 450, were visible at the capsid surface (Figures 3b and 4b). If the missing 30 aa were to form a loop, it would radiate further outwards than the three-fold protrusions (VR-I and VR-III). However, given that two unrelated cell lines, feline cells [28] and insect cells, resulted in the same cleavage event, it may be that the DLLD/G caspase cleavage site [34] is cut in minks as well. Thus, VR-VII might have a flexible, linear amino acid element on the capsid surface. AlphaFold 2 predictions of the 30 aa stretch suggest a helix-turn-helix motif for this sequence [35]. More research to determine the importance of the VR-VII sequence, including the potential helix-turn-helix for the viral life cycle, is needed.

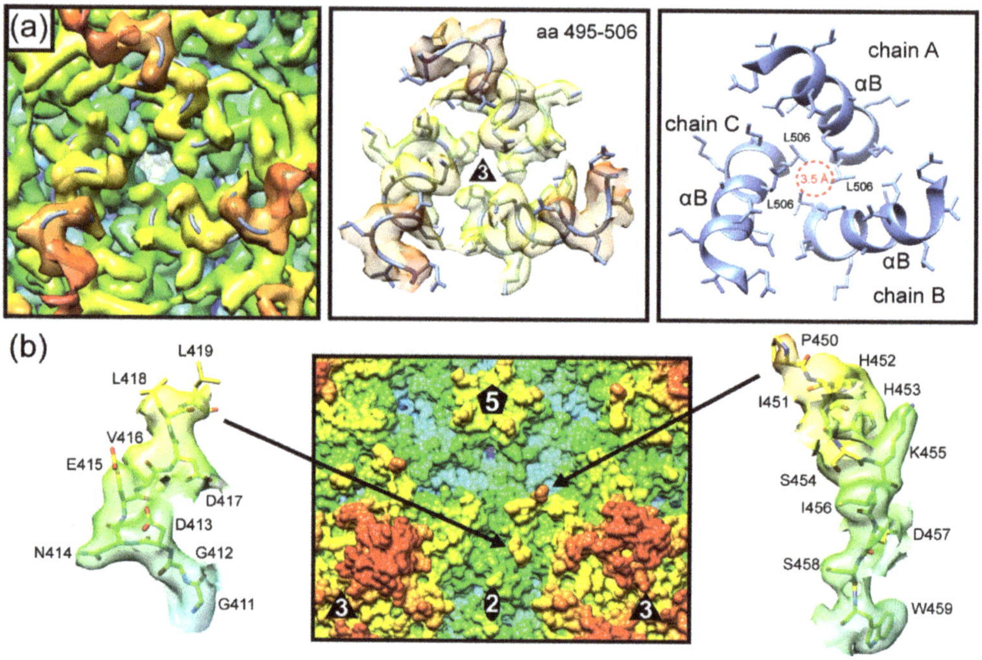

Figure 4. Unique capsid features of AMDV. (**a**) The α-helices B of three symmetry-related monomers are positioned around the three-fold symmetry axis. Left and center panel: the ribbon diagram of aa 495–506 fitted into the density map of AMDV (center panel with amino acid side chains). Right panel: The ribbon diagrams are shown without the map. Leucine 506 is located near the center, surrounding a pore approximately 3.5 Å in diameter. (**b**) AMDV's cleaved VR-VII is located at the two/five-fold wall. The N-terminal end (leucine 419), shown inside the density map (left), is located closer to the two-fold symmetry axis, while the C-terminal arm of the loop (right model inside the density map) is located closer to the five-fold symmetry axis. No density was observed for aa 420 to 449.

3.4. Inter-Genus Sequence and Structural Comparisons

For capsid sequence and structural comparison of PARV4 and AMDV with the subfamily *Parvovirinae*, representative members of the genera were chosen for which structural data were available. At the time of this study, capsid structures were available for four of the ten *Parvovirinae* genera. The representative members that were selected for the genera members used were as follows: for the *Bocaparvovirus* genus, HBoV1; for the *Dependoparvovirus* genus, AAV2; for the *Erythroparvovirus* genus, B19; and for the *Protoparvovirus* genus, CPV. Overall, the capsid amino acid sequence identities of viruses from different genera were low, irrespective of the genera compared. They ranged from 13% (AMDV vs. PARV4) to 34% (AMDV vs. CPV) (Figure 5a). In a previous study characterizing distant members of the *Protoparvovirus* genus, even intra-genus capsid sequence identity was as low as 30% [10]. Thus, AMDV showed a close relationship to the *Protoparvovirus* genus (34% to CPV) and PARV4 showed a close relationship to the *Erythroparvovirus* genus (29% to B19). This also translated to a high structural similarity of 68% for the AMDV capsid structure aligned with the capsid structure of CPV (Figure 5a,b).

(a)

amino acid sequence identity of major VP (in %)

	CPV	AMDV	HBoV1	PARV4	AAV2	B19
CPV		34	19	16	18	16
AMDV	68		18	13	16	14
HBoV1	52	41		20	24	21
PARV4	46	42	57		20	29
AAV2	58	47	63	66		24
B19	44	36	52	63	63	

structurally aligned amino acids: Cα distance < 2 Å (in %)

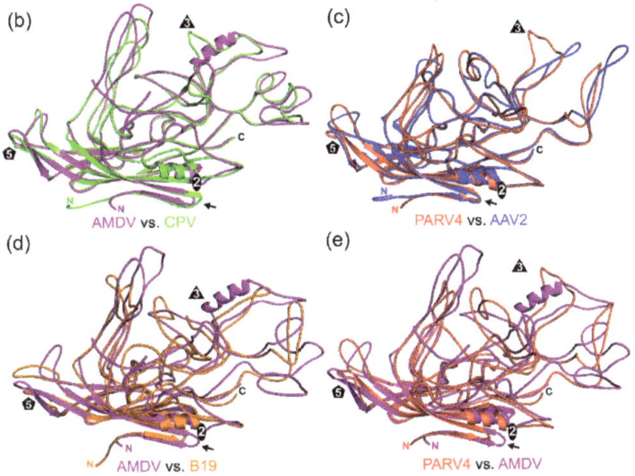

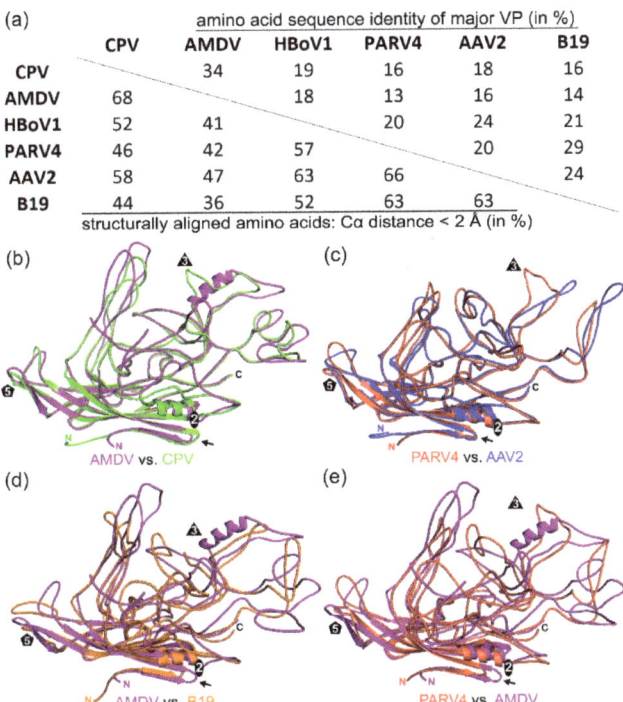

Figure 5. Sequence and structural comparison. (**a**) Amino acid sequence identity comparison of the major VPs (top right) between CPV, AMDV, HBoV1, PARV4, AAV2, and B19 (in %). Structural similarity (bottom left) was defined as the percentage of aligned Cα atoms of the amino acid chain within 2 Å distance when the capsid structures were superposed. (**b**) Superposition of AMDV (purple) and CPV (green). The N- and C-termini and the approximate icosahedral two-, three-, and five-fold axes are indicated. (**c**) Superposition of PARV4 (red) and AAV2 (blue). (**d**) Superposition of AMDV (purple) and B19 (orange). (**e**) Superposition of PARV4 (red) and AMDV (purple). Arrows indicate the position of the AB loop.

Common features between the AMDV and CPV capsids include the three-fold protrusions formed by VR-I and VR-III, VR-V not being surface-exposed, and the extended AB loop on the inside of the capsid, which has been shown to be involved in nucleotide binding for the protoparvoviruses [36]. For PARV4 and B19, the 29% sequence identity translated to 63% structural similarity (Figure 5a). However, despite only having a sequence identity of 20%, the AAV2 capsid had the highest structural similarity to the PARV4 capsid (Figure 5c). Common features between the PARV4 and AAV2 capsids include the three-fold protrusions formed by VR-IV, VR-V, and VR-VIII and the two-/five-fold wall formed by VR-I, VR-III, and VR-IX [3]. Furthermore, while the capsids of PARV4 and CPV are not very similar, both viruses possess a similar subloop in VR-VIII leading towards the three-fold symmetry axis, which results in the fused appearance of the three-fold protrusions (compare the green ribbon in Figure 5b with the red ribbon in Figure 5c).

The AMDV capsid showed the lowest structural similarity to the B19 capsid, with 36% structurally aligned residues (Figure 5a,d), and the PARV4 capsid showed the lowest structural similarity to the AMDV capsid, with 42% structural similarity (Figure 5a,e). In these structural comparisons, the only region that aligned was the core jelly-roll motif.

3.5. Unusual Length of AMDV VP1u, VP2, and VR-VII

Members of the genus *Amdoparvovirus* (and *Aveparvovirus*) differ from most viruses in the subfamily in that they do not possess the common PLA_2 sequence motif in the VP1u region (Figure 6a). Furthermore, their VP1u is short (only 43 aa) in comparison to other viruses of the *Parvovirinae* (Table 2). For most viruses, the VP1u region is ~100–200 amino acids longer. In the case of PARV4 the VP1 open reading frame codes for a 362 aa VP1u region. However, the exact start codon for VP1 is still debated [14,37]. In contrast to AMDV's short VP1u, its major capsid protein is among the largest in the subfamily. Compared with other members of the *Parvovirinae*, it displays multiple significant insertions and some deletions, resulting in a ~60 to 120 aa larger VP2 (Table 2). At the N-terminus it possesses the longest glycine-rich region of the family [3]. However, most insertions are located at the capsid surface. In fact, AMDV has the longest loop for VR-I, VR-III, VR-IV, and VR-VII among natural *Parvovirinae* isolates for which structures have been determined (Table 2). The only major deletion is located in VR-V, which is shared with CPV and other protoparvoviruses, as this loop is not surface-exposed in these viruses [3]. Given the differences in the lengths of VP1u and VP2 relative to other viruses, it may be possible that some functions of the VP1u region are conducted by the major capsid protein. One such region that may exhibit additional functions could be VR-VII. This loop in AMDV is 31–42 aa longer than in any other genus (Table 2). Furthermore, one side of the loop is cleaved directly at the capsid surface (Figure 4b), which may allow the remaining loop to fold according to its function. The sequence in this region is specific to the genus *Amdoparvovirus*, and structural predictions suggest a helix-turn-helix motif (Figure 6b).

Table 2. VP and loop amino acid length comparison of AMDV with other members of the *Parvovirinae*.

AMDV vs.	VP1u	Major VP	VR I	VR II	VR III	VR IV	VR V	VR VI	VR VII	VR VIII	HI loop	VR IX
CPV	−95 #	+61 #	+6	+1	+7	+8	0	+5	+35	−4	−2	+6
HBoV1	−86 *	+105	+14	+4	+11	+22	−25	+12	+42	+21	+2	−1
AAV2	−159 *	+114	+14	+4	+25	+13	−20	+5	+39	+9	−3	+4
PARV4	−319	+95	+15	+4	+18	+19	−16	−4	+31	+5	−2	−4
B19	−184	+93	+3	+3	+16	+21	−20	+3	+39	+13	−1	−5

Example: AMDV has 95 aa less than CPV in VP1u and 61 aa more in the major VP. * Including the VP1/2 common region.

Helix-turn-helix motifs are predicted to be present in the PLA_2 domains of the VP1u for most viruses of the *Parvovirinae* (Figure 6). Despite low amino acid sequence identities for the PLA_2 domains ranging from 30–50%, the predicted α-helices of the different viruses are well superposable. In addition to the PLA_2 domain, some viruses may have other functional domains in their VP1u and/or VP1/2 common regions. Both HBoV1 and CPV possess α-helices near their C-termini (Figure 6b,c). CPV's α-helix in this region has high sequence similarity to the only α-helix in AMDV VP1u (Figure 6a). AAV2, B19, and PARV4 display α-helices near the N-terminus of VP1u (Figure 6d–f). For Parvovirus B19, the presence of a receptor-binding domain at the N terminus, which is predominantly α-helical, has been described before [6,38]. A recent study showed that AAV2 and other AAV serotypes are dependent on a G protein-coupled receptor, GPR108, for effective transduction and that the interaction is dictated by the VP1u region [39]. While the exact amino acids in VP1u for the interaction have not been determined, it is possible that the N-terminal region including the α-helix (aa 9–24) are involved (Figure 6d). PARV4, with its very long VP1u region, displays a substantial α-helical region near the N-terminus. Five α-helices (aa 15–121) were predicted, which could represent a receptor-binding domain (Figure 6f). To date, no receptor has been identified for PARV4. Due to the size, it is highly likely that most, if not all, of the VP1u region of PARV4 is localized on the exterior side of the capsid, similar to that of Parvovirus B19 [40], which would enable PARV4 to bind its receptor with its potential VP1u RBD.

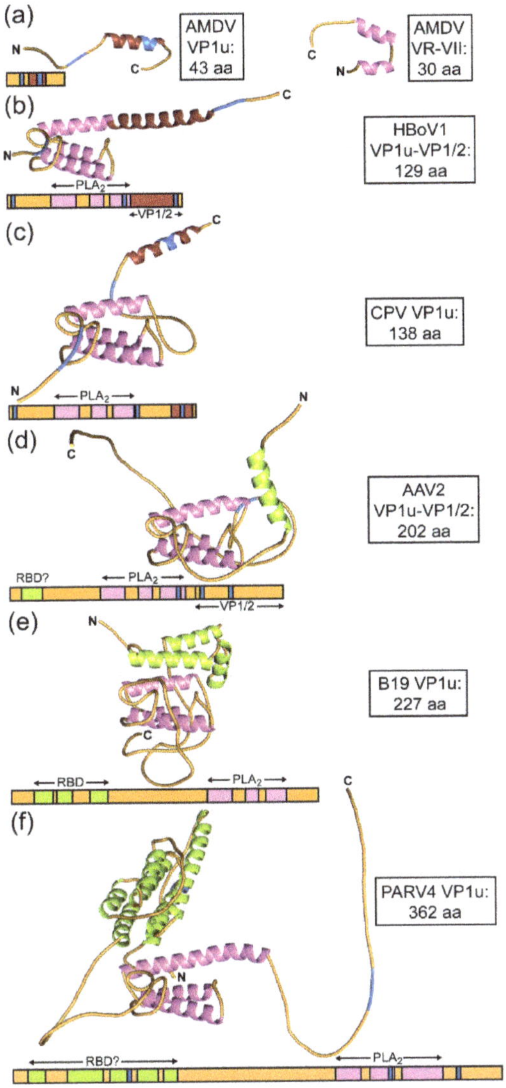

Figure 6. Structural prediction for VP1u. Alphafold [35] predictions utilizing the primary sequences of (**a**) the AMDV VP1u and VR-VII regions, (**b**) the HBoV1 VP1u and VP1/2 common region, (**c**) the CPV VP1u, (**d**) the AAV2 VP1u and VP1/2 common region, (**e**) the B19 VP1u, and (**f**) the PARV4 VP1u. The helices of the PLA2 domains are colored magenta, the helices of (potential) receptor-binding domains (RBD) light green, the C-terminal helices dark red, and the basic regions blue. The N- and C-termini are indicated.

4. Conclusions

This study extends the available capsid structural atlas of the subfamily *Parvovirinae* to six of the ten genera (Figure 7). The newly added structures of AMDV and PARV4 will provide and add to the structural platform for functional annotation of these viruses. Currently, the cellular receptors and many steps of the viral life cycle for these viruses are unknown, and elucidation of the capsid structures may help to understand their disease mechanisms at a molecular level.

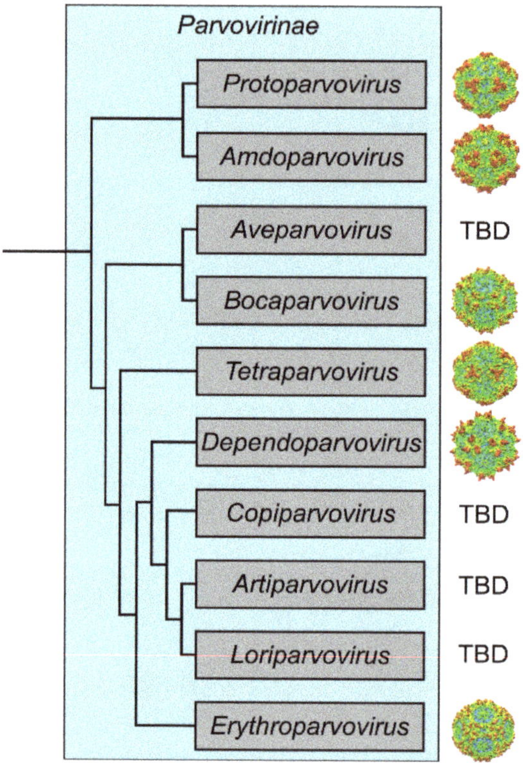

Figure 7. Cladogram of the *Parvovirinae* subfamily based on Penzes et al. [2]. The representative members of the genera for which capsid structures have been determined are CPV (*Protoparvovirus*), AMDV (*Amdoparvovirus*), HBoV1 (*Bocaparvovirus*), PARV4 (*Tetraparvovirus*), AAV2 (*Dependoparvovirus*), and B19 (*Erythroparvovirus*). Radially colored capsid surface representations (blue to red) are viewed along the two-fold axis and were generated using Chimera [25]. TBD: to be determined.

In the case of AMDV, similar to B19 and HBoV1, antibody-dependent enhancement (ADE) of infection was described as a form of entry to host cells for this virus, complicating vaccination strategies [41–44]. The capsid structure of AMDV may help to identify the epitopes of the antibodies, as in studies on other parvoviruses [45]. Alternatively, if ADE post-vaccination cannot be prevented, the capsid structures may help in the development of therapeutics directly targeting the capsid.

Author Contributions: Conceptualization, M.M., M.S.-V. and R.M.; methodology, R.L. and M.M.; validation, M.M. and R.M.; formal analysis, R.L. and M.M.; investigation, R.L., M.M. and A.J.Y.; resources, P.C., J.Q., M.S.-V. and X.F.; data curation, R.L. and M.M.; writing—original draft preparation, R.L. and M.M.; writing—review and editing, R.L., M.M., R.M., J.Q. and M.S.-V.; visualization, R.L. and M.M.; supervision, R.M.; project administration, R.M.; funding acquisition, and R.M. All authors have read and agreed to the published version of the manuscript.

Funding: The study was funded by the NIH grant R01 NIH GM082946 (to R.M.). Data collection at Florida State University through the Southeastern Consortium for Microscopy of Macro Molecular Machines (SECM4) was made possible by NIH grants S10OD018142-01, S10RR025080-01, and U24GM116788.

Institutional Review Board Statement: Not applicable.

Informed Consent Statement: Not applicable.

Data Availability Statement: The PARV4 and AMDV cryo-EM-reconstructed density maps and models built for their capsids were deposited in the Electron Microscopy Data Bank (EMDB) with the accession numbers EMD-28522/PDB ID 8EP9 (PARV4), EMD-28514/PDB ID 8EP2 (AMDV VP1/2), and EMD-28514 (AMDV-VP2).

Acknowledgments: The authors wish to thank the late Mavis Agbandje-McKenna for initiating this research project and for her pioneering studies of parvovirus capsid structures. The authors also want to thank the UF-ICBR Electron Microscopy Core (RRID:SCR_019146) for access to electron microscopes utilized for cryo-electron micrograph screening.

Conflicts of Interest: The authors declare no conflict of interest.

References

1. Cotmore, S.F.; Agbandje-McKenna, M.; Canuti, M.; Chiorini, J.A.; Eis-Hubinger, A.M.; Hughes, J.; Mietzsch, M.; Modha, S.; Ogliastro, M.; Penzes, J.J.; et al. ICTV Virus Taxonomy Profile: Parvoviridae. *J. Gen. Virol.* **2019**, *100*, 367–368. [CrossRef] [PubMed]
2. Pénzes, J.J.; Söderlund-Venermo, M.; Canuti, M.; Eis-Hübinger, A.M.; Hughes, J.; Cotmore, S.F.; Harrach, B. Reorganizing the family Parvoviridae: A revised taxonomy independent of the canonical approach based on host association. *Arch. Virol.* **2020**, *165*, 2133–2146. [CrossRef] [PubMed]
3. Mietzsch, M.; Penzes, J.J.; Agbandje-McKenna, M. Twenty-Five Years of Structural Parvovirology. *Viruses* **2019**, *11*, 362. [CrossRef] [PubMed]
4. Zadori, Z.; Szelei, J.; Lacoste, M.C.; Li, Y.; Gariepy, S.; Raymond, P.; Allaire, M.; Nabi, I.R.; Tijssen, P. A viral phospholipase A2 is required for parvovirus infectivity. *Dev. Cell* **2001**, *1*, 291–302. [CrossRef]
5. Grieger, J.C.; Snowdy, S.; Samulski, R.J. Separate basic region motifs within the adeno-associated virus capsid proteins are essential for infectivity and assembly. *J. Virol.* **2006**, *80*, 5199–5210. [CrossRef]
6. Leisi, R.; di Tommaso, C.; Kempf, C.; Ros, C. The Receptor-Binding Domain in the VP1u Region of Parvovirus B19. *Viruses* **2016**, *8*, 61. [CrossRef]
7. Snijder, J.; van de Waterbeemd, M.; Damoc, E.; Denisov, E.; Grinfeld, D.; Bennett, A.; Agbandje-McKenna, M.; Makarov, A.; Heck, A.J. Defining the stoichiometry and cargo load of viral and bacterial nanoparticles by Orbitrap mass spectrometry. *J. Am. Chem. Soc.* **2014**, *136*, 7295–7299. [CrossRef]
8. Nonnenmacher, M.; Weber, T. Intracellular transport of recombinant adeno-associated virus vectors. *Gene Ther.* **2012**, *19*, 649–658. [CrossRef]
9. Mietzsch, M.; Jose, A.; Chipman, P.; Bhattacharya, N.; Daneshparvar, N.; McKenna, R.; Agbandje-McKenna, M. Completion of the AAV Structural Atlas: Serotype Capsid Structures Reveals Clade-Specific Features. *Viruses* **2021**, *13*, 101. [CrossRef]
10. Mietzsch, M.; McKenna, R.; Vaisanen, E.; Yu, J.C.; Ilyas, M.; Hull, J.A.; Kurian, J.; Smith, J.K.; Chipman, P.; Lasanajak, Y.; et al. Structural Characterization of Cuta- and Tusavirus: Insight into Protoparvoviruses Capsid Morphology. *Viruses* **2020**, *12*, 653. [CrossRef]
11. Yu, J.C.; Mietzsch, M.; Singh, A.; Jimenez Ybargollin, A.; Kailasan, S.; Chipman, P.; Bhattacharya, N.; Fakhiri, J.; Grimm, D.; Kapoor, A.; et al. Characterization of the GBoV1 Capsid and Its Antibody Interactions. *Viruses* **2021**, *13*, 330. [CrossRef] [PubMed]
12. Kronenberg, S.; Bottcher, B.; von der Lieth, C.W.; Bleker, S.; Kleinschmidt, J.A. A conformational change in the adeno-associated virus type 2 capsid leads to the exposure of hidden VP1 N termini. *J. Virol.* **2005**, *79*, 5296–5303. [CrossRef] [PubMed]
13. Ilyas, M.; Mietzsch, M.; Kailasan, S.; Vaisanen, E.; Luo, M.; Chipman, P.; Smith, J.K.; Kurian, J.; Sousa, D.; McKenna, R.; et al. Atomic Resolution Structures of Human Bufaviruses Determined by Cryo-Electron Microscopy. *Viruses* **2018**, *10*, 22. [CrossRef] [PubMed]
14. Qiu, J.; Soderlund-Venermo, M.; Young, N.S. Human Parvoviruses. *Clin. Microbiol. Rev.* **2017**, *30*, 43–113. [CrossRef] [PubMed]
15. Jones, M.S.; Kapoor, A.; Lukashov, V.V.; Simmonds, P.; Hecht, F.; Delwart, E. New DNA viruses identified in patients with acute viral infection syndrome. *J. Virol.* **2005**, *79*, 8230–8236. [CrossRef] [PubMed]
16. Prakash, S.; Shukla, S.; Ramakrishna, V.; Mishra, H.; Bhagat, A.K.; Jain, A. Human Parvovirus 4: A harmless bystander or a pathogen of severe acute respiratory illness. *Int. J. Infect. Dis.* **2020**, *90*, 21–25. [CrossRef]
17. Benjamin, L.A.; Lewthwaite, P.; Vasanthapuram, R.; Zhao, G.; Sharp, C.; Simmonds, P.; Wang, D.; Solomon, T. Human parvovirus 4 as potential cause of encephalitis in children, India. *Emerg. Infect. Dis.* **2011**, *17*, 1484–1487. [CrossRef]
18. Pan, Y.; Wang, Y.; Wang, M.; Zhang, Q.; Baloch, A.R.; Zhou, J.; Ma, J.; Kashif, J.; Xu, G.; Wang, L.; et al. First detection and genetic characterization of ungulate tetraparvovirus 2 and ungulate tetraparvovirus 4 in special livestock on the Qinghai-Tibet Plateau in China. *Virol. J.* **2019**, *16*, 56. [CrossRef]
19. Canuti, M.; Pénzes, J.J.; Lang, A.S. A new perspective on the evolution and diversity of the genus *Amdoparvovirus* (family *Parvoviridae*) through genetic characterization, structural homology modeling, and phylogenetics. *Virus Evol.* **2022**, *8*, veac056. [CrossRef]
20. Markarian, N.M.; Abrahamyan, L. AMDV Vaccine: Challenges and Perspectives. *Viruses* **2021**, *13*, 1833. [CrossRef]
21. Zheng, S.Q.; Palovcak, E.; Armache, J.P.; Verba, K.A.; Cheng, Y.; Agard, D.A. MotionCor2: Anisotropic correction of beam-induced motion for improved cryo-electron microscopy. *Nat. Methods* **2017**, *14*, 331–332. [CrossRef] [PubMed]

22. Grant, T.; Rohou, A.; Grigorieff, N. cisTEM, user-friendly software for single-particle image processing. *eLife* **2018**, *7*, e35383. [CrossRef] [PubMed]
23. Waterhouse, A.; Bertoni, M.; Bienert, S.; Studer, G.; Tauriello, G.; Gumienny, R.; Heer, F.T.; de Beer, T.A.P.; Rempfer, C.; Bordoli, L.; et al. SWISS-MODEL: Homology modelling of protein structures and complexes. *Nucleic Acids Res.* **2018**, *46*, W296–W303. [CrossRef] [PubMed]
24. Ho, P.T.; Montiel-Garcia, D.J.; Wong, J.J.; Carrillo-Tripp, M.; Brooks, C.L., 3rd; Johnson, J.E.; Reddy, V.S. VIPERdb: A Tool for Virus Research. *Annu. Rev. Virol.* **2018**, *5*, 477–488. [CrossRef] [PubMed]
25. Pettersen, E.F.; Goddard, T.D.; Huang, C.C.; Couch, G.S.; Greenblatt, D.M.; Meng, E.C.; Ferrin, T.E. UCSF Chimera—A visualization system for exploratory research and analysis. *J. Comput. Chem.* **2004**, *25*, 1605–1612. [CrossRef]
26. Emsley, P.; Lohkamp, B.; Scott, W.G.; Cowtan, K. Features and development of Coot. *Acta Crystallogr. D Biol. Crystallogr.* **2010**, *66*, 486–501. [CrossRef]
27. Adams, P.D.; Afonine, P.V.; Bunkoczi, G.; Chen, V.B.; Davis, I.W.; Echols, N.; Headd, J.J.; Hung, L.W.; Kapral, G.J.; Grosse-Kunstleve, R.W.; et al. PHENIX: A comprehensive Python-based system for macromolecular structure solution. *Acta Crystallogr. D Biol. Crystallogr.* **2010**, *66*, 213–221. [CrossRef]
28. Cheng, F.; Chen, A.Y.; Best, S.M.; Bloom, M.E.; Pintel, D.; Qiu, J. The capsid proteins of Aleutian mink disease virus activate caspases and are specifically cleaved during infection. *J. Virol.* **2010**, *84*, 2687–2696. [CrossRef]
29. McKenna, R.; Olson, N.H.; Chipman, P.R.; Baker, T.S.; Booth, T.F.; Christensen, J.; Aasted, B.; Fox, J.M.; Bloom, M.E.; Wolfinbarger, J.B.; et al. Three-dimensional structure of Aleutian mink disease parvovirus: Implications for disease pathogenicity. *J. Virol.* **1999**, *73*, 6882–6891. [CrossRef]
30. Subramanian, S.; Organtini, L.J.; Grossman, A.; Domeier, P.P.; Cifuente, J.O.; Makhov, A.M.; Conway, J.F.; D'Abramo, A., Jr.; Cotmore, S.F.; Tattersall, P.; et al. Cryo-EM maps reveal five-fold channel structures and their modification by gatekeeper mutations in the parvovirus minute virus of mice (MVM) capsid. *Virology* **2017**, *510*, 216–223. [CrossRef]
31. Tan, Y.Z.; Aiyer, S.; Mietzsch, M.; Hull, J.A.; McKenna, R.; Grieger, J.; Samulski, R.J.; Baker, T.S.; Agbandje-McKenna, M.; Lyumkis, D. Sub-2 A Ewald curvature corrected structure of an AAV2 capsid variant. *Nat. Commun.* **2018**, *9*, 3628. [CrossRef] [PubMed]
32. Mietzsch, M.; Kailasan, S.; Garrison, J.; Ilyas, M.; Chipman, P.; Kantola, K.; Janssen, M.E.; Spear, J.; Sousa, D.; McKenna, R.; et al. Structural Insights into Human Bocaparvoviruses. *J. Virol.* **2017**, *91*, e00261-17. [CrossRef] [PubMed]
33. Bleker, S.; Pawlita, M.; Kleinschmidt, J.A. Impact of capsid conformation and Rep-capsid interactions on adeno-associated virus type 2 genome packaging. *J. Virol.* **2006**, *80*, 810–820. [CrossRef]
34. Han, M.H.; Jiao, S.; Jia, J.M.; Chen, Y.; Chen, C.Y.; Gucek, M.; Markey, S.P.; Li, Z. The novel caspase-3 substrate Gap43 is involved in AMPA receptor endocytosis and long-term depression. *Mol. Cell Proteom.* **2013**, *12*, 3719–3731. [CrossRef] [PubMed]
35. Laurents, D.V. AlphaFold 2 and NMR Spectroscopy: Partners to Understand Protein Structure, Dynamics and Function. *Front. Mol. Biosci.* **2022**, *9*, 906437. [CrossRef] [PubMed]
36. Chapman, M.S.; Rossmann, M.G. Single-stranded DNA-protein interactions in canine parvovirus. *Structure* **1995**, *3*, 151–162. [CrossRef]
37. Lou, S.; Xu, B.; Huang, Q.; Zhi, N.; Cheng, F.; Wong, S.; Brown, K.; Delwart, E.; Liu, Z.; Qiu, J. Molecular characterization of the newly identified human parvovirus 4 in the family Parvoviridae. *Virology* **2012**, *422*, 59–69. [CrossRef]
38. Lakshmanan, R.V.; Hull, J.A.; Berry, L.; Burg, M.; Bothner, B.; McKenna, R.; Agbandje-McKenna, M. Structural Dynamics and Activity of B19V VP1u during the pHs of Cell Entry and Endosomal Trafficking. *Viruses* **2022**, *14*, 1922. [CrossRef]
39. Dudek, A.M.; Zabaleta, N.; Zinn, E.; Pillay, S.; Zengel, J.; Porter, C.; Franceschini, J.S.; Estelien, R.; Carette, J.E.; Zhou, G.L.; et al. GPR108 Is a Highly Conserved AAV Entry Factor. *Mol. Ther.* **2020**, *28*, 367–381. [CrossRef]
40. Kaufmann, B.; Chipman, P.R.; Kostyuchenko, V.A.; Modrow, S.; Rossmann, M.G. Visualization of the externalized VP2 N termini of infectious human parvovirus B19. *J. Virol.* **2008**, *82*, 7306–7312. [CrossRef]
41. Aasted, B.; Alexandersen, S.; Christensen, J. Vaccination with Aleutian mink disease parvovirus (AMDV) capsid proteins enhances disease, while vaccination with the major non-structural AMDV protein causes partial protection from disease. *Vaccine* **1998**, *16*, 1158–1165. [CrossRef]
42. Kanno, H.; Wolfinbarger, J.B.; Bloom, M.E. Aleutian mink disease parvovirus infection of mink macrophages and human macrophage cell line U937: Demonstration of antibody-dependent enhancement of infection. *J. Virol.* **1993**, *67*, 7017–7024. [CrossRef] [PubMed]
43. Pyöriä, L.; Toppinen, M.; Mäntylä, E.; Hedman, L.; Aaltonen, L.M.; Vihinen-Ranta, M.; Ilmarinen, T.; Söderlund-Venermo, M.; Hedman, K.; Perdomo, M.F. Extinct type of human parvovirus B19 persists in tonsillar B cells. *Nat. Commun.* **2017**, *8*, 14930. [CrossRef] [PubMed]
44. Xu, M.; Perdomo, M.F.; Mattola, S.; Pyöriä, L.; Toppinen, M.; Qiu, J.; Vihinen-Ranta, M.; Hedman, K.; Nokso-Koivisto, J.; Aaltonen, L.M.; et al. Persistence of Human Bocavirus 1 in Tonsillar Germinal Centers and Antibody-Dependent Enhancement of Infection. *mBio* **2021**, *12*, e03132-20. [CrossRef] [PubMed]
45. Emmanuel, S.N.; Mietzsch, M.; Tseng, Y.S.; Smith, J.K.; Agbandje-McKenna, M. Parvovirus Capsid-Antibody Complex Structures Reveal Conservation of Antigenic Epitopes Across the Family. *Viral Immunol.* **2021**, *34*, 3–17. [CrossRef]

viruses

MDPI

Article

Structural Characterization of Canine Minute Virus, Rat and Porcine Bocavirus

Michael Velez [1], Mario Mietzsch [1,*], Jane Hsi [1], Logan Bell [1], Paul Chipman [1], Xiaofeng Fu [2] and Robert McKenna [1,*]

1 Department of Biochemistry & Molecular Biology, University of Florida, Gainesville, FL 32610, USA
2 Biological Science Imaging Resource, Department of Biological Sciences, Florida State University, Tallahassee, FL 32306, USA
* Correspondence: mario.mietzsch@ufl.edu (M.M.); rmckenna@ufl.edu (R.M.)

Abstract: *Bocaparvovirus* is an expansive genus of the *Parvovirinae*, with a wide range of vertebrate hosts. This study investigates Canine minute virus (CnMV), Rat bocavirus (RBoV), and Porcine bocavirus 1 (PBoV1). Both CnMV and PBoV1 have been found in gastrointestinal infections in their respective hosts, with CnMV responsible for spontaneous abortions in dogs, while PBoV has been associated with encephalomyelitis in piglets. The pathogenicity of the recently identified RBoV is currently unknown. To initiate the characterization of these viruses, their capsids structures were determined by cryo-electron microscopy at resolutions ranging from 2.3 to 2.7 Å. Compared to other parvoviruses, the CnMV, PBoV1, and RBoV capsids showed conserved features, such as the channel at the fivefold symmetry axis. However, major differences were observed at the two- and threefold axes. While CnMV displays prominent threefold protrusions, the same region is more recessed in PBoV1 and RBoV. Furthermore, the typical twofold axis depression of parvoviral capsids is absent in CnMV or very small in PBoV and RBoV. These capsid structures extend the structural portfolio for the *Bocaparvovirus* genus and will allow future characterization of these pathogens on a molecular level. This is important, as no antivirals or vaccines exist for these viruses.

Keywords: parvovirus; bocavirus; capsid; cryo-EM; pathogen; CnMV; PBoV; RBoV

Citation: Velez, M.; Mietzsch, M.; Hsi, J.; Bell, L.; Chipman, P.; Fu, X.; McKenna, R. Structural Characterization of Canine Minute Virus, Rat and Porcine Bocavirus. *Viruses* **2023**, *15*, 1799. https://doi.org/10.3390/v15091799

Academic Editor: Giorgio Gallinella

Received: 4 August 2023
Revised: 18 August 2023
Accepted: 22 August 2023
Published: 24 August 2023

1. Introduction

Parvoviridae is a family of small, non-enveloped viruses with a linear single-stranded (ss) DNA genome of around 4–6 kb [1]. The family is divided into three subfamilies, *Parvovirinae*, *Densovirinae*, and *Hamaparvovirinae*. Members of the *Parvovirinae* exclusively infect vertebrates, *Densovirinae* infect invertebrates, whereas the *Hamaparvovirinae* subfamily contains members that infect either vertebrates or invertebrates [2]. Within the *Parvovirinae* subfamily, the *Bocaparvovirus* genus is the largest, with currently 31 described member species, containing a large number of pathogenic viruses [3].

Bocaviruses possess a ~5.5 kb ssDNA genome with two flanking terminal repeats at either end, involved in replication and genome packaging [4]. Located between these repeats are three major open reading frames (ORFs), NS1, NP1, VP, and a single promoter. Unique to bocaviruses is the NP1 ORF located between the NS1 and VP ORF [5], which was shown to play a role in mRNA processing and subsequent capsid protein expression [5]. The NS1 ORF contains the *ns* gene coding for non-structural protein 1 (NS1), which is responsible for replication and DNA packaging [6]. The VP ORF contains the *cap* gene, which expresses the structural or viral proteins VP1 and VP2 (in addition, some bocaviruses also express a third, VP3) [1,7]. The VPs overlap at their C-termini, with VP2 completely contained in VP1. VP1 possesses a unique N-terminal region (VP1u) with an enzymatic phospholipase A_2 motif, needed for endosomal/lysosomal escape during infection [8], and is expressed approximately tenfold less compared to VP2. Thus, the assembled T = 1 icosahedral capsid, consisting of 60 VPs, is primarily composed of VP2 [7,9].

To date, the capsid structures of six bocaviruses have been determined, either by X-ray crystallography in the case of bovine parvovirus (BPV) [10] or by cryo-electron microscopy (cryo-EM) in the case of the human bocaviruses 1–4 (HBoV1-4) and gorilla bocavirus 1 (GBoV1) [11–13]. Their VP structures contain a conserved eight-stranded jelly roll motif (βB-βI), an additional beta-strand antiparallel to βB, and two alpha helices. The connecting loops between the β-strands are named based on the flanking beta-strands (e.g., DE-loop). These loops form the capsid surface of the virus and display the highest sequence and structural variability within the genus and to other parvoviruses. Ten variable regions (VRs) have been defined for the bocaviruses [14]. In the icosahedral capsid, the 60 VPs assemble via two-, three-, and fivefold symmetry-related VP interactions, resulting in pores at the fivefold symmetry axes, protrusions surrounding the threefold axes, and depressions at the twofold axes [9].

Canine Minute Virus (CnMV) was first isolated from German military dogs in 1967 and was initially thought to be non-pathogenic [15]. Later, it was found to be pathogenic in newborn puppies and fetuses, as the virus was found in the lungs and intestines of nursing puppies, leading to lesions, diarrhea, and death [16]. The CnMV infections were also found to be responsible for abortions of fetuses in dogs [17]. Furthermore, the virus has recently been indicated as a cause for hepatitis in dogs [18]. The capsid (VP1) amino acid sequence identity is 40% and 45% to BPV and HBoV1, respectively.

The first porcine bocavirus (PBoV) was identified in Swedish pigs in 2009 [19]. It was found to be a co-infective agent with Porcine circovirus 2 (PCV2) in postweaning multisystemic wasting syndrome. It has since then been identified in pigs globally, disproportionally affecting piglets aged 3–6 months [20]. It is often found in co-infections of piglets with PCV2, Porcine Torque teno virus (PTTV), Porcine reproductive and respiratory syndrome virus (PRRSV), Classical swine fever virus (CSFV), Porcine epidemic diarrhea virus (PEDV), Porcine kobuvirus (PKoV), Group A rotavirus (GARV), and Transmissible gastroenteritis virus (TGEV) [21–24]. PBoV is usually associated with diarrhea and upper respiratory tract infections in piglets, but a case study in 2016 associated PBoV with a case of encephalomyelitis in a 6-week-old piglet in Germany [24]. Noteworthy, PBoV infections are not exclusive to pigs. In 2018, PBoV was isolated from an upper respiratory infection in a 3-year-old child in northeastern Iran [25], raising public health concerns, considering the fact that these animals are found in close proximity with humans, and these viruses have the capacity to jump to a human host. There are a large number of PBoV strains, which exhibit significant genetic variability [26]. The capsid (VP1) amino acid sequence identity of PBoV1 is 42% and 47% for BPV and HBoV1, respectively.

Rodents are a large and diverse order of mammals living in close proximity to humans, making them an optimal reservoir for emerging pathogens [27]. This characteristic makes identifying pathogens in rodent populations a necessary precaution for public health. In 2017, rat bocavirus (RBoV) was identified from brown rats in China. As a recent addition to the *Bocaparvovirus* genus, its pathogenicity is still unknown, but has been shown to have broad tissue tropism [28]. Its capsid (VP1) amino acid sequence identity is 37% and 41% for BPV and HBoV1, respectively.

The goal of this study was to structurally characterize the capsids of CnMV, PBoV1, and RBoV to obtain further insights into the structural repertoire of this genus of the *Parvovirinae*. The high-resolution structures for these virus capsids, determined using cryo-electron microscopy (cryo-EM) and 3D image reconstruction, are reported. The capsids shared features characteristic of all parvoviruses, such as the fivefold channel and threefold protrusion, but CnMV and RBoV diverge from the other bocaviruses, as they lack a twofold depression. The VP2 monomer of all three viruses exhibited the conserved features observed in other major capsid proteins within the genus, such as the 8-stranded beta-sheet, but also varied, with an additional alpha helix (αC) observed. High variance was observed in VR III and IX, which appeared to translate to the lack of the twofold depression in the CnMV and RBoV capsid. Additionally, insertions in VR IV, V, and VIII are responsible for a change in the phenotype of the threefold protrusions for these viruses.

These observations help establish a structural platform for further research into these viruses and the *Bocaparvovirus* genus.

2. Materials and Methods

2.1. Virus-like Production and Purification

Virus-like particles (VLPs) of CnMV, PBoV, and RBoV were expressed using the Bac-to-Bac baculovirus system, as described previously and following the manufacturer's protocol [29]. The open reading frames for VP2 were synthesized (Azenta/Genewiz) and inserted into the pFastBac plasmid (CnMV: nt 3329-5044, accession # NC_004442.1; PBoV1: nt 3417-5120, accession # NC_024453.2; RBoV: nt 32624965, accession # NC_029133.1). For VLP production, suspension Sf9 insect cells were cultured in Sf-900 II SFM media and infected with the recombinant baculoviruses at a multiplicity of infection of 5 plaque-forming units. The cells were harvested 72 h post infection and pelleted by centrifugation at 1000× *g* for 20 min at 4 °C. The Sf9 cell pellets were resuspended in TNTM buffer (25 mM Tris-HCl, 100 mM NaCl, 0.2% Triton X-100, 2 mM $MgCl_2$, pH 8.0) and subjected to three freeze–thaw cycles. The lysates were benzonase-treated (125 U/mL) for 1 h at 37 °C and clarified by centrifugation at 12,000× *g* for 30 min to remove cell debris. The supernatant was loaded onto a 20% sucrose cushion (*w*/*v* sucrose in TNTM buffer) and centrifuged at 45,000 rpm, using a Ti70 rotor for 3 h at 4 °C. The resulting pellet was resuspended in TNTM buffer, loaded onto a 10–40% sucrose step gradient (*w*/*v* sucrose in TNTM buffer), and centrifuged using a SW41 rotor for 3 h at 4 °C. Individual fractions were recovered from the gradient and analyzed by SDS-PAGE. Fractions containing the expected VP2 band at ~60 kDa were dialyzed in phosphate-buffered saline (PBS), concentrated to > 0.5 mg/mL using Apollo concentrators (Orbital Biosciences, Topsfield, MA, USA), and stored at −20 °C. The integrity of the capsids was analyzed via negative stain electron microscopy using a Tecnai G2 Spirit electron microscope at 200 kV, as described previously [30].

2.2. Cryo-EM Data Collection

Aliquots of the purified CnMV, PBoV1, and RBoV samples were applied to glow discharged, holey carbon grids and the grids vitrified in liquid ethane using a Vitrobot Mark 4 (FEI) at 95% humidity and 4 °C. The grids were screened for the VLP's particle distribution using a Tecnai G2 F20-TWIN transmission electron microscope (FEI) at 200 kV under low-dose conditions (20 $e^-/Å^2$) at a magnification of 82,500-fold on a 16-megapixel charge-coupled device (CCD) camera. High-resolution data for the CnMV sample were collected at the Florida State University through the Southeastern Consortium for Microscopy of Macro Molecular Machines (SECM4), using a Titan Krios electron microscope with a DE-64 detector. The microscope was run at 300 kV, with a total dose of 59 $e^-/Å^2$ to collect 52 frames per micrograph. Data for RBoV and PBoV were collected at the Stanford-SLAC Cryo-EM Center (S^2C^2), using a Titan Krios (FEI) electron microscope operated at 300 kV, equipped with a Falcon 4 direct electron detector (Thermo Fisher). A total of 50 movie frames were collected per micrograph at a total electron dose of ~50 $e^-/Å^2$. The movie frames were aligned using MotionCor2, as described previously [31].

2.3. Three-Dimensional Particle Reconstruction

The software package cisTEM was used to reconstruct the individual two-dimensional images to three-dimensional electron density maps of the reported viruses, as reported previously [32]. Briefly, the aligned micrographs were imported and their contrast transfer functions (CTFs) calculated. Micrographs of poor quality were removed and capsids automatically picked using a characteristic particle radius of 125 Å. The individual capsid images were sorted via 2D classification into 20 classes. Classes containing impurities were discarded. The Ab-Initio 3D function was utilized to generate an initial map from 10% of the particles. This map was further refined using the automatic refinement function with default settings. The resolutions of the reported maps were determined at a Fourier shell correlation (FSC) criterion threshold of 0.143. The final electron density maps were sharpened using the pre-cut off B-factor value of −90 Å^2 and variable post-cut off B-factor values of 0, 20, and 50 Å^2.

2.4. Model Building and Structure Refinement

Initial atomic VP models for CnMV, RBoV, and PBoV1 were generated with SWISS-MODEL, using their primary amino acid sequences and the capsid structure of HBoV1 as a template [33]. Full capsid models (60 copies of VP2) were created using VIPERdb2 oligomer generator [34]. These models were fitted in their respective density map in UCSF-Chimera [35] and their pixel size adjusted using MAPMAN [36]. The EM density maps and monomer models of the viruses were then imported into Coot, where manual model building and real-space refinement tools were used to improve the capsid models to better fit their electron density maps [37]. Finally, the 60-mer capsid models were automatically refined, using the real-space-refine subroutine in PHENIX with default settings, which also provided refinement statistics [38] (Table 1).

Table 1. Summary of data collection, image processing, and refinement statistics.

Parameter	CnMV	PBoV1	RBoV
Total no. of micrographs	653	7949	7616
Defocus range (µm)	0.5–2.0	0.8–2.1	0.8–2.1
Electron dose (e^-/Å^2)	59	50	50
No. of frames/micrograph	52	50	50
Pixel size (Å/pixel)	0.92	0.95	0.95
No. of particles used for final map	50,866	98,388	9199
Resolution of final map (Å)	2.72	2.31	2.52
PHENIX model refinement statistics			
Map CC	0.84	0.88	0.88
RMSD Bonds (Å)	0.01	0.01	0.01
RMSD Angles (°)	0.83	0.90	0.82
All-atom clash score	9.34	7.81	7.95
Ramachandran plot (%)			
Favored	97.8	97.9	98.5
Allowed	2.2	2.1	1.5
Outliers	0.0	0.0	0.0
Rotamer outliers	0.0	0.0	0.0
No. of C_β deviations	0	0	0

2.5. Structural Comparison

The capsid surface morphology of CnMV, RBoV, PBoV, and HBoV1 were visually compared using Chimera, while the VP2 models of these viruses were superposed in Coot to obtain overall paired RMSDs between Cα positions and to identify regions of structural similarities and differences. Deviations between non-overlapping Cα positions, because of residue deletion/insertions, were measured using the distance tool in Coot. Regions of two or more adjacent amino acids with ≥2.0 Å difference in superposed VP2 Cα position were considered to be structurally diverse and assigned to the previously described VRs. This information was also used for a structure-based sequence alignment, and to calculate the structural identity (in %) that was defined as the number of aligned residues (≤2.0 Å apart) divided by the total number of residues. Amino acid sequence alignments of the different bocaparvoviruses were performed utilizing the sequence alignment option in VectorNTI (Invitrogen, Waltham, MA, USA).

3. Results and Discussion

3.1. Expression and Purification of VLPs of CnMV, PBoV, and RBoV

To expand the structural repertoire of determined capsid structures for the diverse Bocaparvovirus genus, viruses infecting dogs (CnMV), pigs (PBoV1), and rats (RBoV) were selected. The ORFs of these viruses coding for the major capsid protein VP2 were cloned into the pFastBac1 plasmid to enable the production of the virus-like particles (VLPs), using the Bac-to-Bac expression system in insect Sf9 cells. Following the production and purification of the VLPs, the samples were analyzed for their purity by SDS-PAGE. For all of the three viruses, a band consistent with VP2, migrating at ~60 kDa, was observed (Figure 1). Further analysis of these samples by cryo-EM showed intact capsids of approximately 25 nm in diameter, and thus, they were deemed suitable for high-resolution cryo-EM data collection.

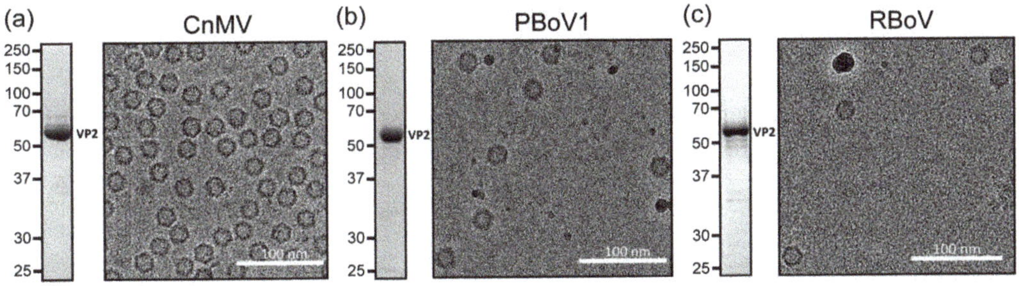

Figure 1. Expression and purification of CnMV, RBoV, and PBoV VLPs. (**a**) An SDS-PAGE of CnMV showing a band at 60 kDa consistent with VP2. To the right, a cryo-EM micrograph of the same sample shows intact capsids of ~25 nm in diameter. (**b**) Depiction as in (**a**) for PBoV1 and for (**c**) RBoV.

3.2. Determination of the CnMV, PBoV1, and RBoV Capsid Structures

Following cryo-EM data collection, three-dimensional-image reconstruction of the capsids, utilizing 50,866 (CnMV), 98,388 (PBoV1), and 9199 (RBoV) individual capsid images, resulted in a resolution of 2.72, 2.31, and 2.52 Å, respectively (Table 1). The reconstructed capsids all exhibited a conserved channel at the fivefold symmetry axes surrounded by a depression (Figure 2a). This feature is found in all capsids of the *Bocaparvovirus* genus, as well as other genera of the subfamily determined [9,32]. In contrast, significant differences among these viruses were observed at the two- and threefold regions to each other and to other bocavirus capsids. A depression at the icosahedral twofold axis is a common feature of capsids in the Parvovirinae subfamily. However, for the viruses characterized in this study, the twofold depressions are either insignificant (PBoV1) or non-existent (CnMV). At the threefold axes, typically protrusions are found for the *Parvovirinae*. Capsid structures previously determined for the *Bocaparvovirus* genus showed disperse protrusions surrounding the threefold axis that do not significantly extend radially from the capsid surface [10–13]. In contrast, the CnMV capsid shows very prominent threefold protrusions, while PBoV1 and RBoV follow the previously described characteristics of the genus (Figure 2a). These differences also result in the CnMV capsid having a larger max. diameter of 289 Å, compared to RBoV1 and RBoV with 275 and 277 Å, respectively. Another feature previously observed for the bocaviruses, with the exception of GBoV1, was the presence of density extending into the interior of the capsid below the fivefold channel [10–13]. This density was also seen for CnMV, but is absent in the PBoV1 and RBoV capsids (Figure 2b). The region below the fivefold channel is also the location of the N-termini of the ordered VP structure for all parvoviruses. It is characterized by a glycine-rich sequence that is hypothesized to act as a hinge for the externalization of the VP1u to utilize its PLA2 activity [39,40]. In CnMV 16, in PBoV1 20, and in RBoV 19, glycines are found within the first ~40 amino acids. However, the number of glycines does not correlate with the presence of the density below the fivefold channel, as BPV, HBoV1-4, and GBoV1 possess only 10–13 glycines in the corresponding region.

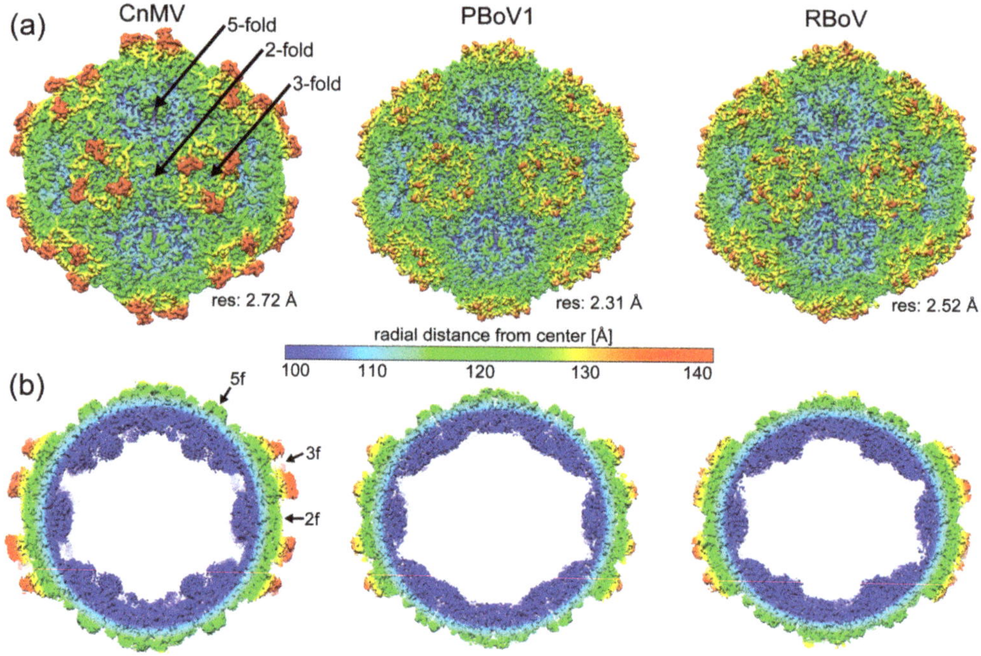

Figure 2. Determination of the CnMV, PBoV1, and RBoV capsid structures. (**a**) Capsid surface density maps of CnMV, PBoV1, and RBoV contoured at a 2 sigma (σ) threshold level. The maps are radially colored (blue to red) according to distance to the capsid center, as indicated by the scale bar in the center. The approximate icosahedral two-, three-, and fivefold axes are indicated. (**b**) Cross-sectional views of the CnMV, PBoV1, and RBoV density map at a 0.5σ threshold.

3.3. *CnMV, PBoV1, and RBoV Possess an Additional Surface α-Helix*

The high resolution of the cryo-EM maps allowed the building of reliable atomic models, starting from amino acids 34, 41, and 42 (VP2 numbering) at the N-terminus for CnMV, PBoV1, and RBoV, respectively. Structural order was observed at the C-terminus with highly ordered amino acid side-chain densities (Figure 3a). In the case of PBoV1 and RBoV, the cryo-EM maps for the most part also showed densities for the carbonyl groups of the main-chain and densities for a specific rotamer for the individual amino acids, guiding the model building for these viruses. The overall models showed good refinement statistics and high map correlation coefficients (CC) of 0.84 to 0.88 (Table 1).

The VP structures of CnMV, PBoV1, and RBoV conserve the features previously described for other bocaviruses, which comprise the eight-stranded jelly roll motif (βB-βI), including the additional beta-strand A and two alpha helices (αA and αB). While the α-helix A (10 amino acids) is part of the core capsid and found in all parvoviruses, α-helix B (8 amino acids) is located at the surface in the VR-III-loop and specific for the *Bocaparvovirus* genus. In the structures described here, an additional α-helix C (seven amino acids) is present in the VR-V loop (Figure 3b). Currently, the only other virus of the *Parvovirinae* with an α-helix at the capsid surface is the Aleutian Mink Disease Virus (AMDV) of the *Amdoparvovirus* genus [32]. However, unlike for the bocaviruses, AMDV's α-helix is located in the VR-VIII loop.

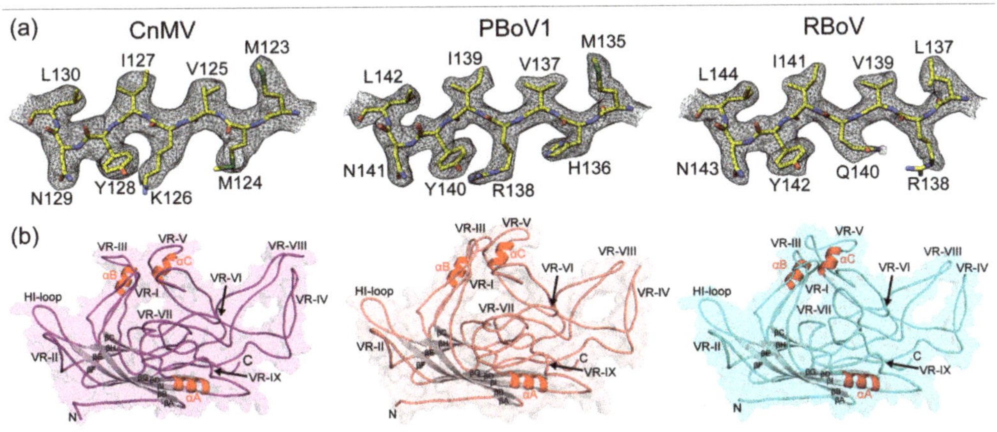

Figure 3. The VP structure of CnMV, PBoV1, and RBoV. (**a**) Amino acid residues modeled for the βD strand are shown inside their density maps at a sigma (σ) threshold of 2.5 (in black). The amino acid residues are labeled and shown as stick representations and colored according to atom type: C = yellow, O = red, N = blue, S = green. These images were generated using UCSF-Chimera [35]. (**b**) The VP structures are shown as ribbon diagrams inside transparent surface representations. The secondary structure elements (α-helices in red, β-strands in gray), the N- and C-termini, and variable regions (VRs) are labeled.

3.4. Structural Differences among the Bocaviruses Are Localized to the Variable Regions

In order to obtain an overview of the structural repertoire within the *Bocaparvovirus* genus, CnMV, PBoV1, and RBoV were compared to each other, but also to previously determined capsids structures of BPV and HBoV1 (Figure 4a). The amino acid sequence identity among these viruses for the structural ordered VP ranges from 41 to 54% (Figure 4b). HBoV1 acts as representative for the other HBoV genotypes and GBoV1 since their sequence identities are in the 77–90% range [12]. As expected, the capsid cores for all bocaviruses are nearly perfectly superposable (Figure 4a). It is also the region where the highest level of sequence conservation is found. In contrast, low sequence identities and significant structural differences were observed in the previously defined VRs for this genus when comparing these five viruses, resulting in overall structural similarities of 76–91% [10]. The least variability is found in the fivefold region with VR-II and the HI-loop (also known as VR-VIIIB). In VR-II, none of the viruses possess an insertion or deletion, and only HBoV1's loop shows some structural divergence, with a max. Cα-Cα distance of ~6 Å compared to CnMV (Figure 4a). The HI-loop is structurally conserved among the bocaviruses, with the exception of BPV due to a 2 aa deletion in this virus compared to the other bocaviruses. The greater structural conservation of the fivefold region among viruses of the same genus is also observed for the *Dependoparvovirus* and *Protoparvovirus* genera [41,42], likely because the Rep or NS proteins, which usually show higher conservation compared to the capsid, bind to this region during genome packaging [39]. For viruses of different genera, the fivefold regions show significant structural variability [32], possibly reflecting differences between the NS or Rep proteins.

The other capsid surface loops show much higher structural variability. The threefold region is primarily composed of VR-IV, -V, and -VIII (Figure 5). The more prominent threefold protrusions of CnMV are the result of significant insertions into VR-IV (+1 aa vs. BPV, +2 aa vs. PBoV1 and HBoV1, +4 aa vs. RBoV) and VR-VIII (+12 aa vs. PBoV1, +13 aa vs. RBoV, +15 aa vs. BPV, +17 aa vs. HBoV1) (Figure 4). Between the threefold protrusions, CnMV's VR-V is considerably more extensive in all of the newly determined bocaviruses (−3 aa vs. RBoV, −2 aa vs. PBoV1, +17 aa vs. BPV, +18 aa vs. HBoV1). Thus, the presence of α-helix C exclusively in CnMV, PBoV1, and RBoV (Figure 3b) is the result of the additional amino acids in this loop. The threefold region has been shown to display epitopes for neutralizing antibodies and receptor binding sites in other parvoviruses [43,44]. Currently, O-linked α2-3 sialic acid attached to glycophorin A is the only described receptor for BPV in the genus *Bocaparvovirus* [45,46]. However, its binding site has not been determined yet.

(a)

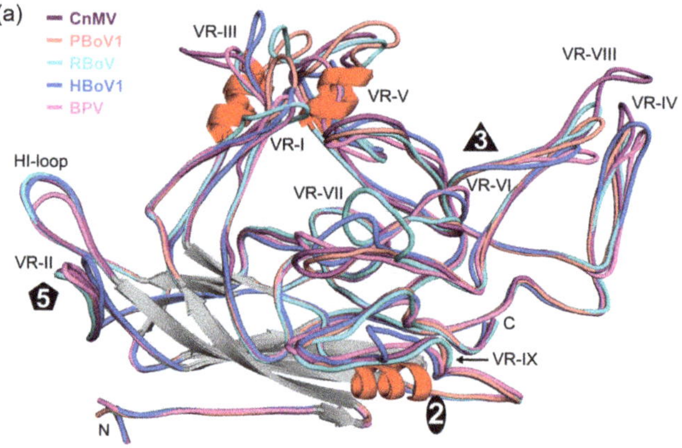

(b)

amino acid sequence identity of VP structure (in %)

	CnMV	PBoV1	RBoV	HBoV1	BPV
CnMV		54	44	45	42
PBoV1	91		50	50	45
RBoV	85	85		49	41
HBoV1	82	80	76		48
BPV	84	81	78	85	

structurally aligned amino acids: Cα distance < 2 Å (in %)

Figure 4. Sequence and structure comparison within the *Bocaparvovirus* genus. (**a**) Superposition of CnMV (purple), PBoV1 (salmon), RBoV (cyan), HBoV1 (blue), and BPV (pink). The variable regions, the N- and C-termini, and the approximate location of the icosahedral two-, three-, and fivefold axes are shown. (**b**) Amino acid sequence identity comparison of the structurally ordered VP region for the given viruses (top right, in %). The structural similarity is shown in the bottom left corner and was defined as the percentage of aligned Cα atoms of the amino acid chain within 2 Å distance when the capsid structures were superposed.

The twofold symmetry axis is surrounded by VR-I, VR-III, VR-VI, VR-VII, and VR-IX. Usually, VR-I, VR-III, and parts of VR-IX form the two–fivefold wall on the capsid [10,11]. However, due to the lack of a significant depression at the twofold axis, this capsid feature is absent in the newly determined bocavirus capsids. The lack of any twofold depression in CnMV is caused by an insertion in VR-III (+2 aa vs. HBoV1, +3 aa vs. PBoV1, + 6 aa vs. RBoV and BPV) and its loop conformation advancing towards the twofold symmetry axis (Figure 5). In PBoV1 and RBoV, the shorter VR-III does not cover the entire twofold region, but their loop also advances the twofold axis and restricts the size of the depression. Additionally, a different loop confirmation of VR-IX in CnMV, PBoV1, and RBoV compared to HBoV1 and BPV near the twofold axis (Figure 4a) further causes an increase in the radial capsid surface in this region. Previously, a seven amino acid insertion of HBoV1 in VR-IX (aa 505–511, Figure 4a) was suggested to be a host determinant. None of the newly determined capsid structures possess this insertion, and therefore, this feature currently remains specific for primate bocaviruses.

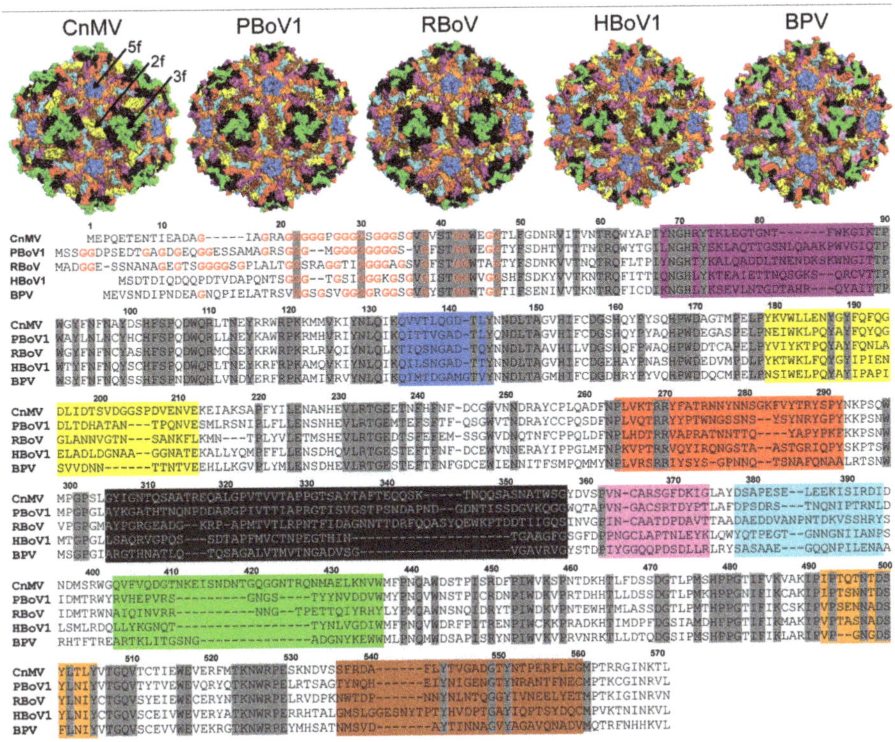

Figure 5. Location of the VRs on the capsid surface. Capsid surface representations of the bocaviruses with the VRs colored (VR-I = purple, VR-II = blue, VR-III = yellow, VR-IV = red, VR-V = dark gray, VR-VI = pink, VR-VII = cyan, VR-VIII = green, HI-loop = orange, VR-IX = brown). The approximate icosahedral two- (2f), three- (3f), and fivefold (5f) axes are indicated on the CnMV capsid. These images were generated using PyMol [47]. The residue range of the colored VRs is shown in the amino acid sequence alignment below. Amino acid numbering, based on the CnMV sequence, is shown above the alignment. Conserved amino acids are highlighted in gray and the glycines near the N-terminus colored red.

In contrast to VR-III, CnMV's VR-I is the shortest loop in comparison to the other bocaviruses (−3 aa vs. BPV, −4 aa vs. HBoV1, −6 aa vs. PBoV1 and RBoV) and is located between the threefold protrusion and the fivefold region (Figure 5). The VR-VI loop, while being only 1 aa shorter in CnMV, PBoV1, and RBoV compared to HBoV1 and BPV, is not surface-exposed in the former viruses caused by the much longer VR-V loop situated above this loop. The VR-VII loop is located at the base of the threefold protrusion in CnMV. Probably due to the different appearance of the threefold region, this loop also displays high structural heterogeneity among the bocaviruses (Figure 4a). The longest loop is found in RBoV (+2 aa vs. CnMV and HBoV1, +4 aa vs. PBoV1), with an up to 13 Å Cα-Cα distance.

To date, most bocavirus capsids have not been studied on a molecular level. However, recent studies have analyzed the impact of natural-occurring and engineered capsid variants of HBoV1 on infectivity and antigenicity due to the interest of using bocaviral vectors for gene therapy applications [48]. The previously mapped monoclonal antibodies to the HBoV capsids [43] are unlikely to bind to CnMV, PBoV1, or RBoV capsids, as the loops vary significantly in structure and amino acid sequence, as described above. However, natural exposure to these viruses may result in some seroprevalence in the human population, as the hosts of these viruses live in close proximity to humans. Consequently, a PBoV strain was isolated from an upper respiratory infection in a 3-year-old child in northeastern Iran in 2018 [25]. Similar crossings of species have been shown previously for parvoviruses.

For example, the emergence of Canine parvovirus (CPV) in the 1970s was a result of cross-species transfer from Feline panleukopenia virus (FPV), resulting in a deadly pandemic in canines [49]. Thus, studying these viruses is not only of interest for the health of livestock and pets, but also a public health concern.

4. Conclusions

The *bocaparvovirus* genus contains a large group of virus species in the *Parvovirinae* subfamily, with members infecting a wide range of vertebrate hosts. Prior to this study, only the primate bocaviruses, HBoV1-4 and GBoV1, and bovine parvovirus, BPV, had been structurally characterized, covering only a small number of the viruses host diversity of this extensive genus. The determination of the CnMV, PBoV1, and RBoV capsid structure expands the structural atlas for this genus. For other genera, such as the *Protoparvovirus* genus, viruses infecting the same hosts have been described, such as CPV, porcine parvovirus, or H-1 parvovirus. However, no significant structural similarities, except for the capsid core, which is shared among all parvoviruses, were observed, and the amino acid sequence identities among the viruses of the same host range from 17 to 23%.

Compared to the previously published bocavirus capsid structures, the CnMV, PBoV1, and RBoV capsids show a higher level of structural heterogeneity (Figure 6). However, currently, many of these viruses are poorly understood. Thus, the capsid structures will help future characterization of these pathogens on a molecular level, in particular, in the absence of antivirals or vaccines.

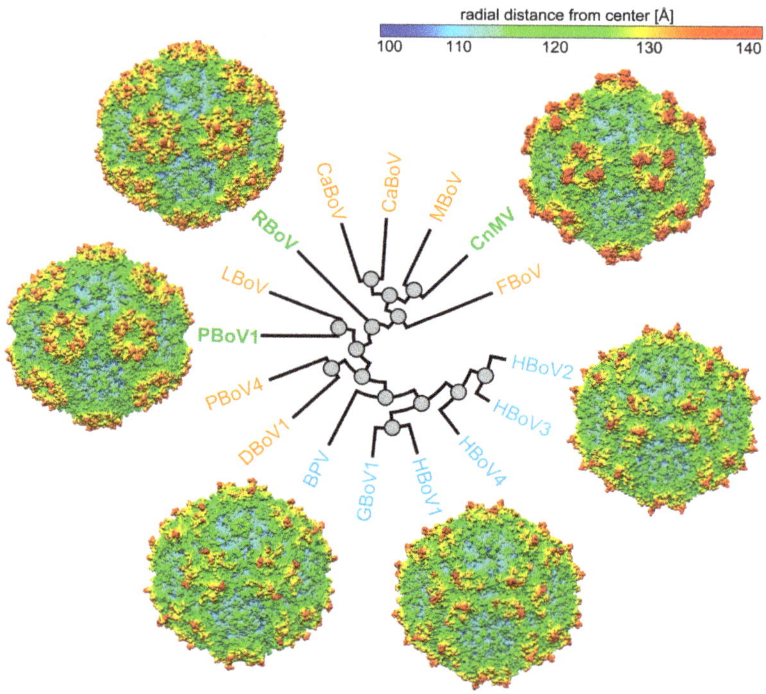

Figure 6. Capsid structures of the genus *Bocaparvovirus*. Radial dendrogram of selected bocaviruses using their VP2 amino acid sequence, generated at https://ngphylogeny.fr/ (accessed on 12 July 2023). The viruses for which capsid structures were previously determined are colored blue, those that are determined in this study are colored green, and the viruses without a known capsid structure are orange. Capsid surface maps based on the atomic model are shown for CnMV,

HBoV2, HBoV1, BPV, PBoV1, and RBoV (ordered clockwise). The maps are radially colored (blue to red) according to distance to the capsid center, as indicated by the scale bar. DBoV: dromedary camel bocavirus, LBoV: rabbit bocavirus, MBoV: mink bocavirus, CslBoV: California sea lion bocavirus, CaBoV: canine bocavirus, FBoV: feline bocavirus.

Author Contributions: Conceptualization, M.M. and R.M.; investigation, M.V., J.H. and L.B.; resources, P.C. and X.F.; writing—original draft preparation, M.V. and M.M.; writing—review and editing, M.M. and R.M.; visualization, M.V. and M.M..; supervision, M.M. and R.M.; project administration, R.M.; funding acquisition, R.M. All authors have read and agreed to the published version of the manuscript.

Funding: This study was funded by the NIH grant R01 NIH GM082946 (to R.M.). Data collection at Florida State University through the Southeastern Consortium for Microscopy of Macro Molecular Machines (SECM4) was made possible by NIH grants S10OD018142-01, S10RR025080-01, and U24GM116788.

Institutional Review Board Statement: Not applicable.

Informed Consent Statement: Not applicable.

Data Availability Statement: The CnMV, PBoV1, and RBoV cryo-EM-reconstructed density maps and models built for their capsids were deposited in the Electron Microscopy Data Bank (EMDB) with the accession numbers EMD-41614/PDB ID 8TU0 (CnMV), EMD-41615/PDB ID 8TU01 (PBoV1), and 41616/PDB ID 8TU2 (RBoV).

Acknowledgments: The authors wish to thank the late Mavis Agbandje-McKenna for initiating this research project and for her pioneering studies of parvovirus capsid structures. The authors also want to thank the UF-ICBR Electron Microscopy Core (RRID:SCR_019146) for access to electron microscopes utilized for cryo-electron micrograph screening. Some of this work was performed at the Stanford-SLAC Cryo-EM Center (S^2C^2), which is supported by the National Institutes of Health Common Fund Transformative High-Resolution Cryo-Electron Microscopy program (U24 GM129541). The content is solely the responsibility of the authors and does not necessarily represent the official views of the National Institutes of Health.

Conflicts of Interest: The authors declare no conflict of interest.

References

1. Cotmore, S.F.; Agbandje-McKenna, M.; Canuti, M.; Chiorini, J.A.; Eis-Hubinger, A.M.; Hughes, J.; Mietzsch, M.; Modha, S.; Ogliastro, M.; Penzes, J.J.; et al. ICTV Virus Taxonomy Profile: Parvoviridae. *J. Gen. Virol.* **2019**, *100*, 367–368. [CrossRef] [PubMed]
2. Penzes, J.J.; Soderlund-Venermo, M.; Canuti, M.; Eis-Hubinger, A.M.; Hughes, J.; Cotmore, S.F.; Harrach, B. Reorganizing the family Parvoviridae: A revised taxonomy independent of the canonical approach based on host association. *Arch. Virol.* **2020**, *165*, 2133–2146. [CrossRef] [PubMed]
3. Jager, M.C.; Tomlinson, J.E.; Lopez-Astacio, R.A.; Parrish, C.R.; Van de Walle, G.R. Small but mighty: Old and new parvoviruses of veterinary significance. *Virol. J.* **2021**, *18*, 210. [CrossRef] [PubMed]
4. Shao, L.; Shen, W.; Wang, S.; Qiu, J. Recent Advances in Molecular Biology of Human Bocavirus 1 and Its Applications. *Front. Microbiol.* **2021**, *12*, 696604. [CrossRef] [PubMed]
5. Zou, W.; Cheng, F.; Shen, W.; Engelhardt, J.F.; Yan, Z.; Qiu, J. Nonstructural Protein NP1 of Human Bocavirus 1 Plays a Critical Role in the Expression of Viral Capsid Proteins. *J. Virol.* **2016**, *90*, 4658–4669. [CrossRef] [PubMed]
6. Shen, W.; Deng, X.; Zou, W.; Cheng, F.; Engelhardt, J.F.; Yan, Z.; Qiu, J. Identification and Functional Analysis of Novel Nonstructural Proteins of Human Bocavirus 1. *J. Virol.* **2015**, *89*, 10097–10109. [CrossRef] [PubMed]
7. Qiu, J.; Soderlund-Venermo, M.; Young, N.S. Human Parvoviruses. *Clin. Microbiol. Rev.* **2017**, *30*, 43–113. [CrossRef]
8. Qu, X.W.; Liu, W.P.; Qi, Z.Y.; Duan, Z.J.; Zheng, L.S.; Kuang, Z.Z.; Zhang, W.J.; Hou, Y.D. Phospholipase A2-like activity of human bocavirus VP1 unique region. *Biochem. Biophys. Res. Commun.* **2008**, *365*, 158–163. [CrossRef]
9. Mietzsch, M.; Penzes, J.J.; Agbandje-McKenna, M. Twenty-Five Years of Structural Parvovirology. *Viruses* **2019**, *11*, 362. [CrossRef]
10. Kailasan, S.; Halder, S.; Gurda, B.; Bladek, H.; Chipman, P.R.; McKenna, R.; Brown, K.; Agbandje-McKenna, M. Structure of an enteric pathogen, bovine parvovirus. *J. Virol.* **2015**, *89*, 2603–2614. [CrossRef]
11. Mietzsch, M.; Kailasan, S.; Garrison, J.; Ilyas, M.; Chipman, P.; Kantola, K.; Janssen, M.E.; Spear, J.; Sousa, D.; McKenna, R.; et al. Structural Insights into Human Bocaparvoviruses. *J. Virol.* **2017**, *91*, e00261-17. [CrossRef] [PubMed]
12. Yu, J.C.; Mietzsch, M.; Singh, A.; Jimenez Ybargollin, A.; Kailasan, S.; Chipman, P.; Bhattacharya, N.; Fakhiri, J.; Grimm, D.; Kapoor, A.; et al. Characterization of the GBoV1 Capsid and Its Antibody Interactions. *Viruses* **2021**, *13*, 330. [CrossRef] [PubMed]

13. Luo, M.; Mietzsch, M.; Chipman, P.; Song, K.; Xu, C.; Spear, J.; Sousa, D.; McKenna, R.; Söderlund-Venermo, M.; Agbandje-McKenna, M. pH-Induced Conformational Changes of Human Bocavirus Capsids. *J. Virol.* **2021**, *95*, e02329-20. [CrossRef] [PubMed]
14. Gurda, B.L.; Parent, K.N.; Bladek, H.; Sinkovits, R.S.; DiMattia, M.A.; Rence, C.; Castro, A.; McKenna, R.; Olson, N.; Brown, K.; et al. Human bocavirus capsid structure: Insights into the structural repertoire of the parvoviridae. *J. Virol.* **2010**, *84*, 5880–5889. [CrossRef] [PubMed]
15. Binn, L.N.; Lazar, E.C.; Eddy, G.A.; Kajima, M. Recovery and characterization of a minute virus of canines. *Infect. Immun.* **1970**, *1*, 503–508. [CrossRef] [PubMed]
16. Harrison, L.R.; Styer, E.L.; Pursell, A.R.; Carmichael, L.E.; Nietfeld, J.C. Fatal disease in nursing puppies associated with minute virus of canines. *J. Vet. Diagn. Investig.* **1992**, *4*, 19–22. [CrossRef] [PubMed]
17. Carmichael, L.E.; Schlafer, D.H.; Hashimoto, A. Pathogenicity of minute virus of canines (MVC) for the canine fetus. *Cornell Vet.* **1991**, *81*, 151–171. [PubMed]
18. Choi, J.W.; Jung, J.Y.; Lee, J.I.; Lee, K.K.; Oem, J.K. Molecular characteristics of a novel strain of canine minute virus associated with hepatitis in a dog. *Arch. Virol.* **2016**, *161*, 2299–2304. [CrossRef]
19. Blomström, A.L.; Belák, S.; Fossum, C.; McKillen, J.; Allan, G.; Wallgren, P.; Berg, M. Detection of a novel porcine boca-like virus in the background of porcine circovirus type 2 induced postweaning multisystemic wasting syndrome. *Virus Res.* **2009**, *146*, 125–129. [CrossRef]
20. Zhai, S.; Yue, C.; Wei, Z.; Long, J.; Ran, D.; Lin, T.; Deng, Y.; Huang, L.; Sun, L.; Zheng, H.; et al. High prevalence of a novel porcine bocavirus in weanling piglets with respiratory tract symptoms in China. *Arch. Virol.* **2010**, *155*, 1313–1317. [CrossRef]
21. Zhang, H.B.; Huang, L.; Liu, Y.J.; Lin, T.; Sun, C.Q.; Deng, Y.; Wei, Z.Z.; Cheung, A.K.; Long, J.X.; Yuan, S.S. Porcine bocaviruses: Genetic analysis and prevalence in Chinese swine population. *Epidemiol. Infect.* **2011**, *139*, 1581–1586. [CrossRef] [PubMed]
22. Zhang, Q.; Hu, R.; Tang, X.; Wu, C.; He, Q.; Zhao, Z.; Chen, H.; Wu, B. Occurrence and investigation of enteric viral infections in pigs with diarrhea in China. *Arch. Virol.* **2013**, *158*, 1631–1636. [CrossRef] [PubMed]
23. Cságola, A.; Lőrincz, M.; Cadar, D.; Tombácz, K.; Biksi, I.; Tuboly, T. Detection, prevalence and analysis of emerging porcine parvovirus infections. *Arch. Virol.* **2012**, *157*, 1003–1010. [CrossRef] [PubMed]
24. Pfankuche, V.M.; Bodewes, R.; Hahn, K.; Puff, C.; Beineke, A.; Habierski, A.; Osterhaus, A.D.; Baumgärtner, W. Porcine Bocavirus Infection Associated with Encephalomyelitis in a Pig, Germany(1). *Emerg. Infect. Dis.* **2016**, *22*, 1310–1312. [CrossRef] [PubMed]
25. Safamanesh, S.; Azimian, A.; Shakeri, A.; Ghazvini, K.; Jamehdar, S.A.; Khosrojerdi, M.; Youssefi, M. Detection of Porcine Bocavirus From a Child With Acute Respiratory Tract Infection. *Pediatr. Infect. Dis. J.* **2018**, *37*, e338–e339. [CrossRef] [PubMed]
26. Aryal, M.; Liu, G. Porcine Bocavirus: A 10-Year History since Its Discovery. *Virol. Sin.* **2021**, *36*, 1261–1272. [CrossRef]
27. Meerburg, B.G.; Singleton, G.R.; Kijlstra, A. Rodent-borne diseases and their risks for public health. *Crit. Rev. Microbiol.* **2009**, *35*, 221–270. [CrossRef]
28. Lau, S.K.; Yeung, H.C.; Li, K.S.; Lam, C.S.; Cai, J.P.; Yuen, M.C.; Wang, M.; Zheng, B.J.; Woo, P.C.; Yuen, K.Y. Identification and genomic characterization of a novel rat bocavirus from brown rats in China. *Infect. Genet. Evol. J. Mol. Epidemiol. Evol. Genet. Infect. Dis.* **2017**, *47*, 68–76. [CrossRef]
29. Berger, I.; Poterszman, A. Baculovirus expression: Old dog, new tricks. *Bioengineered* **2015**, *6*, 316–322. [CrossRef]
30. Ilyas, M.; Mietzsch, M.; Kailasan, S.; Vaisanen, E.; Luo, M.; Chipman, P.; Smith, J.K.; Kurian, J.; Sousa, D.; McKenna, R.; et al. Atomic Resolution Structures of Human Bufaviruses Determined by Cryo-Electron Microscopy. *Viruses* **2018**, *10*, 22. [CrossRef]
31. Zheng, S.Q.; Palovcak, E.; Armache, J.P.; Verba, K.A.; Cheng, Y.; Agard, D.A. MotionCor2: Anisotropic correction of beam-induced motion for improved cryo-electron microscopy. *Nat. Methods* **2017**, *14*, 331–332. [CrossRef] [PubMed]
32. Lakshmanan, R.; Mietzsch, M.; Jimenez Ybargollin, A.; Chipman, P.; Fu, X.; Qiu, J.; Söderlund-Venermo, M.; McKenna, R. Capsid Structure of Aleutian Mink Disease Virus and Human Parvovirus 4: New Faces in the Parvovirus Family Portrait. *Viruses* **2022**, *14*, 2219. [CrossRef]
33. Waterhouse, A.; Bertoni, M.; Bienert, S.; Studer, G.; Tauriello, G.; Gumienny, R.; Heer, F.T.; de Beer, T.A.P.; Rempfer, C.; Bordoli, L.; et al. SWISS-MODEL: Homology modelling of protein structures and complexes. *Nucleic Acids Res.* **2018**, *46*, W296–W303. [CrossRef]
34. Ho, P.T.; Montiel-Garcia, D.J.; Wong, J.J.; Carrillo-Tripp, M.; Brooks, C.L., 3rd; Johnson, J.E.; Reddy, V.S. VIPERdb: A Tool for Virus Research. *Annu. Rev. Virol.* **2018**, *5*, 477–488. [CrossRef] [PubMed]
35. Pettersen, E.F.; Goddard, T.D.; Huang, C.C.; Couch, G.S.; Greenblatt, D.M.; Meng, E.C.; Ferrin, T.E. UCSF Chimera—A visualization system for exploratory research and analysis. *J. Comput. Chem.* **2004**, *25*, 1605–1612. [CrossRef] [PubMed]
36. Kleywegt, G.J.; Jones, T.A. xdlMAPMAN and xdlDATAMAN—Programs for reformatting, analysis and manipulation of biomacromolecular electron-density maps and reflection data sets. *Acta Crystallogr. D Biol. Crystallogr.* **1996**, *52 Pt 4*, 826–828. [CrossRef] [PubMed]
37. Emsley, P.; Cowtan, K. Coot: Model-building tools for molecular graphics. *Acta Crystallogr. D Biol. Crystallogr.* **2004**, *60 Pt 12 Pt 1*, 2126–2132. [CrossRef]
38. Adams, P.D.; Afonine, P.V.; Bunkoczi, G.; Chen, V.B.; Davis, I.W.; Echols, N.; Headd, J.J.; Hung, L.W.; Kapral, G.J.; Grosse-Kunstleve, R.W.; et al. PHENIX: A comprehensive Python-based system for macromolecular structure solution. *Acta Crystallogr. D Biol. Crystallogr.* **2010**, *66 Pt 2*, 213–221. [CrossRef]

39. Bleker, S.; Sonntag, F.; Kleinschmidt, J.A. Mutational analysis of narrow pores at the fivefold symmetry axes of adeno-associated virus type 2 capsids reveals a dual role in genome packaging and activation of phospholipase A2 activity. *J. Virol.* **2005**, *79*, 2528–2540. [CrossRef]
40. Stahnke, S.; Lux, K.; Uhrig, S.; Kreppel, F.; Hosel, M.; Coutelle, O.; Ogris, M.; Hallek, M.; Buning, H. Intrinsic phospholipase A2 activity of adeno-associated virus is involved in endosomal escape of incoming particles. *Virology* **2011**, *409*, 77–83. [CrossRef]
41. Mietzsch, M.; Jose, A.; Chipman, P.; Bhattacharya, N.; Daneshparvar, N.; McKenna, R.; Agbandje-McKenna, M. Completion of the AAV Structural Atlas: Serotype Capsid Structures Reveals Clade-Specific Features. *Viruses* **2021**, *13*, 101. [CrossRef] [PubMed]
42. Mietzsch, M.; McKenna, R.; Vaisanen, E.; Yu, J.C.; Ilyas, M.; Hull, J.A.; Kurian, J.; Smith, J.K.; Chipman, P.; Lasanajak, Y.; et al. Structural Characterization of Cuta- and Tusavirus: Insight into Protoparvoviruses Capsid Morphology. *Viruses* **2020**, *12*, 653. [CrossRef] [PubMed]
43. Kailasan, S.; Garrison, J.; Ilyas, M.; Chipman, P.; McKenna, R.; Kantola, K.; Soderlund-Venermo, M.; Kucinskaite-Kodze, I.; Zvirbliene, A.; Agbandje-McKenna, M. Mapping Antigenic Epitopes on the Human Bocavirus Capsid. *J. Virol.* **2016**, *90*, 4670–4680. [CrossRef]
44. Meyer, N.L.; Chapman, M.S. Adeno-associated virus (AAV) cell entry: Structural insights. *Trends Microbiol.* **2022**, *30*, 432–451. [CrossRef] [PubMed]
45. Blackburn, S.D.; Cline, S.E.; Hemming, J.P.; Johnson, F.B. Attachment of bovine parvovirus to O-linked alpha 2,3 neuraminic acid on glycophorin A. *Arch. Virol.* **2005**, *150*, 1477–1484. [CrossRef]
46. Johnson, F.B.; Fenn, L.B.; Owens, T.J.; Faucheux, L.J.; Blackburn, S.D. Attachment of bovine parvovirus to sialic acids on bovine cell membranes. *J. Gen. Virol.* **2004**, *85 Pt 8*, 2199–2207. [CrossRef] [PubMed]
47. DeLano, W.L. *The PyMOL Molecular Graphics System*; DeLano Scientific: San Carlos, CA, USA, 2002.
48. Fakhiri, J.; Linse, K.P.; Mietzsch, M.; Xu, M.; Schneider, M.A.; Meister, M.; Schildgen, O.; Schnitzler, P.; Soderlund-Venermo, M.; Agbandje-McKenna, M.; et al. Impact of Natural or Synthetic Singletons in the Capsid of Human Bocavirus 1 on Particle Infectivity and Immunoreactivity. *J. Virol.* **2020**, *94*, e00170-20. [CrossRef] [PubMed]
49. Parrish, C.R.; Kawaoka, Y. The origins of new pandemic viruses: The acquisition of new host ranges by canine parvovirus and influenza A viruses. *Annu. Rev. Microbiol.* **2005**, *59*, 553–586. [CrossRef]

viruses

MDPI

Article

A Conserved Receptor-Binding Domain in the VP1u of Primate Erythroparvoviruses Determines the Marked Tropism for Erythroid Cells

Cornelia Bircher [1], Jan Bieri [1], Ruben Assaraf [1], Remo Leisi [1,2] and Carlos Ros [1,*]

1 Department of Chemistry, Biochemistry and Pharmaceutical Sciences, University of Bern, 3012 Bern, Switzerland; cornelia.bircher@uzh.ch (C.B.); jan.bieri@unibe.ch (J.B.); ruben.assaraf@unibe.ch (R.A.); remo.leisi@cslbehring.com (R.L.)
2 CSL Behring AG, 3000 Bern, Switzerland
* Correspondence: carlos.ros@unibe.ch

Abstract: Parvovirus B19 (B19V) is a human pathogen with a marked tropism for erythroid progenitor cells (EPCs). The N-terminal of the VP1 unique region (VP1u) contains a receptor-binding domain (RBD), which mediates virus uptake through interaction with an as-yet-unknown receptor (VP1uR). Considering the central role of VP1uR in the virus tropism, we sought to investigate its expression profile in multiple cell types. To this end, we established a PP7 bacteriophage-VP1u bioconjugate, sharing the size and VP1u composition of native B19V capsids. The suitability of the PP7-VP1u construct as a specific and sensitive VP1uR expression marker was validated in competition assays with B19V and recombinant VP1u. VP1uR expression was exclusively detected in erythroid cells and cells reprogrammed towards the erythroid lineage. Sequence alignment and in silico protein structure prediction of the N-terminal of VP1u (N-VP1u) from B19V and other primate erythroparvoviruses (simian, rhesus, and pig-tailed) revealed a similar structure characterized by a fold of three or four α-helices. Functional studies with simian parvovirus confirmed the presence of a conserved RBD in the N-VP1u, mediating virus internalization into human erythroid cells. In summary, this study confirms the exclusive association of VP1uR expression with cells of the erythroid lineage. The presence of an analogous RBD in the VP1u from non-human primate erythroparvoviruses emphasizes their parallel evolutionary trait and zoonotic potential.

Keywords: parvovirus B19; B19V; VP1u; VP1uR; receptor; tropism; primate erythroparvovirus; simian erythroparvovirus; rhesus erythroparvovirus; pig-tailed erythroparvovirus

Citation: Bircher, C.; Bieri, J.; Assaraf, R.; Leisi, R.; Ros, C. A Conserved Receptor-Binding Domain in the VP1u of Primate Erythroparvoviruses Determines the Marked Tropism for Erythroid Cells. *Viruses* **2022**, *14*, 420. https://doi.org/10.3390/v14020420

Academic Editor: Giorgio Gallinella

Received: 11 January 2022
Accepted: 15 February 2022
Published: 17 February 2022

1. Introduction

Human parvovirus B19 (B19V), also known as primate erythroparvovirus 1, is a small, nonenveloped icosahedral virus classified within the genus *Erythroparvovirus* of the family *Parvoviridae* [1]. B19V infections are typically associated with the childhood rash disease *erythema infectiosum*, also known as fifth disease [2]. In adults, B19V infection causes an expanding range of syndromes, and factors influencing the severity of the infection are poorly understood. In individuals with underlying immune or hematologic disorders, B19V may cause severe cytopenias, myocarditis, vasculitis, glomerulonephritis, and encephalitis [3]. Although rare, B19V may also cause lethal infections [4]. The infection has been frequently associated with arthropathies in adults and represents a risk factor for maternal–fetal transmission, causing fetal anemia, non-immune fetal hydrops, and fetal death [5,6]. B19V is transmitted primarily through the respiratory route by aerosol droplets [7]. The virus can also be transmitted vertically to the developing fetus, via blood transfusion, contaminated plasma-derived therapeutic products, and organ transplantation [8–11]. Following the main entry through the respiratory route, the virus targets and productively exclusively infects erythroid precursor cells (EPCs) in bone marrow. The damage caused to the infected EPCs leads to the erythroid disorders during infection [12]. The internalization of B19V by antibody-dependent enhancement [13,14] may explain the presence of viral components in nonerythroid tissue [15], as well as the possible association of B19V infection with cardiovascular disease [16,17].

The nonenveloped B19V capsid is a compact T = 1 icosahedral particle composed of two structural proteins, VP1 and VP2, that share the same C-terminal sequence [18]. VP1 has an additional N-terminal extension, the so-called "VP1 unique region" (VP1u). The most N-terminal region of VP1u harbors a cluster of epitopes that are targeted by neutralizing antibodies [19–21], indicating the importance of this region in viral infection. VP1u is not accessible to antibodies in virions circulating in the blood [22]; however, this region becomes accessible upon interaction with the target cells, a process that is required for virus uptake [23,24]. In earlier studies, we revealed that this region specifically binds a receptor, herein named VP1uR, which is required for B19V uptake and productive infection [25]. VP1uR is expressed in erythroid cells and coincides with the homing of BFU-E cells to erythroblastic islands in bone marrow, as well as the subsequent differentiation to the immobilized CFU-E stage, proerythroblasts and early basophilic erythroblasts [26]. The receptor-binding domain (RBD) in the N-terminal region of VP1u spans amino acids 5-80. By introducing specific mutations, we identified the critical residues required for a functional RBD. Structural predictions and mutational studies reveal an RBD consisting of a spatial configuration of three consecutive α-helices. Although VP1u monomers were functional, their dimerization promoted receptor interaction and internalization [27].

The genus *Erythroparvovirus* comprises three additional non-human primate viruses, i.e., primate erythroparvovirus 2 (simian parvovirus (SPV)); primate erythroparvovirus 3 (rhesus macaque parvovirus (RhMPV)); and primate erythroparvovirus 4 (pig-tailed macaque parvovirus (PtMPV)). SPV was identified in cynomolgus monkeys with anemia [28,29]. PtMPV and RhMPV were identified in anemic pig-tailed macaques and rhesus monkeys, respectively [30]. The genomic organization of all primate erythroparvoviruses is very similar. The predicted non-structural protein 1 (NS1) and VP1 of SPV share 50% and 62% similarity with B19V, respectively. Similar to B19V, there is a putative splice acceptor site for the VP2 and 67% homology with B19 VP2. Equivalent protein sizes and homologies are estimated for RhMPV and PtMPV based on sequence information [31].

Epidemiologic studies suggest that SPV transmission occurs horizontally, probably through the respiratory tract, as seen for B19 infections in humans [32]. Experimental infection of cynomolgus macaques with SPV produced transient viremia, reticulocytopenia, and typical changes of erythroid cells in the bone marrow [33]. When SPV was discovered, the affected macaques were coinfected with immunosuppressive type D simian retrovirus (SRV). Only macaques dually infected with SPV and SRV became anemic [32], suggesting that most SPV infections are asymptomatic, which complicates the determination of their prevalence. Infection rates for both PtMPV and RhMPV are also undetermined [31]. The significant anemia induced by SPV, PtMPV, and RhMPV in immunosuppressed animals suggests a similar tropism for erythroid progenitor cells in bone marrow, as observed for B19V. In line with this hypothesis, SPV showed high tropism for erythroid progenitor cells, as identified by in vitro infection of cynomolgus bone marrow cells [31].

SPV VP2 immunoblotting of sera from monkey handlers appeared to indicate a correlation between exposure to SPV-positive macaques and the presence of SPV antibodies in human blood [34]. However, possible cross-reactivity with B19V antibodies has not been excluded. SPV can replicate, although moderately, in human bone marrow in vitro [34], and evidence of B19V replication in cynomolgus bone marrow cells was revealed by in situ hybridization and immunofluorescent microscopy [35]. These experimental observations suggest that SPV and probably RhMPV and PtMPV may be able to infect humans.

Considering the important function of VP1u-RBD in B19V tropism and cell entry, we sought to examine the expression profile of the VP1u cognate receptor in cells from different tissues and to explore the presence of an analog motif in non-human primate erythroparvoviruses. In previous studies, we used a recombinant VP1u and an empty

MS2 bacteriophage-VP1u bioconjugate to detect VP1uR expression in various cell types by immunofluorescence [25,26,36]. In this study, we incorporated the VP1u region of B19V on the surface of *Pseudomonas aeruginosa* bacteriophage PP7 by click chemistry. The PP7-VP1u bioconjugate shares the size and VP1u composition of native B19V but lacks the entire VP2. This approach allowed for a more sensitive and quantitative determination of the expression profile of VP1uR in multiple cell types, as well as the possibility to study VP1uR-dependent virus uptake by RT-qPCR. This study confirms the strong association of VP1uR expression with cells of the erythroid lineage and identifies an equivalent RBD in the N-VP1u from non-human primate erythroparvoviruses.

2. Materials and Methods

2.1. Cells, Viruses, and Bacteria

UT7/Epo cells were cultured in MEM with 5% fetal calf serum (FCS) and 2 U/mL recombinant human erythropoietin (Epo). KU812Ep6 cells were cultured in RPMI 1640 with 10% FCS and 6 U/mL Epo. HepG2 and MRC-5 cells were cultured in DMEM with 10% FCS. K562 and KG1a cells were cultured in IMDM with 10% FCS. HeLa, HEK 293, NB324K, and A549 cells were cultured in DMEM with 5% FCS. REH cells were cultured in RPMI 1640 with 20% FCS. Erythroid progenitor cells (EPCs) were cultured in IMDM supplemented with 20% BIT 9500, 100 ng/mL SCF, 5 µg/mL IL-3, 1 µM hydrocortisone, and 3 U/mL rhEpo to induce differentiation toward the erythroid lineage. HiDEP and HuDEP cells were cultured in IMDM with 15% BIT 9500, 50 ng/mL SCF, 3 U/mL Epo, 1 µM dexamethasone, and 1 µg/mL doxycycline. HUVEC cells were cultured in vascular cell basal medium (ATCC PCS-100-030) supplemented with the endothelial cell growth kit-VEGF (ATCC PCS-100-041) containing 5 ng/mL rh VEGF, 5 ng/mL rh EGF, 5 ng/mL rh FGF basic, 15 ng/mL rh IGF-1, 10 mM L-glutamine, 0.75 U/mL heparin sulfate, 1 µg/mL hydrocortisone, 50 µg/mL ascorbic acid, and 2% FCS. Human dermal fibroblasts were cultured in fibroblast basal medium (ATCC PCS-201-030) supplemented with fibroblast growth kit-serum-free (ATCC PCS-201-040) containing 500 µg/mL human serum albumin (HSA), 0.6 mM linoleic acid, 0.6 µg/mL lecithin, 7.5 mM L-glutamine, 5 ng/mL rh FGF basic, 5 ng/mL rh EGF/TGF-1 supplements, 5 µg/mL rh insulin, 1 µg/mL hydrocortisone, and 50 µg/mL ascorbic acid. All culture media were supplemented with L-glutamine and 50 U/mL penicillin-streptomycin. B19V- and B19-infected human plasmas were obtained from CSL Behring AG, Charlotte, NC, USA. *Pseudomonas aeruginosa* and *Pseudomonas aeruginosa* bacteriophage PP7 were obtained from ATCC; 15692 and 15692-B4, respectively.

2.2. PP7 production

A volume of 100 µL of densely grown *P. aeruginosa* starter culture was infected with 0.1 µL of a PP7 stock in 18 mL soft agar (37 °C), composed of LB broth and LB agar Miller (7.5 g/l agar) in a 1:1 ratio. The inoculated soft agar was poured on a Petri dish (165 cm^2) and incubated overnight at 37 °C. The soft agar was scraped off and transferred to a 50 mL falcon tube. After the addition of 10 mL PBS, the tube was vortexed and centrifuged at 3000× *g* for 25 min at RT. The supernatant was transferred to a new tube and centrifuged again at 3000× *g* for 10 min. The supernatant, containing the PP7, was filtered through a 0.22 µm filter. In the last step, PP7 was purified by ultracentrifugation through a 20% sucrose cushion (150,000× *g*, 4 h at 4 °C). Plaque-forming units and protein concentrations were quantified by plaque assay and SDS-PAGE, respectively.

Plaque assays of PP7 were carried out with the host bacteria *P. aeruginosa*. A volume of 10 µL of a densely grown bacteria starter culture was mixed with 2.5 mL soft agar and poured onto a prepared agar plate. Ten-fold dilutions of PP7 were prepared in LB broth and then evenly distributed on top of the solidified soft agar. The plates were incubated overnight at 37 °C. Plaques were counted the next day, and the results were expressed as plaque-forming units per milliliter (PFU/mL).

2.3. B19V and Simian VP1u Expression

B19V VP1u cloning and expression were carried out as previously described [26]. The DNA fragment-encoding simian VP1u was amplified from a pET-21(+) vector (Twist Bioscience, San Francisco, CA, USA) with restriction-site overhang primers (*Hin*dIII forward, 5′-CGA AAG CTT AGT GAG CCT GCT TCC AAA A-3′; *Kpn*I reverse, 5′-CGA GGT ACC ACA GTC TCT AAC CAC TTG T-3′). The amplicon was cloned into the pT7-FLAG-MAT Tag-2 expression vector (Sigma, St Louis, MO, USA), verified by sequencing, and transformed into *E. coli* XL10 Gold. Protein expression was carried out in *E. coli* BL21(DE3) cells induced with 1 mM isopropyl-β-D-thiogalactopyranoside (IPTG) at an OD_{600} of 0.6 for 4 h at 37 °C. The recombinant VP1u was purified twice with Ni-NTA magnetic agarose beads (Invitrogen, Carlsbad, CA, USA) under native conditions.

2.4. PP7-VP1u Bioconjugation

B19V and simian VP1u were bioconjugated to PP7 capsids following the same protocol. The bifunctional crosslinker trans-cyclooctene-PEG_4-NHS ester (TCO-NHS; Jena Bioscience, Thuringia, Germany) was dissolved in DMSO and added to the PP7 capsids (2 mg/mL) to a final concentration of 50 µM. Crosslinking between the NHS ester and accessible lysines was carried out for 1 h at room temperature in PBS. Subsequently, lysine-reactive fluorescent dye NHS-Atto488 was dissolved in DMSO and added to the PP7-TCO capsids to obtain a final concentration of 100 µM. The fluorescent-labelling reaction was carried out for 1 h at room temperature in PBS (pH 7.4). The reaction was quenched with the addition of 50 mM Tris (pH 8). Non-coupled crosslinker and fluorescent dye were separated from the TCO capsids by centrifugation through 20% sucrose (150,000× *g*, 2 h, 4 °C). In a second step, VP1u was reduced with 1 mM TCEP. After reduction, TCEP was removed using a 0.5 mL Amicon 10 kDa filter device. The bifunctional crosslinker methyl-tetrazine-PEG_4-maleimide (MeTz-Mal) was dissolved in DMSO and added to the previously reduced VP1u in a 20x molar excess. The crosslinking reaction was incubated for 2h at room temperature. Non-coupled crosslinker was separated from VP1u-MeTz with a 0.5 mL Amicon 10 kDa filter (washed 3x with PBS). The concentration of VP1u-MeTz and PP7-TCO was quantified with an SDS-PAGE, as well as Coomassie staining and densitometric analysis. The final click reaction between PP7-TCO and VP1u-MeTz was carried out by incubation of PP7-TCO with a 5x molar excess of VP1u-MeTz for 1h at room temperature. Non-coupled VP1u-MeTz was separated from PP7-VP1u bioconjugates by centrifugation through 20% sucrose (150,000× *g*, 2 h, 4 °C). The final PP7-VP1u stock concentration was quantified by PCR and SDS-PAGE.

2.5. SDS-PAGE and Western blot

SDS-PAGE was performed to analyze the purity of the expressed VP1u variants and to verify the efficiency of the PP7-VP1u coupling. For Western blot, the proteins in the gel were blotted on a PVDF membrane and blocked overnight with 5% milk. For detection, a rat anti-FLAG antibody was used, followed by an HPR-coupled secondary antibody. Detection was performed with SuperSignal West Dura Extended Duration Substrate (Thermo Fisher, Waltham, MA, USA) and visualized with a photo film.

2.6. Detection of PP7-VP1u and B19V Uptake by qPCR and Confocal Microscopy

The different cell types (3×10^5) were resuspended in 200 µL PBS and incubated with 10^{10} PP7-VP1u bioconjugates (B19V or simian) or B19V from human plasma (10^{10}) at 37 °C for 30 min. Subsequently, cells were washed twice with 1 mL PBS, trypsinized for 4 min (0.25% trypsin/EDTA solution (Sigma, St. Louis, MO, USA) diluted to 50% in PBS) at 37 °C, and washed twice more with 1 mL PBS. For PP7-VP1u quantification, cells were lysed in 140 µL lysis buffer (0.5% Tween-20 in PBS). The cell debris was removed by centrifugation, and the supernatant was transferred to a new tube. The phage RNA of the internalized bioconjugates was extracted with a QIAamp Viral RNA Mini Kit (Qiagen, Hilden, Germany) and quantified by RT-PCR with iTaq SybrGreen qPCR (BioRad, Hercules, CA, USA) and

PP7-specific primers; forward, 5′-GGC AAC TGA GCA TAA CGG CAC-3′; reverse, 5′-GCT CCA TAG CGA TGA AGC GAA C-3′. For B19V quantification, intracellular B19V genomes were extracted from the cell pellet with a DNeasy Blood and Tissue Kit (Qiagen) and quantified by PCR with iTaq SybrGreen qPCR (BioRad) and B19V-specific primers; forward (nt 413-433), 5′-GGG CAG CCA TTT TAA GTG TTT-3′; reverse (nt 534-552), 5′-CCA GGA AAA AGC AGC CCA G-3′. Results were normalized by quantification of the β-actin gene and expressed as a percentage of maximal uptake.

To visualize internalized virus, the infected cells were resuspended in 20 µL PBS, spotted on coverslips, fixed with acetone/methanol (1:1) at −20 °C for 4 min, and allowed to dry. Samples incubated with Atto488-labeled PP7-VP1u bioconjugates were directly mounted with Mowiol containing DAPI. Immunofluorescence detection of B19V was carried out with MAb 860-55D (Mikrogen, Neuried, Germany) against intact capsids, followed by a goat anti-human Alexa Fluor 549 (Agilent Technologies, Santa Clara, CA, USA). Internalized viruses were visualized by confocal microscopy (LSM 880, Zeiss, Jena, Germany) using a 63x oil-immersion objective.

2.7. Detection of Recombinant VP1u in Cells by Confocal Microscopy

Recombinant VP1u constructs (50 ng) were incubated with a rat anti-FLAG antibody for 1 h at 37 °C. Subsequently, the VP1u constructs were incubated with cells (3×10^5) in 200 µL PBS at 4 °C for 40 min to allow binding or at 37 °C to allow binding and internalization. Cells were processed for immunofluorescence as described above. Detection of recombinant VP1u constructs was carried out with a secondary goat anti-rat antibody, Alexa Fluor 488, or a goat anti-rabbit antibody, Alexa Fluor 594 (Agilent Technologies, Santa Clara, CA, USA), and visualized by confocal microscopy.

2.8. Competition and Neutralization Assays

The internalization of PP7-VP1u constructs and native B19V were examined in the presence of recombinant VP1u or PP7-VP1u. Cells were resuspended in 200 µL PBS and incubated with 500 ng of recombinant VP1u or a 10x molar excess of PP7-VP1u for 40 min at 4 °C prior to incubation with PP7-VP1u or B19V at 37 °C for 30 min. Subsequently, samples were processed for qPCR and/or immunofluorescence microscopy as specified above.

The capacity of a human antibody against the N-VP1u of B19V (MAb 1418-1; aa 30 to 42) [37,38] to recognize and block the uptake of human and simian VP1u was examined. PP7-VP1u bioconjugates were incubated with a 200x molar excess of MAb 1418-1 for 1 h at 4 °C. After incubation, PP7-VP1u uptake was examined in UT7/Epo cells by RT-qPCR as described above.

2.9. In Silico Predictions

VP1u sequence alignments were carried out with the Clustal Omega multiple sequence alignment program [39]. Ab initio tertiary structure prediction of the RBDs was performed using the QUARK server (https://zhanggroup.org/QUARK/, accessed on 12 September 2020) [40]. The structures were visualized and analyzed with PyMOL molecular graphics software (version 2.5.0).

3. Results

3.1. PP7-VP1u Bioconjugation

PP7-VP1u bioconjugates were assembled by bio-orthogonal click chemistry (Figure 1A). PP7 was coupled to the heterobifunctional crosslinker TCO-NHS, and VP1u was crosslinked to the heterobifunctional crosslinker MeTz-Mal. Subsequently, PP7-TCO and VP1u-MeTz were crosslinked by inverse-electron-demand Diels–Alder reaction. SDS-PAGE was performed to verify the purity of PP7, PP7-TCO, and PP7-VP1u. The PP7 bacteriophage capsid protein is visible at 13.9 kDa. Additionally, the capsid-associated maturation protein is slightly visible at 50.8 kDa (Figure 1B). Sensitive Western blot analysis showed that approximately three VP1u units were crosslinked to one PP7 capsid and that non-coupled VP1u was effectively removed after the crosslinking reaction (Figure 1C).

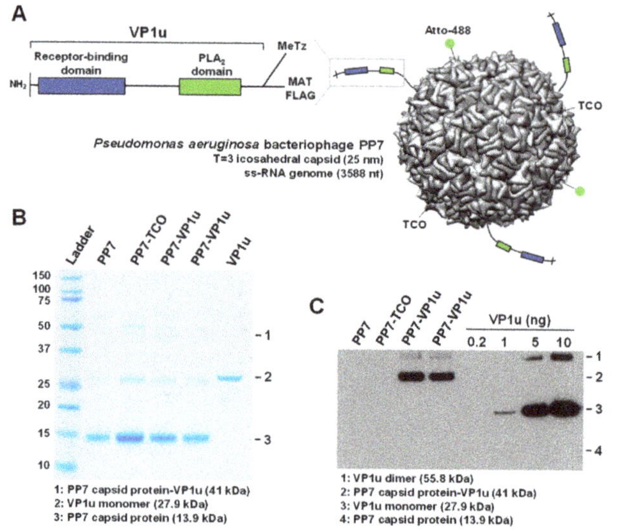

Figure 1. PP7-VP1u bioconjugation. (**A**) Schematic depiction of the PP7-VP1u construct, consisting of a bacteriophage PP7 capsid and three VP1u units of B19V. VP1u contains a C-terminal MAT tag for purification, a C-terminal FLAG tag for detection, and a unique cysteine for crosslinking. Additionally, the capsid was labeled with NHS-Atto488. (**B**) SDS-PAGE and (**C**) Western blot analysis of PP7 capsids, recombinant VP1u, and PP7-VP1u construct (two replicates). VP1u and PP7-VP1u conjugates were detected with an anti-FLAG antibody.

3.2. PP7-VP1u Is Internalized into UT7/Epo Cells and Competes with B19V

The capacity of the PP7-VP1u bioconjugate to bind and internalize UT7/Epo cells was tested by RT-qPCR. Following incubation for 30 min at 37 °C, the cells were briefly trypsinized to remove non-internalized PP7-VP1u particles. The sample incubated at 4°C served as a control of the trypsinization treatment. Internalized PP7-VP1u constructs were quantified by RT-PCR. The result showed that only the VP1u-bioconjugated construct incubated at 37 °C was able to internalize. Competition with recombinant VP1u efficiently inhibited PP7-VP1u uptake, confirming that the construct internalizes following interaction with VP1uR (Figure 2A). When added to the cells before native B19V, the PP7-VP1u particles interfered significantly with B19V uptake, although less efficiently than the recombinant VP1u (Figure 2B). The internalization kinetics of B19V and PP7-VP1u were examined in parallel at 5 min intervals. The results revealed a similar uptake profile between the native virus and the bioconjugate phage capsid (Figure 2C).

The capacity of PP7-VP1u to internalize UT7/Epo cells was also tested by fluorescence microscopy. Following incubation for 30 min at 37 °C, the cells were washed, trypsinized to remove non-internalized particles, fixed, and examined by fluorescence microscopy. B19V- and PP7-TCO-infected cells were used as a positive and negative control, respectively. At 37 °C, PP7-VP1u particles appear with the typical clustered intracellular distribution similar to that observed in cells infected with B19V. Binding but not uptake is observed at 4 °C (Figure 2D). Taken together, PP7-VP1u internalized into UT7/Epo cells with comparable efficiency as native B19V, confirming its suitability as a sensitive and quantitative VP1uR marker.

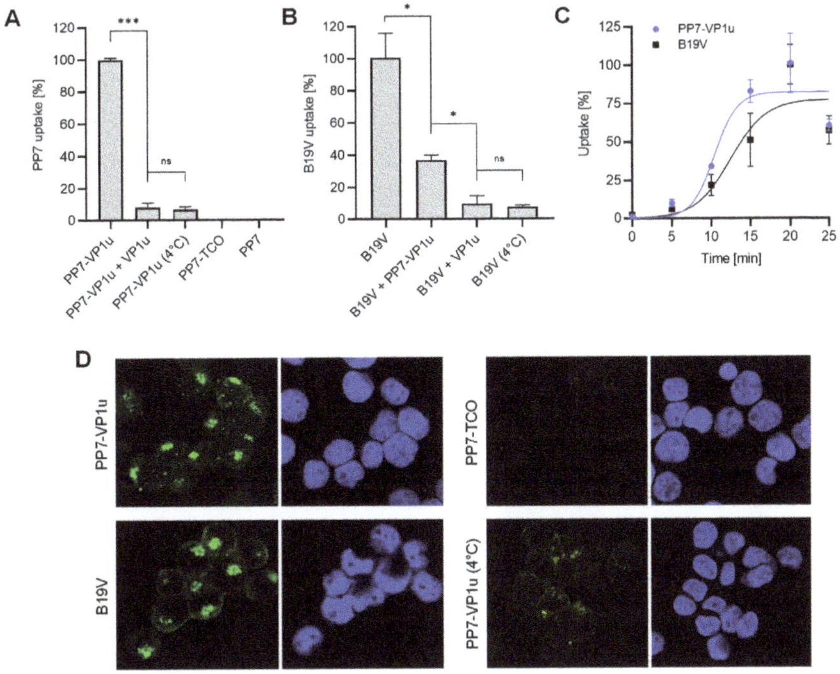

Figure 2. PP7-VP1u uptake into UT7/Epo cells. (**A**) PP7-VP1u uptake was quantified by RT-qPCR. For the competition, recombinant VP1u (500 ng) was added to the cells at 4 °C 40 min before incubation with PP7-VP1u. (**B**) Internalization of native B19V into UT7/Epo cells was quantified by PCR. For the competition, PP7-VP1u (10x molecular excess) or recombinant VP1u (500 ng) was added to the cells at 4 °C for 40 min before infection with B19V. The sample at 4 °C served as a negative control (no internalization). (**C**) Internalization kinetics determined by RT-qPCR (PP7-VP1u) or qPCR (B19V) at 5 min intervals. (**D**) Binding and uptake of Atto488-labeled PP7-VP1u constructs and native B19V. B19V was detected with human MAb 860-55D against capsids and stained with secondary Alexa-Fluor 488 anti-human antibody. PP7-TCO served as a negative control. The quantitative RT-PCR results are presented as the mean ± SD of three independent experiments. *** $p < 0.001$; * $p < 0.05$; ns, not significant.

3.3. VP1uR Expression is Restricted to Epo-Dependent Erythroid Cells

The capacity of PP7-VP1u to bind and internalize UT7/Epo cells with similar efficiency as B19V validates the use of the phage bioconjugate as a sensitive marker for the quantitative determination of VP1uR expression. We first examined the expression of VP1uR in non-hematopoietic cells. To this end, PP7-VP1u was incubated with cells from the lung (A549 and MRC-5), kidney (HEK 293T and NB324), liver (HepG2), and cervix (HeLa). In contrast to UT7/Epo cells, which served as a positive control, no significant signal of internalized PP7 RNA or capsid fluorescence signal was detected in any non-hematopoietic cells tested, confirming the restricted expression profile of VP1uR (Figure 3A,B).

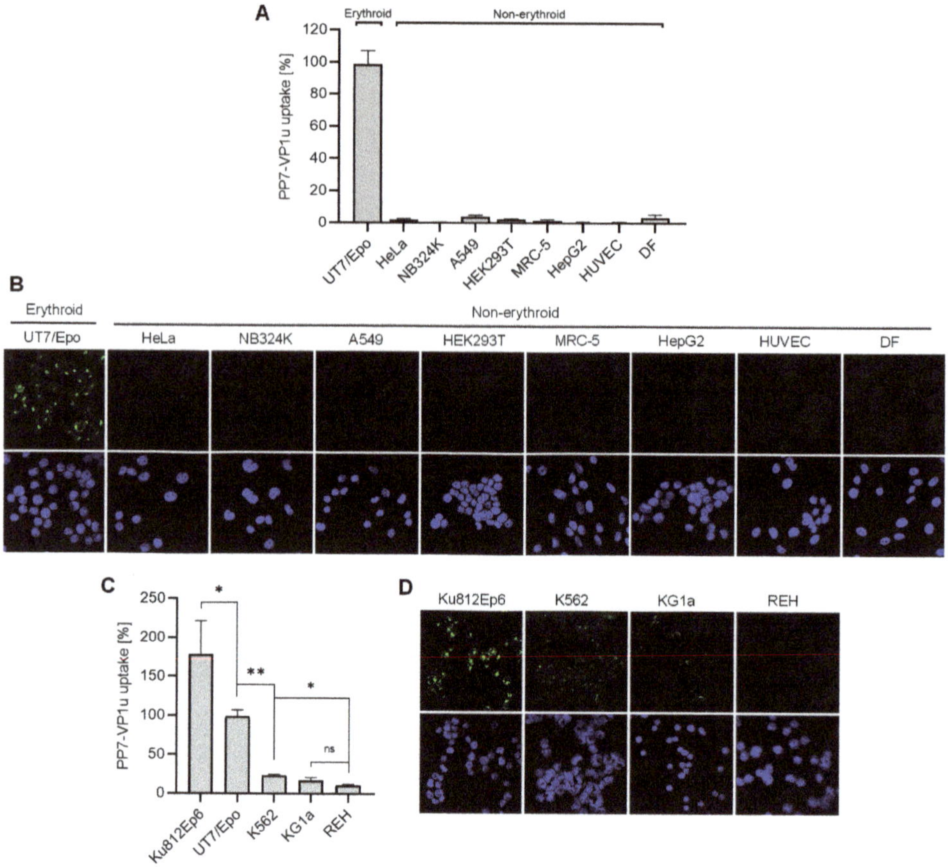

Figure 3. Expression profile of VP1uR in erythroid and non-erythroid cells. PP7-VP1u was incubated with different human cell types derived from non-erythroid tissues for 30 min at 37 °C. UT7/Epo served as a positive control. The internalized constructs were quantified by RT-PCR (**A**) and detected by fluorescence confocal microscopy (**B**). PP7-VP1u was incubated with different human hematopoietic cell lines for 30 min at 37 °C. UT7/Epo served as a positive control. The internalized constructs were quantified by RT-PCR (**C**) and detected by fluorescence confocal microscopy (**D**). All samples were treated with trypsin before RNA extraction to remove bound but not internalized constructs. The quantitative RT-PCR results are presented as the mean ± SD of three independent experiments. ** $p < 0.01$; * $p < 0.05$.

We next tested cell lines originating from distinct differentiation stages of the hematopoietic hierarchy roadmap, i.e., lymphopoiesis (REH cells), granulo- and monocytopoiesis (KG1a and Ku812Ep6), erythropoiesis (UT7/Epo), and multipotent hematopoietic stem cell (K562). For comparability, the internalization assay with PP7-VP1u was performed in the same way as described above for non-hematopoietic cells. As quantified by RT-PCR (Figure 3C), only cells involved in Epo-dependent erythroid differentiation, Ku812Ep6 and UT7/Epo, expressed VP1uR abundantly. Whereas K562 had a low but detectable expression, reaching approximately 20% of that observed in UT7/Epo cells, KG1a and lymphoid REH cells did not show a significant expression of VP1uR. The corresponding fluorescence microscopy images confirm the predominant VP1uR expression in the Epo-dependent erythroid cell lines with a clear intracellular signal, a weak signal in K562, a weak pericellular signal in KG1a cells, and no signal in REH cells (Figure 3D).

3.4. Quantification of VP1uR Expression at Progressive Erythroid Differentiation Stages

To accurately resolve the expression profile of VP1uR and erythroid differentiation, CD34+ hematopoietic stem cells were cultured in erythroid differentiation medium containing Epo and tested daily for PP7-VP1u uptake. The results show that after induction of erythroid differentiation, VP1uR expression increases until day 8 and decreases thereafter (Figure 4A). The quantitative data are supported by the fluorescence microscopy images, which show PP7-VP1u internalization after 3 and 8 days of differentiation. Immunostaining with a glycophorin A antibody confirmed the commitment and differentiation of the cells toward the erythroid lineage (Figure 4B). These findings confirm that VP1uR expression is upregulated in EPCs upon Epo stimulation.

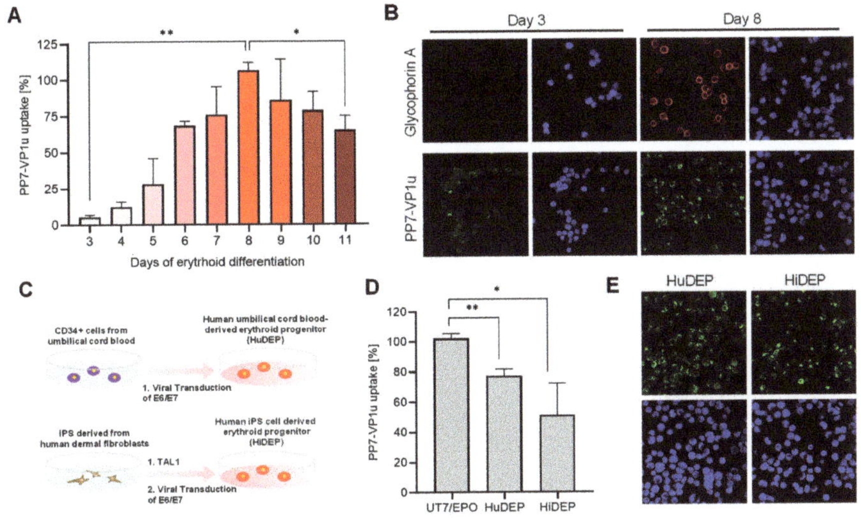

Figure 4. VP1uR expression is upregulated during erythroid differentiation. (**A**) EPCs at progressive differentiation phases were incubated with PP7-VP1u for 30 min at 37 °C and quantified by RT-PCR. (**B**) Confocal microscopy images of EPCs at days 3 and 8 of erythroid differentiation. Cells were incubated with PP7-VP1u or immunostained with a glycophorin A antibody. (**C**) Schematic depiction of the erythroid reprogramming strategy [41]. (**D**) PP7-VP1u bioconjugates were incubated with HuDEP and HiDEP cells for 30 min at 37 °C. Internalization was quantified by RT-qPCR and compared with UT7/Epo cells. (**E**) Representative images of HuDEP and HiDEP cells incubated with PP7-VP1u and visualized by confocal microscopy. The quantitative RT-PCR results are presented as the mean ± SD of two (**A**) or three (**D**) independent experiments. ** $p < 0.01$; * $p < 0.05$.

3.5. VP1uR Expression Can Be Induced by Cellular Reprogramming towards Erythroid lineage

HuDEP and HiDEP cells were established from umbilical cord blood CD34+ cells and iPS derived from human fibroblasts, respectively (Figure 4C). These cells express erythroid-specific markers, which are upregulated after the induction of differentiation [41]. Neither CD34+ blood cells [26] nor human fibroblast cells (Figure 3A,B), used as precursor cells, express VP1uR. In clear contrast, VP1uR expression was detected following cellular reprogramming towards erythroid lineage (Figure 4D). The quantitative RT-PCR result was confirmed by fluorescence microscopy with the PP7-VP1u construct (Figure 4E).

3.6. Structural Comparison of the RBD of B19V and Related Primate Erythroparvoviruses

The receptor-binding domain (RBD) in the N-terminal region of VP1u of B19V was characterized in detail in our previous studies. It was shown that the B19V RBD has a well-defined structure of a three-helix fold, which forms a spatial cluster of internalization-important amino acids at the interface of helices 1 and 3 [27]. Considering the importance of the N-VP1u RBD in B19V tropism and the infection similarities between B19V and related primate erythroparvoviruses, we sought to compare the sequence and predicted structure of their N-VP1u.

As shown in Figure 5A, the primate erythroparvoviruses cluster in a monophyletic group within the genus Erythroparvovirus. Multiple sequence alignment shows significant differences in the N-VP1u amino acid sequence from primate erythroparvoviruses (Figure 5B). Only a few amino acids are conserved in the RBD of B19V, SPV, RhMPV, and PtMPV. Interestingly, amino acids F25 and L59, which were characterized as internalization-relevant for B19V VP1u [27], are also conserved in the other primate erythroparvoviruses. Further internalization-relevant amino acids of B19V VP1u are not conserved by identical amino acids, but they are replaced by amino acids with comparable properties. For example, in helix 1, the polar amino acid glutamine is conserved in B19V (Q22) and PtMPV (Q25), whereas it is replaced by glutamate in SPV (E25) and RhMPV (E27). Similarly, internalization-important hydrophobic amino acids of B19V are replaced by analogous hydrophobic amino acids within other primate erythroparvoviruses.

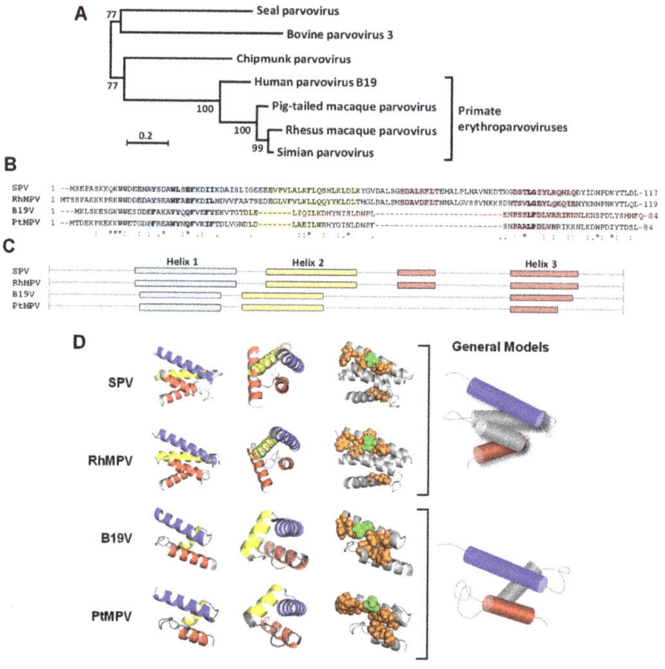

Figure 5. N-VP1u from primate erythroparvoviruses. (**A**) Phylogenetic tree of the genus Erythroparvovirus. VP1 sequences were aligned with MUSCLE configured for the highest accuracy [42], and the tree was reconstructed using the maximum-likelihood method implemented in the PhyML program [43]. Bootstrap values are indicated. (**B**) N-VP1u sequences were aligned using the Clustal Omega multiple sequence alignment program. Relevant amino acids for VP1u internalization are highlighted in bold letters. (**C**) Helix distribution according to secondary structure prediction in QUARK modeling. Helix 1 is blue, helix 2 is yellow, and helix 3 is red. (**D**) The RBDs (SPV AA 14-117, RhMPV AA 15-119, B19V 14-84, and PtMPV AA 14-84) were modeled by QUARK and visualized with PyMOL, showing similar high-confidence structure predictions of the different viruses. First column: front view with the N-terminus top left and the C-terminus in the lower part; second column: side view of the models; third column: spatial cluster of the important amino acids as spheres in the helical structure (green: polar; orange: hydrophobic). A schematic representation of the two models of helix configuration is shown on the right. SPV: simian parvovirus; RhMPV; rhesus macaque parvovirus; B19V: parvovirus B19; PtMPV: pig-tailed macaque parvovirus.

Secondary and tertiary protein structure predictions of N-VP1u were performed with the QUARK server [40]. Although the sequences are barely conserved, the predicted helix distribution and the tertiary structure of N-VP1u of primate erythroparvoviruses show striking similarities (Figure 5C). The RBDs of human B19V and PtMPV is composed of three helices. Both RBDs show an identical helix distribution, leading to a very similar 3D structure. The three-helix fold forms a spatial cluster of important amino acids at the interface of helices 1 and 3. The RBDs of SPV and RhMPV harbors four helices, both folding to a virtually identical 3D structure. The additional helix is located between helices 2 and 3, encoded by an additional sequence that is not present in the sequence of B19V and PtMPV. The four-helix fold builds a spatial cluster of important amino acids that are located on the interface of helices 1 and 3 (Figure 5D). Taken together, the internalization-important amino acids show a remarkably conserved structural arrangement within the RBDs of all primate erythroparvoviruses, and the phylogenetic relationship between the viruses correlates well with the similarity in their predicted RBD models.

3.7. N-VP1u of SPV Harbors a Functional RBD, Mediating Virus Uptake into Erythroid Cells

The striking similarity observed between the predicted N-VP1u structure of B19V and that of other primate erythroparvoviruses suggests a common RBD function. To verify the presence of a functional RBD in the VP1u of non-human primate erythroparvoviruses, we generated a simian PP7-VP1u bioconjugate following the same approach as that used for B19V (Figure 1). Incubation of the simian PP7-VP1u bioconjugate with non-hematopoietic (HeLa), hematopoietic (KG1a), and erythropoietic (UT7/Epo) cell lines at 37 °C for 1h showed strong internalization of simian PP7-VP1u into UT7/Epo but not into HeLa or KG1a cells (Figure 6A,B). This finding confirms the presence of a functional RBD in the N-VP1u of SPV that is able to mediate virus uptake into human erythroid cells.

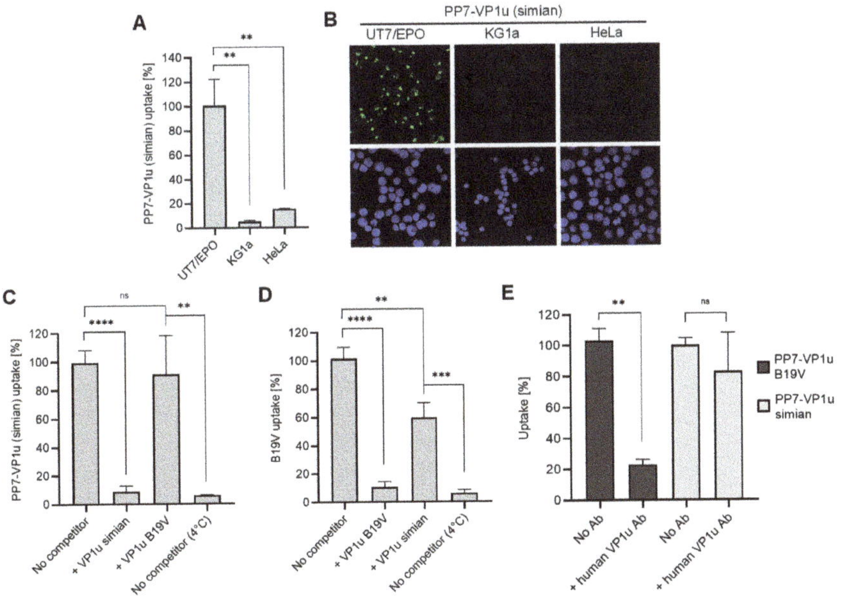

Figure 6. Uptake of simian PP7-VP1u into human cells. Simian PP7-VP1u was incubated with UT7/Epo, KG1a, and HeLa cells for 30 min at 37 °C. The internalized constructs were quantified by RT-PCR (**A**) and detected by fluorescence confocal microscopy (**B**). (**C**,**D**) Internalization of simian

PP7-VP1u and native B19V into UT7/Epo cells in the presence of competitors. Samples incubated without competitors at 37 °C and 4 °C served as a reference for maximal internalization and complete block, respectively. (**E**) B19V and simian PP7-VP1u internalization into UT7/Epo cells was carried out in the absence or presence of a 200-fold molecular excess of MAb 1418-1 against B19V VP1u. Internalized bioconjugates were quantified by RT-PCR. The quantitative RT-PCR results are presented as the mean ± SD of three independent experiments. **** $p < 0.0001$; *** $p < 0.001$; ** $p < 0.01$; ns, not significant.

Furthermore, the uptake of simian PP7-VP1u was tested in competition with recombinant VP1u of SPV and B19V. Whereas simian VP1u was able to efficiently block internalization of the bioconjugate, the inhibitory effect of B19V VP1u on simian PP7-VP1u was not significant (Figure 6C). On the other hand, simian VP1u was able to disturb the internalization of native B19V but not as efficiently as the B19 VP1u (Figure 6D). These results suggest that SPV and B19V binding to VP1uR may involve neighboring domains of the receptor, resulting in a partial competition between the two species.

During B19V viremia, antibodies produced against RBDs in N-VP1u are crucial to clearing the infection. An antibody targeting N-VP1u (aa 30 to 42; MAb 1418-1) obtained from a B19V-infected patient was shown to efficiently neutralize B19V infection [37,38]. Considering the zoonotic potential of SPV, we tested the capacity of MAb 1418-1 to block simian PP7-VP1u uptake in UT7/Epo cells. Whereas the antibody effectively inhibited B19 PP7-VP1u uptake, simian PP7-VP1u internalization remained undisturbed (Figure 6E), suggesting that the differences in structure and sequence within the RBD allow SPV to evade recognition by human antibodies.

4. Discussion

4.1. Expression Profile of VP1uR

The N terminal of VP1u of B19V harbors an RBD required for virus uptake [25,27]. The VP1u cognate receptor, herein named VP1uR, has not yet been identified, but its expression profile seems restricted to the few cell types that B19V can infect, i.e., EPCs at Epo-dependent differentiation stages and the erythroid cell lines UT7/Epo and Ku812Ep6 [26,36]. Considering its central role in infection, a detailed characterization of the expression profile of VP1uR is needed to better understand the tropism and pathogenesis of B19V.

In this study, we developed a PP7 bacteriophage-VP1u bioconjugate as a sensitive and quantitative marker to analyze VP1uR expression by fluorescence microscopy and RT-qPCR. The PP7-VP1u construct allowed for the study of VP1u-dependent uptake without the involvement of other interacting domains within the B19V capsid. The PP7 capsid has a similar size as that of B19V, does not bind to eukaryotic cells, and contains a specific RNA genome that was used for quantification. Functional assays confirmed that the PP7-VP1u construct can bind and internalize erythroid cells with similar efficiency as native B19V (Figure 2C,D). Competition assays with recombinant VP1u showed that PP7-VP1u internalization is mediated exclusively by VP1u and its cognate receptor, without the engagement of additional receptor molecules (Figure 2A,B). Accordingly, the PP7-VP1u bioconjugate appeared as a sensitive method to detect and quantify VP1uR expression.

VP1uR expression was systematically investigated in hematopoietic and non-hematopoietic cells derived from different tissues. The functional receptor was exclusively detected in the erythroid cell lines UT7/Epo and Ku812Ep6 (Figure 3), in EPCs at Epo-dependent differentiation stages, and in cells reprogrammed towards the erythroid lineage (Figure 4). These results confirm that VP1uR expression is tightly linked to erythropoiesis, determining the marked erythroid tropism of B19V. VP1uR expression was significantly increased in Ku812Ep6 cells compared to the reference cell line, UT7/Epo. Ku812 cells were established from a patient with a blastic crisis of chronic myelogenous leukemia [44]. Differentiation toward the erythroid lineage in the presence of Epo led to the clone Ku812Ep6, which displayed a significantly increased susceptibility to B19V [45]. Epo-independent hematopoietic cell lines, such as KG1a and K562, show a low but detectable VP1uR expression (Figure 3C,D), suggesting that Epo per se does not induce VP1uR expression but rather supports the survival and proliferation of the erythroid cell population that expresses VP1uR.

The stimulation of isolated CD34+ cells with erythropoiesis-supporting cytokines triggered erythroid differentiation, which was evidenced by the expression of glycophorin A (GPA). VP1uR expression was upregulated during the first days of differentiation, reaching the highest level after eight days, and downregulated during the terminal erythroid differentiation stages (Figure 4). These results confirm previous studies wherein a direct correlation between B19V uptake and erythroid differentiation was observed [26,46].

VP1uR expression was detected in cells reprogrammed towards the erythroid lineage. HuDEP and HiDEP cells are immortalized EPCs established from umbilical cord blood CD34+ cells and induced pluripotent stem (iPS) cells (derived from fibroblasts) expressing TAL1, respectively [41]. TAL1 is essential in early hematopoiesis and erythroid differentiation [47,48]. Immortalization was achieved by the induction and expression of HPV16-E6/E7. HuDEP and HiDEP cells express the erythroid-specific marker GPA, whereas CD36 and c-KIT (CD117), which are markers of immature erythroid cells, are detected at very low levels [41]. PP7-VP1u was able to internalize HuDEP and HiDEP cells, although to a lesser extent compared to UT7/Epo cells. These cells exhibit gene expression patterns characteristic of terminal erythroid differentiation stages [49], which correspond with the observed downregulation of VP1uR expression during erythroblast stages.

4.2. Characterization of RBDs from Non-Human Primate Erythroparvoviruses

B19V is closely related to three other primate erythroparvoviruses, i.e., SPV, RhMPV, and PtMPV [29,30,32]. The tropisms and clinical features observed in natural and experimental infections with these viruses resemble those of B19V and suggest their possible zoonotic potential [31–35]. Considering that the marked erythroid tropism of B19V is mediated by the RBD in N-VP1u, we hypothesized that a similar RBD might be present in N-VP1u from other primate erythroparvoviruses.

Previous investigations revealed that the B19V RBD has a well-defined structure of a three-helix fold, which forms a spatial cluster of internalization-relevant amino acids at the interface of helices 1 and 3 [27]. We compared the primary sequences located in the putative RBD within the VP1u region, and modulated in silico the RBD with the computer algorithm QUARK (Figure 5). The predicted RBD model of PtMPV exhibited a remarkable resemblance to that of B19V. The SPV and RhMPV RBD differed from the B19V RBD by an additional α-helix between helices 2 and 3. Although the primary amino acid sequences of primate VP1u regions were moderately conserved, the in silico modulations exhibited a similar spatial arrangement of helices 1 and 3. Internalization-important amino acids that were previously identified for B19V [27] were conserved by either identical amino acids or conservative replacements, resulting in a comparable spatial arrangement for all primate erythroparvoviruses.

The remarkable similarity of the predicted N-VP1u structure from the different primate erythroparvoviruses suggests a common function as an RBD required for virus uptake into erythroid progenitor cells. In line with this hypothesis, simian VP1u was able to specifically internalize into human UT7/Epo cells (Figure 6A,B), confirming its function as an RBD for virus uptake into erythroid cells. The close homology of all four primate erythroparvoviruses and the similar structure and function of their RBDs suggest that the uptake mechanism of these viruses is evolutionarily conserved. One possible evolutionary scenario is the infection of humans by an ancestor of SPV and the deletion of the additional helix in the RBD during the adaptive course of evolution, which resulted in the characteristic three-helix cluster of B19V. However, it is also conceivable that PtMPV represents an intermediate evolutionary step between SPV and B19V. Taken together, primate erythroparvoviruses could have a zoonotic potential for humans and be of particular concern for immunocompromised persons or pregnant women. Nevertheless, the results of this study are limited to the step of virus attachment and internalization and do not allow for conclusions about the permissiveness of human erythroid cells to non-human primate erythroparvoviruses.

The question remains whether B19V and the related non-human primate viruses rely on the same receptor structure for internalization. The fact that B19V VP1u was not able to interfere with simian PP7-VP1u uptake and simian VP1u only partially competed with B19V internalization (Figure 6C,D) suggests that B19V and SPV interaction with VP1uR may involve different binding sites. The possibility of two unrelated receptors, however, appears rather unlikely, since the RBD of SPV and B19V showed a similar structure with a comparable spatial cluster of internalization-important amino acids, as well as the same extraordinary specificity for erythroid cell types. B19V and SPV may recognize distinctive surface glycosylation patterns of the same receptor, where the steric hindrance of the additional helix in the RBD of SPV could play a key role. Finally, the internalization of simian VP1u was not affected in presence of MAb 1418-1 (Figure 6E). The differences in the structure and sequence of the RBD of SPV allow the simian virus to escape the neutralizing human antibody while maintaining the capacity to recognize VP1uR. Accordingly, SPV VP1u could be exploited for the therapeutic targeting of human erythroid cells without the limitation of pre-existing B19V-neutralizing antibodies.

5. Conclusions

The RBD in the N-VP1u of B19V interacts with VP1uR for virus internalization into susceptible cells. VP1uR expression was systematically analyzed in cells from different tissues by using a specific and sensitive marker based on a phage-VP1u bioconjugate. The receptor was exclusively detected in cells of the erythroid lineage, explaining the marked erythroid tropism of B19V. Structural and functional studies of N-VP1u from related non-human primate erythroparvoviruses revealed the presence of an analogous RBD-mediating virus internalization into human erythroid cells. These findings underline the close evolutionary relationship among human and animal erythroparvoviruses and further substantiate their zoonotic potential.

Author Contributions: Conceptualization, C.B., J.B., R.L. and C.R.; methodology, C.B., J.B. and R.A.; formal analysis, C.B., J.B., R.L. and C.R.; investigation, C.B., J.B., R.A., R.L. and C.R.; writing—original draft preparation, C.B. and C.R.; writing—review and editing, C.B., J.B., R.A., R.L. and C.R.; supervision, R.L. and C.R.; project administration, C.R.; funding acquisition, C.R. All authors have read and agreed to the published version of the manuscript.

Funding: This research was funded by the Swiss National Science Foundation (SNSF), grant number 31003A_179384.

Institutional Review Board Statement: Not applicable.

Informed Consent Statement: Not applicable.

Data Availability Statement: The data presented in this study are available on request from the corresponding author.

Acknowledgments: We are grateful to Y. Nakamura (Ibaraki, Japan) for kindly providing the HuDEP and HiDEP cells. We thank E. Morita (Tohoku University School of Medicine, Japan) and N. Ikeda (Fujirebio, Inc., Tokyo, Japan) for kindly providing the UT7/Epo and the KU812Ep6 cell line, respectively.

Conflicts of Interest: The authors declare no conflict of interest. The funders had no role in the design of the study; in the collection, analyses, or interpretation of data; in the writing of the manuscript, or in the decision to publish the results.

References

1. Cotmore, S.F.; Agbandje-McKenna, M.; Canuti, M.; Chiorini, J.A.; Eis-Hubinger, A.-M.; Hughes, J.; Mietzsch, M.; Modha, S.; Ogliastro, M.; Pénzes, J.J.; et al. ICTV Virus Taxonomy Profile: Parvoviridae. *J. Gen. Virol.* **2019**, *100*, 367–368. [CrossRef] [PubMed]
2. Qiu, J.; Söderlund-Venermo, M.; Young, N.S. Human Parvoviruses. *Clin. Microbiol. Rev.* **2017**, *30*, 43–113. [CrossRef] [PubMed]
3. Survey, J.T.; Reamy, B.V.; Hodge, J. Clinical presentations of parvovirus B19 infection. *Am. Fam. Physician* **2007**, *75*, 75.

4. Papadogiannakis, N.; Tolfvenstam, T.; Fischler, B.; Norbeck, O.; Broliden, K. Active, Fulminant, Lethal Myocarditis Associated with Parvovirus B19 Infection in an Infant. *Clin. Infect. Dis.* **2002**, *35*, 1027–1031. [CrossRef] [PubMed]
5. Giorgio, E.; De Oronzo, M.A.; Iozza, I.; Di Natale, A.; Cianci, S.; Garofalo, G.; Giacobbe, A.M.; Politi, S. Parvovirus B19 during pregnancy: A review. *J. Prenat. Med.* **2010**, *4*, 63–66.
6. Ornoy, A.; Ergaz, Z. Parvovirus B19 infection during pregnancy and risks to the fetus. *Birth Defects Res.* **2017**, *109*, 311–323. [CrossRef]
7. Heegaard, E.D.; Brown, K.E. Human Parvovirus B19, Clin. *Microbiol. Rev.* **2002**, *15*, 485–505. [CrossRef]
8. Brown, K.E.; Young, N.S.; Alving, B.M.; Barbosa, L.H. Parvovirus B19: Implications for transfusion medicine. Summary of a workshop. *Transfus.* **2001**, *41*, 130–135. [CrossRef]
9. Eid, A.J.; Brown, R.A.; Patel, R.; Razonable, R.R. Parvovirus B19 Infection after Transplantation: A Review of 98 Cases. *Clin. Infect. Dis.* **2006**, *43*, 40–48. [CrossRef]
10. Parsyan, A.; Candotti, D. Human erythrovirus B19 and blood transfusion? An update. *Transfus. Med.* **2007**, *17*, 263–278. [CrossRef]
11. Stramer, S.L.; Dodd, R.Y.; Subgroup, D. Transfusion-transmitted emerging infectious diseases: 30 years of challenges and progress. *Transfus.* **2013**, *53*, 2375–2383. [CrossRef] [PubMed]
12. Ganaie, S.S.; Qiu, J. Recent Advances in Replication and Infection of Human Parvovirus B19. *Front. Cell. Infect. Microbiol.* **2018**, *8*, 166. [CrossRef] [PubMed]
13. Munakata, Y.; Kato, I.; Saito, T.; Kodera, T.; Ishii, K.K.; Sasaki, T. Human parvovirus B19 infection of monocytic cell line U937 and antibody-dependent enhancement. *Virology* **2006**, *345*, 251–257. [CrossRef] [PubMed]
14. Von Kietzell, K.; Pozzuto, T.; Heilbronn, R.; Gröss, L.T.; Fechner, H.; Weger, S. Antibody-Mediated Enhancement of Parvovirus B19 Uptake into Endothelial Cells Mediated by a Receptor for Complement Factor C1q. *J. Virol.* **2014**, *88*, 8102–8115. [CrossRef]
15. Adamson-Small, L.A.; Ignatovich, I.V.; Laemmerhirt, M.G.; Hobbs, J.A. Persistent parvovirus B19 infection in non-erythroid tissues: Possible role in the inflammatory and disease process. *Virus Res.* **2014**, *190*, 8–16. [CrossRef]
16. Schenk, T.; Enders, M.; Pollak, S.; Hahn, R.; Huzly, D. High Prevalence of Human Parvovirus B19 DNA in Myocardial Autopsy Samples from Subjects without Myocarditis or Dilative Cardiomyopathy. *J. Clin. Microbiol.* **2009**, *47*, 106–110. [CrossRef]
17. Verdonschot, J.; Hazebroek, M.; Merken, J.; Debing, Y.; Dennert, R.; Rocca, H.-P.B.-L.; Heymans, S. Relevance of cardiac parvovirus B19 in myocarditis and dilated cardiomyopathy: Review of the literature. *Eur. J. Hear. Fail.* **2016**, *18*, 1430–1441. [CrossRef]
18. Cotmore, S.F.; McKie, V.C.; Anderson, L.J.; Astell, C.R.; Tattersall, P. Identification of the major structural and nonstructural proteins encoded by human parvovirus B19 and mapping of their genes by procaryotic expression of isolated genomic fragments. *J. Virol.* **1986**, *60*, 548–557. [CrossRef]
19. Saikawa, T.; Anderson, S.; Momoeda, M.; Kajigaya, S.; Young, N.S. Neutralizing linear epitopes of B19 parvovirus cluster in the VP1 unique and VP1-VP2 junction regions. *J. Virol.* **1993**, *67*, 3004–3009. [CrossRef]
20. Anderson, S.; Momoeda, M.; Kawase, M.; Kajigaya, S.; Young, N.S. Peptides derived from the unique region of B19 parvovirus minor capsid protein elicitneutralizing antibodies in rabbits. *Virology* **1995**, *206*, 626–632. [CrossRef]
21. Zuffi, E.; Manaresi, E.; Gallinella, G.; Gentilomi, G.A.; Venturoli, S.; Zerbini, M.; Musiani, M. Identification of an Immunodominant Peptide in the Parvovirus B19 VP1 Unique Region Able to Elicit a Long-Lasting Immune Response in Humans. *Viral Immunol.* **2001**, *14*, 151–158. [CrossRef] [PubMed]
22. Ros, C.; Gerber, M.; Kempf, C. Conformational Changes in the VP1-Unique Region of Native Human Parvovirus B19 Lead to Exposure of Internal Sequences That Play a Role in Virus Neutralization and Infectivity. *J. Virol.* **2006**, *80*, 12017–12024. [CrossRef] [PubMed]
23. Bönsch, C.; Kempf, C.; Ros, C. Interaction of Parvovirus B19 with Human Erythrocytes Alters Virus Structure and Cell Membrane Integrity. *J. Virol.* **2008**, *82*, 11784–11791. [CrossRef] [PubMed]
24. Bönsch, C.; Zuercher, C.; Lieby, P.; Kempf, C.; Ros, C. The Globoside Receptor Triggers Structural Changes in the B19 Virus Capsid That Facilitate Virus Internalization. *J. Virol.* **2010**, *84*, 11737–11746. [CrossRef]
25. Leisi, R.; Ruprecht, N.; Kempf, C.; Ros, C. Parvovirus B19 Uptake Is a Highly Selective Process Controlled by VP1u, a Novel Determinant of Viral Tropism. *J. Virol.* **2013**, *87*, 13161–13167. [CrossRef]
26. Leisi, R.; Von Nordheim, M.; Ros, C.; Kempf, C. The VP1u Receptor Restricts Parvovirus B19 Uptake to Permissive Erythroid Cells. *Viruses* **2016**, *8*, 265. [CrossRef]
27. Leisi, R.; Di Tommaso, C.; Kempf, C.; Ros, C. The Receptor-Binding Domain in the VP1u Region of Parvovirus B19. *Viruses* **2016**, *8*, 61. [CrossRef]
28. O'Sullivan, M.G.; Anderson, D.C.; Fikes, J.D.; Bain, F.T.; Carlson, C.S.; Green, S.W.; Young, N.S.; Brown, K.E. Identification of a novel simian parvovirus in cynomolgus monkeys with severe anemia. A paradigm of human B19 parvovirus infection. *J. Clin. Investig.* **1994**, *93*, 1571–1576. [CrossRef]
29. Brown, K.E.; Green, S.W.; O'Sullivan, M.; Young, N.S. Cloning and Sequencing of the Simian Parvovirus Genome. *Virology* **1995**, *210*, 314–322. [CrossRef]
30. Green, S.W.; Malkovska, I.; O'Sullivan, M.; Brown, K.E. Rhesus and Pig-Tailed Macaque Parvoviruses: Identification of Two New Members of the Erythrovirus Genus in Monkeys. *Virology* **2000**, *269*, 105–112. [CrossRef]
31. Brown, K.E.; Young, N.S. The simian parvoviruses. *Rev. Med. Virol.* **1997**, *7*, 211–218. [CrossRef]
32. O'Sullivan, M.G.; Anderson, D.K.; Lund, J.E.; Brown, W.P.; Green, S.W.; Young, N.S.; Brown, K.E. Clinical and epidemiological features of simian parvovirus infection in cynomolgus macaques with severe anemia. *Lab. Anim. Sci.* **1996**, *46*, 291–297. [PubMed]

33. O'Sullivan, M.G.; Anderson, D.K.; Goodrich, J.A.; Tulli, H.; Green, S.W.; Young, N.S.; Brown, K.E. Experimental infection of cynomolgus monkeys with simian parvovirus. *J. Virol.* **1997**, *71*, 4517–4521. [CrossRef] [PubMed]
34. Brown, K.E.; Liu, Z.; Gallinella, G.; Wong, S.; Mills, I.P.; O'Sullivan, M.G. Simian Parvovirus Infection: A Potential Zoonosis. *J. Infect. Dis.* **2004**, *190*, 1900–1907. [CrossRef] [PubMed]
35. Gallinella, G.; Anderson, S.M.; Young, N.S.; Brown, K.E. Human parvovirus B19 can infect cynomolgus monkey marrow cells in tissue culture. *J. Virol.* **1995**, *69*, 3897–3899. [CrossRef] [PubMed]
36. Leisi, R.; Von Nordheim, M.; Kempf, C.; Ros, C. Specific Targeting of Proerythroblasts and Erythroleukemic Cells by the VP1u Region of Parvovirus B19. *Bioconjugate Chem.* **2015**, *26*, 1923–1930. [CrossRef]
37. Gigler, A.; Dorsch, S.; Hemauer, A.; Williams, C.; Kim, S.; Young, N.S.; Zolla-Pazner, S.; Wolf, H.; Gorny, M.K.; Modrow, S. Generation of Neutralizing Human Monoclonal Antibodies against Parvovirus B19 Proteins. *J. Virol.* **1999**, *73*, 1974–1979. [CrossRef]
38. Dorsch, S.; Kaufmann, B.; Schaible, U.; Prohaska, E.; Wolf, H.; Modrow, S. The VP1-unique region of parvovirus B19: Amino acid variability and antigenic stability. *J. Gen. Virol.* **2001**, *82*, 191–199. [CrossRef]
39. Sievers, F.; Wilm, A.; Dineen, D.; Gibson, T.J.; Karplus, K.; Li, W.; Lopez, R.; McWilliam, H.; Remmert, M.; Söding, J.; et al. Fast, scalable generation of high-quality protein multiple sequence alignments using Clustal Omega. *Mol. Syst. Biol.* **2011**, *7*, 539. [CrossRef]
40. Xu, D.; Zhang, Y. Ab initio protein structure assembly using continuous structure fragments and optimized knowledge-based force field. *Proteins: Struct. Funct. Bioinform.* **2012**, *80*, 1715–1735. [CrossRef]
41. Kurita, R.; Suda, N.; Sudo, K.; Miharada, K.; Hiroyama, T.; Miyoshi, H.; Tani, K.; Nakamura, Y. Establishment of Immortalized Human Erythroid Progenitor Cell Lines Able to Produce Enucleated Red Blood Cells. *PLoS ONE* **2013**, *8*, e59890. [CrossRef]
42. Edgar, R.C. MUSCLE: Multiple sequence alignment with high accuracy and high throughput. *Nucleic Acids Res.* **2004**, *32*, 1792–1797. [CrossRef]
43. Guindon, S.; Gascuel, O. A Simple, Fast, and Accurate Algorithm to Estimate Large Phylogenies by Maximum Likelihood. *Syst. Biol.* **2003**, *52*, 696–704. [CrossRef] [PubMed]
44. Kishi, K. A new leukemia cell line with philadelphia chromosome characterized as basophil precursors. *Leuk. Res.* **1985**, *9*, 381–390. [CrossRef]
45. Miyagawa, E.; Yoshida, T.; Takahashi, H.; Yamaguchi, K.; Nagano, T.; Kiriyama, Y.; Okochi, K.; Sato, H. Infection of the erythroid cell line, KU812Ep6 with human parvovirus B19 and its application to titration of B19 infectivity. *J. Virol. Methods* **1999**, *83*, 45–54. [CrossRef]
46. Takahashi, T.; Ozawa, K.; Asano, S.; Takaku, F. Susceptibility of human erythropoietic cells to B19 parvovirus in vitro increases with differentiation. *Blood* **1990**, *75*, 603–610. [CrossRef] [PubMed]
47. Robb, L.; Lyons, I.; Li, R.; Hartley, L.; Kontgen, F.; Harvey, R.; Metcalf, D.; Begley, C.G. Absence of yolk sac hematopoiesis from mice with a targeted disruption of the scl gene. *Proc. Natl. Acad. Sci. USA* **1995**, *92*, 7075–7079. [CrossRef]
48. Hall, M.A.; Curtis, D.; Metcalf, D.; Elefanty, A.; Sourris, K.; Robb, L.; Göthert, J.; Jane, S.M.; Begley, C.G. The critical regulator of embryonic hematopoiesis, SCL, is vital in the adult for megakaryopoiesis, erythropoiesis, and lineage choice in CFU-S12. *Proc. Natl. Acad. Sci. USA* **2003**, *100*, 992–997. [CrossRef]
49. Masuda, T.; Wang, X.; Maeda, M.; Canver, M.C.; Sher, F.; Funnell, A.P.W.; Fisher, C.; Suciu, M.; Martyn, G.E.; Norton, L.J.; et al. Transcription factors LRF and BCL11A independently repress expression of fetal hemoglobin. *Science* **2016**, *351*, 285–289. [CrossRef]

viruses

MDPI

Article

Oncolytic H-1 Parvovirus Hijacks Galectin-1 to Enter Cancer Cells

Tiago Ferreira [1], Amit Kulkarni [2], Clemens Bretscher [1], Petr V. Nazarov [3], Jubayer A. Hossain [4], Lars A. R. Ystaas [4], Hrvoje Miletic [4,5], Ralph Röth [6,7], Beate Niesler [6,7] and Antonio Marchini [1,2,*,†]

1 Laboratory of Oncolytic Virus Immuno-Therapeutics, German Cancer Research Centre, Im Neuenheimer Feld 242, 69120 Heidelberg, Germany; bt_tiago@hotmail.com (T.F.); c.bretscher@gmx.de (C.B.)
2 Laboratory of Oncolytic Virus Immuno-Therapeutics, Luxembourg Institute of Health, 84 Val Fleuri, L-1526 Luxembourg, Luxembourg; amitkulkar@gmail.com
3 Bioinformatics Platform and Multiomics Data Science Research Group, Department of Cancer Research, Luxembourg Institute of Health, L-1526 Luxembourg, Luxembourg; petr.nazarov@lih.lu
4 Department of Biomedicine, University of Bergen, 5007 Bergen, Norway; jubayer.hossain@uib.no (J.A.H.); larsystaas@gmail.com (L.A.R.Y.); hrvoje.miletic@uib.no (H.M.)
5 Department of Pathology, Haukeland University Hospital, 5021 Bergen, Norway
6 nCounter Core Facility, Institute of Human Genetics, University of Heidelberg, 69120 Heidelberg, Germany; ralph.roeth@med.uni-heidelberg.de (R.R.); beate.niesler@med.uni-heidelberg.de (B.N.)
7 Department of Human Molecular Genetics, University of Heidelberg, 69120 Heidelberg, Germany
* Correspondence: a.marchini@dkfz.de; Tel.: +49-6221-424969
† Present address: European Commission, Joint Research Centre (JRC), 2440 Geel, Belgium.

Abstract: Clinical studies in glioblastoma and pancreatic carcinoma patients strongly support the further development of H-1 protoparvovirus (H-1PV)-based anticancer therapies. The identification of cellular factors involved in the H-1PV life cycle may provide the knowledge to improve H-1PV anticancer potential. Recently, we showed that sialylated laminins mediate H-1PV attachment at the cell membrane. In this study, we revealed that H-1PV also interacts at the cell surface with galectin-1 and uses this glycoprotein to enter cancer cells. Indeed, knockdown/out of *LGALS1*, the gene encoding galectin-1, strongly decreases the ability of H-1PV to infect and kill cancer cells. This ability is rescued by the re-introduction of *LGALS1* into cancer cells. Pre-treatment with lactose, which is able to bind to galectins and modulate their cellular functions, decreased H-1PV infectivity in a dose dependent manner. In silico analysis reveals that *LGALS1* is overexpressed in various tumours including glioblastoma and pancreatic carcinoma. We show by immunohistochemistry analysis of 122 glioblastoma biopsies that galectin-1 protein levels vary between tumours, with levels in recurrent glioblastoma higher than those in primary tumours or normal tissues. We also find a direct correlation between *LGALS1* transcript levels and H-1PV oncolytic activity in 53 cancer cell lines from different tumour origins. Strikingly, the addition of purified galectin-1 sensitises poorly susceptible GBM cell lines to H-1PV killing activity by rescuing cell entry. Together, these findings demonstrate that galectin-1 is a crucial determinant of the H-1PV life cycle.

Keywords: oncolytic virus immunotherapy; protoparvovirus H-1PV; virus host interactions; virus cell entry; galectin-1; laminin γ1

Citation: Ferreira, T.; Kulkarni, A.; Bretscher, C.; Nazarov, P.V.; Hossain, J.A.; Ystaas, L.A.R.; Miletic, H.; Röth, R.; Niesler, B.; Marchini, A. Oncolytic H-1 Parvovirus Hijacks Galectin-1 to Enter Cancer Cells. *Viruses* **2022**, *14*, 1018. https://doi.org/10.3390/v14051018

Academic Editor: Giorgio Gallinella

Received: 13 April 2022
Accepted: 7 May 2022
Published: 11 May 2022

1. Introduction

Oncolytic viruses selectively infect and destroy cancer cells while sparing normal tissues [1]. They can also stimulate strong anti-tumour immune responses and destroy tumour vasculature [2]. No fewer than 40 oncolytic viruses are currently under evaluation in clinical trials as treatments against a variety of cancers. Among them is H-1 rat protoparvovirus (H-1PV), a member of the *Parvoviridae* family in the genus *Protoparvovirus* [3,4]. This genus in addition to H-1PV includes Kilham rat virus, LuIII virus, minute virus of mice (MVM), mouse parvovirus, tumour virus X and rat minute virus [5,6], which are also evaluated at the preclinical level as oncolytic viruses.

The H-1PV genome is a linear, single-stranded DNA molecule of around 5 kb containing the P4 and P38 promoters. The P4 promoter regulates the expression of the non-structural (NS) gene unit encoding the NS1 and NS2 proteins. The P38 promoter controls the expression of the structural VP gene unit, which encodes the VP1 and VP2 capsid proteins and the non-structural small alternatively translated protein [4]. NS1 is the major regulator of viral DNA replication and gene transcription and is the major effector of virus oncotoxicity [7,8].

Preclinical studies in a number of cellular and animal models indicate that H-1PV can target a large variety of tumour cell lines from different tumour entities [4]. This preclinical evaluation paved the way for the clinical evaluation of H-1PV in patients with glioblastoma (GBM) [9] or pancreatic carcinoma [10]. In early-phase clinical trials, H-1PV treatment was shown to be safe and well-tolerated. Virus treatment was also associated with the first evidence of efficacy, including (i) the ability to cross the blood–brain barrier after intravenous delivery; (ii) effective distribution and expression in the tumour bed; (iii) immunoconversion of the tumour microenvironment; and (iv) improved progression-free survival and overall survival in comparison to historical controls [9]. However, treatment with H-1PV, like other oncolytic viruses, was unable to eradicate tumours in patients with the regimes used [9]. Therefore, there is an urgent need to improve the clinical outcome of H-1PV oncolytic therapy. A promising approach is the identification of host cell factors that modulate the H-1PV life cycle. This knowledge could provide hints to which drugs or treatment modalities might be combined with the virus in order to enhance its oncotoxicity. In addition, a deeper understanding of the H-1PV life cycle could help to identify biomarkers capable of predicting which patients would most likely benefit from virus treatment [11].

The first step of the virus life cycle is the virus recognition of receptor (s), co-receptor (s) or other co-factors on the cell surface modulating host cell entry. In the case of H-1PV and other protoparvoviruses, sialic acid is essential for virus–cell attachment [12–14]. Recently, we performed a druggable genome-wide siRNA library screen to identify putative modulators of H-1PV infection. The screen identified *LAMC1*, encoding the laminin $\gamma 1$ chain, as a positive modulator of virus transduction. Characterisation of the interaction between H-1PV and laminin $\gamma 1$ revealed that laminins, and in particular those containing laminin $\gamma 1$, play a key role in mediating H-1PV attachment at the cell surface and subsequent entry into cancer cells. H-1PV binding to laminin is dependent on the sialic acid moieties in these molecules [14]. We have also shown that H-1PV cell uptake occurs through clathrin-mediated endocytosis and that the virus then passes through early to late endosomes prior to entering the nucleus. These events are dependent on dynamin activity and low endosomal pH [15].

The siRNA library screen also identified *LGALS1*, the gene encoding galectin-1 (Gal-1), as a leading activator of H-1PV infection. Interestingly, galectins are known to interact with laminins [16,17]. To date, 15 galectins have been identified in mammals [18]. They are widely expressed in various cell types and are involved in a variety of physiological functions including cell migration, mediation of cell–cell interactions, cell–matrix adhesion, transmembrane signalling, inflammation, and the immune response [19]. All galectins share a highly conserved carbohydrate-recognition domain, which binds to β-galactosides in N-linked and O-linked glycoproteins [20]. However, despite their similarities, galectins have notably different binding properties. Galectins are increasingly recognised as mediators of viral infections. However, the specific outcome of a galectin-virus interaction depends heavily on the particular galectin, the cell type, the virus, and the surrounding microenvironment. For instance, Gal-1 stabilises the binding of the human immunodeficiency virus (HIV)-1 to the host CD4 receptor on the surface of T cells by crosslinking CD4 and viral gp120 [21]. By contrast, Gal-1 inhibits Influenza A virus infection by interacting directly with the viral envelope glycoproteins [22]. In the context of protoparvoviruses, Gal-3 promotes MVM cell uptake and infection [23,24].

In view of the potential use of H-1PV as an anti-cancer therapeutic, our goal is to characterise the early events of H-1PV infection. In this study, we demonstrate that Gal-1 plays a key role in H-1PV infection at the level of virus entry.

2. Materials and Methods

2.1. Cells

Cervical carcinoma-derived HeLa, pancreatic ductal adenocarcinoma-derived BxPC3, glioma-derived, NCH125, NCH37, U251, LN308, T98G, and A172-MG cell lines were maintained in-house [14]. The NCH125 LGALS1 KO and NCH125 CRISPR Control cell lines were established in this study (see below-*Generation of LGALS1 knockout cell line*). HeLa Control and HeLa LAMC1 KD cells were established in a previous study [14]. All cells were cultured in Dulbecco's modified Eagle's medium (DMEM) supplemented with 10% FBS, 100 units/mL penicillin, 100 μg/mL streptomycin and 2 mM L-glutamine (all from Gibco, Thermo Fischer Scientific, Darmstadt, Germany) in a humidified incubator at 37 °C and 5% CO_2. All cancer cell lines were regularly tested for mycoplasma contamination using a VenorGEM OneStep Mycoplasma contamination kit (Minerva Biolabs, Berlin, Germany) and tested by a human cell authentication test (Multiplexion GmbH, Mannheim, Germany).

2.2. Viruses

Both wild-type H-1PV and recombinant H-1PV harbouring the green fluorescent protein-encoding gene (recH-1PV-EGFP) were produced, purified and titrated as previously described [25,26].

2.3. siRNA-Mediated Knockdown

Cells were seeded at a density of 4 x 10^4 cells/well in 24-well plates and grown in 500 μL of normal growth medium. After 24 h, cells were transfected with 10 nM siRNA using Lipofectamine RNAiMAX (Thermo Fisher Scientific, Carlsbad, CA, USA) according to the manufacturer's instructions. The following siRNAs were used for the galectins study (all purchased from Life Technologies, Paisley, UK: Silencer Select *LGALS1* siRNA (Cat. N. 4390824), Silencer *LGALS3* siRNA (Cat. N. 11332) and Silencer Select Negative Control #2 siRNA (Cat. N. 4390846). The siRNA targeting the *LAMC1* gene (Cat. N. SI00035742) and the AllStars Negative siRNA (Cat. N. SI03650318) used as a negative control were purchased from Qiagen (Hilden, Germany). After 24 h, the medium was replaced, and cells were grown for an additional 24 h to allow efficient gene silencing.

2.4. Viral Transduction Assay

Depending on the experiment, after 48 h siRNA transfection or 24 h after seeding or after pre-treatment with chemical for 30 min, cells were infected for 24 h with recH-1PV-EGFP at 0.3–0.5 TU/cell. Cells were then washed once with PBS and processed for fluorescence microscopy as described below. At least three independent experiments, each performed in duplicate, were performed for every condition.

2.5. Fluorescence Microscopy

Cells washed once with PBS were fixed with 3.7% paraformaldehyde on ice for 15 min, permeabilised with 1% Triton X-100 for 10 min and stained with 4′,6-diamidin-2-phenylindol (DAPI). Fluorescence images of enhanced green fluorescent protein (EGFP)-positive cells were acquired using a BZ-9000 fluorescence microscope (Keyence Corporation, Osaka, Japan) with a 10X objective. DAPI staining was used to visualise the cell nuclei.

2.6. Lactose Pre-treatment for H-1PV Transduction Analysis

β-lactose was purchased from Sigma-Aldrich Chemie GmbH Darmstadt, Germany (Cat. No. L-3750). Lactose stock solution was freshly prepared before treatment of the cells. HeLa cells were seeded at a density of 4×10^4 cells/well in 24-well plates and then pre-treated with increasing amounts (50, 100, 150, and 200 mM) of lactose for 30 min and then cells were infected with recH-1PV-EGFP for 4 h and grown for an additional 20 h. Cells were then processed as described in viral transduction assay and fluorescent microscopy sections. Numbers represent the arithmetic mean percentage of EGFP-positive cells relative to the number of EGFP-positive cells observed in untreated cells, which was arbitrarily set as 100%.

2.7. Western Blotting

Standard Western blotting was performed as described previously [15]. Immunoblotting was carried out with the following antibodies: rabbit polyclonal anti-galectin-1 (HPA000646) at 1:1000 dilution, and mouse anti-β-tubulin (T8328) (both purchased from Sigma-Aldrich, Hamburg, Germany) at 1:4000 dilution; rabbit polyclonal anti-laminin gamma 1 (PA5-36300; Thermo Fisher Scientific, Carlsbad, CA, USA) at dilution 1:1000; rabbit anti-NS1 SP8 antiserum [27] and rabbit anti-VP1/2 antiserum [28] at 1:5000 dilution. Thereafter, the membrane was incubated with horseradish peroxidase-conjugated secondary antibodies (Santa Cruz, Heidelberg, Germany) used at 1:1000 dilution.

2.8. Generation of the LGALS1 Knockout Cell Line

CRISPR/Cas9-mediated knockout of *LGALS1* in NCH125 was accomplished using galectin-1 Double Nickase Plasmid ([h]sc-400941-NIC), whereas the CRISPR/Cas9 negative control was obtained using the Control CRISPR/Cas9 Plasmid (sc-418922; both from Santa Cruz). NCH125 cells were seeded in a 6-well plate at about 70% confluency. After 24 h, 2 μg of DNA were transfected using Lipofectamine LTX (Thermo Fisher Scientific, Carlsbad, CA, USA) according to the vendor's protocol. Transfected cells were selected in normal growth medium containing 1 μg/mL puromycin (Thermo Fisher Scientific, Shanghai, China) for 72 h. Individual clones were obtained by limiting dilution. Knockout was confirmed by Western blotting.

2.9. Plasmid Transfection

To rescue *LGALS1* expression, the plasmid encoding *LGALS1* gene was used (SC118705; OriGene Technologies, Inc. Rockville, MD, USA). NCH125 Control and LGALS1 KO cells were seeded at a density of 3×10^5 cells/well in a 6-well plate. The next day, cells were transfected with 2.5 μg of DNA using Lipofectamine LTX or mock-transfected for 48 h.

2.10. Confocal Microscopy

Cells were seeded at a density of 3.5×10^3 cells/spot on spot slides and grown in 50 μL of complete cellular medium. The next day, cells were infected with wild-type H-1PV at an MOI of 500 pfu/cell in a total of 70 μL of 5% fetal bovine serum (FCS)-containing medium. At 2 h post-infection, cells were fixed with 3.7% paraformaldehyde on ice for 15 min and permeabilised with 1% Triton X-100 for 10 min. Immunostaining was carried out with the following antibodies, all used at 1:500 dilution for 1 h: mouse monoclonal anti-H-1PV capsid [29] and rabbit polyclonal anti-galectin-1 (HPA000646; Sigma-Aldrich, Darmstadt, Germany). Anti-mouse Alexa Fluor 594 IgG (A11005; Thermo Fisher Scientific, Carlsbad, CA, USA) or anti-rabbit Alexa Fluor 488 IgG (A11008; Thermo Fisher Scientific, Carlsbad, CA, USA) were used as secondary antibodies. Nuclei were stained with DAPI. Images of randomly assigned cells in the green channel (galectin-1), red channel (H-1PV), or blue channel (DAPI) were acquired with a confocal microscope (Leica TCS SP5 II, Wetzlar, Germany). Picture analysis was carried out using the LAS X Software (Leica, Wetzlar, Germany).

2.11. MTT Viability Assay

To determine cell viability after virus infection, the conversion of 3-(4,5-dimethylthiazol-2-yl)-2,5-diphenyl-2H-tetrazolium bromide (MTT) (Sigma-Aldrich Chemie GmbH, Steinheim, Germany) was measured. For this purpose, cells were seeded on a 96-well plate at a density of 2000 cells/well in 50 µL of culture medium supplemented with 10% FCS. The next day, 50 µL of serum-free medium containing wild-type H-1PV were added on top of the cells. In rescue experiments, cells were treated with H-1PV at an MOI of 5 pfu/cell, or 5 µg/mL of recombinant galectin-1 (ab50237; Abcam, Cambridge, UK), or both simultaneously. Every 24 h post-treatment, for a total of 4 time points, 10 µL of 5 mg/mL MTT were added and subsequently incubated for 2 h at 37 °C. Thereafter, the supernatant was aspirated, and the plates were air-dried at 37 °C overnight. To solubilise the formazan product, cells were then incubated with 100 µL of isopropanol for 20 min with moderate shaking and the absorbance was read with an ELISA reader at 570 nm. Viability of treated cells was expressed as a ratio of the measured absorbance (arithmetic mean of three replicates per condition) to the corresponding absorbance of untreated cells (arbitrarily defined as 100%).

2.12. *Binding-Only and Binding and Entry Assays*

First, the culture medium was removed and replaced with 200 µL serum-free medium containing H-1PV at an MOI of 5 pfu/cell (or H-1PV at an MOI of 5 pfu/cell and 5 µg/mL of recombinant galectin-1 simultaneously in rescue experiments). Infection was performed for 1 h at 4 °C to allow only cell surface virus binding or for 4 h at 37 °C to also allow virus cell internalisation. Thereafter, cells were extensively washed with PBS, trypsinised for 5 min, quenched with serum-containing medium and subjected to three snap freeze-thaw cycles to release cell-associated viral particles. Viral DNA was purified from cell lysates using the QiAamp MinElute Virus Spin kit (Qiagen, Hilden, Germany) according to the manufacturer's instructions. Cell-associated H-1PV genomes were quantified by following a parvovirus-specific quantitative PCR (qPCR) protocol, as previously described [12]. A minimum of three independent experiments were performed in triplicate for every condition tested.

2.13. *Flow Cytometry*

Cells were seeded at a density of 5×10^5 cells/well in a 6-well plate. The next day, cells were infected with H-1PV at an MOI of 25 pfu/cell for 1 h at 4 °C. Cells were washed with ice-cold PBS and then gently scraped off with a cell lifter on ice. Cells were then fixed with 2% formaldehyde for 15 min at 4 °C and blocked with 2.5% albumin bovine fraction V (BSA; SERVA Electrophoresis, Heidelberg, Germany)/PBS for 20 min at 4 °C. Cells were then incubated with H-1PV anti-capsid antibody (dilution 1:500) for 30 min at 4 °C, and subsequently with Alexa Fluor 488 goat α-mouse (1:500) for 30 min at 4 °C. Three washes with 2.5% BSA/PBS were performed between each staining step. Analysis was carried out using a FACS Calibur (BD Biosciences, San Jose, CA, USA).

2.14. *Tissue Microarray*

Patient material for the tissue microarray was derived from paraffin embedded GBM biopsies obtained from the Department of Pathology, Haukeland University Hospital, Bergen, Norway. The project (number 2017/2505) was approved by the Regional Ethics Committee (Bergen, Norway). Control tissues (brain, liver and tonsil) were derived from autopsy material. The microarray included 61 primary GBM and 49 recurrent GBM biopsies, plus 12 biopsies from normal tissues (four each from brain, tonsil and liver). Immunohistochemical staining was carried out as described previously [30] using galectin-1 antibody (sc-166618; Santa Cruz, Santa Cruz, CA, USA) at a dilution of 1:200 followed by a biotinylated anti-mouse antibody (Vector Laboratories, Burlingame, CA, USA) at a dilution of 1:1100. Galectin-1-positive cells were counted via automated counting, as described previously [31].

2.15. Correlation Analysis between Gene Expression of Cancer Cell Lines and H-1PV-Induced Oncolysis

Gene expression data were taken from two databases: 53 cancer cell lines of NCI-60 dataset (https://discover.nci.nih.gov/cellminer, accessed on 23 January 2021, RNAseq data) and the Cancer Cell Line Encyclopedia (CCLE, 52 cancer cell lines) [32]. Simple linear regression models were built for 2 considered genes of interest (*LGALS1* and *LAMC1*) and 2 control genes (*LGALS3* and *GAPDH*), predicting experimentally observed EC50 values. Additionally, a two-variable regression was built predicting EC50 with both genes *LGALS3* and *GAPDH*. Significance of the models was characterised by the p-values (p), coefficients of determination (R^2) and Pearson correlations (R).

2.16. Measurement of Transcript Levels

The mRNA expression levels of the target of interest *LGALS1*, as well as of the reference genes *ACTB*, *GAPDH* and *PGK1*, were quantified at the nCounter Core Facility on a SPRINT Profiler system by nCounter technology (NanoString Technologies (Seattle, WA, USA), as described previously [14]. Accession numbers and target sequences of analysed genes are:

LGALS1 gene (accession number NM_002305.4): GGTGCGCCTGCCCGGGAACATC-CTCCTGGACTCAATCATGGCTTGTGGTCTGGTCGCCAGCAACCTGAATCTCAAACCT GGAGAGTGCCTTCGAGTGCGA

ACTB gene (accession number NM_001101.2): TGCAGAAGGAGATCACTGCCCTG-GCACCCAGCACAATGAAGATCAAGATCATTGCTCCTCCTGAGCGCAAGTACTCCGT GTGGATCGGCGGCTCCATCCT

GAPDH gene (NM_001256799.1): GAACGGGAAGCTTGTCATCAATGGAAATCC-CATCACCATCTTCCAGGAGCGAGATCCCTCCAAAATCAAGTGGGGCGATGCTGGCG CTGAGTACGTCGTG

PGK1 gene (NM_000291.2): GCAAGAAGTATGCTGAGGCTGTCACTCGGGCTAAGC AGATTGTGTGGAATGGTCCTGTGGGGGTATTTGAATGGGAAGCTTTTGCCCGGGGAA CCAAAGC

2.17. xCELLigence

Cell proliferation was monitored in real time through the xCelligence system (ACEA Biosciences Inc. San Diego, CA, USA) according to the manufacturer's instructions. Briefly, 8×10^4 cells per well were seeded in a 96-well E-plate (Roche, Mannheim, Germany) in a total volume of 100 µL of complete DMEM medium. Cells were treated during the cellular growth phase with H-1PV at an MOI of 5 pfu/cell or 5 µg/mL of recombinant galectin-1, or both simultaneously. Cell proliferation was monitored every 30 min in real time. Data are expressed as "Cell index" ($n = 3$) calculated by the RTCA software 1.2.1 (Agilent) as a measure of cell adhesion and, therefore, cell viability.

2.18. Statistical Analysis

Results are shown as the arithmetic mean of biological replicates ± standard deviation (SD) from a representative experiment. Statistical significance was determined by a paired two-tailed Student's t-test, unless stated otherwise, using Microsoft Excel 365 and/or GraphPad Prism version 8. Only values below 0.05 were considered significant: $p \leq 0.05$ (*), $p \leq 0.01$ (**) and $p \leq 0.001$ (***).

3. Results

3.1. Knockdown of LGALS1, but Not LGALS3, Hampers H-1PV Infection

To identify cellular modulators of the H-1PV life cycle, we previously carried out a high-throughput siRNA library screening in cervical carcinoma-derived HeLa cells using a siRNA library targeting the human druggable genome (6961 genes, each targeted by a pool of four siRNAs/gene) [14]. This led to the identification of laminins, in particular those containing the laminin γ1 chain, as factors used by H-1PV to attach at the cell surface and to enter cancer cells [14]. In the same screening, *LGALS1*—the gene encoding Gal-1—

emerged as another top activator of H-1PV transduction, as its silencing decreased H-1PV transduction by approximately 70% [14]. These findings, along with the fact that galectins interact with laminins [17], prompted us to hypothesise that Gal-1 is involved in H-1PV infection at the level of cell entry. This hypothesis was also supported by the discovery that MVM (a closely related protoparvovirus) requires Gal-3 to efficiently infect mouse cells [23,24].

We confirmed the results of the siRNA library screening by performing a knockdown of *LGALS1* using an independent siRNA. Given the role of Gal-3 in host cell entry by MVM, we also investigated the effect of siRNA-mediated silencing of *LGALS3*. A recombinant H-1PV expressing the *EGFP* reporter gene (recH-1PV-EGFP) was used for these experiments [25]. This non-replicative parvovirus shares the same capsid of the wild type but harbours the *EGFP* gene under the control of the natural P38 late promoter, whose activity is regulated by the NS1 viral protein. Therefore, the EGFP signal directly correlates with the ability of the virus to reach the nucleus and initiate its own gene transcription.

Cervical cancer-derived HeLa, glioma-derived NCH125 and pancreatic carcinoma-derived BxPC3 cell lines were transfected with siRNAs targeting *LGALS1* or *LGALS3*, or a scrambled siRNA. After 48 h, cells were infected with recH-1PV-EGFP and grown for a further 24 h. Efficient gene silencing was achieved for both genes in cells transfected with their respective siRNAs (Figure S1). However, only the siRNA targeting *LGALS1* significantly decreased H-1PV transduction (by more than 55%). As opposed to the role of Gal-3 in MVM infection, silencing of *LGALS3* did not significantly alter H-1PV transduction when compared with scramble controls (Figure 1). These results confirm the results of our siRNA library screening, which indicated that Gal-1, but not Gal-3, plays a key role in H-1PV infection in the cell lines tested.

3.2. Pre-Treatment with Lactose Inhibits H-1PV Infection

Gal-1 is a member of the galectins which belongs to a sub-family of lectins, defined by their highly conserved carbohydrate recognition domain (CRD) with the ability to bind to a number of beta-galactosides. Among the beta-galactosides, lactose is known to modulate the function of Gal-1 by directly binding to the CRD [33]. Hence, we hypothesised that treatment with lactose may interfere with H-1PV infectivity by competing with the virus for the interaction with Gal-1. To test this hypothesis, HeLa cells were pre-treated with increasing concentrations of soluble β-lactose before being infected with recH-1PV-EGFP. Pre-treatment with lactose decreased H-1PV transduction in a dose dependent manner (Figure 2). These results provide further evidence that H-1PV interaction with Gal-1 plays a crucial role in modulating H-1PV infectivity.

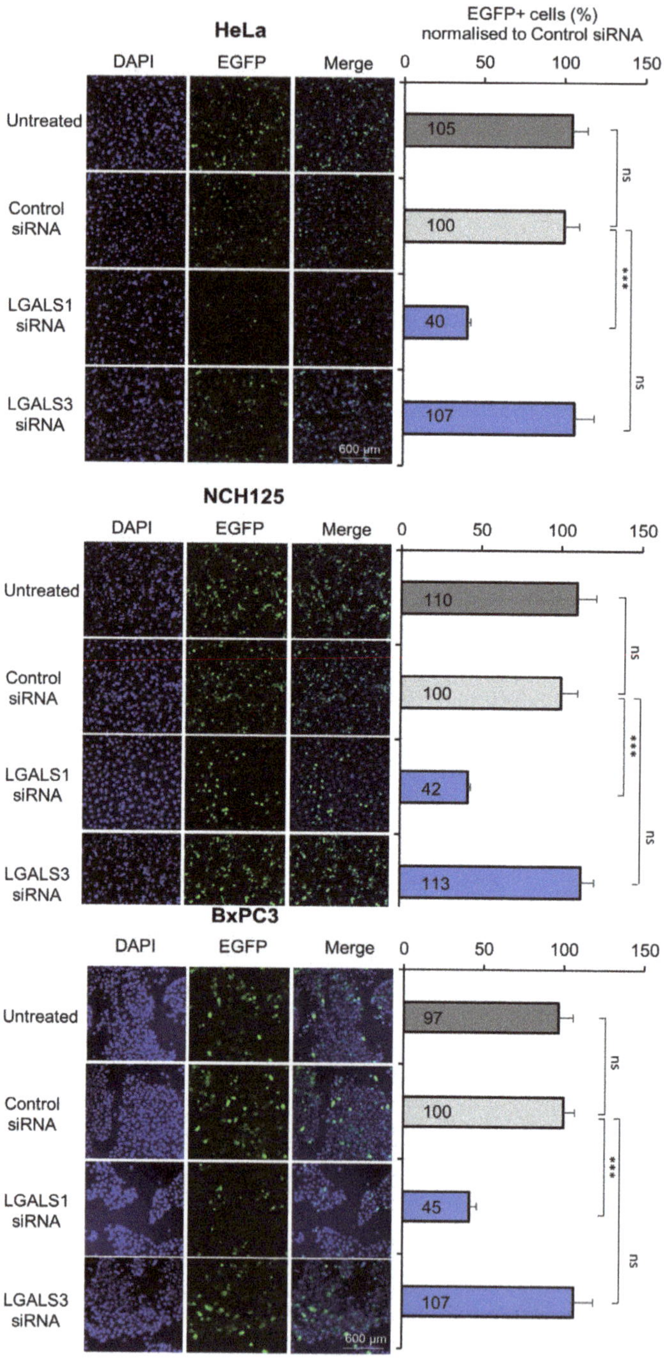

Figure 1. H-1PV transduction is reduced in *LGALS1*, but not *LGALS3*, knockdown cell lines. HeLa, NCH125 and BxPC3 cells were transfected with siRNAs targeting *LGALS1* or *LGALS3* or with a scrambled siRNA. At 48 h post-transfection, cells were infected with recH-1PV-EGFP for 4 h and grown for an additional 20 h. Cells were then processed as described in the Materials and Methods.

Numbers represent the arithmetic mean percentage of EGFP-positive cells relative to the number of EGFP-positive cells observed in cells transfected with control siRNA, which was arbitrarily set as 100%. The independent experiment shown was repeated thrice each with three biologically independent samples (*ns–not significant*; *** $p \leq 0.001$, calculated by using a one-way ANOVA).

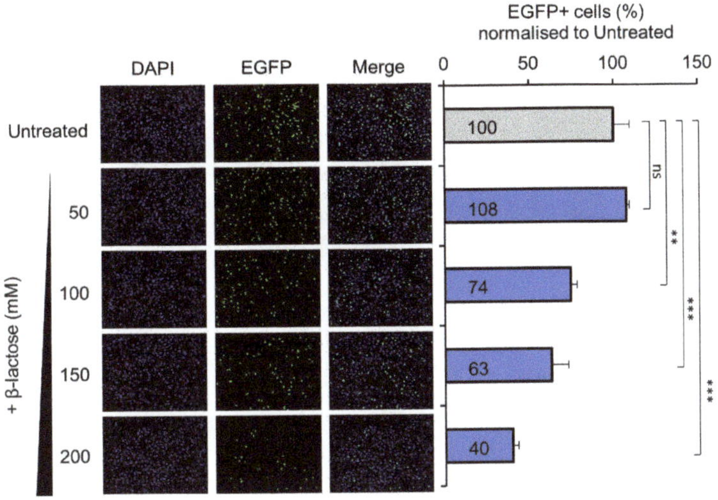

Figure 2. Pre-treatment with lactose decreases H-1PV infection in a dose-dependent manner. HeLa cells were pre-treated with the indicated concentrations of β-lactose for 30 min and then infected with recH-1PV-EGFP for 4 h. At 20 h after infection, cells were then harvested and processed as described in the Materials and Methods section. Numbers represent the arithmetic mean percentage of EGFP-positive cells relative to the number of EGFP-positive cells observed in untreated cells, which was arbitrarily set as 100%. The independent experiment shown was repeated thrice each with three biologically independent samples (*ns–not significant*; ** $p > 0.05$; *** $p \leq 0.001$, calculated by using a one-way ANOVA).

3.3. *Galectin-1 Knockout Impairs H-1PV Infection in NCH125 Cells*

To further investigate the biological role of Gal-1 in H-1PV infection, we took advantage of the CRISPR-Cas9 technology and established the NCH125 *LGALS1* knockout cell line (LGALS1 KO). We also established the NCH125 control cell line (Control) using a non-targeting guide RNA control sequence. Given that H-1PV requires S-phase factors expressed in proliferating cells for a productive infection [8], we evaluated the proliferation of LGALS1 KO versus Control cells. Both cell lines proliferated at a similar rate, as shown by real-time monitoring of cell growth and viability via xCELLigence (Figure S2).

We infected LGALS1 KO and Control cell lines with wild-type H-1PV and analysed the number of internalised virus particles by immunofluorescence using a specific anti-capsid antibody [29]. Two hours post-infection, fluorescence was significantly lower in LGALS1 KO cells than in Control cells (Figure 3A). Then, we evaluated the levels of viral proteins 48 h post-infection with the wild-type H-1PV. In agreement with previous results, Western blotting analysis revealed that NS1 and VP1 protein levels were lower in LGALS1 KO cells than in Control cells (Figure 3B). Finally, we analysed H-1PV transduction efficiency by infecting both cell lines with recH-1PV-EGFP. Consistent with reduced H-1PV entry, a significant decrease in transduction activity was found in LGALS1 KO cells (47%) in comparison with Control cells (Figure 3C). Strikingly, transient transfection of LGALS1 KO cells with a plasmid encoding *LGALS1* 48 h prior to infection, by re-establishing Gal-1 protein levels to values similar to those observed in Control cells (Figure 3C: Western blotting analysis), rescued the reduction in H-1PV transduction in these cells (Figure 3C).

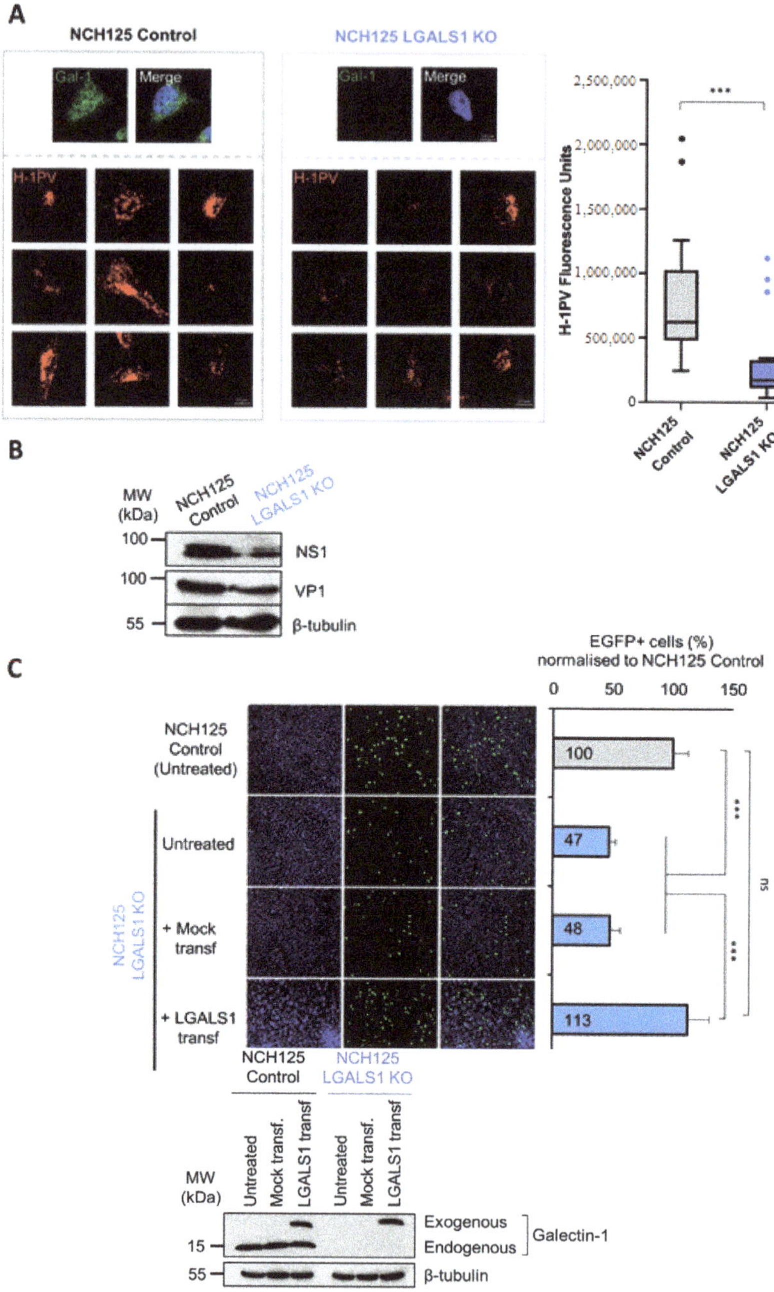

Figure 3. H-1PV infectivity is reduced in NCH125 LGALS1 KO cells. (**A**) H-1PV entry decreases in NCH125 LGALS1 KO cells. Control and LGALS1 KO cells were infected with H-1PV at an MOI of 50 pfu/cell for 2 h at 37 °C and prepared for confocal microscopy analysis. Gal-1 (green) and H-1PV

capsid (red) were detected using specific antibodies, while DAPI (blue) was used to stain nuclei. As expected, Gal-1 was readily detected in Control cells, while it fell below detection limits in LGALS1 KO cells. The lower panel shows representative examples of H-1PV-infected cells. Quantification of the H-1PV fluorescence signal is shown on the right. This was retrieved from two independent experiments in which the fluorescence intensity was quantified in 25 randomly identified cells using ImageJ. Box plot depicts the median with a centre line, and the Tukey–Whiskers plots indicate variability outside the upper and lower quartiles ($n = 25$, *** $p \leq 0.001$). (**B**) Control and LGALS1 KO cells were infected with H-1PV at an MOI of 2 pfu/cell for 48 h, and NS1 and VP1 protein levels were assessed by Western blotting. Beta-tubulin was used as a loading control. (**C**) H-1PV transduction is decreased in LGALS1 KO cells and re-established by transfecting the cells with a plasmid carrying *LGALS1*. LGALS1 KO cells were transfected with a plasmid encoding *LGALS1*, treated only with lipofectamine LTX (mock transfection) or left untreated. In addition, 48 h post-transfection, cells were infected with recH-1PV-EGFP for 24 h. Control cells were also included, and the level of virus transduction was set arbitrarily at 100%. The independent experiment shown was repeated twice each with four biologically independent samples (*ns*: $p > 0.05$; *** $p \leq 0.001$, calculating using a one-way ANOVA). On the right side, Western blotting analysis shows the levels of Gal-1 at the time of infection. Beta-tubulin was used as a loading control.

3.4. Galectin-1 Knockout Decreases H-1PV Oncolytic Activity in NCH125 Cells

As *LGALS1* knockdown/out decreased the overall amount of internalised H-1PV, we assessed whether this would result in reduced oncolytic activity. For this purpose, we assessed the susceptibility of LGALS1 KO and Control cell lines to H-1PV infection in a time course experiment in which viability of infected cells was assessed every 24 h for a total of 96 h. Whereas the viability of Control cells decreased progressively over time, the viability of LGALS1 KO cells, which were less sensitive to H-1PV infection, remained high throughout the experiment (above 75%; Figure 4A). Remarkably, the susceptibility of LGALS1 KO cells to H-1PV oncotoxicity was re-established by infecting the cells together with human recombinant Gal-1. Indeed, the viability of LGALS1 KO cells infected with H-1PV dropped from 74% to 18% in the presence of Gal-1; a control experiment showed that the protein itself was not toxic to the cells at the concentrations used (Figure 4B). Together, these results highlight the critical role of Gal-1 in H-1PV infection in NCH125 cells.

3.5. Galectin-1 Plays a Role in H-1PV Virus Entry Rather Than Cell Surface Attachment

The results shown above indicate that Gal-1 is involved in the early steps of H-1PV infection. However, whether Gal-1 is required for H-1PV attachment at the cell surface, internalisation, or both events, remains to be determined. To elucidate the role of Gal-1 in H-1PV infection, we first performed virus binding and entry assays. LGALS1 KO and Control cell lines were infected with wild-type H-1PV at 37 °C for different times (0.5, 1, 2 and 4 h) and then cell-associated viral DNA was quantified by PCR. In agreement with previous results, we observed less cell-associated H-1PV DNA in LGALS1 KO cells than in Control cells (Figure 5A). The addition of recombinant Gal-1 increased the number of cell-associated H-1PV genomes in LGALS1 KO cells to values that were similar to those found in H-1PV-infected Control cells (Figure 5B). These results confirm the role of Gal-1 in H-1PV binding and/or entry.

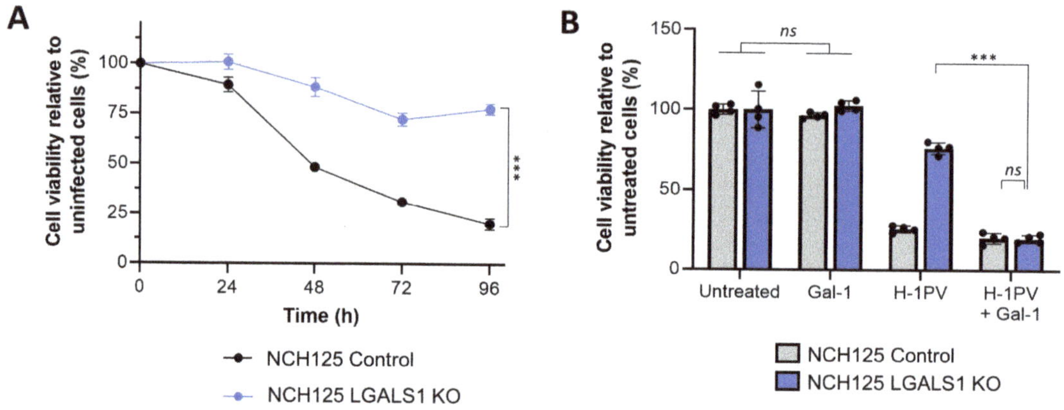

Figure 4. H-1PV has reduced oncolytic activity in NCH125 LGALS1 KO cells, which is rescued by supplementing with recombinant Gal-1 protein; (**A**) H-1PV oncolytic activity is reduced in NCH125 LGALS1 KO cells. Control and LGASL1 KO cells were infected with H-1PV at an MOI of 1 pfu/cell. Cell viability was assessed by MTT every 24 h for a total of 96 h. The curve plot depicts the mean ± standard deviation for each time point expressed as a percentage of cell viability compared to corresponding uninfected cells. The independent experiment shown was repeated thrice each with four biologically independent samples (*** $p \leq 0.001$). (**B**) Purified Gal-1 rescues H-1PV oncolytic activity in NCH125 LGALS1 KO cells. Control and LGASL1 KO cells were infected (or not) with H-1PV at an MOI of 1 pfu/cell, in the presence or absence of 5 µg/mL of human recombinant Gal-1. Cell viability was assessed at 72 h post-infection by MTT. Columns depict the percentage (mean value) of cell viability compared to uninfected cells ± standard deviation bars. The independent experiment shown was repeated twice each with four biologically independent samples (*ns:* $p > 0.05$; *** $p \leq 0.001$, calculated using a one-way ANOVA).

Concerning the possible involvement of Gal-1 in H-1PV cell surface attachment, LGALS1 KO and Control cell lines were inoculated with H-1PV at 4 °C for 1 h. Under these conditions, only virus attachment at the cell surface virus occurs, while cell entry is prevented [14]. After removing unbound H-1PV particles, those that remained attached to the cell surface were stained with an anti-capsid antibody and Flow cytometry analysis was performed. No significant differences in the fluorescence signal (H-1PV binding) were observed between the LGALS1 KO and Control cells (Figure 5C). The same findings were obtained by quantitative PCR analysis (Figure 5D). These results speak for an involvement of Gal-1 in H-1PV entry rather than in H-1PV binding to the cell surface.

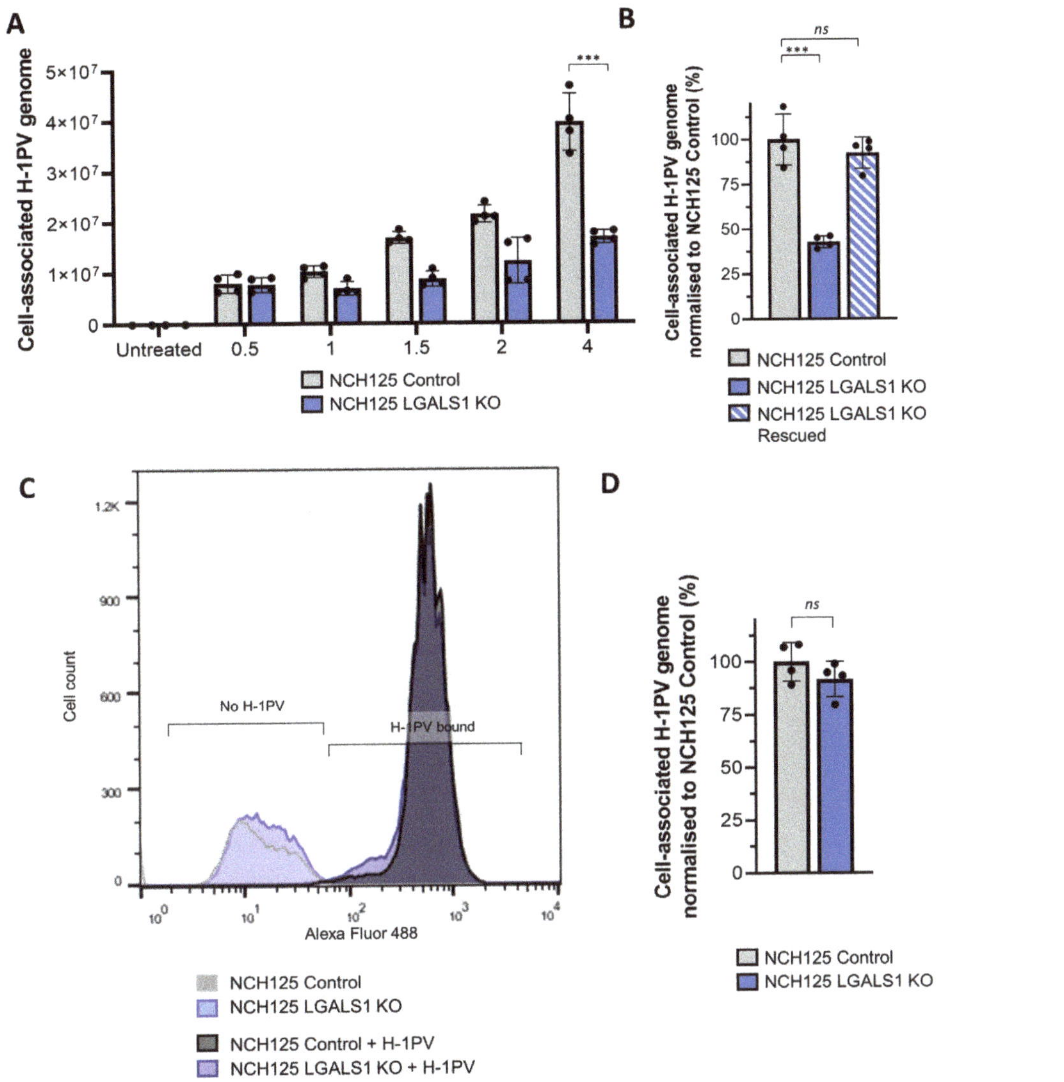

Figure 5. H-1PV cell entry, but not cell attachment, is reduced in NCH125 LGALS1 KO cells. (**A**) H-1PV binding and entry assay assessed by qPCR. NCH125 Control and LGALS1 KO cells were infected with H-1PV at an MOI of 5 pfu/cell for 0.5, 1, 1.5, 2 and 4 h at 37 °C. Cells were then extensively washed and harvested, and encapsidated viral DNA was extracted and subjected to qPCR. Columns in the graph show the number of copies of the cell-associated H-1PV genome with relative standard deviations (*** $p \leq 0.001$). The independent experiment shown was repeated thrice; $n = 3$ biologically independent samples. (**B**) Binding and entry is rescued by the addition of purified recombinant Gal-1. At the time of H-1PV infection (at an MOI of 5 pfu/cell), Gal-1 was added (or not) to the culture medium. Infection was carried out for 4 h. Numbers indicate the percentage of cell-associated genomes relative to NCH125 Control cells infected with H-1PV arbitrarily set as 100% The independent experiment shown was repeated twice each with four biologically independent samples (*ns*: $p > 0.05$; *** $p \leq 0.001$, calculated using a one-way ANOVA). (**C**) H-1PV cell surface binding assessed by Flow cytometry. A representative flow cytometry histogram with overlay of Control (black) and LGALS1 KO cells (blue) shows no difference in H-1PV-associated cells. Cells were

either mock- or H-1PV-infected (at an MOI of 25 pfu/cell) for 1 h at 4 °C. Cells were not permeabilised for the Flow cytometry analysis, and cell surface-bound H-1PV particles were detected with a specific anti-capsid antibody. The independent experiment shown was repeated twice each with two biologically independent samples. (**D**) H-1PV binding only, assessed by qPCR. Control and LGALS1 KO cells were infected with H-1PV (at an MOI of 5 pfu/cell) for 1 h at 4 °C. Cells were then washed and harvested, and extracted encapsidated viral DNA was quantified by qPCR. The independent experiment shown was repeated thrice each with three biologically independent samples.

3.6. Gal-1 Cooperates with Laminins in Mediating H-1PV Infection

Given that laminins containing the γ1 chain play determinant roles in H-1PV attachment at the cell surface as well as in H-1PV cell entry, we asked whether siRNA-mediated silencing of *LAMC1* in LGALS1 KO cells would further decrease H-1PV infection (Figure S3). In agreement with the results shown above, reduced H-1PV cell uptake was observed in LGALS1 KO cells. Furthermore, given the important role of laminins in H-1PV cell attachment and entry, knockdown of *LAMC1* gene expression also strongly reduced cell-associated H-1PV genomes in NCH125 cells. The reduction observed upon *LAMC1* knockdown was not significantly different between LGALS1 KO cells and Control cells, indicating that, in the absence of Gal-1, the depletion of *LAMC1* does not further reduce H-1PV cell uptake (Figure 6A). To confirm these results, we repeated the double knock-down experiment in HeLa cells (Figure S3). To this end, we silenced *LGALS1* gene expression in the previously established HeLa LAMC1 KD cell line (in which the *LAMC1* gene was knocked down via CRISPR-Cas9) [14]. In agreement with published results, infection of HeLa LAMC1 KD cells presented a 40% reduction in cell-associated H-1PV genomes in comparison with Control cells. The silencing of *LGALS1* also decreased H-1PV cell uptake in HeLa cells, yet no significant difference was observed between HeLa control and HeLa LAMC1 KD cell lines (Figure 6B). The fact that removal/reduction of both laminin γ1 and Gal-1 does not synergistically inhibit infection suggests that the two factors may act on the same H-1PV entry pathway. At the same time, the finding that, under these conditions, a fraction of viral particles is still able to penetrate cells supports the idea that H-1PV may also use alternative pathways and exploit other cellular factors to infect cells.

3.7. Gal-1 Is a Marker of Bad Prognosis in Various Tumour Types including GBM

Growing evidence indicates that overexpression of *LGALS1* is associated with metastasis formation, tumour recurrence and poor tumour prognosis [34]. Our analysis of brain tumour expression datasets using the GlioVis web application (http://gliovis.bioinfo.cnio.es/, accessed on 23 January 2021) revealed that *LGALS1* overexpression is associated with worse overall survival for brain tumours. Focusing particularly on GBM, we observed that these tissues have significantly higher expression of *LGALS1* in comparison to those from healthy individuals (Figure S4A) and *LGALS1* levels increase with the severity of the malignancy from WHO grade II to IV (Figure S4B). High *LGALS1* expression is associated with poor prognosis in glioma (Figure S5).

Next, we investigated whether Gal-1 protein levels varied between normal tissues, primary and recurrent GBM tissues. To this end, we used an in-house protein tissue microarray including a cohort of 110 GBM patient biopsies (61 primary and 49 recurrent GBM) and 12 biopsies from normal tissues (four each from brain, liver, and tonsil) and performed immunohistochemistry using an anti-galectin-1 antibody. Levels of Gal-1 were higher overall in GBM biopsies than in normal tissues. Among the GBM biopsies, we found a diversified Gal-1 expression profile with recurrent GBM tissues expressing significantly higher levels of Gal-1 than primary GBM tissues (45% of recurrent GBM tissues expressed medium or high levels of Gal-1, compared with 20% of primary GBM tissues; Figure 7).

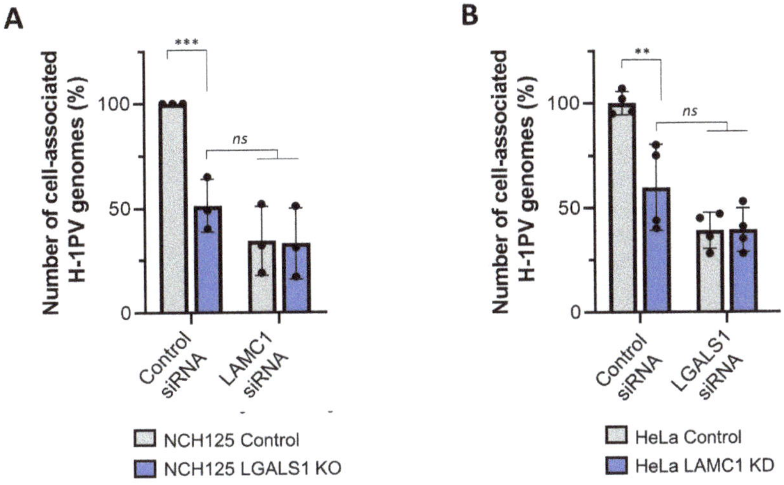

Figure 6. Effect on H-1PV binding and entry upon depletion of both *LAMC1* and *LGALS1* in NCH125 and HeLa cells. (**A**) NCH125 Control and LGALS1 KO cells were transfected with a siRNA targeting *LAMC1* or a negative control siRNA. At 48 h post-transfection, cells were infected with H-1PV at an MOI of 5 pfu/cell for 4 h at 37 °C. Cells were then extensively washed and harvested, and encapsidated viral DNA was extracted and subjected to qPCR. Columns in the graph show the number of copies of the cell-associated H-1PV genome with relative standard deviations (*ns*: $p > 0.05$; *** $p \leq 0.001$, calculated using a one-way ANOVA). The independent experiment shown was repeated thrice each with threebiologically independent samples. (**B**) HeLa Control and HeLa LAMC1 KD cells were transfected with a siRNA targeting *LGALS1* or a negative control siRNA. After 48 h siRNA transfection, cells were infected with H-1PV at an MOI of 5 pfu/cell for 4 h at 37 °C. Cells were then processed as per **A**. The experiment was performed with four biologically independent samples (** $p \leq 0.01$, calculated using a one-way ANOVA).

3.8. *LGALS1* Expression Profile of NCI-60 Cells Positively Correlates with H-1PV Oncotoxicity

Given the important role of Gal-1 in H-1PV infection, we looked for a putative correlation between *LGALS1* expression levels and H-1PV oncotoxicity. To this end, we screened 53 cancer cell lines from the NCI-60 panel for their susceptibility to H-1PV [14]. The gene expression profiles of these cell lines are fully characterised and publicly available [35]. We assessed virus-mediated oncotoxicity by monitoring cell viability in real time using xCELLigence [14]. We calculated the viral MOI responsible for killing 50% of the cell population at 72 h post-infection (EC50). Using gene expression data from NCI-60 and the Cancer Cell Line Encyclopedia (CCLE), we found that *LGALS1* mRNA expression levels anti-correlated with EC50 values, suggesting that cells expressing higher levels of *LGALS1* may be more susceptible to virus killing activity (Figure 8).

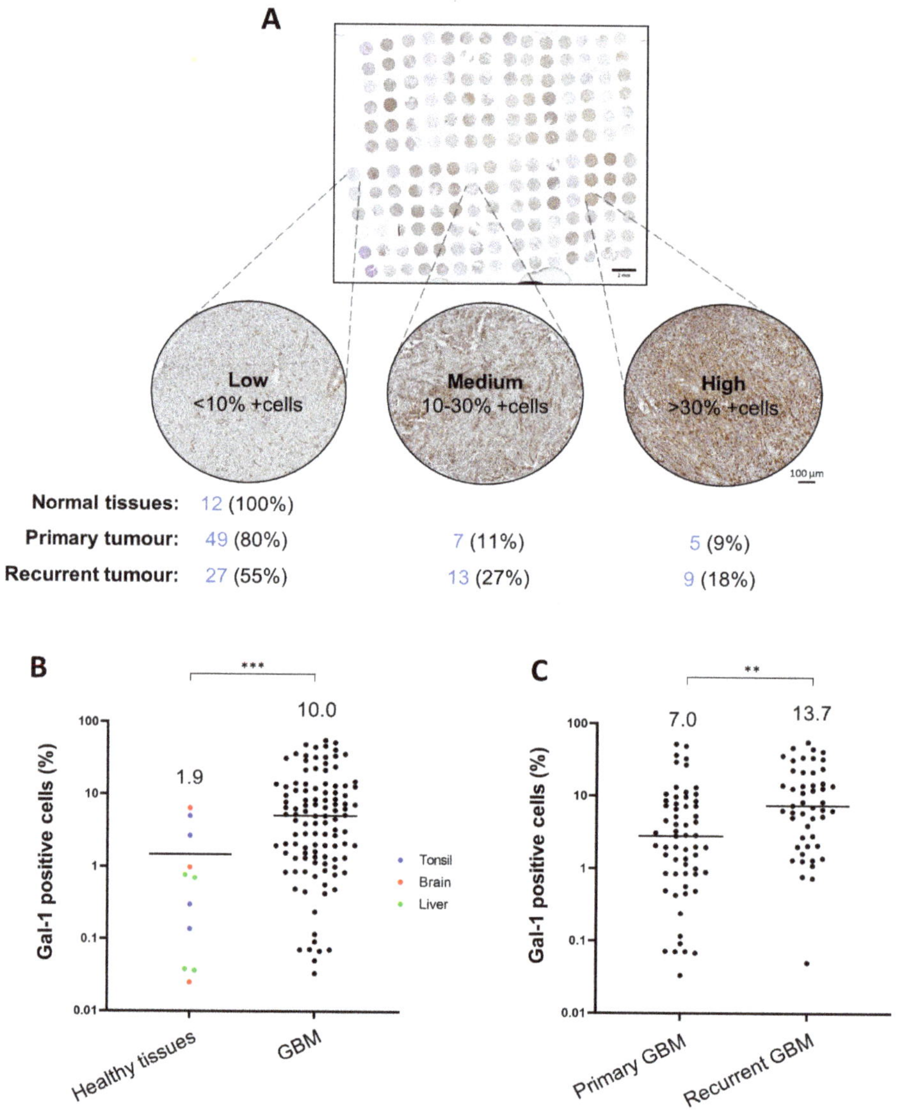

Figure 7. Differential expression of Gal-1 in normal tissues and in primary and recurrent GBM biopsies. (**A**) overview of the tissue microarray. This study included biopsies from normal tissue ($n = 12$), primary GBM biopsies ($n = 61$) and recurrent GBM biopsies ($n = 49$). Biopsies were categorised based on Gal-1 expression after immunostaining with anti-galectin-1 antibody: low (<10% positive cells), medium (10–30% positive cells) or high expression (>30% positive cells). The number of biopsies in each category are indicated under each representative image. The staining was performed twice in each normal sample and thrice on tumour tissues. Quantification of Gal-1-positive cells (%) was performed as described in the Materials & Methods section using in-house software; (**B**) comparative analysis of Gal-1 expression between healthy tissues and GBM biopsies (primary and recurrent); (**C**) comparative analysis of Gal-1 expression between primary and recurrent GBM biopsies. The arithmetic mean of Gal-1-positive cells is indicated with a horizontal line and by the number above (** $p \leq 0.01$; *** $p \leq 0.001$).

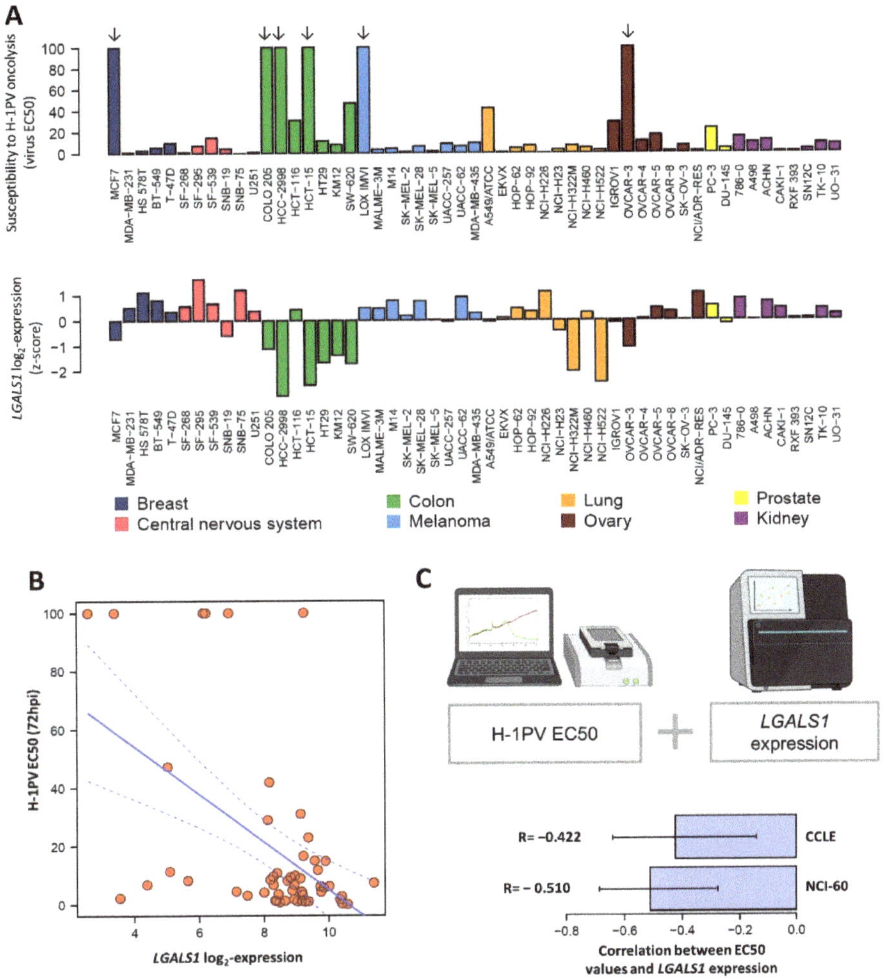

Figure 8. Correlation between *LGALS1* gene expression of cancer cell lines and their susceptibility to H-1PV-induced oncolysis. (**A**) *LGALS1* gene expression was retrieved from the National Cancer Institute (NCI)-60 database. Fifty-three cancer cell lines from the NCI-60 panel were tested for their susceptibility to H-1PV infection by xCELLigence. H-1PV EC50 values were calculated as the viral MOI that kills 50% of the cell population at 72 h post-infection (72hpi), measured by xCELLigence (see also [14]). Six cancer cell lines (MCF7, COLO 205, HCC-2998, HCT-15, LOX IMVI, OVCAR-3 (indicated by arrows) were found to be resistant to cell lysis even at the maximum tested concentrations of H-1PV (MOI 50 pfu/cell). Therefore, as EC50 values could not be calculated for those cell lines, their values were arbitrarily fixed as 100; (**B**) *LGALS1* expression versus H-1PV EC50. Each blue dot corresponds to a cell line and the grey line corresponds to a linear regression. (**C**) *LGALS1* levels are moderately anti-correlated with H-1PV EC50. *LGALS1* gene expression measurements were retrieved from the NCI-60 (53 cell lines) and Cancer Cell Line Encyclopedia (CCLE) (52 cell lines). Bar plot depicts the correlation between the gene expression from each dataset and the EC50 values (Pearson's correlation). Significant anti-correlation was observed for both NCI-60 and CCLE datasets with $R = -0.510$, C.I. (−0.685, −0.277), $p < 0.001$ and −0.422, C.I. (−0.641, −0.139), $p < 0.01$ respectively (in both cases, the null hypothesis: $R = 0$).

A similar anti-correlation was previously shown for *LAMC1* [14]. Therefore, we asked whether we could better predict the susceptibility of a certain cancer cell to H-1PV infectivity and cell killing by analysing the expression levels of the two genes together. As negative controls, *LGALS3* (selected for showing no apparent role in H-1PV infection) and *GAPDH* were chosen. Using both NCI-60 and the CCLE databases, we found that a slight increase in predictability of EC50 may be achieved by combining *LAMC1* and *LGALS1* in a single linear regression model. For NCI-60, R^2 of the combined model was 0.313 ($p = 8.3 \times 10^{-5}$), while simple models gave R^2 of 0.188 (*LAMC1*, $p = 1.2 \times 10^{-3}$, $R = -0.433$) and 0.260 (*LGALS1*, $p = 9.8 \times 10^{-5}$, $R = -0.510$). Control genes show no significant linear relation (*LGALS3*: $R^2 = 0.015$, $p = 0.38$, *GAPDH*: $R^2 = 0.018$, $p = 0.34$) (Figure S6). Similar results were obtained using the CCLE dataset (Figure S7). These results are in line with the important role that laminin $\gamma 1$ and Gal-1 play in H-1PV cell surface recognition and entry.

3.9. *LGALS1 Expression Positively Correlates with H-1PV Oncolysis in Glioma Cell Lines*

Glioma cancer cell lines are generally susceptible to H-1PV oncolysis [36]. However, not all cancer cell lines respond similarly to H-1PV oncolysis: they range from highly to lowly permissive, or are even resistant. We recently described four glioma cell lines that are semi-permissive to H-1PV infection, namely U251, LN308, T98G and A172-MG, which all express low levels of *LAMC1* mRNA [14]. However, it is possible that other cell components may account for the poor susceptibility of these cell lines to virus infection. Using the NanoString technology, we found that *LGALS1* mRNA levels were lower in the four aforementioned cell lines, as well as in the control normal human astrocytes, than in two H-1PV-sensitive glioma cell lines (NCH125 and NCH37) (Figure 9A). Monitoring of cell viability in real time by xCELLigence confirmed our previous results showing that NCH125 and NCH37 cell lines are efficiently killed by H-1PV at an MOI of 5 (pfu/cell). By contrast, U251, LN308, T98G, A172-MG cell lines as well as control normal human astrocytes were not. Remarkably, susceptibility of the four semi-permissive glioma cell lines to H-1PV oncotoxicity was substantially enhanced by the addition of human recombinant Gal-1 (Figure 9B). Consistent with our previous results, the addition of exogenous Gal-1 promoted H-1PV entry in the four glioma cell lines leading to an increase in the number of cell-associated viral genomes by 1.5- to 2.8-fold (Figure 9D), while not interfering with viral binding to the cell surface (Figure 9C). Together, these results confirm that Gal-1 plays a critical role in H-1PV infection at the level of virus entry and provide evidence that Gal-1 levels can determine the outcome of H-1PV infection. These results further support the importance of Gal-1 to H-1PV oncolytic activity and pave the way for its use in predicting the success of H-1PV infection.

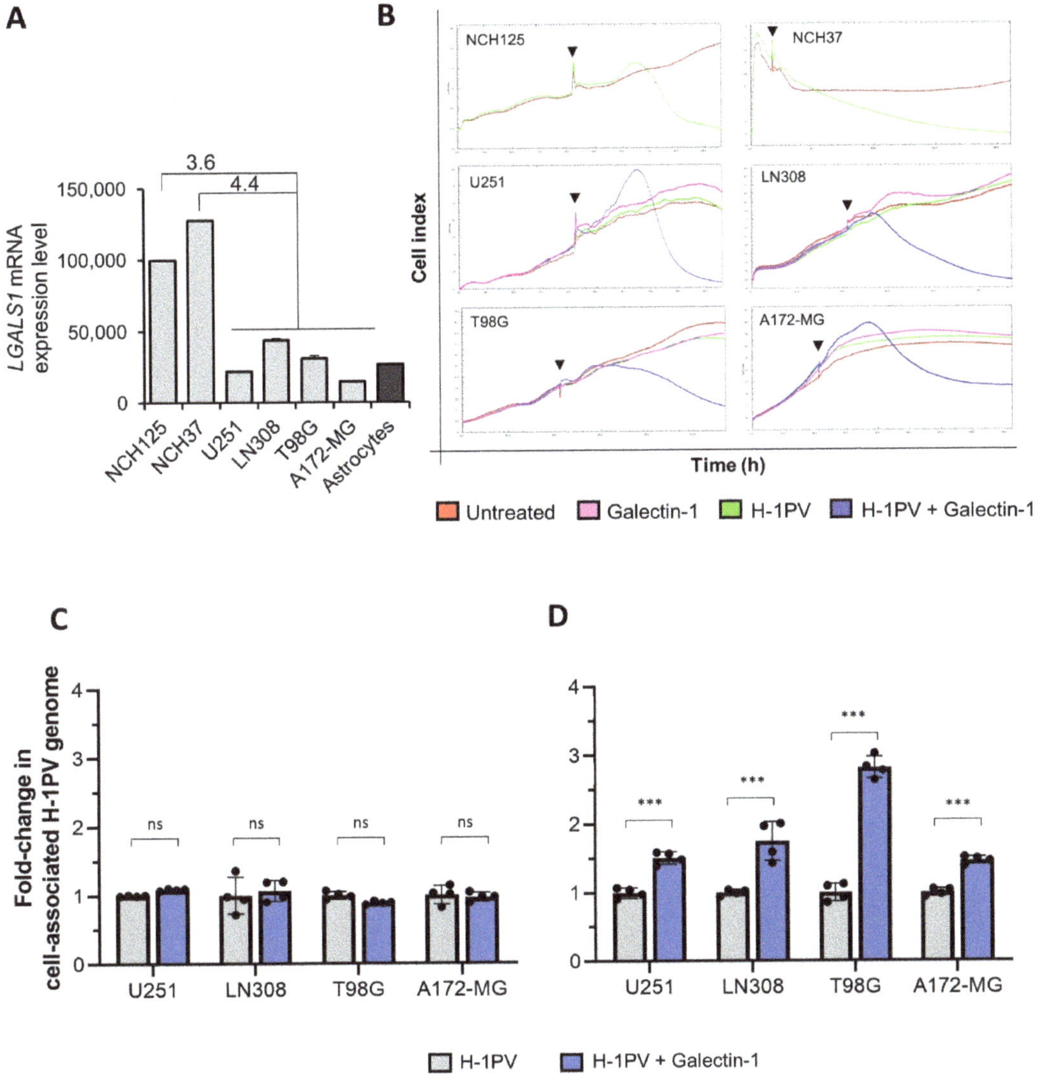

Figure 9. Galectin-1 levels in glioma cell lines determine the success of H-1PV infection. (**A**) Total mRNA was isolated from glioma cell lines susceptible (NCH125; NCH37) or semi-permissive (U251; LN308; T98G; A172-MG) to H-1PV infection, and *LGALS1* mRNA transcripts were measured using nCounter analysis. Bar graph depicts the *LGALS1* transcript counts; numbers on the top of the columns indicate gene expression fold changes between susceptible and semi-permissive cancer cell lines. The independent experiment is shown; n = 1 (NCH125, NCH37, U251 and A172-MG); n = 2 (LN308 and T98G); n = 3 (human astrocytes) biologically independent samples. (**B**) NCH125 and NCH37 cell lines were either infected with H-1PV at an MOI of 5 pfu/cell (green) or left untreated (red). Semi-permissive cell lines were infected with H-1PV at an MOI of 5 pfu/cell (green), incubated with 5 µg/mL of human recombinant Gal-1 (pink), H-1PV and Gal-1 simultaneously (blue), or left untreated (red). Cell viability was assessed by xCELLigence every 30 min in real time. The curve shows the "Cell index" mean of three biologically independent samples (n = 3) at any given time, which is proportional to the viability of the cell population. Black arrows indicate the time of treatment. (**C**) H-1PV binding at the cell surface is not affected by Gal-1 addition. U251, LN308, T98G

and A172-MG cells were incubated with H-1PV alone at an MOI of 5 pfu/cell or with H-1PV and Gal-1. Incubations were carried out for 1 h at 4 °C (binding only). Cells were then washed and harvested, and encapsidated viral DNA was extracted and subsequently quantified by qPCR. Columns in the graph show the fold change of number of copies of cell-associated H-1PV genome relative to the virus-infected cells arbitrarily set as 1, with respective standard deviations. The independent experiment shown was performed with four biologically independent samples (*ns*: $p > 0.05$; *** $p \leq 0.001$, calculated using a one-way ANOVA). (**D**) H-1PV entry is rescued upon Gal-1 addition. U251, LN308, T98G and A172-MG cells were incubated with H-1PV alone at an MOI of 5 pfu/cell or with H-1PV and Gal-1. Incubations were carried out either for 4 h at 37 °C (binding and entry). Cells were processed and results analysed as described in C.

4. Discussion

Following more than five decades of preclinical research, H-1PV monotherapy has been evaluated in patients with recurrent GBM and pancreatic carcinoma in early-phase clinical trials. H-1PV treatment was demonstrated to be safe, well tolerated and associated with surrogate evidence of anticancer efficacy, including immunoconversion of the tumour microenvironment and improved progression-free survival and overall survival in comparison with historical controls [9]. These promising results have motivated research aiming at further improving H-1PV efficacy [11,37].

The virus life cycle is a multistep process that is heavily dependent on the presence and abundance of viral (co-)receptors, processing enzymes and proteins required for a productive infection. The levels and activities of these components may vary in different cancer cells, determining their susceptibility to a particular virus. We anticipate that a better understanding of the H-1PV life cycle may provide the cues to further develop H-1PV-based therapies. For instance, this knowledge may help to identify new drugs that enhance H-1PV replication in cancer cells and/or oncolytic activity by modulating H-1PV-related cellular pathways. Furthermore, the cellular factors involved in the H-1PV life cycle may also serve as biomarkers to predict whether a certain tumour is susceptible or resistant to H-1PV infection.

Recently, we found that H-1PV enters cancer cells via clathrin-mediated endocytosis, a process that involves dynamin and requires a low pH in the endocytic compartments [15]. We also reported that laminins, in particular those containing the laminin $\gamma 1$ chain, act as attachment factors at the cell surface for a successful H-1PV infection [14]. In particular, we found that sialic acid moieties in the laminins provide a docking place for the virus to anchor to at the cell surface [14]. Laminin $\gamma 1$ was originally identified as a modulator of the H-1PV life cycle in a siRNA screening using a druggable-genome library performed in HeLa cells. The same screening revealed Gal-1 as another top activator of H-1PV infection. Indeed, silencing of *LGALS1* impaired H-1PV virus transduction by approximately 70% in HeLa cells. These results prompted us to explore whether Gal-1 is involved in the early steps of H-1PV infection.

In the present study, we show that Gal-1 plays a central role in H-1PV infection at the level of H-1PV cell entry but not cell attachment, indicating a role that is distinct from that of laminins in the virus cell cycle. By contrast, knockdown of *LGALS3* did not impair H-1PV infection (Figure 1), further supporting the specificity of the interaction between H-1PV and Gal-1.

Until the present study, Gal-3 was the only galectin that had been implicated in a protoparvovirus infection. Indeed, knockdown of *LGALS3* rendered LA9 mouse fibroblasts less susceptible to MVM infection. This phenotype was not due to reduced binding to the cell surface; instead, Gal-3 was responsible for promoting efficient virus uptake [24]. Our results indicate that Gal-1 is essential for a productive H-1PV infection at the level of cell entry, with no evidence of its requirement in viral binding to the plasma membrane in NCH125 cell lines. Therefore, these findings suggest that the mechanisms through which Gal-1 mediates H-1PV entry are similar to those of Gal-3 in MVM infection [23]. The fact that our results do not support an involvement of Gal-3 or clathrin-independent endocytosis in the H-1PV entry process [15] suggests that H-1PV and MVM engage different galectins for their entry processes which may contribute to their different tropism. At this point, we cannot also exclude that, in addition to Gal-1, other members of the galectin family may participate in the H-1PV entry process.

Based on our results, we envision a model in which H-1PV interacts with different classes of molecules, rather than with a single cell surface receptor, in order to enter cancer cells. Laminins containing γ1 chains would accumulate virus in the vicinity of the cell surface via sialic acid, while Gal-1 would promote the efficient internalisation of virus particles into a clathrin-coated pit. After engagement of these factors, H-1PV would penetrate the cells preferentially via clathrin-mediated endocytosis [15].

One possibility arises that H-1PV hijacks extracellular Gal-1 to enter the cells together with the protein. Our results support this idea by showing that the addition of exogenous purified Gal-1 boosts H-1PV infection at the level of virus entry, thereby sensitising semi-permissive cancer cells to H-1PV-mediated oncolysis. On the other hand, we cannot exclude that Gal-1 may play additional roles at post-entry levels, including viral trafficking and DNA uncoating.

Galectins are known to be synthesised in the cytoplasm and accumulate there until they are secreted via a poorly characterised pathway [38]. The exact mechanism through which galectin(s) translocate across the cell membrane remains also poorly understood [39]. However, previous research has shown that inhibition of the lipid raft-dependent pathway does not impede Gal-1 internalisation; instead, a total block of Gal-1 internalisation was observed only when both clathrin-mediated endocytosis and lipid rafts were disrupted, demonstrating that Gal-1 enters cells through various mechanisms, including clathrin-mediated endocytosis [40,41]. Therefore, it may be possible that H-1PV uses Gal-1 to enter cancer cells through clathrin-mediated endocytosis.

Alternatively, Gal-1 could mediate the binding of H-1PV to other cellular factors involved in its entry, e.g. a transmembrane receptor or a co-receptor. A number of studies have shown that the multivalent binding activity of Gal-1 and other galectins is able to cross-link carbohydrates and glycoconjugates [42,43]. For instance, Gal-1 cross-linking has the ability to massively redistribute a diverse population of glycoproteins on the cell surface of T cells and segregate them into membrane microdomains [44]. Gal-1 has also been associated with the assembly and remodelling of the extracellular matrix [45], and has been shown to bind to various components present there, especially those containing polylactosamine chains, such as laminins [45,46]. In this respect, *LAMC1* knockdown in NCH125 LGALS1 KO cells, or *LGALS1* knockdown in HeLa LAMC1 KD cells did not further decrease H-1PV cell uptake (Figure 6), suggesting that laminins and Gal-1 may cooperate in the early steps of H-1PV infection presumably by performing overlapping roles. However, as there is still residual internalisation of H-1PV (Figure 3C), it is likely that H-1PV may use alternative pathways to enter cells and that other unidentified cell factors are involved in this process. On the other hand, other laminins with or without the laminin-γ1 chain may contribute to residual H-1PV entry, independently from Gal-1. Future studies are needed to further characterize the pathways involved in H-1PV cell binding-entry and to determine whether other cellular factors besides laminins and Gal-1 are involved in these events.

Gal-1 and galectins in general have been described as playing important roles in different aspects of various viral infections, leading to their promotion or inhibition. For instance, Gal-1 stabilised the binding of HIV-1 to $CD4^+$ T cells by cross-linking the viral gp120 and the host CD4 receptor, thereby helping HIV-1 to infect these cells [21]. Furthermore, soluble Gal-1 enhanced the uptake of HIV-1 by monocyte-derived macrophages, whereas Gal-3 had no effect on infection [47]. Enterovirus 71 is another example where Gal-1 has a supporting role. Gal-1 facilitates infection by interacting with the carbohydrate residues in VP1 and VP3 domains, leading to a more efficient release and dissemination of virus to other cells [48]. During Nipah virus (NiV) infection, Gal-1 enhances virus cell attachment to primary human endothelial cells [49]. However, later in the NiV replication cycle, Gal-1 seems to exert an inhibitory effect. Indeed, Gal-1 specifically binds to the viral glycoproteins NiV-F and NiV-G, which are responsible for cell-cell fusion and syncytia formation, thus blocking virus infection [50,51]. The inhibitory effect of Gal-1 is also observed in Influenza A infection, both in vitro and in vivo. Gal-1 binds directly to the envelope glycoproteins, stopping influenza from inducing hemagglutination and thereby impairing infectivity. Accordingly, influenza infection led to poorer survival rates in *LGALS1* KO mice than in wild-type mice [22].

Apart from their role in virus infections, galectins are also linked to apoptosis, angiogenesis, cell migration and tumour-immune escape [52]. In particular, high levels of Gal-1 are associated with cancer progression, poor prognosis and recurrence (reviewed in [34]). Several cancer types have been implicated, including gastric cancer [53], ovarian cancer [54], pancreatic cancer [55] and GBM [56]. In agreement with previous studies, our in silico analysis revealed that GBM presents significantly higher levels of *LGALS1* than normal tissues, and that *LGALS1* expression increases from grade II to IV gliomas (Figure S4). In terms of survival, high *LGALS1* expression is associated with a poor prognosis in glioma (Figure S5). To complement the bioinformatic analysis, we assessed a cohort of 122 patient biopsies by immunohistochemistry. We showed that Gal-1 protein levels vary across GBM with higher levels found in biopsies from patients with recurrent versus primary GBM, while in normal tissues the levels were relatively low (Figure 7). These findings corroborate previous studies showing that elevated levels of Gal-1 are associated with GBM progression [57–59]. They also further support the use of H-1PV to treat GBM, especially those cases with high Gal-1 protein content, given the key role that this protein has in virus entry and oncolysis.

We also found a correlation between *LGALS1* expression levels and the ability of H-1PV to induce oncolysis in 59 cancer cell lines (Figures 8 and 9). These results suggest that tumours with elevated *LGALS1* expression levels are likely to be more susceptible to H-1PV oncolytic activity. Building on these findings, we show that, while virus attachment is unaffected, virus entry is enhanced in the U251, LN308, U87 and A172-MG semi-permissive cell lines when H-1PV is administrated together with recombinant Gal-1 (Figure 9). Under these conditions (2 h from infection), H-1PV is still likely at the very early stages of infection, strongly supporting that Gal-1 plays a role in the H-1PV cell entry process. In agreement with enhanced infection, we found that susceptibility of these semi-permissive glioma cells to H-1PV oncolytic activity increases upon addition of exogenous Gal-1, suggesting that a certain level of Gal-1 is required for an efficient and productive H-1PV infection. Together, these findings support the idea that Gal-1 may represent a limiting factor for H-1PV oncolysis, and therefore, that tumours with high Gal-1 expression are more likely to respond to H-1PV treatment.

A similar correlation was previously shown for *LAMC1* where cell lines highly expressing this gene were found to be more susceptible to H-1PV oncotoxicity [14]. Anti-correlation analysis of *LAMC1* obtained in the previous work (Pearson correlation $R = -0.52$, $R^2 = 0.27$) stated a slightly higher anti-correlation than the one obtained in this re-analysis (*LAMC1* $R = -0.433$, $R^2 = 0.188$). Using the current datasets, *LGALS1* anti-correlation (*LGALS1*, $R = -0.510$, $R^2 = 0.260$) is moderately higher than that of *LAMC1*. Update of the datasets with acquisition of novel mRNA sequencing data may account for these differences. Interestingly, the anti-correlation is strongest when the *LGALS1* and *LAMC1* expression levels are analysed together, suggesting that their combined expression analysis may better predict the success of H-1PV infection against a certain tumour. This is in line with the concept that both genes play an important role in H-1PV infectivity. Our results also present new scenarios for treatment in which exogenous administration of recombinant Gal-1 could constitute a promising adjunct in H-1PV-based therapies. However, given the role of Gal-1 in carcinogenesis [60], its possible use with H-1PV must be carefully evaluated.

Supplementary Materials: The following are available online at https://www.mdpi.com/article/10.3390/v14051018/s1, Figure S1: LGALS1 and LGALS3 knockdown in HeLa, NCH125 and BxPC3 cell lines. Figure S2: Cell proliferation of NCH125 Control versus NCH125 LGALS1 KO. Figure S3:

Depletion of both *LAMC1* and *LGALS1* in NCH125 and HeLa cells. Figure S4: *LGALS1* overexpression in high-grade GBM. Figure S5: Higher levels of *LGALS1* are associated with poor prognosis in glioma. Figure S6: NCI60 database retrieved *LGALS1* and *LAMC1* expression levels showed anti-correlation with EC50 values and a slight increase in the ability to predict susceptibility to H-1PV induced oncotoxicity. Figure S7: CCLE database that retrieved *LGALS1* and *LAMC1* expression levels showed anti-correlation with EC50 values and showed a slight increase in the ability to predict susceptibility to H-1PV induced oncotoxicity.

Author Contributions: T.F. and A.K. designed, performed experiments and analysed the data; C.B. performed confocal microscopy analysis; J.A.H., L.A.R.Y. and H.M. provided and performed the GBM tissue microarray; R.R. and B.N. carried out the Nanostring analysis. P.V.N. performed correlation analysis. T.F., A.K. and A.M. wrote the manuscript and prepared figures. A.M. designed, secured funding, participated in data analysis, coordinated and supervised the research. All authors have read and agreed to the published version of the manuscript.

Funding: This study was supported initially by a seeding grant from Institut National du Cancer (INCA) and at later stages by a grant from ORYX GmbH to A.M. Our deepest gratitude also goes to André Welter, the Luxembourg Cancer Foundation and Télévie for supporting oncolytic virus immuno-therapy.

Institutional Review Board Statement: The tissue microarray prepared from GBM biopsies was approved by the Regional Ethics Committee of Bergen, (Norway) with the number 2017/2505.

Informed Consent Statement: Informed consent was obtained from all subjects involved in the study.

Data Availability Statement: All relevant data supporting the findings of this study are available within the paper and its Supplementary material. All other data are available from the corresponding author on request. Figure 8, Figure S6 and Figure S7 were generated employing the data sets publicly available at the CellMiner™ (https://discover.nci.nih.gov/cellminer, accessed on 23 January 2021) and at The Cancer Cell Line Encyclopedia portals (https://portals.broadinstitute.org/ccle, accessed on 23 January 2021). Figures S4 and S5 were generated using the Glio-Vis data portal (http://gliovis.bioinfo.cnio.es/, accessed on 23 January 2021).

Acknowledgments: We thank Barbara Leuchs (DKFZ, Heidelberg, Germany) for kindly providing the H-1PV capsid monoclonal antibody. We would also like to show our gratitude to Tiina Marttila for producing both the H-1PV wild-type and the recH-1PV-EGFP viruses and Anabel Grewenig for technical assistance in Western blot analysis. We thank Jean Rommelaere, Assia Angelova and Marcelo Ehrlich for fruitful discussion. We are also grateful to Caroline Hadley (INLEXIO) for critically reading the manuscript.

Conflicts of Interest: An international patent application protecting some of the results described in this article was submitted in November 2018 with T.F., A.K. and A.M. as co-inventors. A.M. is an inventor of several H-1PV-related patents/patent applications.

References

1. Marchini, A.; Scott, E.M.; Rommelaere, J. Overcoming barriers in oncolytic virotherapy with HDAC inhibitors and immune checkpoint blockade. *Viruses* **2016**, *8*, 9. [CrossRef] [PubMed]
2. Marchini, A.; Daeffler, L.; Pozdeev, V.I.; Angelova, A.; Rommelaere, J. Immune Conversion of Tumor Microenvironment by Oncolytic Viruses: The Protoparvovirus H-1PV Case Study. *Front. Immunol.* **2019**, *10*, 1848. [CrossRef] [PubMed]
3. Cotmore, S.F.; Tattersall, P. Parvoviral host range and cell entry mechanisms. *Adv. Virus Res.* **2007**, *70*, 183–232. [PubMed]
4. Bretscher, C.; Marchini, A. H-1 parvovirus as a cancer-killing agent: Past, present, and future. *Viruses* **2019**, *11*, 562. [CrossRef]
5. Cotmore, S.F.; Agbandje-McKenna, M.; Chiorini, J.A.; Mukha, D.V.; Pintel, D.J.; Qiu, J.; Soderlund-Venermo, M.; Tattersall, P.; Tijssen, P.; Gatherer, D. The family parvoviridae. *Arch. Virol.* **2014**, *159*, 1239–1247. [CrossRef]
6. Ros, C.; Bayat, N.; Wolfisberg, R.; Almendral, J.M.J.V. Protoparvovirus cell entry. *Viruses* **2017**, *9*, 313. [CrossRef]
7. Hristov, G.; Kramer, M.; Li, J.; El-Andaloussi, N.; Mora, R.; Daeffler, L.; Zentgraf, H.; Rommelaere, J.; Marchini, A. Through Its Nonstructural Protein NS1, Parvovirus H-1 Induces Apoptosis via Accumulation of Reactive Oxygen Species. *J. Virol.* **2010**, *84*, 5909–5922. [CrossRef]
8. Nuesch, J.P.; Lacroix, J.; Marchini, A.; Rommelaere, J. Molecular pathways: Rodent parvoviruses–mechanisms of oncolysis and prospects for clinical cancer treatment. *Clin. Cancer Res.* **2012**, *18*, 3516–3523. [CrossRef]

9. Geletneky, K.; Hajda, J.; Angelova, A.L.; Leuchs, B.; Capper, D.; Bartsch, A.J.; Neumann, J.O.; Schoning, T.; Husing, J.; Beelte, B.; et al. Oncolytic H-1 Parvovirus Shows Safety and Signs of Immunogenic Activity in a First Phase I/IIa Glioblastoma Trial. *Mol. Ther.* **2017**, *12*, 2620–2634. [CrossRef]
10. Hajda, J.; Leuchs, B.; Angelova, A.L.; Frehtman, V.; Rommelaere, J.; Mertens, M.; Pilz, M.; Kieser, M.; Krebs, O.; Dahm, M.; et al. Phase 2 Trial of Oncolytic H-1 Parvovirus Therapy Shows Safety and Signs of Immune System Activation in Patients With Metastatic Pancreatic Ductal Adenocarcinoma. *Clin. Cancer Res.* **2021**, *27*, 5546–5556. [CrossRef]
11. Hartley, A.; Kavishwar, G.; Salvato, I.; Marchini, A. A Roadmap for the Success of Oncolytic Parvovirus-Based Anticancer Therapies. *Ann. Rev. Virol* **2020**, *7*, 537–557. [CrossRef] [PubMed]
12. Allaume, X.; El-Andaloussi, N.; Leuchs, B.; Bonifati, S.; Kulkarni, A.; Marttila, T.; Kaufmann, J.K.; Nettelbeck, D.M.; Kleinschmidt, J.; Rommelaere, J.; et al. Retargeting of rat parvovirus H-1PV to cancer cells through genetic engineering of the viral capsid. *J. Virol.* **2012**, *86*, 3452–3465. [CrossRef] [PubMed]
13. Halder, S.; Nam, H.J.; Govindasamy, L.; Vogel, M.; Dinsart, C.; Salome, N.; McKenna, R.; Agbandje-McKenna, M. Structural characterization of H-1 parvovirus: Comparison of infectious virions to empty capsids. *J. Virol.* **2013**, *87*, 5128–5140. [CrossRef] [PubMed]
14. Kulkarni, A.; Ferreira, T.; Bretscher, C.; Grewenig, A.; El-Andaloussi, N.; Bonifati, S.; Marttila, T.; Palissot, V.; Hossain, J.A.; Azuaje, F.; et al. Oncolytic H-1 parvovirus binds to sialic acid on laminins for cell attachment and entry. *Nat. Commun.* **2021**, *12*, 3834. [CrossRef]
15. Ferreira, T.; Kulkarni, A.; Bretscher, C.; Richter, K.; Ehrlich, M.; Marchini, A. Oncolytic H-1 Parvovirus Enters Cancer Cells through Clathrin-Mediated Endocytosis. *Viruses* **2020**, *12*, 1199. [CrossRef]
16. Vandenbrule, F.; Buicu, C.; Baldet, M.; Sobel, M.E.; Cooper, D.N.; Marschal, P.; Castronovo, V. Galectin-1 modulates human melanoma cell adhesion to laminin. *Biochem. Biophys. Res. Commun.* **1995**, *209*, 760–767. [CrossRef]
17. Cousin, J.M.; Cloninger, M.J. The role of galectin-1 in cancer progression, and synthetic multivalent systems for the study of galectin-1. *Int. J. Mol. Sci.* **2016**, *17*, 1566. [CrossRef]
18. Vasta, G.R.; Ahmed, H.; Bianchet, M.A.; Fernández-Robledo, J.A.; Amzel, L.M. Diversity in recognition of glycans by F-type lectins and galectins: Molecular, structural, and biophysical aspects. *Ann. N. Y. Acad. Sci.* **2012**, *1253*, E14. [CrossRef]
19. Johannes, L.; Jacob, R.; Leffler, H. Galectins at a glance. *J. Cell Sci* **2018**, *131*, jcs208884. [CrossRef]
20. Wang, W.H.; Lin, C.Y.; Chang, M.R.; Urbina, A.N.; Assavalapsakul, W.; Thitithanyanont, A.; Chen, Y.H.; Liu, F.T.; Wang, S.F. The role of galectins in virus infection—A systemic literature review. *J. Microbiol. Immunol Infect.* **2020**, *53*, 925–935. [CrossRef]
21. Ouellet, M.; Mercier, S.; Pelletier, I.; Bounou, S.; Roy, J.; Hirabayashi, J.; Sato, S.; Tremblay, M.J. Galectin-1 acts as a soluble host factor that promotes HIV-1 infectivity through stabilization of virus attachment to host cells. *J. Immunol.* **2005**, *174*, 4120–4126. [CrossRef] [PubMed]
22. Yang, M.-L.; Chen, Y.-H.; Wang, S.-W.; Huang, Y.-J.; Leu, C.-H.; Yeh, N.-C.; Chu, C.-Y.; Lin, C.-C.; Shieh, G.-S.; Chen, Y.-L. Galectin-1 binds to influenza virus and ameliorates influenza virus pathogenesis. *J. Virol.* **2011**, *85*, 10010–10020. [CrossRef] [PubMed]
23. Garcin, P.O.; Nabi, I.R.; Pante, N. Galectin-3 plays a role in minute virus of mice infection. *Virology* **2015**, *481*, 63–72. [CrossRef]
24. Garcin, P.; Cohen, S.; Terpstra, S.; Kelly, I.; Foster, L.J.; Panté, N. Proteomic analysis identifies a novel function for galectin-3 in the cell entry of parvovirus. *J. Proteom.* **2013**, *79*, 123–132. [CrossRef] [PubMed]
25. El-Andaloussi, N.; Endele, M.; Leuchs, B.; Bonifati, S.; Kleinschmidt, J.; Rommelaere, J.; Marchini, A. Novel adenovirus-based helper system to support production of recombinant parvovirus. *Cancer Gene Ther.* **2011**, *18*, 240–249. [CrossRef] [PubMed]
26. El-Andaloussi, N.; Leuchs, B.; Bonifati, S.; Rommelaere, J.; Marchini, A. Efficient recombinant parvovirus production with the help of adenovirus-derived systems. *J. Vis. Exp.* **2012**, *62*, e3518. [CrossRef] [PubMed]
27. Bodendorf, U.; Cziepluch, C.; Jauniaux, J.-C.; Rommelaere, J.; Salomé, N. Nuclear export factor CRM1 interacts with nonstructural proteins NS2 from parvovirus minute virus of mice. *J. Virol.* **1999**, *73*, 7769–7779. [CrossRef] [PubMed]
28. Kestler, J.; Neeb, B.; Struyf, S.; Damme, J.V.; Cotmore, S.F.; D'Abramo, A.; Tattersall, P.; Rommelaere, J.; Dinsart, C.; Cornelis, J.J. cis requirements for the efficient production of recombinant DNA vectors based on autonomous parvoviruses. *Hum. Gene Ther.* **1999**, *10*, 1619–1632. [CrossRef]
29. Leuchs, B.; Roscher, M.; Muller, M.; Kurschner, K.; Rommelaere, J. Standardized large-scale H-1PV production process with efficient quality and quantity monitoring. *J. Virol. Methods* **2016**, *229*, 48–59. [CrossRef]
30. Hossain, J.A.; Riecken, K.; Miletic, H.; Fehse, B. Cancer suicide gene therapy with TK. 007. In *Suicide Gene Therapy*; Springer: Berlin/Heidelberg, Germany, 2019; pp. 11–26.
31. Hossain, J.A.; Latif, M.A.; Ystaas, L.A.; Ninzima, S.; Riecken, K.; Muller, A.; Azuaje, F.; Joseph, J.V.; Talasila, K.M.; Ghimire, J. Long-term treatment with valganciclovir improves lentiviral suicide gene therapy of glioblastoma. *J. Neurooncol.* **2019**, *21*, 890–900. [CrossRef]
32. Barretina, J.; Caponigro, G.; Stransky, N.; Venkatesan, K.; Margolin, A.A.; Kim, S.; Wilson, C.J.; Lehar, J.; Kryukov, G.V.; Sonkin, D.; et al. The Cancer Cell Line Encyclopedia enables predictive modelling of anticancer drug sensitivity. *Nature* **2012**, *483*, 603–607. [CrossRef] [PubMed]
33. Nesmelova, I.V.; Ermakova, E.; Daragan, V.A.; Pang, M.; Menendez, M.; Lagartera, L.; Solis, D.; Baum, L.G.; Mayo, K.H. Lactose binding to galectin-1 modulates structural dynamics, increases conformational entropy, and occurs with apparent negative cooperativity. *J. Mol. Biol.* **2010**, *397*, 1209–1230. [CrossRef] [PubMed]

34. Wu, R.; Wu, T.; Wang, K.; Luo, S.; Chen, Z.; Fan, M.; Xue, D.; Lu, H.; Zhuang, Q.; Xu, X. Prognostic significance of galectin-1 expression in patients with cancer: A meta-analysis. *Cancer Cell Int.* **2018**, *18*, 108. [CrossRef] [PubMed]
35. Shoemaker, R.H. The NCI60 human tumour cell line anticancer drug screen. *Nat. Rev. Cancer* **2006**, *6*, 813–823. [CrossRef] [PubMed]
36. Herrero y Calle, M.; Cornelis, J.J.; Herold-Mende, C.; Rommelaere, J.; Schlehofer, J.R.; Geletneky, K. Parvovirus H-1 infection of human glioma cells leads to complete viral replication and efficient cell killing. *Int. J. Cancer* **2004**, *109*, 76–84. [CrossRef]
37. Angelova, A.; Ferreira, T.; Bretscher, C.; Rommelaere, J.; Marchini, A. Parvovirus-Based Combinatorial Immunotherapy: A Reinforced Therapeutic Strategy against Poor-Prognosis Solid Cancers. *Cancers* **2021**, *13*, 342. [CrossRef]
38. Elola, M.T.; Wolfenstein-Todel, C.; Troncoso, M.F.; Vasta, G.R.; Rabinovich, G.A. Galectins: Matricellular glycan-binding proteins linking cell adhesion, migration, and survival. *Cell Mol. Life Sci.* **2007**, *64*, 1679–1700. [CrossRef]
39. Bänfer, S.; Jacob, R. Galectins in Intra-and Extracellular Vesicles. *Biomolecules* **2020**, *10*, 1232. [CrossRef]
40. Fajka-Boja, R.; Blasko, A.; Kovacs-Solyom, F.; Szebeni, G.; Toth, G.; Monostori, E. Co-localization of galectin-1 with GM1 ganglioside in the course of its clathrin-and raft-dependent endocytosis. *Cell Mol. Life Sci.* **2008**, *65*, 2586–2593. [CrossRef]
41. Lepur, A.; Carlsson, M.C.; Novak, R.; Dumić, J.; Nilsson, U.J.; Leffler, H. Galectin-3 endocytosis by carbohydrate independent and dependent pathways in different macrophage like cell types. *Biochim. Biophy. Acta Gen. Subj.* **2012**, *1820*, 804–818. [CrossRef]
42. Brewer, C.F. Binding and cross-linking properties of galectins. *Biochim. Biophys. Acta Gen. Subj.* **2002**, *1572*, 255–262. [CrossRef]
43. Garner, O.B.; Baum, L.G. Galectin–glycan lattices regulate cell-surface glycoprotein organization and signalling. *Bioch. Soc. Trans.* **2008**, *36*, 1472–1477. [CrossRef] [PubMed]
44. Pace, K.E.; Lee, C.; Stewart, P.L.; Baum, L.G. Restricted receptor segregation into membrane microdomains occurs on human T cells during apoptosis induced by galectin-1. *J. Immunol.* **1999**, *163*, 3801–3811.
45. Moiseeva, E.P.; Williams, B.; Samani, N.J. Galectin 1 inhibits incorporation of vitronectin and chondroitin sulfate B into the extracellular matrix of human vascular smooth muscle cells. *Biochim. Biophys. Acta Gen. Subj.* **2003**, *1619*, 125–132. [CrossRef]
46. Moiseeva, E.P.; Javed, Q.; Spring, E.L.; de Bono, D.P. Galectin 1 is involved in vascular smooth muscle cell proliferation. *Cardiovasc. Res.* **2000**, *45*, 493–502. [CrossRef]
47. Mercier, S.; St-Pierre, C.; Pelletier, I.; Ouellet, M.; Tremblay, M.J.; Sato, S. Galectin-1 promotes HIV-1 infectivity in macrophages through stabilization of viral adsorption. *Virology* **2008**, *371*, 121–129. [CrossRef]
48. Lee, P.-H.; Liu, C.-M.; Ho, T.-S.; Tsai, Y.-C.; Lin, C.-C.; Wang, Y.-F.; Chen, Y.-L.; Yu, C.-K.; Wang, S.-M.; Liu, C.-C. Enterovirus 71 virion-associated galectin-1 facilitates viral replication and stability. *PLoS ONE* **2015**, *10*, e0116278. [CrossRef]
49. Garner, O.B.; Yun, T.; Pernet, O.; Aguilar, H.C.; Park, A.; Bowden, T.A.; Freiberg, A.N.; Lee, B.; Baum, L.G. Timing of galectin-1 exposure differentially modulates Nipah virus entry and syncytium formation in endothelial cells. *J. Virol.* **2015**, *89*, 2520–2529. [CrossRef]
50. Levroney, E.L.; Aguilar, H.C.; Fulcher, J.A.; Kohatsu, L.; Pace, K.E.; Pang, M.; Gurney, K.B.; Baum, L.G.; Lee, B. Novel innate immune functions for galectin-1: Galectin-1 inhibits cell fusion by Nipah virus envelope glycoproteins and augments dendritic cell secretion of proinflammatory cytokines. *J. Immunol.* **2005**, *175*, 413–420. [CrossRef]
51. Garner, O.B.; Aguilar, H.C.; Fulcher, J.A.; Levroney, E.L.; Harrison, R.; Wright, L.; Robinson, L.R.; Aspericueta, V.; Panico, M.; Haslam, S.M. Endothelial galectin-1 binds to specific glycans on nipah virus fusion protein and inhibits maturation, mobility, and function to block syncytia formation. *PLoS Pathog.* **2010**, *6*, e1000993. [CrossRef]
52. Chou, F.-C.; Chen, H.-Y.; Kuo, C.-C.; Sytwu, H.-K.J. Role of galectins in tumors and in clinical immunotherapy. *Int. J. Mol. Sci.* **2018**, *19*, 430. [CrossRef] [PubMed]
53. Chen, J.; Zhou, S.-J.; Zhang, Y.; Zhang, G.-Q.; Zha, T.-Z.; Feng, Y.-Z.; Zhang, K. Clinicopathological and prognostic significance of galectin-1 and vascular endothelial growth factor expression in gastric cancer. *World J. Gastroenterol.* **2013**, *19*, 2073. [CrossRef] [PubMed]
54. Schulz, H.; Schmoeckel, E.; Kuhn, C.; Hofmann, S.; Mayr, D.; Mahner, S.; Jeschke, U. Galectins-1,-3, and-7 are prognostic markers for survival of ovarian cancer patients. *Int. J. Mol. Sci.* **2017**, *18*, 1230. [CrossRef] [PubMed]
55. Martinez-Bosch, N.; Barranco, L.E.; Orozco, C.A.; Moreno, M.; Visa, L.; Iglesias, M.; Oldfield, L.; Neoptolemos, J.P.; Greenhalf, W.; Earl, J. Increased plasma levels of galectin-1 in pancreatic cancer: Potential use as biomarker. *Oncotarget* **2018**, *9*, 32984. [CrossRef]
56. Chou, S.-Y.; Yen, S.-L.; Huang, C.-C.; Huang, E.-Y. Galectin-1 is a poor prognostic factor in patients with glioblastoma multiforme after radiotherapy. *BMC Cancer* **2018**, *18*, 105. [CrossRef]
57. Jung, T.-Y.; Jung, S.; Ryu, H.-H.; Jeong, Y.-I.; Jin, Y.-H.; Jin, S.-G.; Kim, I.-Y.; Kang, S.-S.; Kim, H.-S. Role of galectin-1 in migration and invasion of human glioblastoma multiforme cell lines. *J. Neurosurg.* **2008**, *109*, 273–284. [CrossRef]
58. Verschuere, T.; Van Woensel, M.; Fieuws, S.; Lefranc, F.; Mathieu, V.; Kiss, R.; Van Gool, S.W.; De Vleeschouwer, S. Altered galectin-1 serum levels in patients diagnosed with high-grade glioma. *J. Neurooncol.* **2013**, *115*, 9–17. [CrossRef]
59. Astorgues-Xerri, L.; Riveiro, M.E.; Tijeras-Raballand, A.; Serova, M.; Neuzillet, C.; Albert, S.; Raymond, E.; Faivre, S. Unraveling galectin-1 as a novel therapeutic target for cancer. *Cancer Treat. Rev.* **2014**, *40*, 307–319. [CrossRef]
60. Blanchard, H.; Bum-Erdene, K.; Bohari, M.H.; Yu, X. Galectin-1 inhibitors and their potential therapeutic applications: A patent review. *Expert Opin. Ther. Pat.* **2016**, *26*, 537–554. [CrossRef]

viruses

MDPI

Article

A Functional Minigenome of Parvovirus B19

Alessandro Reggiani, Andrea Avati †, Francesca Valenti ‡, Erika Fasano, Gloria Bua, Elisabetta Manaresi and Giorgio Gallinella *

Department of Pharmacy and Biotechnology, University of Bologna, 40138 Bologna, Italy; alessandro.reggiani5@unibo.it (A.R.); andrea.avati@student.unisi.it (A.A.); francesca.valenti@ior.it (F.V.); erika.fasano2@unibo.it (E.F.); gloria.bua2@unibo.it (G.B.); elisabetta.manaresi@unibo.it (E.M.)

* Correspondence: giorgio.gallinella@unibo.it

† Current Address: Department of Biotechnology, Chemistry and Pharmacy, University of Siena, 53100 Siena, Italy.

‡ Current Address: Department of Surgical Sciences and Technologies, IRCCS Rizzoli, 40136 Bologna, Italy.

Abstract: Parvovirus B19 (B19V) is a human pathogenic virus of clinical relevance, characterized by a selective tropism for erythroid progenitor cells in bone marrow. Relevant information on viral characteristics and lifecycle can be obtained from experiments involving engineered genetic systems in appropriate in vitro cellular models. Previously, a B19V genome of defined consensus sequence was designed, synthesized and cloned in a complete and functional form, able to replicate and produce infectious viral particles in a producer/amplifier cell system. Based on such a system, we have now designed and produced a derived B19V minigenome, reduced to a replicon unit. The genome terminal regions were maintained in a form able to sustain viral replication, while the internal region was clipped to include only the left-side genetic set, containing the coding sequence for the functional NS1 protein. Following transfection in UT7/EpoS1 cells, this minigenome still proved competent for replication, transcription and production of NS1 protein. Further, the B19V minigenome was able to complement B19-derived, NS1-defective genomes, restoring their ability to express viral capsid proteins. The B19V genome was thus engineered to yield a two-component system, with complementing functions, providing a valuable tool for studying viral expression and genetics, suitable to further engineering for purposes of translational research.

Keywords: parvovirus B19; synthetic genome; genetic engineering; replicon unit; functional complementation

Citation: Reggiani, A.; Avati, A.; Valenti, F.; Fasano, E.; Bua, G.; Manaresi, E.; Gallinella, G. A Functional Minigenome of Parvovirus B19. *Viruses* **2022**, *14*, 84. https://doi.org/10.3390/v14010084

Academic Editor: Luis Martinez-Sobrido

Received: 6 December 2021
Accepted: 29 December 2021
Published: 4 January 2022

1. Introduction

Within the family *Parvoviridae* [1], Parvovirus B19 (B19V) is a human pathogenic virus of clinical relevance, responsible for transient or persistent erythroid aplasia, infectious erythema, arthropathies, myocarditis and intrauterine infections, among others [2,3]. The variability in the pathogenetic processes and the resulting clinical outcomes of diverse nature and severity depend on a complex interplay between the viral properties, the characteristics of target cells in the different tissues, and the physiological status and immune response of infected individuals. B19V has a marked tropism for erythroid progenitor cells (EPCs) in the bone marrow, both susceptible and permissive depending on their differentiation and proliferation state [4]. In EPCs, infection normally induces cell cycle arrest and apoptosis [5], thus causing a temporary block in erythropoiesis which can become clinically relevant [6]. Different non-erythroid cell types, including endothelial, stromal, or synovial cells, are also susceptible but mainly non-permissive. In these cells, infection can trigger inflammatory responses and consequent tissue damage [7], and generally results in long-term persistence of viral DNA within tissues [8].

Investigation of viral genetics is fundamental to better understanding of the B19V replication cycle, the virus–cell interaction in different environments, the pathogenetic processes underlying the wide range of associated diseases, and the devising of more efficient antiviral strategies [9,10]. The B19V genome is composed of two inverted, terminal repeated regions (ITR) of imperfect palindromic sequence, 383 nt long, flanking a unique internal region (IR), 4830 nt long, containing all the coding sequences (Figure S1). The role of ITRs is crucial. The ability of palindromic sequences to fold in self-priming, hairpin secondary structures, and the presence of specific cis-recognition sequences acting as origins of replication, allow replication of the viral DNA through a rolling hairpin mechanism [11–13]. The activity of the unique transcription promoter (P_6) at the left end of the internal region also depends critically on regulatory sequences within the upstream ITR [14–18]. Within the IR, distribution of splicing and cleavage-polyadenylation recognition sequences along the genome ensures coordinate processing of the pre-mRNA to a set of mature mRNAs [19–22]. Functionally, these can be divided into a set expressed from the left side of the genome, mainly coding for NS1 protein in an early phase of replication, and a set expressed from the right side of the genome, mainly coding for the structural VP proteins in the late phase of replication [23–25].

NS1 protein is the major non-structural protein, essential to virus replication and central for interaction with host cell components [9]. It is involved in the replication of the B19V genome, by its capacity to bind to specific recognition sites in the terminal regions, and by its endonuclease and helicase activities effecting ITR terminal resolution and strand unwinding. It is involved in viral transcription, enhancing activity of the P_6 promoter by its trans-activating domains, thus promoting overall B19V genome expression. Besides, NS1 is a heterologous trans-activator of cellular genes, therefore inducing alterations in the cellular environment. It has a role in regulating progression through the cell cycle and in inducing apoptosis, therefore contributing to the pathogenesis of B19V infection. Given all this, NS1 is a matter of relevant interest in studying B19V, not least as a pharmacological target [26,27]. Viral capsid proteins VP1 and VP2 assemble to form a capsid shell of 22 nm in diameter, arranged in a T = 1 icosahedral structure [28]. Being translated from the same coding frame, both proteins share a common region that forms the core shell, while the VP1 protein, about 5% in abundance, possesses an additional N-terminal region, VP1u, crucial for cell recognition, attachment and penetration [29,30].

Information can be obtained from experiments involving engineered genetic systems in appropriate in vitro cellular models, since cloned forms of the B19V genome can be competent for replication and constitute an effective tool for studying the viral lifecycle and its interaction with target cells [31,32]. Previously, a model system was established by a novel synthetic strategy [33]. A reference genome of defined consensus sequence was designed, synthesized and cloned in a complete and functional form in a plasmid vector. Such a genome was able to replicate and produce infectious viral particles in a producer/amplifier cell system, the myeloblastoid UT7/EpoS1cells, allowing generation and further propagation of virus in EPC cell cultures. Replicative competence was linked to preservation of sequence integrity and asymmetry within the terminal regions, while preservation of the complete internal region ensured maintenance of the cis-acting signals required for regulation of viral genome expression. Therefore, the full proteome of B19V could be co-ordinately expressed and novel infectious viral particles produced. Further investigation is required to assess the flexibility of this system to genetic manipulation, and its potential as an advanced tool for basic research and translational applications.

With this aim, the main objective of the present experiments was to create a genetic unit derived from the complete, competent cloned B19V genome, simplified to a potential replicon unit. In this minigenome, the terminal regions were maintained in a form able to sustain viral replication, while the internal region was clipped to contain only the left-side genetic set. This would only allow the production of the subset of mRNAs corresponding to the early phase, including the mRNAs for NS1 protein. Following transfection in UT7/EpoS1 cells, replication, transcription and production of NS1 protein were monitored to assess the functional competence of the minigenome. Further, the capacity of this minigenome to complement defective forms of B19 genome rescuing production of viral capsid proteins and the possibility of producing transducing viral particles was also tested.

2. Materials and Methods

2.1. Molecular Cloning

Experiments were carried out on the previously established pCK10 and pCH10 plasmid clones containing the reference B19V EC sequence (GenBank KY940273) [33]. Plasmids pCK10 and pCH10 contain as inserts B19V EC segments, including the complete internal region and extension of both ITRs beyond the sites of dyad symmetry (pCK10, nt. 136–5461) or up to the sites of dyad symmetry (pCH10, nt. 184–5413).

The derived pCK10-pAs1 and pCH10-pAs1 plasmids were obtained by deletion of the genomic segment between nt. 2813–5169. To the purpose, a synthetic segment of appropriate sequence was transferred into pCK10 and pCH10 to replace the original insert by cloning using the XmaI and BssHII sites at positions 2251 and 5413. The derived pCH10-A1.1 and pCH10-A1.2 plasmids were obtained by deletion of the genomic segments between nt. 588–2089 and 588–2209, respectively. Synthetic segments of appropriate sequence were transferred into pCH10 to replace the original insert by cloning using the BssHII sites and BamHI sites at positions 184 and 4076.

Synthetic DNA inserts were obtained from Eurofins Genomics. Restriction endonuclease (RE) and ligase enzymes were obtained from Thermo Fisher Scientific and used according to manufacturer's directions. Plasmid clones were maintained in SURE bacterial cells (Agilent Technologies, Santa Clara, CA, USA) under ampicillin selection and growth in LB medium at 30 °C. Plasmid DNA purification was performed by PureYield Plasmid Midiprep (Promega, Madison, WI, USA). Inserts used for transfection assay were amplified by PCR by using the Expand High Fidelity System (Roche, Basel, Switzerland) as described, further purified by using Wizard SV Gel and PCR clean-up system (Promega) and quantified by UV absorbance determination.

2.2. Cell Culture

UT7/EpoS1 cells, obtained from KE Brown [34], were cultured in IMDM (Cambrex, East Rutherford, NJ, USA), 10% FCS and 2 U/mL Epo α (Eprex, Janssen, Beerse, Belgium), at 37 °C and 5% CO_2. Cells were kept in culture at densities between 2×10^5–1×10^6 cells/mL and used for transfection experiments when at a density of 3×10^5 cells/mL. Erythroid progenitor cells (EPCs) were generated in vitro from peripheral blood mononuclear cells (PBMC) obtained from the leukocyte-enriched buffy coats of healthy blood donors, from the Immunohematology and Transfusion Service, S. Orsola-Malpighi University Hospital, Bologna (http://www.aosp.bo.it/content/immunoematologia-e-trasfusionale; authorization 0070755/1980/2014, issued by Head of Service). Availability was granted under conditions complying with Italian privacy law. Neither specific ethics committee approval nor written consent from donors was required for this research project. In vitro culture was carried out following established protocol [35], and cells were used for infection experiments at day 8 of in vitro growth and differentiation.

2.3. Transfection and Infection

UT7/EpoS1 cells were transfected by using the Amaxa Nucleofection System (Lonza, Basel, Switzerland), with V Nucleofector Reagent and T20 program setting, at a ratio of 1 µg insert DNA for 10^6 cells. Following transfection, the cells were incubated at 37 °C and 5% CO_2 in complete medium at an initial density of 10^6 cells/mL, until collection at the indicated time points. Cells and cell-free supernatants were separated by centrifugation at 4000 rpm for 5 min in microfuge (Eppendorf, Hamburg, Germany), then fractions were used for analysis and/or successive infection experiments.

For infection experiments, cell-free supernatants obtained from transfected UT7/EpoS1 cells were added to EPCs cells at a ratio of 100 µL for 1×10^6 cells. Infection was carried out at 37 °C for 2 h, then cells were washed free of inoculum and expanded in complete medium at 37 °C and 5% CO_2 at an initial density of 10^6 cells/mL, until collection at the indicated time points and subsequent processing as described.

2.4. Quantitative Molecular Analysis

Experimental samples were processed for total nucleic acid purification by using the Viral Total Nucleic Acid kit for the Maxwell 16 extractor (Promega), then quantitative determination of B19V nucleic acids (viral DNA, total mRNA, mRNA subsets) was carried out by qPCR and qRT-PCR according to previously established protocols [23,24]. Genomic DNA coding for 18S rRNA (rDNA) was amplified for calibration with respect to cell copy number. Absolute quantification of both viral DNA and total viral RNA was obtained by using the primer pair R2210–R2355, located in the central exon of B19V genome, while determination of the relative abundance of the different subsets of viral transcripts was obtained by using a selected array of primer pairs, as indicated in Table 1. For the DpnI Assay, DNA previously treated with either EcoRI or EcoRI+DpnI restriction enzymes was amplified by using primers encompassing DpnI site at position 1801 on the B19V genome, and the fraction of DNA not cleaved by the enzyme determined by qPCR analysis and absolute quantitation with respect to an external calibration curve.

Table 1. Primer combinations used in the qPCR and qRT-PCR assays for the detection and quantitative evaluation of B19V nucleic acids. See also Figure S1 for primer location on B19V genome.

Primer	Sense	Primer	Antisense	DNA Target
18Sfor	CGGACAGGATTGACAGATTG	18Srev	TGCCAGAGTCTCGTTCGTTA	Genomic 18S rDNA
R2210	CGCCTGGAACACTGAAACCC	R2355	GAAACTGGTCTGCCAAAGGT	Virus DNA
D1801f	CTTGGTGGTCTGGGATGAAG	D1801r	TACTCCAGGCACAGCTACAC	for DpnI Assay
Primer	**Sense**	**Primer**	**Antisense**	**RNA Target**
R1882	GCGGGAACACTACAACAACT	R2033	GTCCCAGCTTTGTGCATTAC	NS mRNA
R2210	CGCCTGGAACACTGAAACCC	R2355	GAAACTGGTCTGCCAAAGGT	Central exon, total RNA
R4869	ATATGACCCCACAGCTACAG	R5014	TGGGCGTTTAGTTACGCATC	VP1/2 mRNA
R4899	ACACCACAGGCATGGATACG	R5014	TGGGCGTTTAGTTACGCATC	Distal exon, pAd cleaved

2.5. IIF and Cytofluorimetric Analysis

For detection of viral proteins by immunofluorescence, aliquots of 5×10^4 cells were spotted on glass slides and fixed with 1:1 acetone:methanol for 10 min at −20 °C. For detection of NS protein, cells were incubated with the human monoclonal antibody MAb1424 (kindly supplied by Susanne Modrow) (1:100 in PBS/FCS 10%), then with an anti-human FITC-conjugated secondary antibody (Dako, 1:20 in PBS/FCS 10%). For detection of VP proteins, cells were incubated with a monoclonal mouse antibody against VP1 and VP2 proteins (MAb8293, Chemicon, Merck Millipore, Milan, Italy) (1:200 in PBS/BSA 1%), then with AlexaFluor488 anti-mouse secondary antibodies (Life Technologies, Monza, Italy) (1:1000 in PBS/BSA 1%). Cell populations were also analysed for expression of viral proteins by using flow cytometry (FACSCalibur, Becton Dickinson, Milan, Italy). Aliquots of 10^6 cells were fixed in PBS/formaldehyde 0.5% O/N at 4 °C, permeabilized in PBS/saponin 0.2% at RT while rocking for 45 min and incubated in suspension with antibodies diluted in PBS/FCS 2% (1:100 NS primary; 1:40 anti-human FITC secondary). Data were analysed using the Cell Quest Pro Software (Becton Dickinson).

3. Results

3.1. Design and Construction of a B19V Minigenome

In the design of a B19V minigenome with potential replicative activity, the rational requirements were: (i) to preserve both terminal regions up to the sites of dyad symmetry, retaining the capacity of hairpin formation; and (ii) to preserve the internal region extending up to the pAp1 proximal cleavage-polyadenylation signal, as a gene cassette with potential for coding for the NS1 protein, while eliminating the genomic region coding for the viral capsid proteins. To this end, a large deletion was operated in the right-side of genome, and a novel chimeric cleavage-polyadenylation signal created, named pAs1, joining the upstream cis-elements of pAp1 and the downstream cis-elements of pAd (Figure 1).

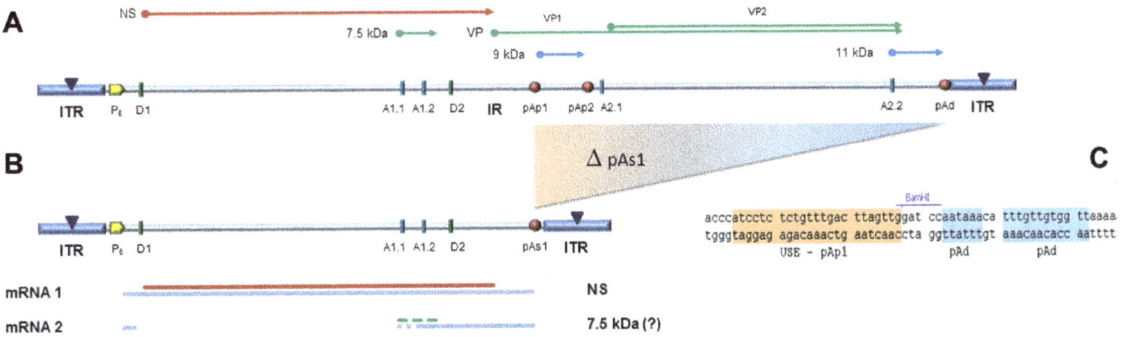

Figure 1. (**A**) Map of B19V genome. ITR: inverted terminal repeats (▼, site of dyad symmetry). IR: internal region and relevant cis-acting functional sites (P_6, promoter; pAp1, pAp2, proximal cleavage-polyadenylation sites; pAd, distal cleavage-polyadenylation site; D1, D2, splice donor sites; A1.1, A1.2, A2.1, A2.2, splice acceptor sites). Coding sequences for viral NS, VP and smaller non-structural proteins are aligned to map. **Δ**: deletion to create a novel cleavage-polyadenylation signal (pAs1). (**B**) Map of B19V derived minigenome; simplified transcription map, indicating the two classes of mRNAs (mRNA 1–2), with alternative splicing forms (dashed lines) and related coding potential. (**C**) Sequence at the novel pAs1 cleavage-polyadenylation site (USE—pAp1, upstream element to pAp1 [19]).

For the construction of the minigenome, a synthetic gene segment encompassing the designed deletion substituted by the novel pAs1 sequence was synthesised and inserted in order to replace the original sequence in the previously established pCK10 and pCH10 plasmids [33]. The viral insert in pCK10 preserves both terminal regions extending beyond the site of dyad symmetry; however, attempts at cloning in pCK10 only yielded unstable plasmid clones, with deletion of the palindromic sequence in the right-hand terminal region. The viral insert in pCH10 preserves both terminal regions extending up to the site of dyad symmetry; in this case, a stable plasmid clone was successfully obtained, named pCH10-pAs1.

3.2. Functional Competence of the B19V Minigenome

From the pCH10 plasmid, three genomic inserts of different extension can be obtained, differing in their functional competence: CH10, corresponding to the whole cloned insert, extending in the terminal regions to the sites of dyad symmetry (nt. 184–5413); CI0, extending in the terminal regions within the sites of dyad symmetry (nt. 245–5474); and CJ0, extending in the terminal regions only to the start of palindromes (nt. 366–5231). From the pCH10-pAs1 plasmid, three genomic inserts of corresponding extension could also be obtained by analogy: CH10-pAs1, CI0-pAs1, and CJ0-pAs1. The biological activity and functional competence of pCH10 and pCH10-pAs1 derived inserts was comparatively analysed following transfection in UT7/EpoS1 cells. Genomic inserts were obtained by means of in vitro amplification, then purified inserts were used to transfect UT7/EpoS1 cells. At 8- and 24-h post-transfection (hpt), aliquots of cell culture were sampled for quantification of viral nucleic acids (DNA, mRNAs) by qPCR and qRT-PCR (Figure 2, Table S1A), and detection of the NS protein by IIF and cytofluorimetric analysis.

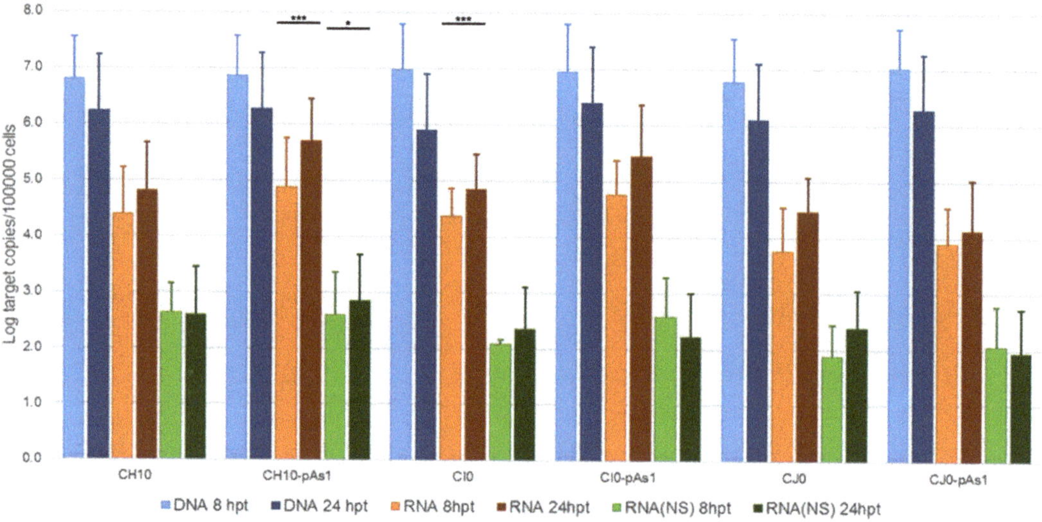

Figure 2. Viral nucleic acids in UT7/EpoS1 cells, transfected with CH10 and CH10-pAs1 derived inserts. Log amounts of target copies (viral DNA, total RNA, NS1 mRNA), normalized to 10^5 cells, at 8 and 24 hpt. Mean and std of duplicate determinations for two different experiments. Two-way ANOVA, Bonferroni post-test: ***, $p < 0.001$; *, $p < 0.05$.

The amount of DNA, either at 8 or 24 hpt, was comparable for all tested inserts, indicating a similar transfection efficiency. Due to the large quantity of input DNA used in transfection, no significant temporal variation in DNA amount was observed for any of the tested inserts, apart from a general decrease from 8 to 24 hpt (mean 0.70 Log, range −1.1–0.57), likely to be due to progressive degradation of exogenous DNA. De novo synthesis of transfected DNA was assessed in a parallel experiment, by transfection of inserts directly excised from plasmids and tested for *Dam* methylation pattern and resistance to DpnI cleavage, both by a qPCR assay and a Southern Blot analysis. In this way, it was possible to investigate CH10 and CH10-pAs1, excised using BssHII, CI0 and CI0-pAs1, excised using AccIII, but not CJ0 and CJ0-pAs1, because of lack of corresponding RE sites.

By qPCR, DNA excised from plasmids was resistant to 1.7% and 1.4% for CH10 and CH10-pAs1, and 1.6% and 1.3% for CI0 and CI0-pAs1. DNA obtained from transfected cells at 24 hpt was resistant to 11.7% and 15.8%, and 8.8% and 19.0%, respectively. By Southern Blot (Figure 3), at 24 hpt, bands corresponding to full-length, DpnI resistant DNA were also observed for all transfected inserts. Data thus obtained are consistent with the maintenance of the replicative competence of transfected inserts, at least for CH10-and CI0-derived inserts, both the complete genomes and the derived minigenomes, a property likely to be due to the preservation of sequence symmetry within the terminal regions and implying a hairpin-independent priming of DNA synthesis.

All transfected inserts showed a sustained transcriptional activity. Viral mRNAs were detected for all inserts at both time-points post-transfection, with a general increase from 8 to 24 hpt of total mRNA (mean 0.56 Log, range −0.01–1.33), and to a lesser extent of NS mRNA (mean 0.08 Log, range −0.36–0.51), significant for CH10-pAs1 only. Although with some variability, overall results attested the early onset and maintenance of viral transcription, implying processing of pre-mRNA at the novel chimeric pAs1 cleavage-polyadenylation site, and preservation of a balanced usage of splicing signals. In fact, a typical ratio of mRNAs pertaining to the left-side genome was produced, including both the unspliced mRNAs coding for NS protein (mRNA 1 in Figure 1), approximately 1% of total viral mRNAs, and the more abundant spliced mRNAs (mRNA 2 in Figure 1), in a pattern analogous to that observed in the early phase of the replicative cycle.

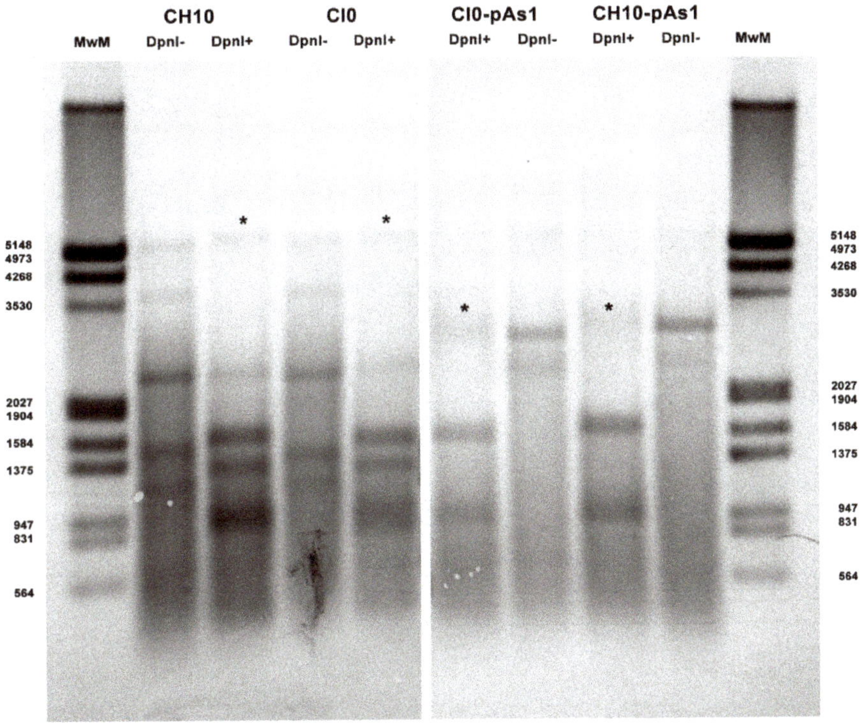

Figure 3. Southern Blot Analysis of B19V DNA obtained from UT7/EpoS1 cells transfected with inserts CH10, CI0 and CH10-pAs1, CI0-pAs1, collected at 24 hpt. Samples were treated by RE DpnI to distinguish de novo synthesized viral DNA (*) based on different *dam* methylation pattern and sensitivity to RE DpnI. MwM: molecular weight marker III, Dig-labelled (Roche). Southern Blotting and hybridization using a full-length digoxigenin-labelled DNA probe was carried out as described [33].

The expression of NS protein was monitored by IIF and cytofluorimetric analysis, sampling transfected cell cultures at 8 and 24 hpt. By IIF (Figure 4), NS protein was already observed at 8 hpt, and at 24 hpt the number of positive cells and signal intensity both increased. Distribution of the protein within the cells showed the same nuclear/cytoplasmic pattern both for all complete or derived minigenome inserts.

By cytofluorimetric analysis (Figure 5), a quantitative assessment of cells expressing NS1 protein was obtained at 24 hpt. The percentage of positive cells was in the range 0.2–1.3% for the complete inserts and increased to 2.6–5.0% for the derived minigenomes, the highest increase was observed for the CI0/CI0-pAs1 combination. Altogether, experiments suggest that the lower genetic complexity of modified genomes promoted progressive expression and accumulation of NS protein in an increasing fraction of the cell population.

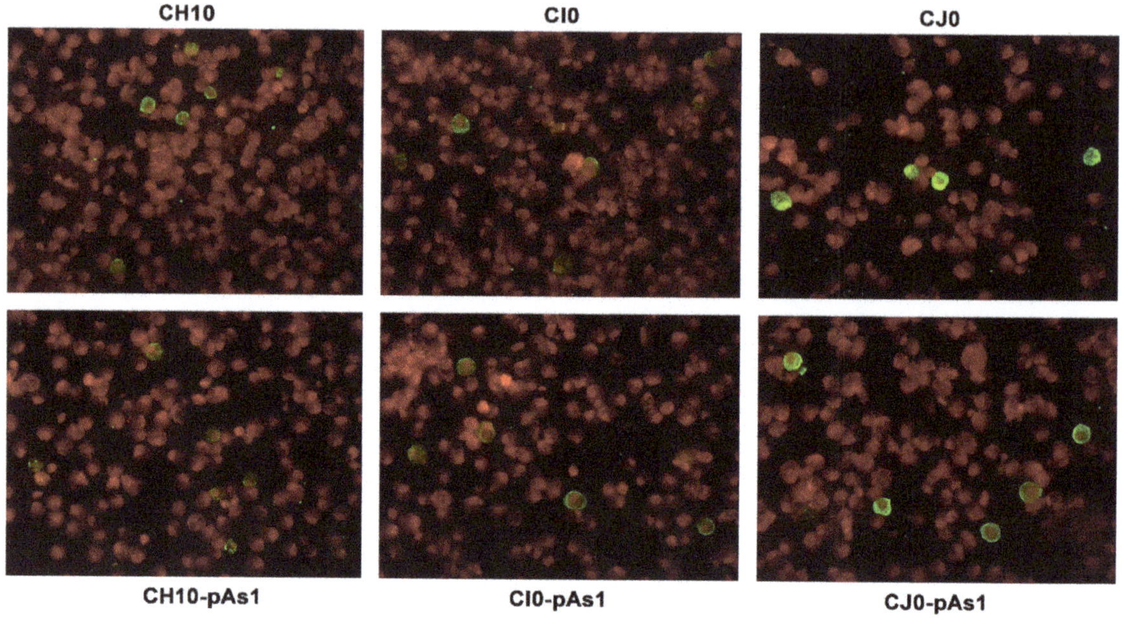

Figure 4. UT7/EpoS1 cells transfected with the indicated inserts were sampled at 24 hpt, and NS1 protein was detected by IIF. Original magnification 400×.

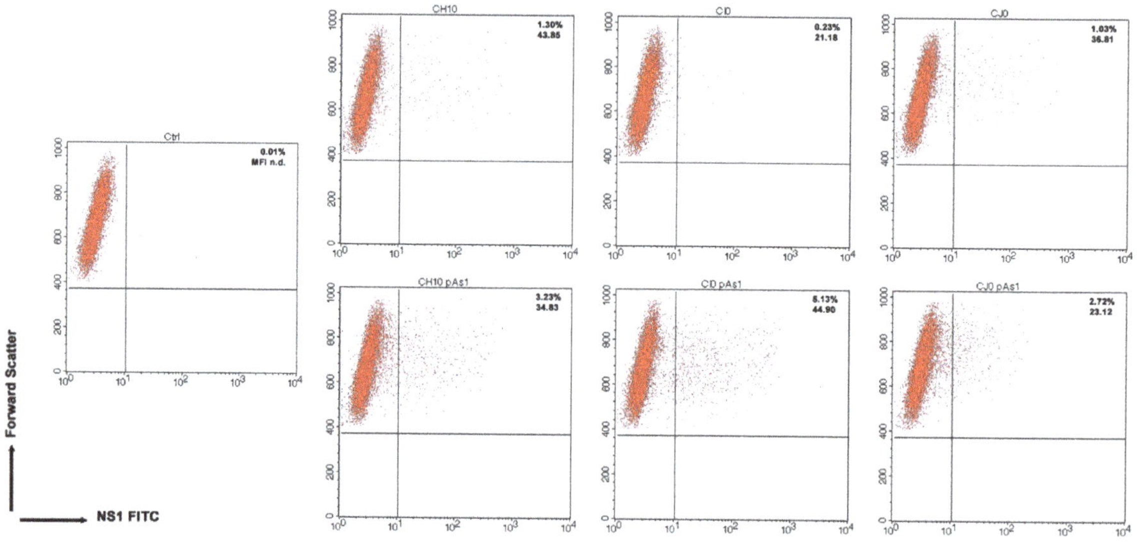

Figure 5. UT7/EpoS1 cells transfected with the indicated inserts (Ctrl, no DNA control) were sampled at 24 hpt, and cell population was analysed by cytofluorimeter to determine the percentage of NS1 expressing cells. Dot plot graph on gated cell population for FSc and NS1 FITC. Reported percentage values of positive cells and geometric mean fluorescence intensity (MFI) for positive subpopulations reported as the average result of two independent determinations.

3.3. Functional Complementation of the B19V Minigenome

The capacity of the CH10-pAs1 minigenome to provide complementing functions through expression of NS1 protein was thereafter tested in a subsequent series of experiments. To the purpose, a set of modified B19V genome clones was designed, defective for the coding sequence of NS protein. In particular, the pCH10 clone was modified by deletion, removing the genomic region corresponding to the first intron within the NS gene, from the splice donor site D1 to the two possible alternative splice acceptor sites A1.1 and A1.2. The obtained plasmids, named CH10-A1.1 and CH10-A1.2, retained the cis-acting sequences directing alternative cleavage-polyadenylation at pAp and pAd sites, sequences regulating alternative splicing of the distal introns at D2 and A2.1/2 sites, and all of the coding sequences for the VP1, VP2 and 11 kDa proteins (Figure 6).

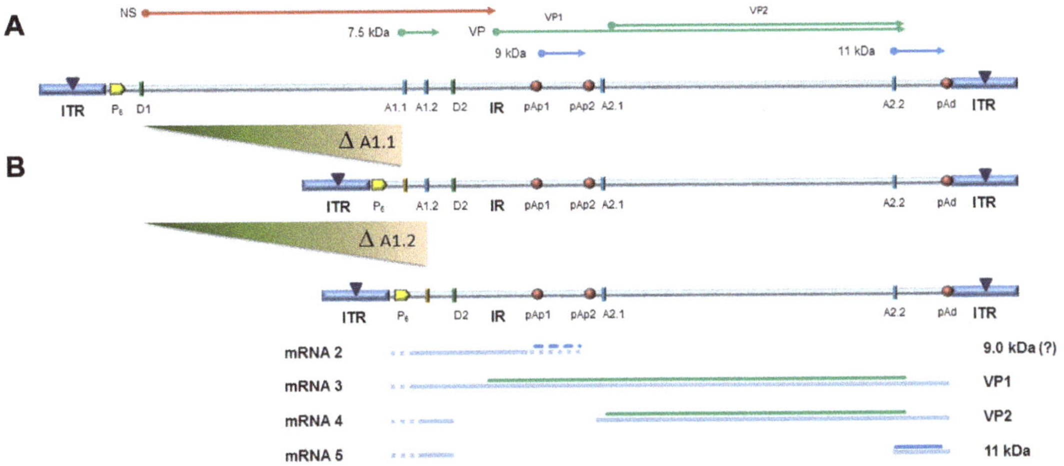

Figure 6. (**A**) Map of B19V genome, see Figure 1. **Δ**: deletion to remove first intron (A1.1/2). (**B**) Map of B19V derived minigenomes; simplified transcription map, indicating the four classes of mRNAs (mRNA 2–5), with alternative splicing/cleavage forms (dashed lines) and related coding potential.

To evaluate the functional competence and possible complementation effects for these defective genomes, inserts obtained by means of in vitro amplification were transfected in UT7/EpoS1 cells, alone or in co-transfection with CH10-pAs1 as helper plasmid. At 24 hpt, aliquots of cell culture were sampled for quantification of viral nucleic acids (DNA, mRNAs) by qPCR and qRT-PCR (Figure 7, Table S1B), and detection of the NS1 and VP proteins by IIF.

No significant differences were observed in the amounts of viral DNA, but relevant information was obtained by quantification of viral RNA. By comparison to the reference CH10 insert, insert CH10-pAs1 confirmed its high transcriptional activity and correct mRNA processing, with an abundance of about 1% unspliced mRNAs coding for NS protein. The NS defective, CH10-A1.1 and -A.2 inserts showed a reduced (−3 Log) basal transcriptional activity, which allowed detection of only the proximally cleaved mRNAs (mRNA 2 in Figure 6), and not of any distally cleaved mRNA (mRNAs 3–5 in Figure 5). Cotransfection of these inserts with CH10-pAs1 inset led to functional complementation, restoring expression from the NS-defective genomes, as shown by the detection of A1.1 and A.2 derived mRNAs, to amounts only about 1 Log lower than what observed for the reference CH10 insert. By composition, the most abundant mRNAs were still the proximally cleaved mRNA species (mRNA 2), which were contributed by both CH10-pAs1 (following splicing) and A1.1/2 (following cleavage at pAp); abundance of NS mRNA (mRNA 1), contributed only by CH10-pAs1, pAd cleaved mRNAs (mRNA 3–5) and VP mRNAs (mRNA 3–4), contributed only by A1.1/2, were in all cases in the order of 1% of total mRNAs.

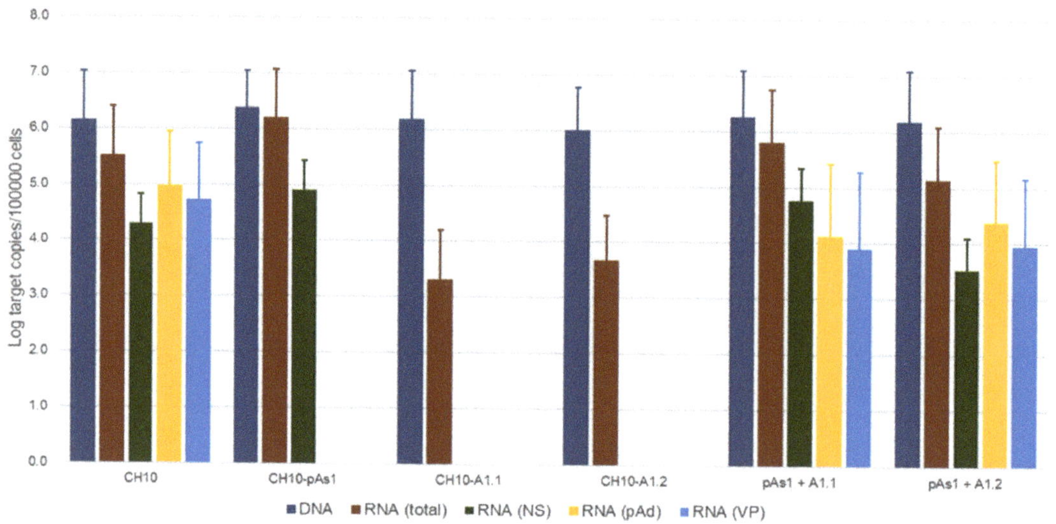

Figure 7. Viral nucleic acids in UT7/EpoS1 cells, transfected/co-transfected with CH10, CH10-pAs1 and CH10-A1.1/2 inserts. Log amounts of target copies (viral DNA, total RNA, NS1 mRNA, pAd cleaved RNA, VP RNA), normalized to 10^5 cells, at 24 hpt. Mean and std of duplicate determinations for two different experiments.

By IIF analysis (Figure 8), expression of both NS and to lesser extents VP proteins was confirmed for the CH10 insert. The expression of NS protein was also confirmed for CH10-pAs1, and not detected in the case of CH10-A1.1/2, as expected. Expression of VP proteins from CH10-A1.1/2 inserts alone was not observed. Cotransfection of CH10-pAs1 and A1.1/2 preserved expression of NS protein from CH10-pAs1 and restored the expression of VP proteins from CH10-A1.1/2, although for the latter detection was limited to a small number of cells. Altogether, data confirm that the NS protein produced by the CH10-pAs1 minigenome is functional in complementation of defective B19V genomes, restoring expression of the late set of mRNAs to a pattern similar to the standard expression profile of B19V genome and allowing production of capsid proteins.

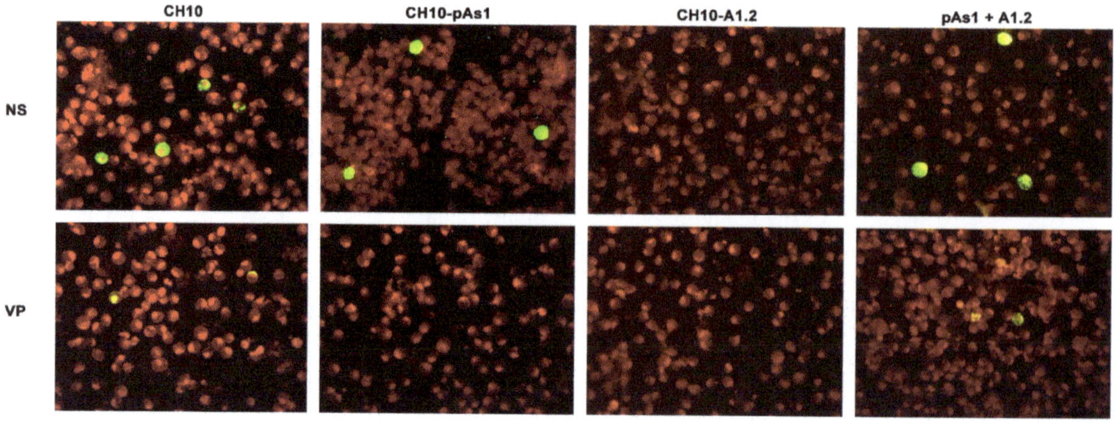

Figure 8. UT7/EpoS1 cells transfected with the indicated inserts were sampled at 24 hpt, and NS1 or VP1/2 proteins were detected by IIF. Results obtained for insert CH10-A1.1 were analogous to what obtained for CH10-A1.2 (not in figure). Original magnification 400×.

3.4. Extracellular Vehiculation of Minigenomes

Following transfection of UT7/EpoS1 cells, measurable amounts of viral DNA were detectable in the cell culture medium until 6 days post-transfection, not associated to cells but partially resistant to nuclease treatment. The possibility that this genetic material could be transferrable to susceptible EPCs was investigated. For the purpose, CH10-pAs1 and CH10-A1.1/2 inserts were transfected in UT7/EpoS1 cells in the different combinations as described, and expression of NS and VP proteins first confirmed for all competent combinations. Then, after a 6 day course, the supernatant of transfected cell cultures was collected and added to in vitro differentiated EPCs cells, as a test system. After a further 48 h course of incubation, EPCs were collected and analysed for any presence of B19V DNA, RNA or expression of NS protein. For all experimental samples, a low measurable amount of DNA was found associated to EPCs (<10^2 copies/10^5 cells). However, no transcriptional activity could be detected in EPCs in any tested combination and no NS protein production could be observed. The obtained results imply that the vehiculation of genetic material from cells transfected with the CH10 derived clones may not be due to the formation of transducing viral particles, and that the process is not functionally relevant to a measurable extent. The hypothesis that such transfer should be attributed to simple carry-over in a nuclease-resistance form, or to the formation of extracellular vesicles or exosomes, and whether a limited number of transducing viral particles is actually produced, requires further investigation.

4. Discussion

In our present work, we designed and produced a B19V minigenome, derived from the complete, competent cloned B19V genome, simplified to a replicon unit. Following transfection in the UT7/EpoS1 cells, this minigenome still proved competent for replication, transcription and production of NS protein. Further, the B19V minigenome was able to complement B19-derived, NS-defective genomes, restoring their ability to express capsid proteins. The unique B19V genome was thus engineered to yield a two-component system, an element expressing the functional NS1 protein, the other the structural capsid proteins, with complementing functions.

In all engineered genetic elements, the terminal regions have been preserved up to the site of dyad symmetry and in opposite flip/flop configurations, thus meeting requirements for maintenance of replicative competence [12,33]. To this respect, interesting information has been obtained by comparing the activity of genomic inserts of different extension within the ITRs. De novo synthesis of transfected DNA could be demonstrated, as previously [33], for the complete CH10 and CI0 inserts, and this property was also conserved for the derived -pAs1 inserts. Hairpin-independent priming of DNA synthesis had been documented in a different experimental setting [11], and it is likely involved here.

The unique P_6 promoter is present in the same position and pattern in all engineered clones, whereas the level of transcription of each one depends on the actual expression of NS protein, due to its strong trans-activating activity on its own promoter [14]. Transcription from the complete CH10, CI0, CJ0, and the derived -pAs1 inserts is detected at high levels already at an early time point (8 hpt), further increasing at a late time point (24 hpt). Transcription levels from the derived -pAs1 inserts is higher than the respective complete clones, but effects depending on the ITR extension are relatively minor. Conversely, sustained transcription from CH10-A.1/2 clones is detectable only upon complementation, and at the late time point.

CH10-pAs1 elements are simplified with respect to pre-mRNA processing. Reduction in the size and complexity of the transcriptional template and the introduction of a novel single cleavage-polyadenylation site at the end of the genome abrogates the early-late transcriptional switch typical of B19V, thus leading to sole accumulation of left-side cassette mRNAs [19,20]. Within these processes, retention of unaltered splicing signals ensures correct processing of pre-mRNAs and unaltered balance of unspliced, NS encoding to spliced mRNAs [25]. Thus, the net effect compared to that observed for complete clones is a sustained accumulation of NS-coding transcripts and overexpression of NS protein in a larger proportion of transfected cells.

Modifications introduced to obtain the defective CH10-A1.1/2 elements have different consequences. Reduction of the genetic template with deletion of the large left-side intron results in the absence of any NS coding mRNA, but both original cleavage-polyadenylation sites are maintained, therefore preserving a possible early-late switch in expression pattern. Moreover, the splicing signals maintained in the right gene cassette still allow alternative splicing events leading to the production of VP1, VP2 and 11 kDa encoding mRNAs [21,22]. In fact, experiments confirmed that such an mRNA set is produced when in the presence of complementing NS protein. However, compared to the complete genome, a relatively higher proportion of short (proximally cleaved, spliced) mRNAs is produced, likely because of the contribution from both transcriptional templates and prevalent pre-mRNA processing. As a consequence, the amount of VP-encoding mRNA obtained from CH10-A.1/2 templates is reduced to suboptimal levels, although enough to achieve production of VP proteins.

The present work reached relevant goals, while showing some critical limitations inherent to the system. A minigenome with characteristics of a replicon has been constructed, able to replicate and overexpress NS protein. Such minigenome may constitute a valuable tool for studying the function of NS protein within a simplified viral genetic contest, mainly its impact on cell functionality, or in the search of molecules with antiviral activity. A functional complementation between defective genomes was obtained, since the minigenome restored the ability of separate genetic units to express capsid proteins. This property opens the possibility of engineering the B19V genome with less stringent structural constraints, allowing for example to modify cis-acting genomic elements, mutagenize or add expression tags to the sequences coding for proteins, or insert heterologous reporter genes, to the purpose of a deeper characterization of B19V replication, expression and interaction in the cellular environment.

Ideally, the compresence in a same cell of two genetic units with complementing functions opens a possibility for packaging and generation of transducing viral particles. However, generation of transducing virus was not shown in our experiments, thus constituting the major limit of the present work. All transfection experiments have been conducted in the UT7/EpoS1 cell line, which is appropriate for research on B19V [36], but at the expense of a very low transfection efficiency. When transfected with a complete genomic insert, de novo produced virus can be subsequently amplified in primary EPCs to yield infectious virus at high titre. In the case of cotransfection of separate complementing units, transducing viral particles would not benefit of any possible subsequent amplification passage. While generation of engineered virus specifically targeting a selected cell population such as EPCs would be of translational interest, further intense research is required to achieve such goal.

Supplementary Materials: The following are available online at https://www.mdpi.com/article/10.3390/v14010084/s1, Figure S1: B19V genome organization, transcription map and primer location. Table S1: Quantitation of viral nucleic acids.

Author Contributions: Conceptualization, A.R., G.B., E.M. and G.G.; Data curation, A.R., G.B. and E.M.; Funding acquisition, G.G.; Investigation, A.R., A.A., F.V. and E.F.; Methodology, A.R., A.A., F.V. and E.F.; Supervision, G.B., E.M. and G.G.; Writing—original draft, A.R. and G.G.; Writing—review & editing, G.G. All authors have read and agreed to the published version of the manuscript.

Funding: This research was funded by Italian Ministry of University and Research, grant PRIN 2017 9JHAMZ_007 to G.G.

Institutional Review Board Statement: Leukocyte-enriched buffy coats of healthy blood donors, were obtained from the Immunohematology and Transfusion Service, S. Orsola-Malpighi University Hospital, Bologna (http://www.aosp.bo.it/content/immunoematologia-e-trasfusionale; authorization 0070755/1980/2014, issued by Head of Service). Availability was granted under conditions complying with Italian privacy law. Neither specific ethics committee approval nor written consent from donors was required for this research project.

Conflicts of Interest: The authors declare no conflict of interest. The funders had no role in the design of the study; in the collection, analyses, or interpretation of data; in the writing of the manuscript, or in the decision to publish the results.

References

1. Cotmore, S.F.; Agbandje-McKenna, M.; Canuti, M.; Chiorini, J.A.; Eis-Hubinger, A.M.; Hughes, J.; Mietzsch, M.; Modha, S.; Ogliastro, M.; Penzes, J.J.; et al. ICTV Virus Taxonomy Profile: Parvoviridae. *J. Gen. Virol.* **2019**, *100*, 367–368. [CrossRef]
2. Gallinella, G. Parvovirus B19 Achievements and Challenges. *ISRN Virol.* **2013**, *2013*, 898730. [CrossRef]
3. Qiu, J.; Soderlund-Venermo, M.; Young, N.S. Human Parvoviruses. *Clin. Microbiol. Rev.* **2017**, *30*, 43–113. [CrossRef] [PubMed]
4. Chisaka, H.; Morita, E.; Yaegashi, N.; Sugamura, K. Parvovirus B19 and the pathogenesis of anaemia. *Rev. Med. Virol.* **2003**, *13*, 347–359. [CrossRef] [PubMed]
5. Chen, A.Y.; Qiu, J. Parvovirus infection-induced cell death and cell cycle arrest. *Future Virol.* **2010**, *5*, 731–743. [CrossRef] [PubMed]
6. Kerr, J.R. A review of blood diseases and cytopenias associated with human parvovirus B19 infection. *Rev. Med. Virol.* **2015**, *25*, 224–240. [CrossRef] [PubMed]
7. Adamson-Small, L.A.; Ignatovich, I.V.; Laemmerhirt, M.G.; Hobbs, J.A. Persistent parvovirus B19 infection in non-erythroid tissues: Possible role in the inflammatory and disease process. *Virus Res.* **2014**, *190*, 8–16. [CrossRef]
8. Bua, G.; Gallinella, G. How does parvovirus B19 DNA achieve lifelong persistence in human cells? *Future Virol.* **2017**, *12*, 549–553. [CrossRef]
9. Ganaie, S.S.; Qiu, J. Recent Advances in Replication and Infection of Human Parvovirus B19. *Front. Cell. Infect. Microbiol.* **2018**, *8*, 166. [CrossRef]
10. Manaresi, E.; Gallinella, G. Advances in the Development of Antiviral Strategies against Parvovirus B19. *Viruses* **2019**, *11*, 659. [CrossRef]
11. Guan, W.; Wong, S.; Zhi, N.; Qiu, J. The genome of human parvovirus B19 can replicate in nonpermissive cells with the help of adenovirus genes and produces infectious virus. *J. Virol.* **2009**, *83*, 9541–9553. [CrossRef]
12. Luo, Y.; Qiu, J. Human parvovirus B19: A mechanistic overview of infection and DNA replication. *Future Virol.* **2015**, *10*, 155–167. [CrossRef]
13. Zou, W.; Wang, Z.; Xiong, M.; Chen, A.Y.; Xu, P.; Ganaie, S.S.; Badawi, Y.; Kleiboeker, S.; Nishimune, H.; Ye, S.Q.; et al. Human Parvovirus B19 Utilizes Cellular DNA Replication Machinery for Viral DNA Replication. *J. Virol.* **2018**, *92*, e01881-17. [CrossRef]
14. Gareus, R.; Gigler, A.; Hemauer, A.; Leruez-Ville, M.; Morinet, F.; Wolf, H.; Modrow, S. Characterization of cis-acting and NS1 protein-responsive elements in the p6 promoter of parvovirus B19. *J. Virol.* **1998**, *72*, 609–616. [CrossRef]
15. Raab, U.; Bauer, B.; Gigler, A.; Beckenlehner, K.; Wolf, H.; Modrow, S. Cellular transcription factors that interact with p6 promoter elements of parvovirus B19. *J. Gen. Virol.* **2001**, *82*, 1473–1480. [CrossRef] [PubMed]
16. Raab, U.; Beckenlehner, K.; Lowin, T.; Niller, H.H.; Doyle, S.; Modrow, S. NS1 protein of parvovirus B19 interacts directly with DNA sequences of the p6 promoter and with the cellular transcription factors Sp1/Sp3. *Virology* **2002**, *293*, 86–93. [CrossRef] [PubMed]
17. Bonvicini, F.; Manaresi, E.; Di Furio, F.; De Falco, L.; Gallinella, G. Parvovirus B19 DNA CpG dinucleotide methylation and epigenetic regulation of viral expression. *PLoS ONE* **2012**, *7*, e33316. [CrossRef] [PubMed]
18. Bua, G.; Tedesco, D.; Conti, I.; Reggiani, A.; Bartolini, M.; Gallinella, G. No G-Quadruplex Structures in the DNA of Parvovirus B19: Experimental Evidence versus Bioinformatic Predictions. *Viruses* **2020**, *12*, 935. [CrossRef] [PubMed]
19. Yoto, Y.; Qiu, J.; Pintel, D.J. Identification and characterization of two internal cleavage and polyadenylation sites of parvovirus B19 RNA. *J. Virol.* **2006**, *80*, 1604–1609. [CrossRef]
20. Guan, W.; Cheng, F.; Yoto, Y.; Kleiboeker, S.; Wong, S.; Zhi, N.; Pintel, D.J.; Qiu, J. Block to the production of full-length B19 virus transcripts by internal polyadenylation is overcome by replication of the viral genome. *J. Virol.* **2008**, *82*, 9951–9963. [CrossRef]
21. Guan, W.; Huang, Q.; Cheng, F.; Qiu, J. Internal polyadenylation of the parvovirus B19 precursor mRNA is regulated by alternative splicing. *J. Biol. Chem.* **2011**, *286*, 24793–24805. [CrossRef]
22. Guan, W.; Cheng, F.; Huang, Q.; Kleiboeker, S.; Qiu, J. Inclusion of the central exon of parvovirus B19 precursor mRNA is determined by multiple splicing enhancers in both the exon and the downstream intron. *J. Virol.* **2011**, *85*, 2463–2468. [CrossRef]
23. Bonvicini, F.; Filippone, C.; Delbarba, S.; Manaresi, E.; Zerbini, M.; Musiani, M.; Gallinella, G. Parvovirus B19 genome as a single, two-state replicative and transcriptional unit. *Virology* **2006**, *347*, 447–454. [CrossRef] [PubMed]
24. Bonvicini, F.; Filippone, C.; Manaresi, E.; Zerbini, M.; Musiani, M.; Gallinella, G. Functional analysis and quantitative determination of the expression profile of human parvovirus B19. *Virology* **2008**, *381*, 168–177. [CrossRef] [PubMed]

25. Bua, G.; Manaresi, E.; Bonvicini, F.; Gallinella, G. Parvovirus B19 Replication and Expression in Differentiating Erythroid Progenitor Cells. *PLoS ONE* **2016**, *11*, e0148547. [CrossRef]
26. Xu, P.; Ganaie, S.S.; Wang, X.; Wang, Z.; Kleiboeker, S.; Horton, N.C.; Heier, R.F.; Meyers, M.J.; Tavis, J.E.; Qiu, J. Endonuclease Activity Inhibition of the NS1 Protein of Parvovirus B19 as a Novel Target for Antiviral Drug Development. *Antimicrob. Agents Chemother.* **2019**, *63*, e01879-18. [CrossRef] [PubMed]
27. Ning, K.; Roy, A.; Cheng, F.; Xu, P.; Kleiboeker, S.; Escalante, C.R.; Wang, J.; Qiu, J. High throughput screening identifies inhibitors for parvovirus B19 infection of human erythroid progenitor cells. *J. Virol.* **2021**, JVI0132621. [CrossRef] [PubMed]
28. Mietzsch, M.; Penzes, J.J.; Agbandje-McKenna, M. Twenty-Five Years of Structural Parvovirology. *Viruses* **2019**, *11*, 362. [CrossRef] [PubMed]
29. Ros, C.; Bieri, J.; Leisi, R. The VP1u of Human Parvovirus B19: A Multifunctional Capsid Protein with Biotechnological Applications. *Viruses* **2020**, *12*, 1463. [CrossRef]
30. Zou, W.; Ning, K.; Xu, P.; Deng, X.; Cheng, F.; Kleiboeker, S.; Qiu, J. The N-terminal 5–68 amino acids domain of the minor capsid protein VP1 of human parvovirus B19 enters human erythroid progenitors and inhibits B19 infection. *J. Virol.* **2021**, *95*, e00466-21. [CrossRef]
31. Zhi, N.; Zadori, Z.; Brown, K.E.; Tijssen, P. Construction and sequencing of an infectious clone of the human parvovirus B19. *Virology* **2004**, *318*, 142–152. [CrossRef]
32. Zhi, N.; Mills, I.P.; Lu, J.; Wong, S.; Filippone, C.; Brown, K.E. Molecular and functional analyses of a human parvovirus B19 infectious clone demonstrates essential roles for NS1, VP1, and the 11-kilodalton protein in virus replication and infectivity. *J. Virol.* **2006**, *80*, 5941–5950. [CrossRef]
33. Manaresi, E.; Conti, I.; Bua, G.; Bonvicini, F.; Gallinella, G. A Parvovirus B19 synthetic genome: Sequence features and functional competence. *Virology* **2017**, *508*, 54–62. [CrossRef]
34. Wong, S.; Brown, K.E. Development of an improved method of detection of infectious parvovirus B19. *J. Clin. Virol.* **2006**, *35*, 407–413. [CrossRef] [PubMed]
35. Filippone, C.; Franssila, R.; Kumar, A.; Saikko, L.; Kovanen, P.E.; Soderlund-Venermo, M.; Hedman, K. Erythroid progenitor cells expanded from peripheral blood without mobilization or preselection: Molecular characteristics and functional competence. *PLoS ONE* **2010**, *5*, e9496. [CrossRef] [PubMed]
36. Ducloux, C.; You, B.; Langele, A.; Goupille, O.; Payen, E.; Chretien, S.; Kadri, Z. Enhanced Cell-Based Detection of Parvovirus B19V Infectious Units According to Cell Cycle Status. *Viruses* **2020**, *12*, 1467. [CrossRef] [PubMed]

viruses

MDPI

Article

Design and Characterization of Mutated Variants of the Oncotoxic Parvoviral Protein NS1

Patrick Hauswirth [1], Philipp Graber [1], Katarzyna Buczak [2], Riccardo Vincenzo Mancuso [3,4], Susanne Heidi Schenk [1], Jürg P. F. Nüesch [5] and Jörg Huwyler [1,*]

1 Division of Pharmaceutical Technology, Department of Pharmaceutical Sciences, University of Basel, 4056 Basel, Switzerland
2 Proteomics Core Facility, Biozentrum, University of Basel, 4056 Basel, Switzerland
3 Division of Clinical Pharmacology & Toxicology, University Hospital of Basel, University of Basel, 4055 Basel, Switzerland
4 Division of Molecular Pharmacy, Department of Pharmaceutical Sciences, University of Basel, 4056 Basel, Switzerland
5 Infection, Inflammation and Cancer Program, Division of Tumor Virology, German Cancer Research Center (DKFZ), 69120 Heidelberg, Germany
* Correspondence: joerg.huwyler@unibas.ch; Tel.: +41-61-207-15-13

Abstract: Oncotoxic proteins such as the non-structural protein 1 (NS1), a constituent of the rodent parvovirus H1 (H1-PV), offer a novel approach for treatment of tumors that are refractory to other treatments. In the present study, mutated NS1 variants were designed and tested with respect to their oncotoxic potential in human hepatocellular carcinoma cell lines. We introduced single point mutations of previously described important residues of the wild-type NS1 protein and a deletion of 114 base pairs localized within the N-terminal domain of NS1. Cell-viability screening with HepG2 and Hep3B hepatocarcinoma cells transfected with the constructed NS1-mutants led to identification of the single-amino acid NS1-mutant NS1-T585E, which led to a 30% decrease in cell viability as compared to NS1 wildtype. Using proteomics analysis, we could identify new interaction partners and signaling pathways of NS1. We could thus identify new oncotoxic NS1 variants and gain insight into the modes of action of NS1, which is exclusively toxic to human cancer cells. Our in-vitro studies provide mechanistic explanations for the observed oncolytic effects. Expression of NS1 variants had no effect on cell viability in NS1 unresponsive control HepG2 cells or primary mouse hepatocytes. The availability of new NS1 variants in combination with a better understanding of their modes of action offers new possibilities for the design of innovative cancer treatment strategies.

Keywords: H1-PV; parvovirus; infection; oncolytic virus; anticancer gene; cancer gene therapy; cancer

Citation: Hauswirth, P.; Graber, P.; Buczak, K.; Mancuso, R.V.; Schenk, S.H.; Nüesch, J.P.F.; Huwyler, J. Design and Characterization of Mutated Variants of the Oncotoxic Parvoviral Protein NS1. *Viruses* **2023**, *15*, 209. https://doi.org/10.3390/v15010209

Academic Editor: Giorgio Gallinella

Received: 3 December 2022
Revised: 30 December 2022
Accepted: 8 January 2023
Published: 11 January 2023

1. Introduction

Whereas most chemotherapeutic agents indiscriminately act on tumor and non-tumor tissue, oncotoxic proteins specifically interact with cancer cells only by suppressing cell growth or inducing apoptosis [1]. Oncotoxic proteins include cytokines, artificially modified secreted proteins, and proteins of viral origin, such as the parvovirus-derived oncotoxic nonstructural protein 1 (NS1) [1,2]. Usually, they are activated in tumor cells only and subsequently modulate pathways involved in cell proliferation, cell cycle control, apoptosis, mitochondrial respiration, and glycolysis [1]. Expression systems encoding for these proteins can be introduced into target cells by a viral or non-viral gene therapy approach [3,4].

The rat parvovirus H1 (H1-PV) shows low pathogenicity in normal human tissues but can infect and kill malignant cells. The natural oncotropism and oncolytic activities were therefore recently explored in phase II clinical trials [5–8]. The H1-PV viral capsid contains the linear, single-stranded DNA genome which encodes two structural and at least six nonstructural proteins, of which the 672 amino acid long NS1 is the major effector for virus propagation and cytotoxicity. The oncotoxic protein NS1 alone is sufficient to induce a strong cytotoxic effect in various human cell lines [3,4,9,10]. In a recent study, NS1 gene delivery using a non-viral vector was proposed to be a promising strategy for an anti-cancer treatment in hepatocellular carcinomas [3]. This is in contrast to viral treatment strategies, which have several drawbacks such as immunogenicity and chromosomal gene insertion [11,12].

In cancer cells, NS1 exploits and activates several distinct pathways within its host cell, not only important for virus propagation but also ultimately leading to cell cycle arrest, apoptosis, necrosis, and lysosomal cell death [2,10]. NS1 activities are modulated by post-translational protein modifications by host cell proteins. In particular, phosphorylation and acetylation of distinct NS1 amino acid residues have been shown to activate or deactivate distinct functions of the protein. In fact, side-directed mutagenesis of NS1 residues S473 and T585 to alanine, which precludes phosphorylation, resulted in a decreased effect of the protein [13,14]. Furthermore, acetylation of residues K85 and K257 of H1-PV NS1 have been shown to increase its cytotoxic effect [15].

It was therefore the aim of the present study to further improve the beneficial properties (i.e., selective killing of cancer cells) of NS1 and to investigate NS1-target cell interactions. We designed single amino acid mutants of selected residues whose modification (i.e., phosphorylation or acetylation) led to altered oncotoxic NS1 activity (Figure 1). We used a phospho-mimetics approach to simulate the phosphorylated state of known serine and threonine phosphorylation sites by replacing serine or threonine to glutamic acid [16]. The acetylation of lysine was simulated by a conversion of lysine to glutamine [17]. Finally, we constructed a NS1 variant previously found in a H1-PV mutant virus, which is characterized by a 114 nucleotide in-frame deletion of NS1. This mutant virus showed increased fitness and infectivity compared to wt-H1-PV [18]. The designed mutants were analyzed with respect to their oncotoxic effects using cell viability assays, which led to the identification of an NS1 mutant (NS1-T585E) with an increased, but still specific oncotoxicity.

Previous experiments using Nanoparticle-mediated gene transfer to target hepatocellular carcinoma cells (HCC) with H-1PV NS1, have shown promising results, not only in tissue culture but in xenotransplants of nude mice as well. However, for an optimal treatment of cancers, it appears necessary to induce a bystander effect. This can be achieved through involvement of the immune-system, breaking the immune-suppressive environment and attracting immune cells through release of cytokines' danger-associated molecular patterns (DAMPS), pathogen-associated molecular patterns (PAMPs), and, potentially, tumor-associated antigens (TAA). The latter has been shown in clinical trials with H-1PV in GBM-treated patients through peptides corresponding to NS1 and VP1, respectively [19]. Although this can be explained by a potential release through the exocytic pathway that becomes usurped in PV-infected cells to transport progeny particles to the plasma-membrane [20], it remains largely unknown whether this pathway is involved in NS1 transduced cancer cells and what kind of DAMPs or TAAs might become exposed at the surface after expression of NS1. To address these questions, the current work determines NS1-association using different proteomics approaches to identify new interaction partners of wild-type NS1 and the most potent phospho-mimetic mutant NS1-T585E of cellular proteins in NS1-transfected Hep3B cells and potential pathways triggered by NS1. Consequently, the obtained results provide significant leads to determine the potential feasibility of an NS1-associated treatment of cancers involving immune-attraction and to obtain a bystander effect.

Although, H-1PV has shown proof-of-concept in a phase I/IIa clinical trial, there are still limitations regarding susceptibility of cancer cells/entities to this virus species. This can, for instance, be overcome through nanoparticle-associated transfer of the cytotoxic NS1 protein and/or NS1-encoding nucleic acids either alone or in combination with other (viral) proteins [10,21]. In addition, there is a large potential to improve efficacy, particularly through engagement of the host immune system in order to induce an anti-tumor immune response through a combination of danger-associated molecular patterns (DAMPs) and pathogen-associated molecular patterns (PAMPs) released from infected/transfected cancer cells. The current manuscript aims to use a virus-free approach to determine the impact of NS1 on the host cell using wildtype and site-directed mutant H1-PV NS1 to identify new cellular targets and interaction partners of NS1. This includes well-established targets necessary for viral replication, such as factors involved in DNA replication and repair, exocytosis, and potential danger-associated molecular patterns associated with cytolysis.

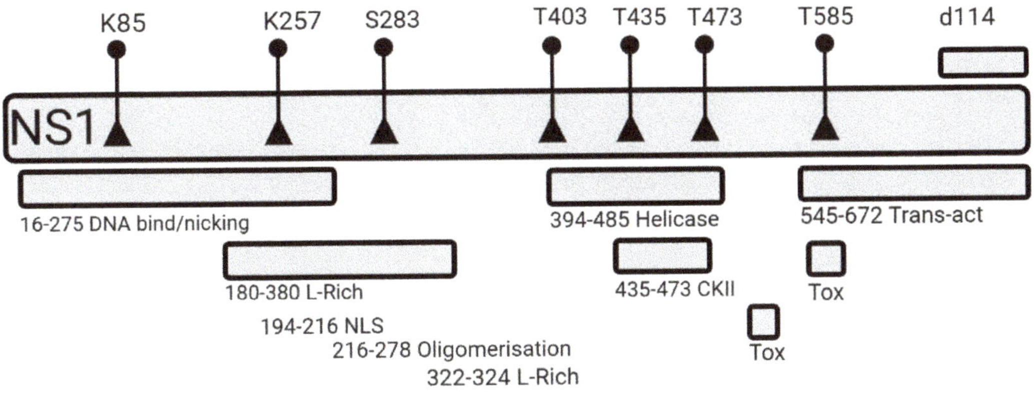

Figure 1. Schematic overview of non-structural protein 1 (NS1) domains and mutation sites. The non-structural parvovirus-derived protein NS1 is comprised of 672 amino acids. Amino acid positions of previously described functional domains within the NS1 protein are summarized: A site-specific DNA binding domain involved in site- and strand-specific nicking (16–275), an L-Rich area which was shown to be crucial for NS1-mediated toxicity (180–380), a nuclear localization signal (194–216), a motif controlling self-assembly into oligomers (216–278), a helicase domain including a NTP-binding pocket (394–485), a region binding CKIIα (435–473), whose interaction is needed for many NS1-signaling pathways, two toxicity domains crucial for NS1 cytotoxicity, and a transactivator domain (545–672), which positively regulates the expression of viral proteins [22]. The locations of specific acetylation [15] and phosphorylation [13,14] sites, where single amino acid mutations and a deletion of 114 nucleotides (d114) [18] were introduced during this work, are indicated. Mutations were introduced by site-directed mutagenesis. For a review see Nüesch et al. [2,10,22].

2. Materials and Methods

2.1. Materials

All chemicals were purchased from Sigma Aldrich (Buchs, Switzerland) and were of analytical grade. Strepatavidin Sepharose High Performance beads were purchased from GE Healthcare (Chicago, IL, USA). cOmplete Protease Inhibitor Cocktail was obtained from Roche (Basel, Switzerland). Dulbecco's phosphate buffered saline (DPBS, without calcium and magnesium), Dulbecco's modified Eagle medium (DMEM, high glucose), 0.25% Trypsin/EDTA, 100 × Penicillin/Streptomycin solution, and poly-D-lysine were obtained from Sigma Aldrich (Buchs, Switzerland). OptiMEM (Gibco) and Lipofectamine 3000 (Invitrogen, Waltham, MA, USA) were obtained from Fisher Scientific AG (Reinach, Switzerland), and foetal calf serum was purchased from Amimed (Bio-concept, Allschwil, Switzerland). Tissue culture plates were purchased from TTP (Trasadingen, Switzerland). Hep3B and HepG2 cells were obtained from ATCC (Manassas, VA, USA). Restriction endonucleases, DNA ligases, and polymerases were obtained from New England Biolabs Inc. (Ipswich, MA, USA). QIAquick PCR Purification Kit, QIAprep Spin Miniprep Kit, and QIAprep Plus Midiprep Kit were purchased from Qiagen (Hilden, Germany). pcDNA3.1+ (Invitrogen) was purchased from Fisher Scientific AG (Reinach, Switzerland), pTagGFP-N was purchased from Evrogen (Moscow, Russia) and MCS-BioID2-HA was purchased from

Addgene (Watertown, MA, USA). E. coli DH5alpha (Invitrogen) were obtained from Fisher Scientific AG (Reinach, Switzerland).

2.2. Cloning of NS1 for Cytotoxicity Studies

Specific NS1-mutants were created by overlap extension PCR and cloned into pcDNA3.1+. pcDNA3.1-NS1 was used as a template for the first round of PCRs. Briefly, two separate overlapping PCR fragments were created using the flanking primers p1 and p2 in combination with the respective mutated reverse or forward primers (see Table S1). The resulting two overlapping PCR products were purified (QIAquick PCR Purification Kit) and subsequently combined at equimolar concentrations to perform an overlap extension PCR, using the outermost primers (p1, p2) to recombine the two mutated fragments. All PCR reactions were carried out using Phusion High-Fidelity DNA Polymerase (New England Biolabs) according to the manufacturer's recommendations. DNA was initially denatured at 98 °C for 30 s followed by 35 cycles of denaturation (98 °C, 10 s), annealing (68 °C, 30 s), and elongation (72 °C, 45 s). Final extension was carried out at 72 °C for 10 min. The final PCR products were digested and ligated into pcDNA3.1+ using BamHI and NotI restriction sites.

2.3. Cloning of Plasmids for Proteomics

For GFP pull down studies, NS1-wt and NS1(T585E) were cloned into pTag-GFP-N Evrogen or pTag-NS1-GFP [3]. pTag-NS1(T585E)-GFP was created by PCR using pcDNA3.1-NS1(T585E) as a template and the flanking primers p1 and p3 as described above. The resulting PCR product was digested and ligated into pTag-GFP using BamHI restriction sites.

For proximity-dependent biotinylation analysis, NS1-wt and NS1(T585E) were amplified by PCR using the respective pcDNA3.1-construct as template and the flanking primers p4, p5. The PCR products were digested and ligated into the MCS-BioID2-HA (Addgene) plasmid using AgeI sites. MCS-BioID2-HA control plasmid was modified to introduce a start codon in the BioID2-gene. Therefore, the original MCS-BioID2-HA plasmid was used as a template and amplified by PCR using primers p22 and p23 as described above. The PCR product (ATG-BioID2-HA) was digested with AgeI and HindIII and ligated into MCS-BioID2-HA, of which the original BioID2 sequence was removed by digestion with the same restriction enzymes.

2.4. Sequencing and Amplification of Plasmid DNA for Transfections

All plasmids were transformed into the chemically competent *E. coli* DH5alpha strain. pDNA from individual colonies was isolated using QIAprepSpin miniprep kit and sequenced to confirm correct sequence and reading frame of the insert. Plasmids that were used for further experiments were purified using the QIAprep Plasmid PlusMidi Kit (Qiagen) in accordance with the manufacturer's recommendations. Plasmids used in the present study are listed in Table 1.

Table 1. Plasmids and Primers used for cloning and mutant design.

Plasmid	PCR Template	Primers	Expressed Protein
pcDNA3.1+	original plasmid (Invitrogen)	-	no protein expression
pcDNA3.1—NS1	Witzigmann et al. [3]	-	NS1-wt
pcDNA3.1—NS1 (K85Q)	pcDNA3.1—NS1	p1, p7; p6, p2	NS1-K85Q
pcDNA3.1—NS1 (K257Q)	pcDNA3.1—NS1	p1, p9; p8, p2	NS1-K257Q
pcDNA3.1—NS1 (S283E)	pcDNA3.1—NS1	p1, p11; p10, p2	NS1-S283E
pcDNA3.1—NS1 (T435E)	pcDNA3.1—NS1	p1, p13; p12, p2	NS1-T435E
pcDNA3.1—NS1 (S473E)	pcDNA3.1—NS1	p1, 15; p14, p2	NS1-S473E
pcDNA3.1—NS1 (T585A)	pcDNA3.1—NS1	p1, 17; p16, p2	NS1-T585A

Table 1. *Cont.*

Plasmid	PCR Template	Primers	Expressed Protein
pcDNA3.1—NS1 (T585E)	pcDNA3.1—NS1	p1, p19; p18, p2	NS1-T585E
pcDNA3.1—NS1 (d114)	pcDNA3.1—NS1	p1, p20; p21, p2	NS1-d114
pTag-GFP-N	original plasmid (Evrogen)	-	GFP
pTag-NS1-GFP	Witzigmann et al. [3]	-	NS1-wt-GFP
pTag-NS1(T585E)-GFP	pcDNA3.1—NS1 (T585E)	p1, p3	NS1-T585E-GFP
MCS-BioID2-HA	original plasmid (Addgene)	-	no protein expression
pBioID2	MCS-BioID2-HA	p22, p23	BioID2
pNS1-BioID2	pcDNA3.1—NS1	p4, p5	NS1-wt-BioID2
pNS1(T585E)-BioID2	(T585E)	p4, p5	NS1-T585E-BioID2

2.5. Cell Culture and Transfection

Hepatocarcinoma cell lines HepG2 and Hep3B were maintained in DMEM high glucose (4.5 g/L), supplemented with 10% fetal calf serum and Penicillin-Streptomycin, referred to as complete culture medium (CCM). Cells were cultured at 37 °C in a humidified CO_2-incubator (5% CO_2). Sub-cultivation was performed twice a week and the cells were kept in culture between passage numbers 22 to 40.

For transfection, cells were seeded at indicated cell densities on poly-D-Lysine (3 µg/cm^2) coated tissue culture plates. Twenty-four hours after seeding, cells were transfected with respective plasmid DNA (pDNA) using Lipofectamine 3000 (Invitrogen) at 2:1 *v*/*w* ratio of plasmid DNA to Lipofectamine 3000. In brief, pDNA was diluted in OptiMEM (Gibco) and mixed with P3000 reagent. Lipofectamine 3000 was diluted with OptiMEM, mixed with the pDNA-P3000-mixture, vortexed, and incubated for 5 min at room temperature before adding dropwise to the cells. To reduce toxic effects of the transfection reagent, the medium was changed 12 h after transfection.

2.6. MTT Cell Viability Assay

In-vitro cell viability was tested using the MTT assay as described [23]. In brief, 8000 cells per well were seeded in 200 µL of CCM into poly-D-lysine coated 96-well plates. Twenty-four hours after seeding, medium was reduced to 150 µL/well, and the cells were transfected with 0.1 µg of pDNA3.1-NS1-constructs as described above. Seventy-two hours post-transfection, the culture medium was reduced to 50 µL per well, and 50 µL of MTT working solution (1 mg/mL) was added. Cells were incubated for 2 h at 37 °C. Formazan crystals were dissolved with DMSO on a shaker in the dark for 30 min at RT. Absorption was measured at 540 nm. Mock transfected cells (i.e., transfections with empty pcDNA3.1+) were used as 100% reference of cell viability.

2.7. Sample Preparation for Phospho- and Total Cell Proteomics

Cells (2 × 10^6 cells) were analyzed 48 h post-transfection. Two mililiters ice-cold DPBS containing cOmplete Protease Inhibitor Cocktail (Roche) was added and cells were harvested on ice with a cell scraper. Cells were collected by centrifugation (115 min at 300× *g*, 4 °C). Washed cells were snap-frozen in liquid nitrogen and stored at −80 °C until use. Cells were lysed in 8 M Urea (Sigma) and 0.1 M ammonium bicarbonate in the presence of phosphatase inhibitors (Sigma) using ultra-sonication (Bioruptor, Diagenode, Belgium). Protein concentration was determined by the BCA assay (Thermo Fisher Scientific, Waltham, MA, USA). Two hundred µg protein was reduced with 5 mM TCEP for 60 min at 37 °C and alkylated with 10 mM chloroacetamide for 30 min at 37 °C. After dilution with 100 mM ammonium bicarbonate buffer to a final urea concentration of 1.6 M, proteins were digested by incubation with sequencing-grade modified trypsin (Promega, Madison, WI, USA) overnight at 37 °C. After acidification using 5% TFA, peptides were desalted on C18 reversed-phase spin columns (Macrospin, Harvard Apparatus, Holliston, MA, USA) and dried under vacuum.

Peptide samples were enriched for phosphorylated peptides using Fe(III)-IMAC cartridges on an AssayMAP Bravo platform as described above [24]. Remaining flow-through fractions of non-phosphorylated peptides were labeled with tandem mass isobaric tags (TMT 16-plex, Thermo Fisher Scientific). Desalted TMT-labeled peptides were fractionated by high-pH reversed phase separation using a XBridge Peptide BEH C18 column (3.5 µm, 130 Å, 1 mm × 150 mm, Waters) on an Agilent 1260 Infinity HPLC system, as described previously [25].

2.8. Sample Preparations for (NS1-)GFP-Pulldowns

GFP pulldown was performed using a GFP-Trap Magnetic Agarose Kit (chromotek). Briefly, cell pellets were resuspended in an ice-cold 10 mM Tris/Cl pH 7.5, 150 mM NaCl, 0.5 mM EDTA, 0.5%, Nonidet P40 Substitute, 0.09% sodium azide, cOmplete protease inhibitor cocktail (Roche). Samples were centrifuged at 17,000× *g* for 10 min at 4 °C, diluted with 10 mM Tris/Cl pH 7.5, 150 mM NaCl, 0.5 mM EDTA, 0.018% sodium azide) supplemented with 1 mM PMSF and protease inhibitor cocktail, and separated from the supernatant with a magnet. Proteins were eluted by on-bead digestion in 1,6 M Urea, 100 mM Ammonium bicarbonate, 5 µg/mL trypsin, pH 8 for 30 min at 27°, followed by reduction in 1.6 M Urea, 100 mM Ammonium bicarbonate, and 1 mM TCEP, pH 8. Reduced sulfhydryl groups were alkylated using chloroacetamide (15 mM) prior to fragmentation of peptides by a second tryptic digest (12 h at 37 °C). The tryptic digest was acidified (pH < 3) using TFA, desalted using C18 reversed phase spin columns (Microspin, Harvard Apparatus), and subjected to LC-MS analysis as described above.

2.9. Sample Preparations for BioID2

BioID protein-proximity labeling in living Hep3B cells was done as described previously [26]. Ten hours after transfection, biotin was added to cells using a final concentration of 50 µM. Forty-eight hours post-transfection, cells were harvested, washed, and lysed. Biotinylated peptides were isolated using streptavidin-Sepharose beads equilibrated in lysis buffer. On-bead digestion was performed as described in the previous section. Peptides were purified and subjected to LC-MS analysis as described above.

2.10. MS Data Acquisition

Phosphorylated peptides were resuspended in 0.1% formic acid and analyzed using Orbitrap Fusion Lumos Mass Spectrometer fitted with an EASY-nLC 1200 (both Thermo Fisher Scientific) and a custom-made column heater set to 60 °C. Peptides were resolved using a RP-HPLC column (75 µm × 36 cm) packed in-house with C18 resin (ReproSil-Pur C18–AQ, 1.9 µm resin; Dr. Maisch GmbH) at a flow rate of 0.2 µL/min. The MS was operated in DDA mode with a cycle time of 3 s. MS1 scans were acquired at a resolution of 120,000 FWHM (at 200 m/z) and a scan range from 375 to 1600 m/z. Precursors were isolated with the isolation window of 1.4 m/z and fragmented with HCD with CE set to 30%. MS2 scans were acquired at a resolution of 30,000 FWHM. Both scans were acquired using Orbitrap.

TMT fractions were resuspended in 0.1% formic acid and analysed using a Q Exactive HF Mass Spectrometer fitted with an EASY-nLC 1000 (both Thermo Fisher Scientific). Column parameters were as above except in length (30 cm). The MS was operated in Top10 DDA mode. MS1 scans were acquired at a resolution of 120,000 FWHM (at 200 m/z) and a scan range from 350 to 1600 m/z. Precursors were isolated with the isolation window of 1.1 m/z and fragmented with HCD with CE set to 30%. MS2 scans were acquired at a resolution of 30,000 FWHM.

Peptides derived from GFP-pull-down and BioID experiment were resuspended in 0.1% formic acid and analysed using LTQ-Orbitrap Elite Mass Spectrometer fitted with an EASY-nLC 1000 (both Thermo Fisher Scientific). Column parameters were as above. The MS was operated in Top20 DDA mode. MS1 scans were acquired using Orbitrap at a resolution of 120,000 FWHM (at 400 m/z). The 20 most abundant precursors were CID fragmented (CE 35%) and analysed in linear ion trap.

2.11. MS Data Analysis

The acquired raw LFQ data-files (PO4 and GFP/BioID) were processed using Progenesis QI software (v2.0, Nonlinear Dynamics Limited) to extract peptide precursor ion intensities. Results were searched against the human proteome database (UNIPROT) using MASCOT, following criteria:mass tolerance of 10 ppm (precursor) and 0.02 Da (fragments)/0.6 Da (fragments) for orbitrap and for ion trap MS2 data, respectively, full tryptic specificity, 3 missed cleavages allowed, carbamidomethylation (C) set as fixed modification and oxidation (M) set as variable modification.

The TMT raw files were searched against human proteome database (UNIPROT) using SpectroMine software (Biognosys). Standard Pulsar search settings for TMTpro were used. Raw reporters ions intensities were exported for further analysis.

Quantitative analysis results from both label-free and TMT quantification were processed using the SafeQuant R package v. 2.3.2. [25], to obtain peptide relative abundances.

2.12. Statistical Analysis

Values are provided as means ± SEM of the indicated number of experiments comprising each $n \geq 3$ measurement. Statistically significant differences in viability between transfected and control cells were identified by ANOVA followed by Student's *t*-test and Bonferroni correction for multiple comparisons. Statistical analysis was done using OriginPro 2018 software (OriginLab, Northampton, MA, USA). The level of significance: 0.05. Proteomics analysis included adjustment of reporter ion intensities, global data normalization by equalizing the total reporter ion intensity across all channels, summation of reporter ion intensities per protein and channel, calculation of protein abundance ratios, and testing for differential abundance using empirical Bayes moderated t-statistics. Calculated q-values were corrected for multiple testing using the Benjamini−Hochberg method. Proteins with a significantly higher abundance in NS1-wt and NS1-T585E compared to control pulldowns, respectively, ($q < 0.05$) were analyzed with Gene Ontology enRIchment anaLysis and visuaLizAtion (GORILLA) tool [27] (background based analysis, background dataset (from uniprot.org), and target datasets were provided at https://doi.org/10.5281/zenodo.6423418), to identify biological processes and cellular compartments, which are affected based on these proteins. Raw data files and statistical values used for analysis are provided in the repository zenodo.org (https://doi.org/10.5281/zenodo.6423418). Data are also available via ProteomeXchange with identifier PXD036350.

3. Results

3.1. Effect of NS1 Mutations on Cytotoxicity

We mutated seven selected amino acid residues within NS1 whose modification (i.e., phosphorylation or acetylation) was suggested to lead to altered oncotoxicity. Lysine residues 85 and 257, whose acetylation had been suggested to increase their oncotoxic effects were mutated to glutamine to mimic their acetylated state. Serine residues 283 and 473 and threonine residues 403, 405, and 585 were mutated to glutamic acid to mimic their phosphorylated state. Additionally, we constructed a NS1 variant previously found in a H1-PV mutant virus, which is characterized by a 114 nucleotide in-frame deletion of NS1-wt residues 1760 to 1873. NS1-wt responsive Hep3B cells were transfected and their effect on cell viability was assessed using the MTT assay 72 h post-transfection. Transfection efficiency was reproducibly shown to be 54%; SD = 0.98% ($n = 3$) after pTag-GFP transfection. Therefore, viability was corrected by 0.5 to compensate for non-transfected cells. Lysine mutants K85Q and K257Q, as well as serine mutation S473E led to a loss of the cytotoxic effect of NS1 and a cell viability not significantly different to mock transfection ($p > 0.05$). NS1 mutants T403E, T435E and S283E showed a significantly lower cytotoxic effect compared to NS1-wt, but a significantly higher cytotoxic effect compared to mock transfection ($p < 0.05$). The 114nt deletion variant (NS1-del-114) led to no significant difference in cell viability compared to NS1-wt in Hep3B cells ($p > 0.05$). However, the NS1 mutant T585E led to a 30% decrease of cell-viability compared to NS1-wt and 63% decrease of cell viability compared to mock-transfection in Hep3B cells ($p < 0.05$). To confirm that the increased cytotoxic effect of NS1-T585E was due to the mutation of threonine 585 to the phosphor-mimetic glutamic acid, the same residue was mutated to alanine (NS1-T585A), which resulted in a lower oncotoxic effect compared to NS1-wt ($p > 0.05$) (Figure 2A). Of note, neither NS1-wt nor NS1-T585E overexpression led to a decrease in cell viability in NS1 unresponsive control HepG2 cells (Figure 2B) or primary mouse hepatocytes (Supplement Figure S3).

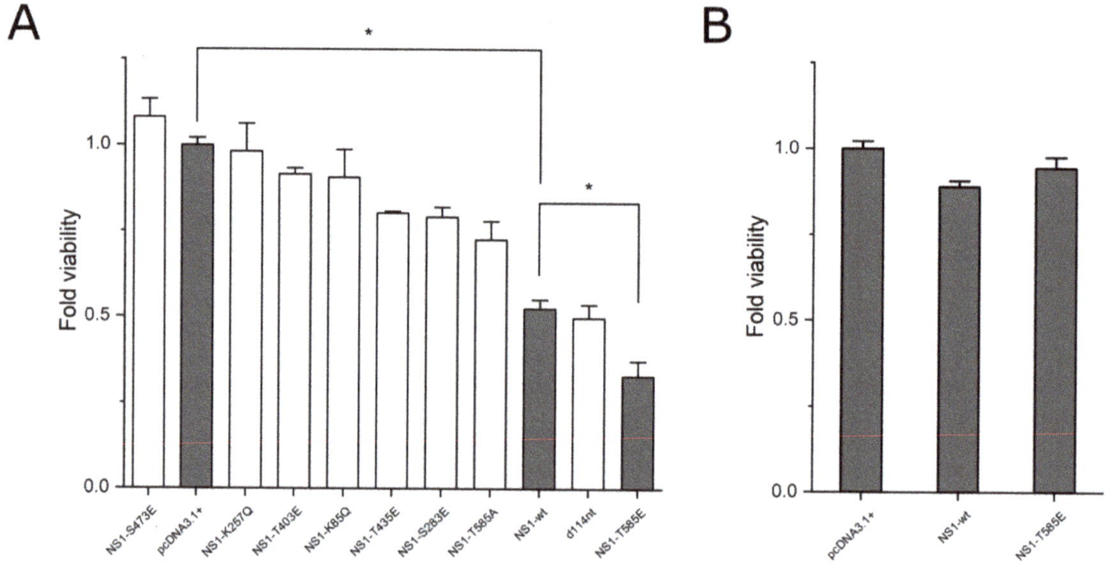

Figure 2. Cell toxicity assays; MTT assays of cells transfected with empty pcDNA3.1+ vector (mock), pcDNA3.1-NS1-wt, or with pcDNA3.1-NS1-mutants. Relative viability was determined 72 h post-transfection and normalized to pcDNA3.1+ (mock) transfection; (**A**) MTT assay using NS1-responsive Hep3B cells; relative viabilities of NS1-wt and NS1-T585E expressing cells are highlighted in grey; (**B**) MTT assay using NS1-unresponsive HepG2 cells (control). Means +/− SEM ($n \geq 5$). *: $p \leq 0.05$. Grey bars: 100% reference, NS1-wt reference, and most potent mutant, respectively.

The increment of mitochondrial reactive oxygen species (ROS) levels within cells after NS1-wt transfection has previously been described [9]. To assess if the elevated cytotoxic effect of NS1-T585E compared to NS1-wt was linked to elevated ROS levels, we transfected NS1-responsive Hep3B cells with either pTag-NS1-wt-GFP, pTag-NS1-T585E-GFP or pTag-GFP-N (control) and compared ROS levels of successfully transfected cells using the MitoSOX assay and FACS analysis. Indeed, Hep3B cells overexpressing NS1-T585E-GFP and NS1-wt-GFP showed a higher ROS level compared to GFP only control cells (Supplement Figure S1). Control experiments with NS1-unresponsive HepG2 cells resulted in no elevated ROS levels (Supplement Figure S2).

3.2. *Proteomics: Effects of NS1-wt and NS1-T585E on the Host-Cell Proteome*

Different proteomic approaches were used to further elucidate and compare the interactions of NS1-wt and mutant NS1-T585E with the host cell proteome, their effects on host-cell protein expression levels, and phosphorylation patterns in NS1-responsive cells. In a first set of experiments, Hep3B cells were transfected with either pcDNA3.1-NS1-wt, pcDNA3.1-NS1-T585E or pcDNA3.1+ (mock transfection). Forty-eight hours post-transfection, the cell proteome was analyzed using mass spectrometry. Three proteins showed a consistently altered expression level across all replicates (q < 0.05) compared to mock transfection in both NS1-wt and NS1-T585E overexpressing cells. NOVA Alternative Splicing Regulator 2 (NOVA2) and

Stearoyl-CoA Desaturase (SCD) were downregulated. Enhanced expression was observed for Small Glutamine Rich Tetratricopeptide Repeat Co-Chaperone Alpha (SGTA) (Figure 3). A list of all differentially regulated genes identified during this study can be found at the repositories zenodo.org (https://doi.org/10.5281/zenodo.6423418) and ProteomeXchange with identifier PXD036350. A volcano plot depicting the changes in the proteome after NS1-wt and NS1-T585E can be found in the supplement (Supplement Figure S4).

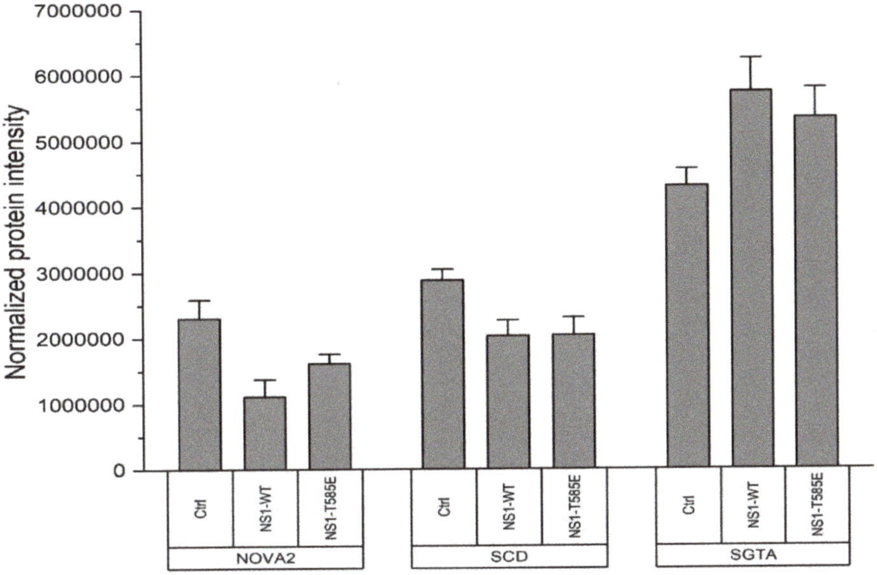

Figure 3. Expression levels of selected proteins after NS1-wt and NS1(T585E) transfection. Hep3B-cells were transfected with pcDNA3.1-NS1-wt, pcDNA3.1-NS1(T585E), or pcDNA3.1+. Normalized protein intensities identified by mass spectrometry for proteins with reproducibly altered expression levels (NOVA2, SDC and SGTA) are shown. Values are means ± SEM, $n = 4$.

3.3. Proteomics: Analysis of Phosphorylation Patterns

Hep3B cells were transfected with either pcDNA3.1-NS1-wt, pcDNA3.1-NS1-T585E or pcDNA3.1+ (mock transfection). Forty-eight hours post transfection, proteins of cell lysates were digested; phosphopeptides were enriched and subsequently quantified by mass spectrometry. NS1-wt overexpression led to a significantly altered ($q < 0.05$) phosphorylation pattern of four proteins: Apoptotic Chromatin Condensation Inducer 1 (ACIN1), Small Glutamine Rich Tetratricopeptide Repeat Co-Chaperone Alpha (SGTA), HIRA Interacting Protein 3 (HIRIP3), and AMMECR Nuclear Protein 1 (AMMECR1).

NS1-T585E overexpression did not lead to any statistically significant differences in phosphorylation patterns compared to mock-plasmid transfection. However, there was a trend towards a higher phosphorylation of ACIN1 at position T254 in cells expressing NS1-T585E. A list of all proteins identified during the phosphor-enrichment experiments can be found at the repositories zenodo.org (https://doi.org/10.5281/zenodo.6423418) and ProteomeXchange with identifier PXD036350. A volcano plot depicting the changes in the phosphorylation patterns after NS1-wt and NS1-T585E can be found in the supplement (Supplement Figure S5).

3.4. Proteomics: Binding of or Close Proximity to NS1

Hep3B-cells were transfected with pTag-NS1-wt-GFP, pTag-NS1-T585E-GFP, or pTag-GFP-N (control-transfection). GFP or NS1-GFP fusion proteins were pulled down with a GFP-Antibody. Subsequently, cellular proteins binding directly or indirectly to NS1 were identified by mass spectrometry. Proteins with a significantly ($q < 0.05$) higher abundance in NS1-wt-GFP and NS1-T585E-GFP compared to GFP-only pulldowns, respectively, were grouped according to selected biological processes and cellular compartments associated with viral infection, stress responses, regulation of gene expression, regulation of the immune system, regulation of the cell cycle, the cytoskeleton, sites of DNA damage, mitochondria, and the ribonucleoprotein complex.

We identified 120 proteins that were significantly enriched using the NS1-wt-GFP approach and 51 using the NS1-T585E-GFP approach. Of these proteins, 16 were significantly enriched in both NS1-wt-GFP and NS1-T585E-GFP pull-downs. The log2 ratios intensities of NS1-wt-GFP/mock or NS1-T585E-GFP/mock of the identified proteins associated with the analyzed biological processes and/or cellular components are shown in Figure 4.

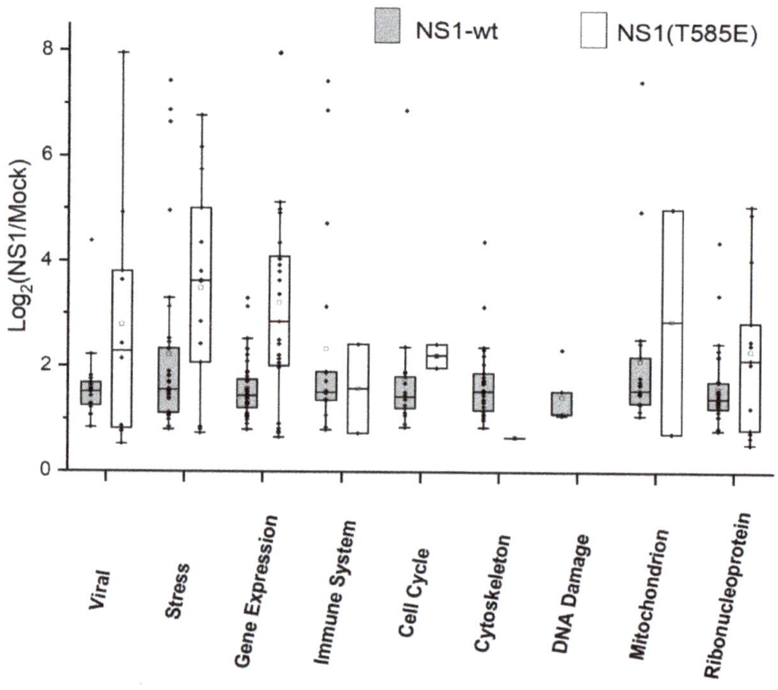

Figure 4. Identification of binding partners of NS1-wt and NS1-T585E by proteomics. Hep3B-cells were transfected with pTag-NS1-wt-GFP, pTag-NS1-T585E-GFP, or pTag-GFP-N. NS1-GFP fusion proteins were pulled down and cellular proteins binding to NS1 were identified by mass spectrometry. Proteins with a significantly higher abundance in NS1-wt-GFP or NS1-T585E-GFP compared to GFP-only pulldown, respectively, are grouped with respect to the indicated biological processes or cellular components. Box plot representation of median, 1st and 3rd quartile, whiskers as quartiles plus 1.5 times the interquartile range (IRQ), and outliers.

In order to identify additional proteins that potentially interact with NS1 or NS1-T585E, we used a proximity-dependent biotinylation technology. Thereby, NS1-wt or NS1-T585E were fused to the N-terminus of the promiscuous biotin ligase BioID2. Hep3B-cells were transfected with pNS1-wt-BioID2-HA, pNS1-T585E-BioID2-HA, or pBioID2-HA (mock transfection). Proteins in close proximity to the biotin ligase and thus to NS1-wt or NS1-T585E were biotinylated, pulled down with streptavidin beads and subsequently identified by mass spectrometry. Proteins with a significantly ($q < 0.05$) higher abundance of NS1-wt-BioID2-HA and NS1-T585E-BioID2-HA compared to GFP-only pulldowns, respectively, were further analyzed using gene ontology enrichment analysis [27] to identify biological processes and cellular compartments, which are associated with the pulled down proteins. As described above, results were grouped. We identified 92 proteins which were significantly enriched using the NS1-wt-BioID2 approach and 267 proteins using the NS1-T585E-BioID2 approach. Results are summarized in Figure 5.

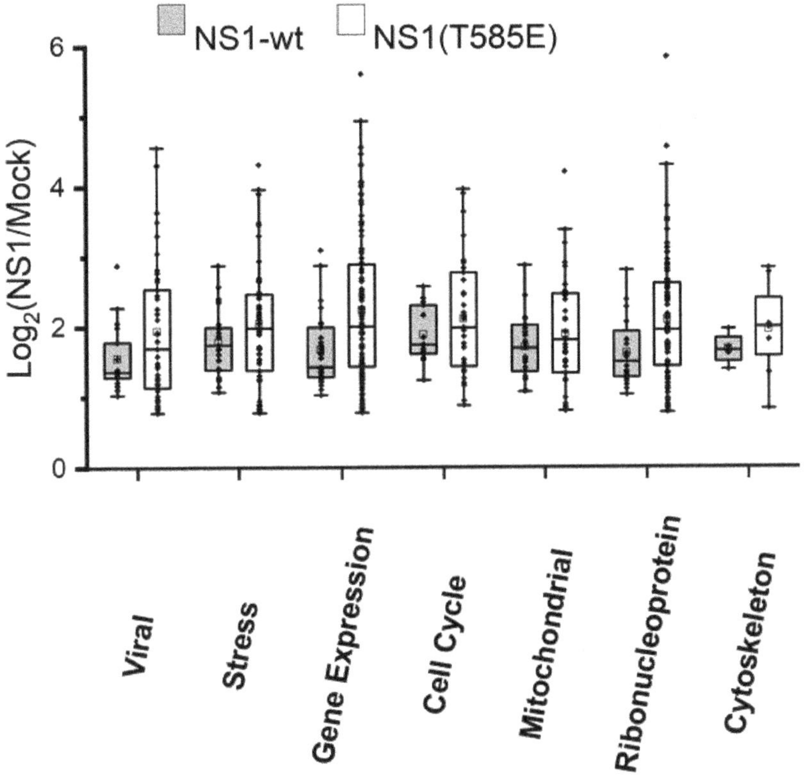

Figure 5. Proteomics-based identification of proteins within close proximity to NS1-wt and NS1-T585E. Hep3B cells were transfected with NS1-wt-BioID2 or NS1-T585E-BioID2 or BioID2 only. Proteins in close proximity and therefore biotinylated by BioID2 were pulled down using streptavidin beads. Proteins identified by mass spectrometry with a significantly higher abundance compared to BioID2-only control are grouped with respect to the indicated biological processes or cellular components. Box plot representation of median, 1st and 3rd quartile, whiskers as quartiles plus 1.5 times the interquartile range (IRQ), and outliers.

Individual proteins identified in both the GFP-trap and the BioID2 approach can be listed as follows: Of the 120 proteins identified in the NS1-wt-GFP pull-down and 92 proteins of the NS1-wt-BioID2 approach, seven proteins were identified by both approaches. These were LIG3, RPL11, HSD17B10, MCM4, RPL9, TUBA1C, and TUBB. Similarly, of the 51 proteins identified in the NS1-T585E-GFP pull-down and 267 proteins of the NS1-T585E-BioID2 approach, 15 proteins were identified by both approaches. These were LIG3, RPL11, BANF1, DDX39A, HIST1H4A, HNRNPU, HSPA9, PRDX1, RBMX, RFC2, RFC4, RNPS1, RPS4X, SRP14, and TRA2B. Of note, only LIG3 and RPL11 were identified in all four experiments. Tubulin seems to be in close proximity to both NS1-wt and NS1-T585E. However, it is only bound to NS1-wt.

4. Discussion

4.1. NS1 Mutant Design

The aim of the present study was to improve the oncotoxic properties of NS1 in view of its potential use in cancer therapy and to study NS1-target cell interactions. We therefore designed eight single amino acid mutants by exchanging NS1 residues, which were previously described as post-translationally modified and thereby as regulating NS1 cancer cell specific NS1 cytotoxicity [13,14,28,29]. Instead of mutating phosphorylation sites (serine or threonine residues) to alanine, as described before [13,14,28,29], we used a phosphomimetic approach, which included the mutation of serine or threonine residues to glutamic acid. The charge and size of the glutamic acid side chain resembles the properties of phosphorylated serine or threonine side chains and may therefore mimic the functional properties of the phosphorylated state of a protein. The validity of this approach to studying the effects of phosphorylated residues on protein functionality has been described in several studies [30–32]. In this study, therefore, we exchanged NS1 residues S283, T403, T435, S473 and T585 with glutamic acid. Acetylation of K85 and K257 has previously been shown to enhance the cytotoxic effect of NS1 [15]. In addition to phosphomimetic mutations, we substituted lysine residues K85 and K257 for glutamine (Q) to simulate an acetylated state of these residues. This acetylation mimicry has also been described previously [33–35]. Last, we introduced a 144nt in-frame deletion to NS1, which has been proposed as leading to an increased viral fitness of H1-PV (i.e., infectivity, viral spread, number of progenitors) in human newborn kidney (NB-324K) cells [18,36].

4.2. Cell Viability Assays

The cytotoxic effect of NS1 is dependent on highly specific host-cell activation and in human cells, therefore, is limited to certain types of cancer cells [3,37]. To investigate if any of the designed mutants has an increased cytotoxic effect in NS1 responding cancer cells, we conducted cell viability assays in NS1 responsive Hep3B hepatocellular carcinoma cells, using unresponsive HepG2 cells as control. NS1 mutant T585E expression led to a 63% lower cell viability compared to the control (mock-transfection) and 30% lower cell-viability as compared to NS1-wt in Hep3B cells. This finding is consistent with the observation that a threonine to alanine mutation of this residue leads to impaired NS1 functionality [13]. It can be concluded that T585 phosphorylation, which occurs at a late stage in the viral life-cycle, is crucial for the cytotoxic functions of NS1 [13]. Indeed, our data confirms a decreased cytotoxicity of NS1-T585A compared to NS1-wt (Figure 2A). The 114nt- deletion in-frame H1-PV mutant, which, it is suggested, leads to an increased viral fitness and an enhanced capability to suppress tumor growth [18,36], showed a cytotoxicity comparable to NS1-wt in our hands. This might indicate that for a beneficial effect of the deletion, an interplay between NS1-d114nt and other viral proteins is needed. The effect of the T585E mutation within the viral genome in regards to the cancer-specific effects of the whole virus should be explored in future studies. Interestingly, all other mutants designed in this study showed, compared to NS1-wt, a decreased cytotoxicity (NS1-S283E and NS1-T435E) or a complete loss of the cytotoxic effect (K85Q, K257Q, T403E, S473E). The impaired functionality of proteins bearing phosphorylation- or acetylation-mimicking mutations might have several reasons. Glutamic acid, for example, does not have the hydration layer and formal charges of phosphate, the mutations might lead to structural alternations of the protein which might affect protein functionality, or phosphor-mimetic mutants might lose a potential ability to act as a kinase [38–40]. Of note, observed cytotoxic effects were paralleled by an increase in reactive oxygen species (ROS). Note that that the mutation of NS1 at residue T585 did not impair its expression. A similar NS1 mutant (S585A) has been introduced into MVMp leading to viruses with reduced toxicity [13]. In addition, NS1-T585E expression was demonstrated by proteomics analysis (see Data at repository (https://doi.org/10.5281/zenodo.6423418)). Analysis of protein expression by proteomics was limited to NS1-T585E because non-active NS1 mutants were of no interest in the present project and were therefore not further investigated.

Importantly, the increased cytotoxic effect of NS1-T585E on NS1-responsive Hep3B cells could not be observed in NS1-unresponsive HepG2 cells or primary mouse hepatocytes, and the associated increase in ROS could also not be observed in HepG2 cells. As described before, NS1-wt is toxic only in certain types of cancers, depending on pathways often activated in transformed cells, whereas other cell types, amongst them untransformed, healthy cells, are unaffected by NS1 cytotoxicity [3]. The same accounts for the whole H1-parvovirus [4,41], which led to the investigation of the virus in phase II clinical studies [8]. It is therefore crucial for any possible application as an anticancer treatment strategy to maintain the specificity of the cytotoxic effect of NS1-mutants. Cytotoxic effects should be limited to certain cancer cell types while non-diseased cells should not be affected [1].

4.3. Induced Changes in the Host-Cell Proteome afterNS1 Expression

A comprehensive study to decipher the interactome of the multifunctional parvoviral non-structural protein NS1 is prone to difficulties, particularly in a cell-free environment. Indeed, to be able to interact directly with several components of a multiprotein-complex, such as the replication machinery or DNA-repair complex, NS1 needs to oligomerize, a process that is dependent on interaction with ATP (or non-hydrolysable ATPs), causing essential conformational alterations [14,28,42]. Therefore, methods to mimic dimerization, such as an N-terminal GST-tag or crosslinking using antibodies [43–45], proved helpful to identify NS1-interaction partners from cellular extracts and to show NS1 interaction with DNA-recognition elements, respectively. Alternatively, proximity-ligation assays could verify the presence of NS1 in the close vicinity of partner proteins in the context of (living) cells.

To get a better understanding on how NS1 exerts its effects on the host cell and why mutant NS1-T585E has an increased effect compared to NS1-wt, we used different proteomic approaches to detect changes in the host cell proteome, including phosphorylation patterns. Furthermore, we identified direct or indirect interaction partners and proteins in close proximity to NS1. On the proteome level, NS1-wt and NS1-T585E expression led to a detectable change of the expression level of only three proteins after 48 h. First, downregulation was observed for NOVA Alternative Splicing Regulator 2 (NOVA2), which is an alternative splicing factor, proposed to also be involved in tumor progression [46]. The extensive involvement of NS1 in the host-cell gene transcription machinery has been previously described [2]. Interestingly, previous work suggests a role for NOVA2, which is upregulated in a variety of cancer cell types, in Wnt signaling. NOVA2 has been proposed to be a positive regulator of β-catenin [47], which, in turn, promotes the expression of a variety of oncogenes, therefore promoting transformation and tumor progression [48]. A downregulation of NOVA2 by NS1 could therefore be a further explanation for the suppression of tumor growth upon NS1 expression. Stearoyl-CoA Desaturase (SCD) is another protein that shows decreased expression levels upon NS1 expression (*wt* and *mutant*). It has been shown that higher SCD levels in cancer cells lead to resistance to ROS induced apoptosis and downregulation of SCD rendered cancer cells that are more sensitive to apoptosis [49]. SCD is overexpressed in different cell lines including liver cancer cell lines such as Hep3B [50].SCD utilizes cytochrome *b*5 electrons and oxygen for fatty acid biosynthesis and is linked to insensitivity to ROS induced apoptosis in certain cancers [50–53]. We speculate that NS1 mediated downregulation of SCD renders Hep3B cells more sensitive to ROS and drug induced apoptosis [49,50], offering an additional explanation of how NS1 exerts its cytotoxic effects. Upregulation was observed for Small Glutamine Rich Tetratricopeptide Repeat Co-Chaperone Alpha (SGTA), which has been previously proposed to interact with and be modified by NS1 of H1-PV [54]. The interaction of NS1 with SGTA is further supported by our observation that SGTA is upregulated upon NS1 (*wt* and *mutant*) expression in Hep3B cells. SGTA has also been shown to be involved in various viral pathways and in protein quality control and localization [55], which is consistent with the extensive involvement of NS1 in the host-cell expression machinery previously described [2].

In the NS1-GFP pull-down experiment, we identified more interaction partners binding to NS1-wt than to the mutant NS1-T585E. This could be explained by a more rigid, less flexible conformation of the mutant NS1-T585E compared to NS1-wt. The latter can adapt its conformation depending on the phosphorylation state of residue T585 and thus interact with a broader variety of proteins. On the other hand, the reduced flexibility of NS1-T585E allows for a more specific and stronger interaction with a given binding partner. It should be noted that the functionality of the NS1-GFP fusion protein was demonstrated and confirmed previously [3].

Because the GFP pull-down reveals only proteins that are tightly associated with NS1, other interaction partners that bind only loosely or in an on/off manner might be lost. Therefore, we used the BioID2 approach to identify proteins in close proximity to NS1-wt or NS1-T585E. Interestingly, in case of the proximity study, not only a larger variety of different proteins but also often a larger ratio of signal intensities of the individual proteins was identified with NS1-T585E compared to NS1-wt. We speculate that the fewer but more stable interactions of NS1-T585E with cellular proteins (as shown in GFP pull-down experiments) facilitate biotinylation of individuals of the same protein in close proximity, thus the higher intensities compared to NS1-*wt*, which has more interaction partners.

We analyzed the proteins identified by the GFP pull-down or the BioID2 approach to determine biological processes that are potentially regulated by NS1-wt and NS-T585E. Amongst the identified biological processes, we focused on biological processes relevant for NS1 activity based on previous publications [2]. This did include viral protein processing biological processes, regulation of gene expression, regulation of the cell cycle, DNA damage repair, stress response, and regulation of the immune system. In addition, proteins were analyzed for their association with cellular compartments, such as the ribonucleoprotein complex, the mitochondrion, and the cytoskeleton.

Surprisingly, analysis of the GFP approach but not the BioID2 approach identified biological processes involved in DNA damage or regulation of the immune system. This might be explained by the C-terminal localization of BioID2 within the NS1-BioID2 fusion protein. The biotinylation radius of BioID2 is restricted to a recommended [56] radius of 20–30 nm. It is therefore possible that certain proteins localized near N-terminal domains might be missed.

As mentioned, NS1-T585E interacts with fewer proteins but seems to bind individuals of one protein more often. Proteins which show a much higher binding-fraction of NS1-T585E/mock compared to NS1-wt/mock include mainly proteins of the gene expression machinery RPL11 (component of the 60S ribosomal subunit), SRSF10 (RNA splicing), and TRA2B (mRNA splicing) as well as cycle progression and DNA replication (namely RFC1 large subunit of the replication factor C), PRIM2 (subunit of DNA primase), and CDK11B (cyclin dependent kinase11)). These findings are in line with the strong involvement of NS1 in the host-cell gene expression machinery and cell cycle progression as described previously. They also support the notion that NS1 mediated disruption of host-cell gene expression and cell cycle arrest partly contributes to the apoptotic effects of NS1 [2,10,57]. Noteworthy is Calmodulin1, which is bound only by NS1-T585E but not by NS1-wt. Calmodulin1 regulates a multitude of physiological processes like cell proliferation, programmed cell death and autophagy and has a major impact on the regulation of several specific cell cycle phases. It is also involved in processes required for tumor progression such as growth, tumor-associated angiogenesis and metastasis [58]. Another interesting protein is Apoptotic Chromatin Condensation Inducer 1 (ACIN1) which is about 7.4 times more abundant in the NS1-T585E-GFP compared to the NS1-wt-GFP pulldown and which also shows a different phosphorylation pattern after both NS1-wt and NS1-T585E expression (see section below). Taken together, these findings may provide an explanation for the stronger cytotoxic effect of NS1-T585E.

4.4. Impact of NS1 on Phosphorylation Patterns

NS1-wt overexpression led to a significantly altered phosphorylation pattern of four proteins: Apoptotic Chromatin Condensation Inducer 1 (ACIN1) is known to induce apoptotic chromatin condensation after activation by caspase-3 [59]. Residue T254 of ACIN1 showed a higher phosphorylation after NS1-T585E and NS1-wt expression compared to mock transfection. This indicates a difference in ACIN1 regulation upon both, NS1-T585E and NS1-wt expression. The lower phosphorylation of residue T254 after NS1-T585E compared to NS1-wt expression might indicate a difference in the regulation of ACIN1. However, as phosphorylation of target proteins can be a highly dynamic process, which may lead to a variety of effects as gain and loss of functions, no conclusion about what exactly the outcome of this difference is can be drawn [38]. ACIN1 is about 7.4 times more abundant in the NS1-T585E-GFP compared to the NS1-wt-GFP pull-down. The protein is activated by caspase 3 upon which it induces apoptotic chromatin condensation [59]. Caspase 3 activation upon NS1-wt expression has previously been described [9]. The direct interaction of NS1-T585E and ACIN1 which is much more pronounced than the interaction of NS1-wt and ACIN1, together with the altered ACIN1 phosphorylation pattern upon NS1 (*wt* and *mutant*) expression might lead to an explanation on how NS1-T585E leads to a much stronger cytotoxic effect.

Phosphorylation of Small Glutamine Rich Tetratricopeptide Repeat Co-Chaperone Alpha (SGTA) is in line with the observed upregulation upon NS1 overexpression and the previously described association with NS1-wt [54].

HIRA Interacting Protein 3 (HIRIP3) is suggested to play a role in histone and chromatin metabolism [60]. HIRIP3 has been proposed as a substrate of CK2 [60]. Interference of NS1 with CK2 signaling has been shown to be important for the cytopathic effects of NS1 [44]. HIRIP3 has also been proposed to be involved in chromatin metabolism and to be dephosphorylated and excluded from the nucleus during chromatin condensation. This could be another indication of an NS1 induced phosphorylation and activation of ACIN1 [61].

The function of AMMECR Nuclear Protein 1 (AMMECR1) has been shown to inhibit apoptosis and to promote cell cycle progression in cancer cells [62]. Its regulation by NS1 could also be linked to the apoptotic effects and cell cycle arrest upon NS1 expression in cancer cells.

We believe that phosphorylations are necessary to expose interfaces for interactions with cell proteins. However, additional features such as the subcellular distribution of the viral protein into microdomains in the cytoplasm are crucial to bring the effector to the target. This is very well controlled upon virus infection rearranging, for instance, the cytoskeleton and in consequence membrane structure [63].

Interestingly, we could show that NS1-wt directly or indirectly binds alpha and beta tubulins. Phosphorylation of tubulins in cells after NS1-expression has been described and a link to cytoskeleton disruption has been proposed [63]. In the case of NS1-T585E, however, close proximity, but not direct or indirect binding to tubulins could be demonstrated.

4.5. Additional NS1 Interaction Partners and Pathways

In the present work, NS1 interaction partners were identified and discussed based on statistical evaluation of proteomics data. They were selected according to two criteria: First, statistical relevance, i.e., a q value of ≤ 0.05 compared to mock transfected control cells. Second, statistical association with a relevant biological process. It should be noted, however, that purely statistical criteria might fail to identify important NS1 partners or biological processes. Subtle upstream modulation of signaling pathways, for example, can have a profound impact on downstream biological processes. Based on literature data, we have therefore reanalyzed the available dataset and manually selected proteins of interest.

Focusing on pathways, identified to contribute to successful infection, progeny particle production and spreading, we found a number of these cell proteins being connected to NS1 after transfection of Hep3B cells. For viral DNA amplification, a reconstituted in-vitro replication system identified, besides polymerase, RPA, RFC, PCNA being essential to drive leading strand synthesis driven by NS1's helicase activity [64]. In addition to these basic replication factors, other NS1-interaction partners identified here, were shown to accumulate in PV-induced replication (APAR-) bodies and others functioning in the DNA-damage response/repair (H2AFY/MCM4) and cell cycle control (cdk11B), processes that were described to contribute to efficient DNA replication and progeny particle production [57,65,66]. Besides strongly validating our results, these findings lead us to suggest that additional interaction partners might provide new insights into the functioning of additional parvoviral mechanisms, such as efficient mRNA processing/splicing regulation for which additional candidates to hnRNPs were identified [67]. Together with the finding of tRNA ligases, potentially facilitating an amber-read-through to generate the proposed non-structural protein NS3, this might enable us to pinpoint the potential functioning of splicing regulation for the generation of viral proteins, particularly in the presence of an innate immune-response (interaction with translation initiation factors).

Interestingly, besides expected NS1-interactions facilitating progeny particle production, there are a number of cellular factors that could serve therapeutic applications using this viral protein as an oncotoxin. Besides factors involved in regulated death-pathways (i.e., interference with the energy metabolism, apoptosis and autophagy) there are more (parvo)viral specific pathways leading to cell disturbances and release of intracellular components modulating cytoskeleton dynamics and exocytosis. The latter is of particular interest, since these factors are indicative for the potential NS1-induced release of DAMPs and PAMPs, in order to induce an anti-tumor immune-response. In addition to chaperones, which were shown to play a significant role for the induction of anti-tumor immune responses, we identified a number of TAAs interacting with NS1 (i.e., TPT1, NUMA1, SPRYD4, SND1, and GNL3). If such polypeptides are released together with NS1, this might significantly contribute to a potential therapy. Indeed, during a first clinical trial using parvovirus H-1PV, immune-activation could be confirmed, including a response against the non-structural protein NS1 [19].

5. Conclusions

Our findings provide an insight into the manifold, multimodal interplay of the NS1 protein and the proteome of NS1-sensitive cancer cells. These findings are instrumental to better understand the tumor-cell specificity and mode of action of NS1. The increased cytotoxic effect of NS1-T585E in NS1-wt-responsive cells, but not in NS1-wt-unresponsive cells, makes NS1-T585E an interesting candidate for the design of safe and efficient NS1-based cancer treatment strategies. The insights on H1-PV—host-cell interactions on a molecular level, provided by this work, will pave the way for further experiments including the development of novel treatment strategies. Such therapeutic approaches might be a combination of viral vector-mediated high-efficiency transduction, stimulation of death pathways, and anti-tumor immune stimulation. Proof-of-concept studies will be carried out using in vivo xenograft murine tumor models.

Supplementary Materials: The following supporting information can be downloaded at: https://www.mdpi.com/article/10.3390/v15010209/s1, Table S1: List of PCR primers, Figure S1: Determination of reactive oxygen species (ROS) production, Figure S2: Determination of reactive oxygen species (ROS) production, Figure S3: Viability of transfected primary mouse hepatocytes, Figure S4: Volcano plot depicting the changes in the proteome after NS1-wt and NS1-T585E expression, Figure S5: Volcano plot depicting the changes of protein phosphorylation after NS1-wt and NS1-T585E expression.

Author Contributions: P.H. contributed to all experiments and writing of the manuscript. P.G. contributed to the BioID proximity assays. K.B. contributed to the proteomics assays (mass spectrometry and data analysis). R.V.M. contributed to the MitoSOX ROS assays (FACS). J.P.F.N. contributed to the proteomics data interpretation and writing of the manuscript. S.H.S. contributed to the experiments and writing of the manuscript. J.H. contributed to the conceptual experimental design and the writing of the manuscript. All authors have read and agreed to the published version of the manuscript.

Funding: This research received no external funding.

Institutional Review Board Statement: Not applicable.

Informed Consent Statement: Not applicable.

Data Availability Statement: Data generated or analysed during this study can be found within the published article and its Supplementary Files. All raw data files and statistical values used for analysis are provided in the repository zenodo.org (https://doi.org/10.5281/zenodo.6423418, accessed on 7 April 2022). Proteomics data are also available via ProteomeXchange with identifier PXD036350.

Acknowledgments: We thank Noëmi Roos and Jens Casper for technical advice, helpful discussions, and for providing primary mouse hepatocytes.

Conflicts of Interest: The authors declare no conflict of interest.

References

1. Lezhnin, Y.N.; Kravchenko, Y.E.; Frolova, E.I.; Chumakov, P.M.; Chumakov, S.P. Oncotoxic Proteins in Cancer Therapy: Mechanisms of Action. *Mol. Biol.* **2015**, *49*, 231–243. [CrossRef]
2. Nüesch, J.P.F.; Lacroix, J.; Marchini, A.; Rommelaere, J. Molecular Pathways: Rodent Parvoviruses—Mechanisms of Oncolysis and Prospects for Clinical Cancer Treatment. *Clin. Cancer Res.* **2012**, *18*, 3516–3523. [CrossRef]
3. Witzigmann, D.; Grossen, P.; Quintavalle, C.; Lanzafame, M.; Schenk, S.H.; Tran, X.-T.; Englinger, B.; Hauswirth, P.; Grünig, D.; van Schoonhoven, S.; et al. Non-Viral Gene Delivery of the Oncotoxic Protein NS1 for Treatment of Hepatocellular Carcinoma. *J. Control. Release* **2021**, *334*, 138–152. [CrossRef]
4. Bretscher, C.; Marchini, A. H-1 Parvovirus as a Cancer-Killing Agent: Past, Present, and Future. *Viruses* **2019**, *11*, 562. [CrossRef]
5. Marchini, A.; Bonifati, S.; Scott, E.M.; Angelova, A.L.; Rommelaere, J. Oncolytic Parvoviruses: From Basic Virology to Clinical Applications. *Virol. J.* **2015**, *12*, 6. [CrossRef]
6. Kaufman, H.L.; Kohlhapp, F.J.; Zloza, A. Oncolytic Viruses: A New Class of Immunotherapy Drugs. *Nat. Rev. Drug Discov.* **2015**, *14*, 642–662. [CrossRef]
7. Rommelaere, J.; Geletneky, K.; Angelova, A.L.; Daeffler, L.; Dinsart, C.; Kiprianova, I.; Schlehofer, J.R.; Raykov, Z. Oncolytic Parvoviruses as Cancer Therapeutics. *Cytokine Growth Factor Rev.* **2010**, *21*, 185–195. [CrossRef]
8. Oryx GmbH & Co. KG. *Phase I/IIa Study of Intratumoral/Intracerebral or Intravenous/Intracerebral Administration of Parvovirus H-1 (ParvOryx) in Patients with Progressive Primary or Recurrent Glioblastoma Multiforme*; Oryx GmbH & Co. KG: Vaterstetten, Germany, 2015.
9. Hristov, G.; Krämer, M.; Li, J.; El-Andaloussi, N.; Mora, R.; Daeffler, L.; Zentgraf, H.; Rommelaere, J.; Marchini, A. Through Its Nonstructural Protein NS1, Parvovirus H-1 Induces Apoptosis via Accumulation of Reactive Oxygen Species. *J. Virol.* **2010**, *84*, 5909–5922. [CrossRef]
10. Nüesch, J.P.F.; Rommelaere, J. Tumor Suppressing Properties of Rodent Parvovirus NS1 Proteins and Their Derivatives. In *Anticancer Genes*; Advances in Experimental Medicine and Biology; Grimm, S., Ed.; Springer: London, UK, 2014; pp. 99–124. ISBN 978-1-4471-6458-6.
11. Kaiser, J. How Safe Is a Popular Gene Therapy Vector? *Science* **2020**, *367*, 131. [CrossRef]
12. Chira, S.; Jackson, C.S.; Oprea, I.; Ozturk, F.; Pepper, M.S.; Diaconu, I.; Braicu, C.; Raduly, L.-Z.; Calin, G.A.; Berindan-Neagoe, I. Progresses towards Safe and Efficient Gene Therapy Vectors. *Oncotarget* **2015**, *6*, 30675–30703. [CrossRef]
13. Daeffler, L.; Hörlein, R.; Rommelaere, J.; Nüesch, J.P.F. Modulation of Minute Virus of Mice Cytotoxic Activities through Site-Directed Mutagenesis within the NS Coding Region. *J. Virol.* **2003**, *77*, 12466–12478. [CrossRef]
14. Corbau, R.; Duverger, V.; Rommelaere, J.; Nüesch, J.P.F. Regulation of MVM NS1 by Protein Kinase C: Impact of Mutagenesis at Consensus Phosphorylation Sites on Replicative Functions and Cytopathic Effects. *Virology* **2000**, *278*, 151–167. [CrossRef] [PubMed]
15. Li, J.; Bonifati, S.; Hristov, G.; Marttila, T.; Valmary-Degano, S.; Stanzel, S.; Schnölzer, M.; Mougin, C.; Aprahamian, M.; Grekova, S.P.; et al. Synergistic Combination of Valproic Acid and Oncolytic Parvovirus H-1PV as a Potential Therapy against Cervical and Pancreatic Carcinomas. *EMBO Mol. Med.* **2013**, *5*, 1537–1555. [CrossRef] [PubMed]
16. Chen, Z.; Cole, P.A. Synthetic Approaches to Protein Phosphorylation. *Curr. Opin. Chem. Biol.* **2015**, *28*, 115–122. [CrossRef] [PubMed]
17. He, M.; Zhang, L.; Wang, X.; Huo, L.; Sun, L.; Feng, C.; Jing, X.; Du, D.; Liang, H.; Liu, M.; et al. Systematic Analysis of the Functions of Lysine Acetylation in the Regulation of Tat Activity. *PLoS ONE* **2013**, *8*, e67186. [CrossRef] [PubMed]
18. Weiss, N.; Stroh-Dege, A.; Rommelaere, J.; Dinsart, C.; Salomé, N. An In-Frame Deletion in the NS Protein-Coding Sequence of Parvovirus H-1PV Efficiently Stimulates Export and Infectivity of Progeny Virions. *J. Virol.* **2012**, *86*, 7554–7564. [CrossRef] [PubMed]
19. Geletneky, K.; Hajda, J.; Angelova, A.L.; Leuchs, B.; Capper, D.; Bartsch, A.J.; Neumann, J.-O.; Schöning, T.; Hüsing, J.; Beelte, B.; et al. Oncolytic H-1 Parvovirus Shows Safety and Signs of Immunogenic Activity in a First Phase I/IIa Glioblastoma Trial. *Mol. Ther.* **2017**, *25*, 2620–2634. [CrossRef]
20. Bär, S.; Rommelaere, J.; Nüesch, J.P.F. Vesicular Transport of Progeny Parvovirus Particles through ER and Golgi Regulates Maturation and Cytolysis. *PLoS Pathog.* **2013**, *9*, e1003605. [CrossRef]

21. Daeffler, L.; Nüesch, J.; Rommelaere, J. Zusammensetzung einer Parvovirus VP1-Proteinvariante und eines arvovirus NS1-Proteins zur Induktion von Zytolyse. 2003.
22. Kerr, J.; Cotmore, S.; Bloom, M.E. *Parvoviruses*; CRC Press: Boca Raton, FL, USA, 2005; ISBN 978-1-4441-1478-2. Available online: https://patents.google.com/patent/DE60124523T2/de (accessed on 9 January 2023).
23. Kiene, K.; Schenk, S.H.; Porta, F.; Ernst, A.; Witzigmann, D.; Grossen, P.; Huwyler, J. PDMS-b-PMOXA Polymersomes for Hepatocyte Targeting and Assessment of Toxicity. *Eur. J. Pharm. Biopharm.* **2017**, *119*, 322–332. [CrossRef]
24. Post, H.; Penning, R.; Fitzpatrick, M.A.; Garrigues, L.B.; Wu, W.; MacGillavry, H.D.; Hoogenraad, C.C.; Heck, A.J.R.; Altelaar, A.F.M. Robust, Sensitive, and Automated Phosphopeptide Enrichment Optimized for Low Sample Amounts Applied to Primary Hippocampal Neurons. *J. Proteome Res.* **2017**, *16*, 728–737. [CrossRef]
25. Ahrné, E.; Glatter, T.; Viganò, C.; von Schubert, C.; Nigg, E.A.; Schmidt, A. Evaluation and Improvement of Quantification Accuracy in Isobaric Mass Tag-Based Protein Quantification Experiments. *J. Proteome Res.* **2016**, *15*, 2537–2547. [CrossRef] [PubMed]
26. Kim, D.I.; Jensen, S.C.; Noble, K.A.; Kc, B.; Roux, K.H.; Motamedchaboki, K.; Roux, K.J. An Improved Smaller Biotin Ligase for BioID Proximity Labeling. *Mol. Biol. Cell* **2016**, *27*, 1188–1196. [CrossRef]
27. Eden, E.; Navon, R.; Steinfeld, I.; Lipson, D.; Yakhini, Z. GOrilla: A Tool for Discovery and Visualization of Enriched GO Terms in Ranked Gene Lists. *BMC Bioinform.* **2009**, *10*, 48. [CrossRef] [PubMed]
28. Nüesch, J.P.; Christensen, J.; Rommelaere, J. Initiation of Minute Virus of Mice DNA Replication Is Regulated at the Level of Origin Unwinding by Atypical Protein Kinase C Phosphorylation of NS1. *J. Virol.* **2001**, *75*, 5730–5739. [CrossRef]
29. Nüesch, J.P.F.; Lachmann, S.; Corbau, R.; Rommelaere, J. Regulation of Minute Virus of Mice NS1 Replicative Functions by Atypical PKCλ In Vivo. *J. Virol.* **2003**, *77*, 433–442. [CrossRef] [PubMed]
30. Guerra-Castellano, A.; Díaz-Moreno, I.; Velázquez-Campoy, A.; De la Rosa, M.A.; Díaz-Quintana, A. Structural and Functional Characterization of Phosphomimetic Mutants of Cytochrome c at Threonine 28 and Serine 47. *Biochim. Biophys. Acta* **2016**, *1857*, 387–395. [CrossRef] [PubMed]
31. Luwang, J.W.; Natesh, R. Phosphomimetic Mutation Destabilizes the Central Core Domain of Human P53. *IUBMB Life* **2018**, *70*, 1023–1031. [CrossRef] [PubMed]
32. Pecina, P.; Borisenko, G.G.; Belikova, N.A.; Tyurina, Y.Y.; Pecinova, A.; Lee, I.; Samhan-Arias, A.K.; Przyklenk, K.; Kagan, V.E.; Hüttemann, M. Phosphomimetic Substitution of Cytochrome C Tyrosine 48 Decreases Respiration and Binding to Cardiolipin and Abolishes Ability to Trigger Downstream Caspase Activation. *Biochemistry* **2010**, *49*, 6705–6714. [CrossRef] [PubMed]
33. Gorsky, M.K.; Burnouf, S.; Dols, J.; Mandelkow, E.; Partridge, L. Acetylation Mimic of Lysine 280 Exacerbates Human Tau Neurotoxicity in Vivo. *Sci. Rep.* **2016**, *6*, 22685. [CrossRef]
34. Wang, X.; Hayes, J.J. Acetylation Mimics within Individual Core Histone Tail Domains Indicate Distinct Roles in Regulating the Stability of Higher-Order Chromatin Structure. *Mol. Cell. Biol.* **2008**, *28*, 227–236. [CrossRef]
35. Kamieniarz, K.; Schneider, R. Tools to Tackle Protein Acetylation. *Chem. Biol.* **2009**, *16*, 1027–1029. [CrossRef]
36. Hashemi, H.; Condurat, A.-L.; Stroh-Dege, A.; Weiss, N.; Geiss, C.; Pilet, J.; Cornet Bartolomé, C.; Rommelaere, J.; Salomé, N.; Dinsart, C. Mutations in the Non-Structural Protein-Coding Sequence of Protoparvovirus H-1PV Enhance the Fitness of the Virus and Show Key Benefits Regarding the Transduction Efficiency of Derived Vectors. *Viruses* **2018**, *10*, 150. [CrossRef]
37. Moehler, M.; Blechacz, B.; Weiskopf, N.; Zeidler, M.; Stremmel, W.; Rommelaere, J.; Galle, P.R.; Cornelis, J.J. Effective Infection, Apoptotic Cell Killing and Gene Transfer of Human Hepatoma Cells but Not Primary Hepatocytes by Parvovirus H1 and Derived Vectors. *Cancer Gene Ther.* **2001**, *8*, 158–167. [CrossRef]
38. Hunter, T. Why Nature Chose Phosphate to Modify Proteins. *Philos. Trans. R. Soc. B Biol. Sci.* **2012**, *367*, 2513–2516. [CrossRef]
39. Pérez-Mejías, G.; Velázquez-Cruz, A.; Guerra-Castellano, A.; Baños-Jaime, B.; Díaz-Quintana, A.; González-Arzola, K.; Ángel De la Rosa, M.; Díaz-Moreno, I. Exploring Protein Phosphorylation by Combining Computational Approaches and Biochemical Methods. *Comput. Struct. Biotechnol. J.* **2020**, *18*, 1852–1863. [CrossRef]
40. Huang, W.; Erikson, R.L. Constitutive Activation of Mek1 by Mutation of Serine Phosphorylation Sites. *Proc. Natl. Acad. Sci. USA* **1994**, *91*, 8960–8963. [CrossRef]
41. Lacroix, J.; Leuchs, B.; Li, J.; Hristov, G.; Deubzer, H.E.; Kulozik, A.E.; Rommelaere, J.; Schlehofer, J.R.; Witt, O. Parvovirus H1 Selectively Induces Cytotoxic Effects on Human Neuroblastoma Cells. *Int. J. Cancer* **2010**, *127*, 1230–1239. [CrossRef]
42. Nüesch, J.P.; Tattersall, P. Nuclear Targeting of the Parvoviral Replicator Molecule NS1: Evidence for Self-Association Prior to Nuclear Transport. *Virology* **1993**, *196*, 637–651. [CrossRef]
43. Nüesch, J.P.; Corbau, R.; Tattersall, P.; Rommelaere, J. Biochemical Activities of Minute Virus of Mice Nonstructural Protein NS1 Are Modulated In Vitro by the Phosphorylation State of the Polypeptide. *J. Virol.* **1998**, *72*, 8002–8012. [CrossRef]
44. Nüesch, J.P.F.; Rommelaere, J. NS1 Interaction with CKIIα: Novel Protein Complex Mediating Parvovirus-Induced Cytotoxicity. *J. Virol.* **2006**, *80*, 4729–4739. [CrossRef]
45. Nüesch, J.P.F.; Rommelaere, J. A Viral Adaptor Protein Modulating Casein Kinase II Activity Induces Cytopathic Effects in Permissive Cells. *Proc. Natl. Acad. Sci. USA* **2007**, *104*, 12482–12487. [CrossRef]
46. Gallo, S.; Arcidiacono, M.V.; Tisato, V.; Piva, R.; Penolazzi, L.; Bosi, C.; Feo, C.V.; Gafà, R.; Secchiero, P. Upregulation of the Alternative Splicing Factor NOVA2 in Colorectal Cancer Vasculature. *Onco Targets Ther.* **2018**, *11*, 6049–6056. [CrossRef]
47. Tang, S.; Zhao, Y.; He, X.; Zhu, J.; Chen, S.; Wen, J.; Deng, Y. Identification of NOVA Family Proteins as Novel β-Catenin RNA-Binding Proteins That Promote Epithelial-Mesenchymal Transition. *RNA Biol.* **2020**, *17*, 881–891. [CrossRef]

48. Shang, S.; Hua, F.; Hu, Z.-W. The Regulation of β-Catenin Activity and Function in Cancer: Therapeutic Opportunities. *Oncotarget* **2017**, *8*, 33972–33989. [CrossRef]
49. Luis, G.; Godfroid, A.; Nishiumi, S.; Cimino, J.; Blacher, S.; Maquoi, E.; Wery, C.; Collignon, A.; Longuespée, R.; Montero-Ruiz, L.; et al. Tumor Resistance to Ferroptosis Driven by Stearoyl-CoA Desaturase-1 (SCD1) in Cancer Cells and Fatty Acid Biding Protein-4 (FABP4) in Tumor Microenvironment Promote Tumor Recurrence. *Redox Biol.* **2021**, *43*, 102006. [CrossRef]
50. Bansal, S.; Berk, M.; Alkhouri, N.; Partrick, D.A.; Fung, J.J.; Feldstein, A. Stearoyl-CoA Desaturase Plays an Important Role in Proliferation and Chemoresistance in Human Hepatocellular Carcinoma. *J. Surg. Res.* **2014**, *186*, 29–38. [CrossRef]
51. Paton, C.M.; Ntambi, J.M. Biochemical and Physiological Function of Stearoyl-CoA Desaturase. *Am. J. Physiol. Endocrinol. Metab.* **2009**, *297*, E28–E37. [CrossRef]
52. Hardy, S.; Langelier, Y.; Prentki, M. Oleate Activates Phosphatidylinositol 3-Kinase and Promotes Proliferation and Reduces Apoptosis of MDA-MB-231 Breast Cancer Cells, Whereas Palmitate Has Opposite Effects. *Cancer Res.* **2000**, *60*, 6353–6358.
53. Chen, L.; Ren, J.; Yang, L.; Li, Y.; Fu, J.; Li, Y.; Tian, Y.; Qiu, F.; Liu, Z.; Qiu, Y. Stearoyl-CoA Desaturase-1 Mediated Cell Apoptosis in Colorectal Cancer by Promoting Ceramide Synthesis. *Sci. Rep.* **2016**, *6*, 19665. [CrossRef]
54. Cziepluch, C.; Kordes, E.; Poirey, R.; Grewenig, A.; Rommelaere, J.; Jauniaux, J.-C. Identification of a Novel Cellular TPR-Containing Protein, SGT, That Interacts with the Nonstructural Protein NS1 of Parvovirus H-1. *J. Virol.* **1998**, *72*, 4149–4156. [CrossRef]
55. Roberts, J.D.; Thapaliya, A.; Martínez-Lumbreras, S.; Krysztofinska, E.M.; Isaacson, R.L. Structural and Functional Insights into Small, Glutamine-Rich, Tetratricopeptide Repeat Protein Alpha. *Front. Mol. Biosci.* **2015**, *2*, 71. [CrossRef]
56. Kim, D.I.; KC, B.; Zhu, W.; Motamedchaboki, K.; Doye, V.; Roux, K.J. Probing Nuclear Pore Complex Architecture with Proximity-Dependent Biotinylation. *Proc. Natl. Acad. Sci. USA* **2014**, *111*, E2453–E2461. [CrossRef]
57. Op De Beeck, A.; Sobczak-Thepot, J.; Sirma, H.; Bourgain, F.; Brechot, C.; Caillet-Fauquet, P. NS1- and Minute Virus of Mice-Induced Cell Cycle Arrest: Involvement of P53 and P21cip1. *J. Virol.* **2001**, *75*, 11071–11078. [CrossRef]
58. Berchtold, M.W.; Villalobo, A. The Many Faces of Calmodulin in Cell Proliferation, Programmed Cell Death, Autophagy, and Cancer. *Biochim. Biophys. Acta (BBA)-Mol. Cell Res.* **2014**, *1843*, 398–435. [CrossRef]
59. Sahara, S.; Aoto, M.; Eguchi, Y.; Imamoto, N.; Yoneda, Y.; Tsujimoto, Y. Acinus Is a Caspase-3-Activated Protein Required for Apoptotic Chromatin Condensation. *Nature* **1999**, *401*, 168–173. [CrossRef]
60. Lorain, S.; Quivy, J.-P.; Monier-Gavelle, F.; Scamps, C.; Lécluse, Y.; Almouzni, G.; Lipinski, M. Core Histones and HIRIP3, a Novel Histone-Binding Protein, Directly Interact with WD Repeat Protein HIRA. *Mol Cell Biol* **1998**, *18*, 5546–5556. [CrossRef]
61. Assrir, N.; Filhol, O.; Galisson, F.; Lipinski, M. HIRIP3 Is a Nuclear Phosphoprotein Interacting with and Phosphorylated by the Serine-Threonine Kinase CK2. *Biol. Chem.* **2007**, *388*, 391–398. [CrossRef]
62. Ge, H.; Cheng, N.; Xu, X.; Yang, Z.; Hoffman, R.M.; Zhu, J. AMMECR1 Inhibits Apoptosis and Promotes Cell-Cycle Progression and Proliferation of the A549 Human Lung Cancer Cell Line. *Anticancer Res.* **2019**, *39*, 4637–4642. [CrossRef]
63. Nüesch, J.P.F.; Lachmann, S.; Rommelaere, J. Selective Alterations of the Host Cell Architecture upon Infection with Parvovirus Minute Virus of Mice. *Virology* **2005**, *331*, 159–174. [CrossRef]
64. Christensen, J.; Tattersall, P. Parvovirus Initiator Protein NS1 and RPA Coordinate Replication Fork Progression in a Reconstituted DNA Replication System. *J. Virol.* **2002**, *76*, 6518–6531. [CrossRef]
65. Bashir, T.; Rommelaere, J.; Cziepluch, C. In Vivo Accumulation of Cyclin A and Cellular Replication Factors in Autonomous Parvovirus Minute Virus of Mice-Associated Replication Bodies. *J. Virol.* **2001**, *75*, 4394–4398. [CrossRef]
66. Adeyemi, R.O.; Landry, S.; Davis, M.E.; Weitzman, M.D.; Pintel, D.J. Parvovirus Minute Virus of Mice Induces a DNA Damage Response That Facilitates Viral Replication. *PLoS Pathog.* **2010**, *6*, e1001141. [CrossRef]
67. Harris, C.E.; Boden, R.A.; Astell, C.R. A Novel Heterogeneous Nuclear Ribonucleoprotein-Like Protein Interacts with NS1 of the Minute Virus of Mice. *J. Virol.* **1999**, *73*, 72–80. [CrossRef]

viruses

MDPI

Article

The Autonomous Parvovirus Minute Virus of Mice Localizes to Cellular Sites of DNA Damage Using ATR Signaling

Clairine I. S. Larsen [1,2,3] and Kinjal Majumder [1,2,3,4,*]

1 Institute for Molecular Virology, University of Wisconsin-Madison, Madison, WI 53706, USA; cilarsen@wisc.edu
2 Cellular and Molecular Biology Graduate Program, University of Wisconsin-Madison, Madison, WI 53706, USA
3 McArdle Laboratory for Cancer Research, University of Wisconsin School of Medicine and Public Health, Madison, WI 53706, USA
4 University of Wisconsin Carbone Cancer Center, University of Wisconsin School of Medicine and Public Health, Madison, WI 53706, USA
* Correspondence: kmajumder@wisc.edu; Tel.: +1-608-890-4888

Abstract: Minute Virus of Mice (MVM) is an autonomous parvovirus of the *Parvoviridae* family that replicates in mouse cells and transformed human cells. MVM genomes localize to cellular sites of DNA damage with the help of their essential non-structural phosphoprotein NS1 to establish viral replication centers. MVM replication induces a cellular DNA damage response that is mediated by signaling through the ATM kinase pathway, while inhibiting induction of the ATR kinase signaling pathway. However, the cellular signals regulating virus localization to cellular DNA damage response sites has remained unknown. Using chemical inhibitors to DNA damage response proteins, we have discovered that NS1 localization to cellular DDR sites is independent of ATM or DNA-PK signaling but is dependent on ATR signaling. Pulsing cells with an ATR inhibitor after S-phase entry leads to attenuated MVM replication. These observations suggest that the initial localization of MVM to cellular DDR sites depends on ATR signaling before it is inactivated by vigorous virus replication.

Keywords: parvoviruses; DNA damage response; Minute Virus of Mice

Citation: Larsen, C.I.S.; Majumder, K. The Autonomous Parvovirus Minute Virus of Mice Localizes to Cellular Sites of DNA Damage Using ATR Signaling. *Viruses* **2023**, *15*, 1243. https://doi.org/10.3390/v15061243

Academic Editor: Giorgio Gallinella

Received: 31 March 2023
Revised: 19 May 2023
Accepted: 23 May 2023
Published: 25 May 2023

1. Introduction

The autonomous parvovirus Minute Virus of Mice (MVM) is lytic in murine hosts and in transformed human cells [1]. The viral genome is single-stranded with inverted terminal repeats (ITRs) at either end that serve as packaging signals and as origins of replication [2]. MVM expresses two non-structural proteins, NS1 and NS2. While NS1 is essential for virus replication, NS2 is required only in murine hosts [3–8]. MVM depends on host cell cycle entry into S-phase to initiate viral replication, utilizing host DNA polymerase delta and alpha to amplify its genome [9,10]. Virus replication proceeds via a partial strand displacement process known as rolling hairpin replication [11]. MVM establishes viral replication centers known as Autonomous Parvovirus-Associated Replication (APAR) bodies in the nuclear environment that colocalize with cellular replication and repair proteins [12–14]. Vigorous MVM replication leads to a potent pre-mitotic cell cycle block at the G2/M border mediated by transcriptional silencing of host Cyclin B1 [15,16].

It has become increasingly clear that DNA viruses associate with host cell DNA damage response (DDR) proteins in the nuclear environment [17,18]. These DDR proteins colocalize with viral replication centers. In particular, DNA viruses like HPV and HBV associate with persistent cellular DDR sites, known as fragile sites [19–22]. Cellular fragile sites are induced by collisions between the host cell replication and transcription machinery and are stabilized by host topoisomerases and cohesin [23–25]. We have previously discovered that MVM genomes localize to cellular DDR sites in order to establish efficient infection [26].

In particular, a subset of cellular fragile sites induced early in S phase (referred to as Early Replicating Fragile sites, or ERFs) are preferred regions for MVM to establish replication centers with the help of NS1 [27]. We have previously discovered that NS1 transports the viral genome to cellular DDR sites by binding to the viral genome and to heterologous DNA molecules containing NS1 binding elements [27]. However, the cellular signaling pathways that drive MVM localization (either NS1 or the viral genome) to cellular DDR sites remain unknown.

DNA viruses modulate the cellular DDR pathways using distinct strategies for their benefit. The related parvovirus Adeno-Associated Virus 2 (AAV2) induces a cellular DDR that is driven by the PI3-kinase-like-kinase DNA-PK [28]. However, DNA-PK signaling does not regulate MVM replication [14]. Instead, the MVM life cycle is dependent on signaling by the ATM kinase pathway [13,14,26]. Perhaps unsurprisingly for a virus that generates single-stranded DNA as it replicates, MVM replication inactivates signaling by the ATR kinase pathway that normally responds to single-stranded DNA breaks [29]. Based on these findings, we have previously proposed that ATR inactivation is a mechanism for MVM pathogenesis, which has evolved to enable MVM to inactivate the cellular signals that sense the single-stranded DNA virus genomes that may inhibit the viral life cycle [29,30].

In this study, we establish NS1 as a proxy marker for cellular DNA damage during MVM infection. Using this marker, we elucidate the cellular DDR pathways that modulate how MVM localizes to cellular sites of DNA damage. Strikingly, we have discovered that MVM localization to sites of cellular damage and early replication is dependent on signaling by the ATR kinase pathway, destined to be inactivated by MVM, and not the ATM or DNA-PK pathways. Our findings suggest that the single-stranded break repair processes aid in the establishment of MVM replication at the onset of infection.

2. Materials and Methods

2.1. Cell Lines and Virus, Viral Infections

Male murine A9 and female human U2OS cells were propagated in 10 percent Serum Plus (Sigma Aldrich) containing DMEM media (Gibco) supplemented with Gentamicin at 37 degrees Celsius and 5 percent carbon dioxide. A9 and U2OS cells were used as representative model systems for these studies because MVMp infects mouse cells and transformed human cells, respectively. Cell lines are routinely authenticated for mycoplasma contamination, and background levels of DNA damage are monitored by γH2AX staining. As A9 cells have smaller nuclei and higher background γH2AX levels relative to U2OS, imaging-based studies of NS1 localization to cellular DDR sites can be difficult to discern microscopically using this system. Therefore, U2OS cells were predominantly used for the laser microirradiation followed by imaging experiments. Wild-type MVMp virus was produced as previously described [26] and genome copies were quantified by Southern blotting [31]. MVMp infection was carried out at a Multiplicity of Infection (MOI) of 25 in all imaging assays. MVMp infection for Western blot analysis was carried out at an MOI of 10. The U2OS and A9 cells lines were obtained from Dr. David Pintel and have been previously published [26,27]. The CMV-NS1 plasmids were obtained from Dr. David Pintel and have also been previously published [14,26,27].

2.2. Cell Synchronization, DNA Damage, and Drug Treatments

A9 cells were parasynchronized in G0 phase of the cell cycle by isoleucine deprivation for 42 h as previously described [32,33]. Cells were infected with MVM upon release into complete DMEM medium (described above) for 16 h for imaging and 24 h for Western analysis. For Western blots, cells were pulsed with ATR inhibitor for 2 h (Berzosertib, Selleckchem S7102) starting at 12 h post-infection. The cells enter S phase approximately 12 h post-release [16]. For immunofluorescence, U2OS cells were infected with MVMp virus or transfected with NS1 expression plasmid for 16 h and treated with inhibitors 30 min prior to laser micro-irradiation unless otherwise indicated. The chemical inhibitors of DNA damage pathways were validated in U2OS cells that had been irradiated with

100 J/m^2 of UV irradiation on a Stratagene crosslinker. Cells were allowed to recover for 30 min in the presence of the indicated DDR inhibitors (Table 1) before being processed for the phospho-specific epitopes described in Table 2. The number of respective DDR foci per nucleus were counted and plotted and are presented in Supplementary Figure S1.

Table 1. Summary of inhibitors used.

Inhibitor	Target	Supplier	Catalog Number	Dosage
Olaparib	PARP	Selleckchem	S1060	1 μM
TDRL-505	RPA binding	Millipore Sigma	5.30535	50 μM
Caffeine	ATM and ATR	Millipore Sigma	W222402	2.5 μM
KU-55933	ATM	Selleckchem	S1092	7 μM
Berzosertib	ATR	Selleckchem	S7102	1 μM and 2 μM
NU7441 (KU-57788)	DNA-PK	Selleckchem	S2638	10 μM
CAS 17374-26-4	CK2	Millipore Sigma	218697	10 μM
CHIR-124	CHK1	Selleckchem	S2683	10 μM

Table 2. Summary table of antibodies used.

Antibody	Supplier	Catalog Number	Application
Tubulin (Clone DM1A)	Sigma	05-829	WB
Mre11	Cell Signaling	4895	WB
RPA phospho-Ser4, Ser8	Thermo Fisher	A300-245A	IF
EXO1 phospho-Ser746	Sigma	ABE1066	IF
CHK1 phospho-Ser345	Cell Signaling	23415	IF
CK2 phospho-Ser/Thr	Cell Signaling	8738	IF
DNAPKcs phospho-Ser2056	Cell Signaling	68716	IF
Poly/Mono-ADP Ribose (E6F6A)	Cell Signaling	83732	IF
ATM phospho-Ser1981	Cell Signaling	13050	IF
ATR phospho-Ser428	Cell Signaling	2853	IF
NBS1 phospho-Ser95	Cell Signaling	3002	IF
MDC1 phospho-T4	Abcam	Ab35967	IF
anti-Mouse-AF568	Thermo Scientific	A11004	IF
anti-Rabbit-AF488	Thermo Scientific	A11034	IF
Anti-mouse IgG, HRP-linked	Cell Signaling	7076	WB
Anti-rabbit IgG, HRP-linked	Cell Signaling	7074	WB

2.3. *Plasmids and Transfections*

The NS1 open reading frame containing a mutation in the splice site for NS2 was cloned into the pcDNA3.1 mammalian expression vector as previously described [14,27]. Plasmids were transfected into U2OS cells for at least 16 h using the LipoD293 transfection reagent (SignaGen Laboratories, Frederick, MD, USA).

2.4. *Laser Micro-Irradiation for Immunofluorescence*

Laser micro-irradiation was performed on 1 million U2OS cells cultured on glass-bottomed dishes (MatTek Corp, Ashland, MA, USA) infected with MVMp at an MOI of 25 or transfected with 1 μg of NS1-expression vectors for 16–20 h. Cells were sensitized with 3.5 μL of Hoechst dye (ThermoFisher Scientific, Madison, WI, USA) 5 min prior to micro-irradiation. Samples were irradiated using a Leica Stellaris DMI8 confocal microscope using 63× oil objective and 2× digital zoom with a 405 nm laser using 25 percent power at 10 Hz frequency for 2 frames per field of view. Regions of interest (ROIs) were selected across the nucleus (edges of the nuclei were demarcated and visualized by Hoechst staining). Samples were processed for immunofluorescence imaging and analysis (described below) immediately after micro-irradiation.

2.5. Immunofluorescence Assays

APAR body imaging was performed on 500,000 U2OS cells plated on glass cover slips and processed as described below. U2OS cells were pre-extracted with CSK Buffer (10 mM PIPES pH 6.8, 100 mM Sodium Chloride, 300 mM Sucrose, 1 mM EGTA, 1 mM Magnesium Chloride) and CSK with 0.5% Triton X-100 for 3 min each before fixation with 4% paraformaldehyde for 10 min at room temperature. Cells were washed in PBS before being permeabilized with 0.5% Triton X-100 in PBS for 10 min at room temperature. Samples were blocked with 3% BSA in PBS for 20 min, incubated with the primary antibody diluted in 3% BSA solution for 20 min, washed in PBS, and incubated with secondary antibody (tagged with the appropriate Alexa-Fluor conjugated fluorophores) for 20 min. Samples were washed in PBS and mounted on glass-bottomed dishes or glass slides with DAPI Fluoromount (Southern Biotech, Birmingham, AL, USA). Images were taken and processed on Leica Stellaris DMI8 Confocal microscope with 63× oil objective lens.

2.6. Image Analysis

Extent of relocalization of NS1 to micro-irradiation sites was quantified by measuring the intensity of NS1 signal along the γH2AX-labeled stripe. Following microirradiation, images were taken and processed on Leica Stellaris DMI8 Confocal microscope with 63× oil objective lens at 1.5× digital zoom. For cells that were NS1-positive by immunofluorescence, the intensity of NS1 signal over the laser micro-irradiated region was quantified using the plot profile tool on FIJI software. Signal intensities were measured at defined intervals from the left end to the right end of the region of interest (ROI) of irradiated nuclei. Values were averaged for 20–40 nuclei in 2–3 biological replicates at each position along the ROI. Quantification of NS1 relocalized to microirradiated sites relative to total NS1 levels in each individual cell was additionally measured by the ratio (NS1 intensity along the microirradiated stripe)/(total NS1 intensity in the nucleus). Images were processed with FIJI and an ROI outlined the nucleus using DAPI channel to measure total intensity of NS1 while another ROI was drawn outlining the microirradiated stripe using the gH2AX channel.

2.7. Cell Cycle Analysis

Cell cycle analysis was performed by staining the total cellular DNA content in A9 fibroblasts with Propidium Iodide stain (Sigma Aldrich, Saint Louis, MO, USA). A9 cells were harvested at the indicated timepoints, washed in 1 mL of PBS, resuspended in 300 µL of PBS, fixed in 700 µL of chilled 100% ethenol overnight at 4 degrees Celsius. Cells were counted, samples were resuspended in 300 µL of PBS, treated with RNAse for 1 h at 37 degrees Celsius, and incubated with Propidium iodide normalized to cell number overnight. Cells were analyzed on a BD LSR Fortessa (University of Wisconsin-Flow Cytometry Laboratory, Madison, WI, USA) on the FL2 channel and assessed for cells in G0/G1, S, and G2/M phases of the cell cycle.

2.8. MVMp Genome Replication Analysis

Cells were harvested at the indicated timepoints, pelleted and resuspended in Cell Lysis Buffer (2% SDS, 0.15 M Sodium chloride, 10 mM Tris pH 8, 1 mM EDTA). Lysed whole-cell extracts were proteinase K (NEB) treated overnight at 37 degrees Celsius. The genomic DNA was sheared with 25 G × 5/8 inch 1 mL needed syringe (BD Biosciences, Franklin Lakes, NJ, USA). The genomic DNA was purified using phenol:chloroform:isoamyl alcohol and precipitated in isopropanol. The DNA was washed in 70% ethanol and resuspended in 100 μL of TE buffer. MVMp genome replication was measured by Taqman-qPCR using forward and reverse primers (F: agccgctgaacttggactaa, R: ctccttggtcaaggctgttc) as well as a Taqman probe that was complementary to the plus strand of the viral genome (ccaaccatcccttaaaccct).

2.9. Salt-Wash Chromatin Immunoprecipitation Combined with Quantitative PCR (swChIP-qPCR)

Salt-wash ChIP-qPCR assays were performed in nuclear extracts from MVMp-infected A9 cells as previously published [34,35]. Briefly, cells were washed with phosphate-buffered saline (PBS) before they were collected with HBE buffer (10 mM HEPES, 5 mM KCl, 1 mM EDTA) into Eppendorf tubes, centrifuged at 1000× *g* for 3 min at room temperature, aspirated, and resuspended in 500 μL HBE. Cells were lysed on ice for 10 min by the addition of 1% NP-40 (to a final concentration of 0.1%); sodium chloride (NaCl) was used to isolate the viral nucleoprotein complexes and crosslinked in 0.1% Formaldehyde for 10 min at room temperature. The crosslinking reactions were quenched in 0.125 M glycine, MVMp-nucleoprotein complexes purified using 3K Amicon Centrifugal Filter Units (Millipore), and purified into PBS and sonicated using a Diagenode Bioruptor Pico for 60 cycles (30 s on and 30 s off per cycle). The samples were incubated overnight at 4 degrees Celsius with the antibodies bound to Protein A Dynabeads (Invitrogen). Samples were washed for 3 min each at 4 degrees Celsius with low salt wash (0.01% SDS, 1% Triton X-100, 2 mM EDTA, 20 mM Tris-HCl pH 8, 150 mM NaCl), high salt wash (0.01% SDS, 1% Triton X-100, 2 mM EDTA 20 mM Tris-HCl pH 8, 500 mM NaCl), lithium chloride wash (0.25 M LiCl, 1% NP40, 1% DOC, 1 mM EDTA, 10 mM Tris HCl pH 8), and twice with TE buffer. Protein-DNA conjugates were eluted with SDS elution buffer (1% SDS, 0.1 M sodium bicarbonate), crosslinks were reversed using 0.2 M NaCl and Proteinase K (NEB) and incubated at 56 degrees Celsius overnight. DNA was purified using PCR Purification Kit (Qiagen) and eluted in 100 μL of Buffer EB (Qiagen). qPCR assays were performed with primers that were complementary to the MVM P4 and P38 promoters that have been previously published [35]. The respective P4 primer sequences were F: tgataagcggttcagggagt and R: ccagccatggttagttggtt, and P38 primer sequences were F: ccgaaaagtacgcctctcag and R: ccgcaacaggagtatttggt.

2.10. Statistical Analysis

Statistical analysis of the imaging studies was performed using Graphpad Prism software. For ChIP-qPCR assays, the statistical significance of ATR association with MVM genome relative to that of IgG pulldown was determined by unpaired Student's *t* test, with statistical significance denoted by ***, $p < 0.001$. For inhibitor treatments, the statistical significance of the number of foci was calculated using unpaired Student's *t*-test with statistical significance denoted by ****, $p < 0.0001$. Statistical significance of MVM replication upon iATR treatment was assessed by unpaired Student's *t*-test with statistical significance denoted by *, $p < 0.05$. For laser micro-irradiation assays, the statistical significance of the difference between NS1 relocalization between different conditions was calculated using one-way ANOVA, multiple comparisons test as previously described [27]. Statistical significance is designated by ****, $p < 0.0001$.

2.11. Western Blot Analysis

Cells were collected at specified time point and pellets were lysed on ice for 15 min in complete Radio-Immuno-Precipitation Assay (RIPA) buffer (20 mM Tris HCL pH 7.5, 150 mM NaCL, 10% glycerol, 1% NP-40, 1% sodium deoxycholate, 0.1% SDS, 1 mM EDTA, 10 mM trisodium pyrophosphate, 20 mM sodium fluoride, 2 mM sodium orthovanadate and 1× protease inhibitor cocktail (MedChemExpress)). Cell lysate was collected following centrifugation for 15 min at 17,000× *g* at 4 degrees Celsius. Protein sample concentration was calculated using BCA assay (Bio-Rad). A 5× protein loading dye (1 M Tris-HCl pH 8,

30% Glycerol, 100 mM DTT, 10 mM EDTA, 350 mM SDS, Bromophenol blue) was added to samples and boiled at 95 °C for 5 min.

Equivalent protein levels were loaded onto a 10% SDS-PAGE gel for electrophoresis and subsequently transferred to a nitrocellulose membrane. Membranes were blocked for 30 min in 5% milk in TBS (20 mM Tris, 150 mM NaCl, pH 7.6) with 0.5% Tween-20. Membranes were incubated with the primary antibody in 5% milk in TBST for 1 h followed by three 5 min washes in TBST prior to incubation with HRP conjugated secondary antibody and ladder conjugate (Bio-Rad) in 5% milk in TBST for 30 min. All incubations were performed at room temperature. The membrane was incubated for 5 min with Clarity Western ECL Blotting Substrate (Bio-Rad) before imaging using a Li-COR-Fortessa scanner and analysis with Image Studio Lite software.

2.12. Antibodies

Primary antibodies were used in immunofluorescence (IF) and Western blot analysis (WB).

The mouse anti-NS1 monoclonal antibody (clone 2C9b) has been previously generated and extensively validated [14,26,27].

3. Results

3.1. NS1 Is a Proxy Marker for Cellular DNA Damage during MVM Infection

Upon infecting host cells, MVM genomes and non-structural proteins localize to pre-existing as well as induced cellular sites of DNA damage [26,27]. This localization is driven by NS1 associating with ACCA motifs on the MVM genome [27]. However, NS1 on its own activates a cytotoxic program in host cells. Therefore, to determine whether activation of this cytotoxic program by ectopic NS1 perturbs the host's ability to recognize cellular DNA breaks, we expressed NS1 by transient transfection and monitored whether host cells recognize induced cellular DNA breaks using laser microirradiation followed by immunofluorescence. Using relocalized NS1 as a marker for induced DNA damage, we monitored the ability of cellular DDR proteins to recognize micro-irradiated sites. As shown in Figure 1A, NS1 relocalized to γH2AX sites, consistent with previously observed findings (Figure 1A, compare panel 1 to 2 [27]). This relocalization was also evident when monitored by staining for phosphorylated NBS1 (Figure 1A, panel 3), phosphorylated MDC1 (Figure 1A, panel 4), and phosphorylated RPA (Figure 1A, panel 5). Therefore, we have extended our observations of NS1 localization during ectopic expression to additional host DDR pathway proteins, finding NS1 relocalized to DDR sites marked by phosphorylated NBS1, MDC1, and RPA. Importantly, this interaction of NS1 with host DDR recognition markers does not impact their ability to recognize additional cellular DNA breaks.

While ectopic NS1 did not perturb the cellular detection of DNA damage, MVM replication is known to utilize ATM kinase signaling and inactivate the ATR kinase pathways [14,29]. To determine whether the actively replicating MVM genome inhibits the recognition of cellular DNA breaks, we analyzed the localization of cellular DDR proteins to laser micro-irradiated stripes during viral infection using NS1 as the DDR marker. As shown in Figure 1B, laser microirradiation of U2OS cells during MVM infection led to relocalization of NS1 to the induced cellular DDR sites marked by γH2AX, consistent with previously published findings (Figure 1B, compare panel 1 to 2 [27]). Using relocalized NS1 as a marker for induced DNA damage, we monitored the ability of cellular DDR proteins to recognize these sites. As shown in Figure 1A, DDR sites monitored by NS1 staining colocalized with DNA break recognition markers such as phosphorylated NBS1 (Figure 1B, panel 3), phosphorylated MDC1 (Figure 1B, panel 4), and phosphorylated RPA (Figure 1B, panel 5). These findings showed that MVM-infected cells still retain the ability to recognize additional cellular DNA breaks.

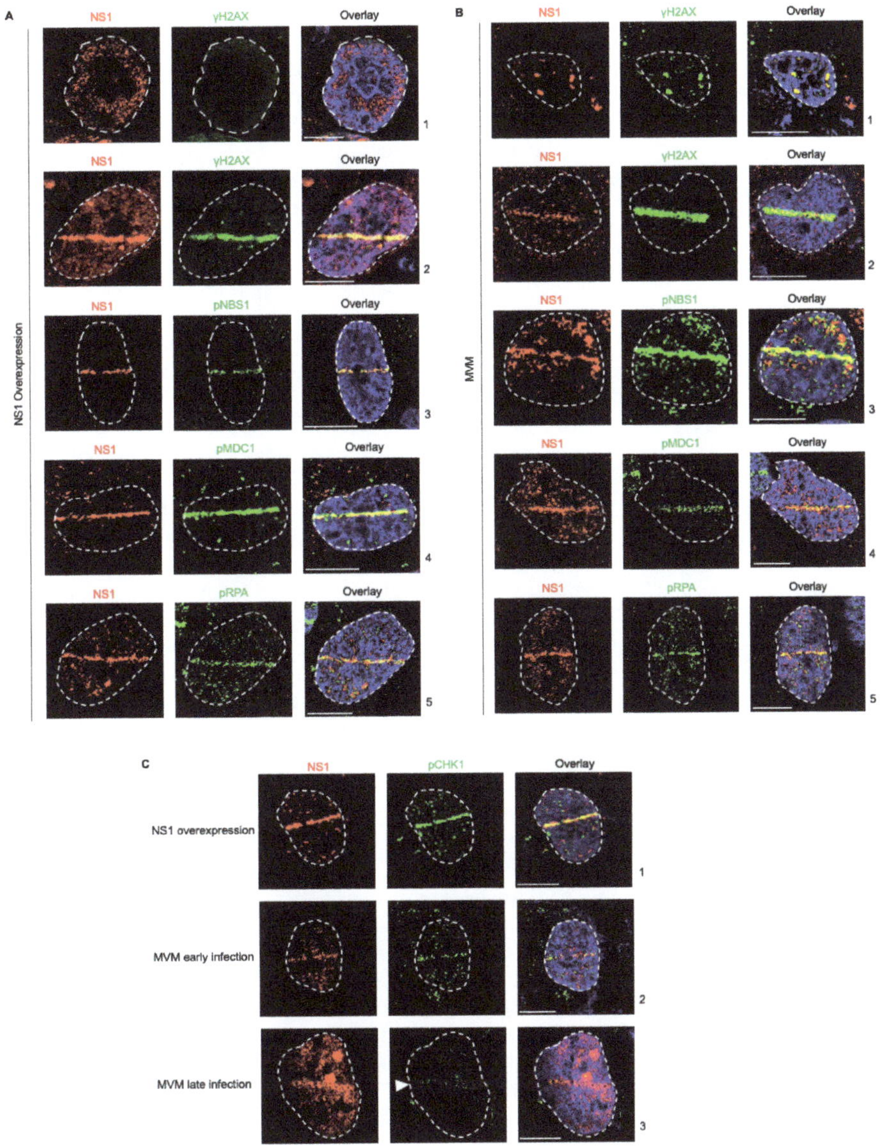

Figure 1. NS1 is a proxy marker for cellular DNA damage during MVM infection. (**A**) U2OS cells transfected with NS1-expressing vectors for 16 h were damaged across the nucleus using laser micro-irradiation and monitored by NS1-DDR staining as indicated. (**B**) U2OS cells infected with MVM at an MOI of 25 for 16 h were damaged across the nucleus using laser micro-irradiation and monitored by NS1-DDR staining as indicated. (**C**) Relocalization of NS1 produced during different stages of MVM infection or ectopic expression were monitored by relocalization to DDR sites marked by phosphorylated CHK1. Viral non-structural protein NS1 (red), respective DDR markers (green), and pan-nuclear content were visualized by DAPI staining (blue). White dashed lines demarcate the nuclear boundaries, white bars represent 10 μm, and white arrowhead in (**C**) panel 3 indicates the location of the laser micro-irradiated stripe. The ratios of NS1 along the laser stripe to that of total nuclear NS1 in 1C are as follows: panel 1 (NS1): 0.404; panel 2 (MVM early): 0.293; and panel 3 (MVM late): 0.197.

MVM infection leads to the inactivation of the ATR kinase pathway by inhibiting the single-stranded break transducer TopBP1 [29]. To confirm that NS1 is an alternative marker for cellular DDR during all stages of MVM infection, we performed laser microirradiation followed by immunofluorescence for NS1 and phosphorylated CHK1, which is activated downstream of ATR/TopBP1 [29]. Ectopically expressed NS1 robustly relocalized with cellular DDR sites that are marked by phospho CHK1 (Figure 1C, panel 1). Similarly, during early infection, when phosphorylation of CHK1 is still possible, NS1 colocalized with phospho CHK1 to mark cellular DDR sites (Figure 1C, panel 2). However, during late stages of infection, which is monitored by high nuclear levels of NS1 associated with inhibition of CHK1 [15], NS1 is still able to relocalize to the cellular DDR sites (Figure 1C, panel 3). These findings indicated that NS1 is a marker for cellular DNA breaks throughout all stages of MVM infection.

3.2. NS1 Localization to Cellular DDR Sites Is Independent of ATM and DNA-PK Signaling but Depends on ATR Signaling

To systematically determine which cellular DDR signals drive the relocalization of NS1 to cellular sites of DNA damage, we used well-characterized DDR inhibitors in U2OS cells transfected with an NS1 expression vector combined with laser micro-irradiation assays ([27]; inhibitors validated in Supplemental Figure S1). We investigated proteins in the ATR, ATM, and DNA-PK DDR pathways to determine which signals drive NS1 relocalization (Figure 2A,B). Inhibition of PARP polymerase that signals the initial activation of cellular DDR signals and local chromatin remodeling [36] did not impact NS1 relocalization (Figure 2C). Similarly, NS1 still relocalized to sites of DDR under inhibition of the single-strand DNA binding protein RPA (Figure 2D). However, in the presence of the pan ATM and ATR inhibitor caffeine, NS1 did not relocalize to sites of DDR (Figure 2H, top left), remaining as diffuse foci around the nucleus. To distinguish if this phenotype was driven distinctly by the ATM or ATR pathways, we used specific small-molecule inhibitors. While inhibition of ATM had no impact on NS1 relocalization (Figure 2H, top right), inhibition of ATR consistently resulted in a loss of relocalization (Figure 2H, lower left, grayscale images in Figure S3A–S3C). This suggested that the ATR signaling pathway is involved in the relocalization of NS1 to sites of DDR. This decrease in NS1 localization relative to γH2AX in the presence of caffeine and iATR was consistently observed in more than 20 nuclei, and was statistically significant (Figure 2H, lower right). These findings were further corroborated by measuring the ratio of NS1 intensity over the microirradiated region to that of the pan-nuclear NS1 that revealed that NS1 relocalization to induced DNA break sites is attenuated in the presence of caffeine and iATR (Supplemental Figure S2). Interestingly, the inhibition of the downstream ATR effector CHK1 did not impact the re-localization of NS1 to the laser micro-irradiated DDR site (Figure 2F).

Surprisingly, although NS1 has been previously shown to interact with the cellular protein kinase CK2 [37] and CK2 interacts with MDC1 to transduce the signals to γH2AX [13,38], inhibition of CK2 activity did not attenuate the relocalization of NS1 to laser-microirradiated γH2AX sites (Figure 2E). Inhibition of DNA-PK signaling did not impact the ability of NS1 to localize to laser micro-irradiated sites (Figure 2G), suggesting NS1 relocalization discriminates between the cellular DDR PI3-kinase-like kinases [17].

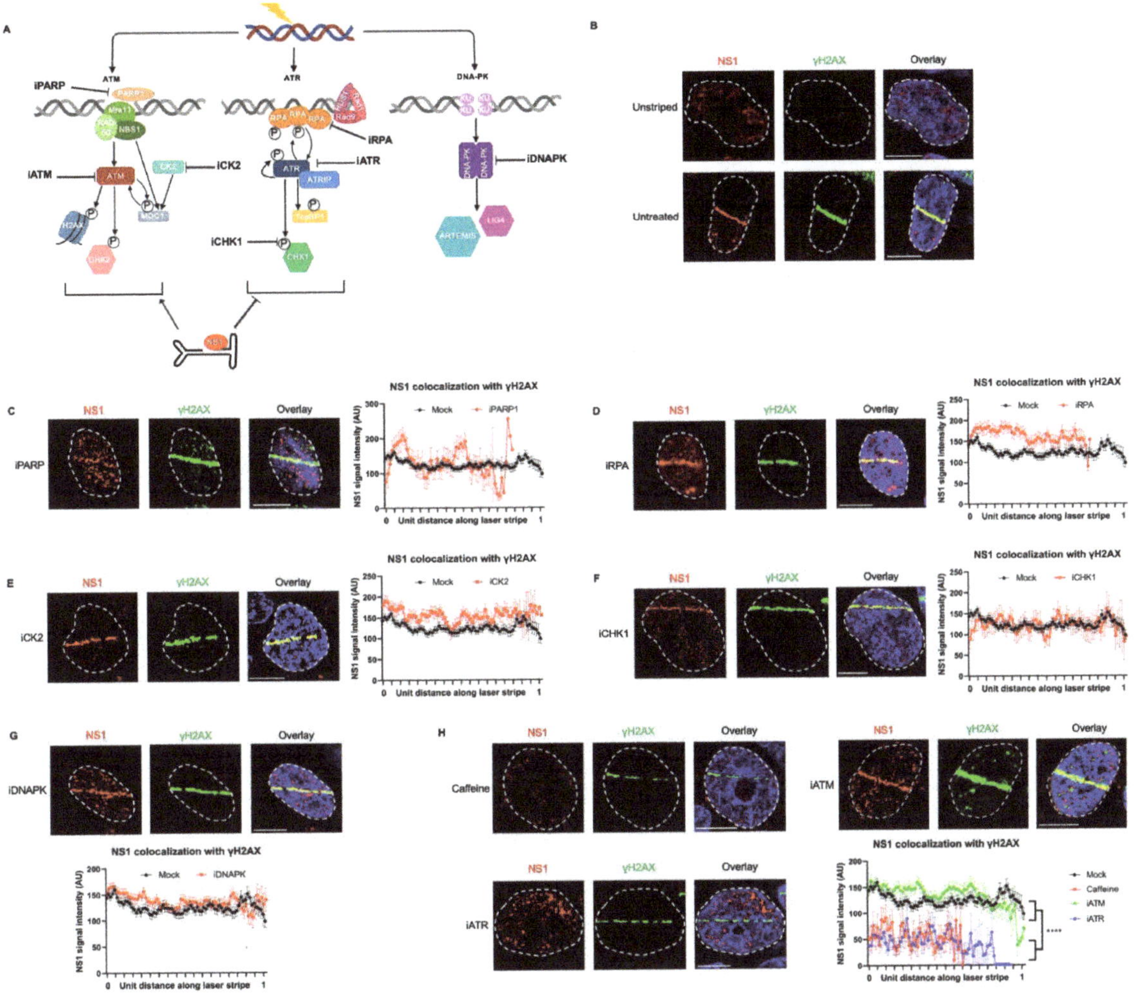

Figure 2. NS1 localization to cellular DDR sites is independent of ATM and DNA-PK signaling but depends on ATR signaling. (**A**) Schematic of cellular DNA damage response mediated by PI3-Kinase-like-Kinases with the relevant proteins inhibited in part (**B–H**) indicated as shown. (**B–H**) U2OS cells were transfected with NS1 overexpression vector for 16 h, treated with the indicated DDR inhibitors 30 min prior to laser micro-irradiation, and processed for NS1-γH2AX colocalization. Viral non-structural protein is depicted by NS1 (red), cellular DDR by γH2AX (green), and pan-nuclear content was visualized by DAPI staining (blue). White dashed lines demarcate the nuclear boundaries and white bars represent 10 μm. The concentrations of the inhibitors used are described in Materials and Methods. Representative relocalization upon laser micro-irradiation of U2OS cells expressing NS1 was compared with relocalization upon (**C**) PARP inhibition, (**D**) RPA inhibition, (**E**) CK2 inhibition, (**F**) CHK1 inhibition, (**G**) DNAPK inhibition, and (**H**) inhibition of the ATM/ATR pathway by caffeine or specific ATM/ATR inhibitors. The average intensity of NS1 localizing to γH2AX-labelled nuclear sites between mock-treated cells and inhibitor-treated cells was averaged over at least 20 independent nuclei, represented in the adjoining profiles with the error bars representing SEM.

3.3. *ATR Associates with the MVM Genome and ATR Signaling Regulates the Early Replication of MVM*

Since it has previously been reported that ATR colocalizes with MVM-NS1 in APAR bodies [29], and we observed that ATR inhibition during NS1 expression attenuated ectopic NS1 localization to cellular DDR sites, we hypothesized that ATR signaling may drive MVM localization during the early stages of infection. To determine whether ATR molecules associate with the MVM genome during infection, we performed chromatin immunoprecipitation assays on nuclear extracts containing the viral genomes that we have recently developed to remove the secondary effects of host-associated cellular DDR sites [34,35]. ChIP-qPCR assays of ATR compared with NS1 pulldowns revealed that ATR molecules associated strongly with the MVM genome at 16 hpi at the P4 (Figure 3A) and P38 promoters (Figure 3B). The pulldown efficiencies of ATR were equivalent to that of NS1, which is known to bind covalently to the 5′ end of the MVM genome and associate with ACCAACCA consensus motifs [3,4,39,40]. To examine whether ATR signaling impacted NS1 localization to cellular sites of DNA damage, we pulsed MVM infected U2OS cells with ATR inhibitor for 30 min prior to laser microirradiation. As shown in Figure 3C, in the presence of ATR inhibitor, MVM-produced NS1 relocalization to induced DDR sites was attenuated at higher concentrations of iATR (grayscale images in Figure S3D). These assays qualitatively suggested that ATR signaling is required for initial localization of NS1 to cellular DDR sites during infection. To determine how ATR signaling regulates MVM life cycle, we treated A9 cells that were synchronized by Isoleucine deprivation and pulsed with ATR inhibitor at 12 h post-release as shown in the schematic (Figure 3D). This strategy of ATR inhibition did not impact A9 cell entry into S phase (which occurs at approximately 12 h post-release into complete media) as determined by cell cycle analysis at 14 hpi (Figure 3E, compare 4 columns on the right). Under these synchronization conditions, in the presence of the ATR inhibitor, MVM-APAR bodies were smaller and formed foci that showed a distinct separation between NS1 and γH2AX (Figure 3F and profiles on the right). To determine the impact of ATR inhibition on MVM replication, the A9 cells were synchronized and pulsed with iATR at 12 hpi, washed at 14 hpi, and harvested at 24 hpi, as schematized in Figure 3G. This led to a decrease in MVM replication, as measured by NS1 levels (Figure 3H, lanes 3 and 4), which also correlated with a decrease in replicating viral genomes (Figure 3I). Taken together, these findings confirmed that inhibition of the ATR signaling pathway attenuates the ability of MVM-NS1 to localize to cellular sites of DNA damage, thereby regulating how viral replication centers are established.

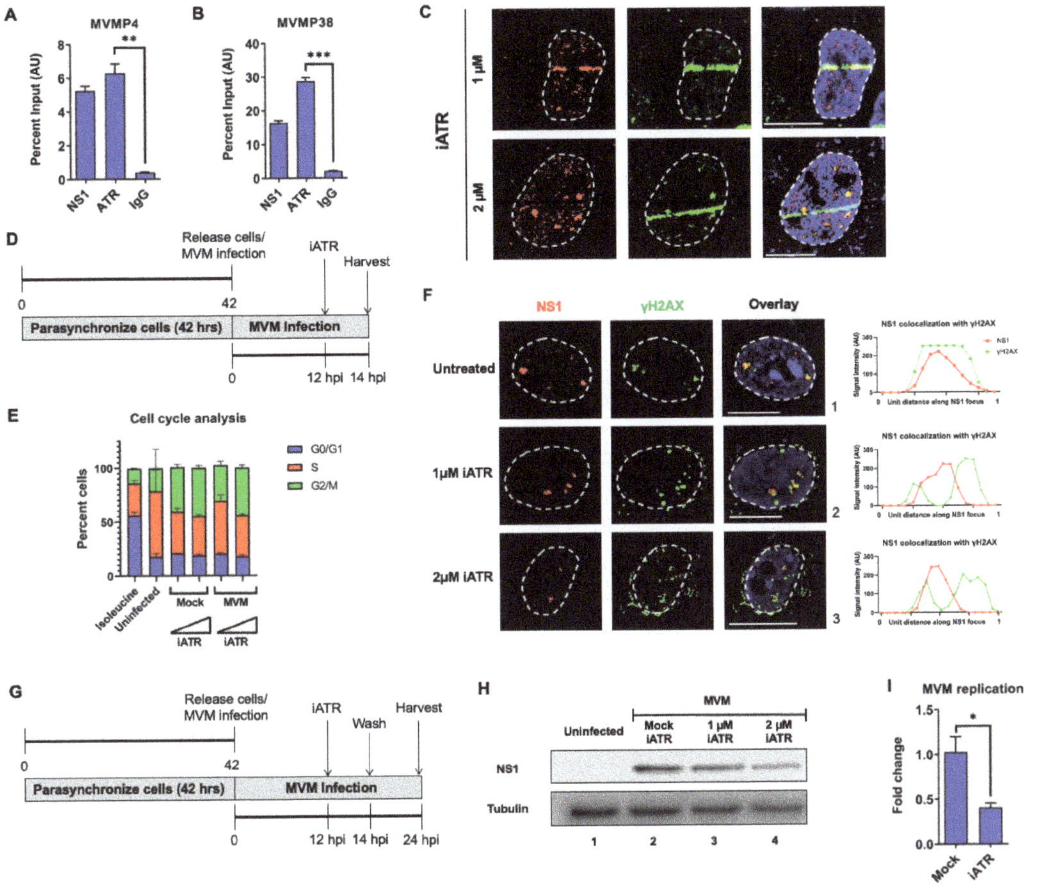

Figure 3. ATR associates with the MVM genome and ATR signaling regulates the early replication of MVM. Parasynchronized A9 cells were infected with MVM at an MOI of 10 for 16 hpi before being processed for salt-wash ChIP-qPCR assays on the viral nucleoprotein extracts for their association with NS1, ATR, and IgG as negative control. The pulldowns were assessed for (**A**) P4 and (**B**) P38 sequences using qPCR analysis. (**C**) U2OS cells infected with MVM for 16 hpi were treated with iATR at concentrations of 1 µM (top panel) and 2 µM (bottom panel) for 30 min prior to laser micro-irradiation before being processed for NS1-γH2AX colocalization. (**D**) Schematic of MVM synchronization for cell cycle analysis and APAR body imaging. A9 cells were synchronized by isoleucine deprivation for 36–42 h (as shown in Figure 3D) before being released into complete DMEM media and infected with MVM at an MOI of 10. At 12 hpi, the cells were pulsed with 1 µM and 2 µM concentrations of iATR for 2 h and harvested at 14 hpi for (**E**) cell cycle analysis and (**F**) APAR body imaging. Viral non-structural protein is depicted by NS1 (red), cellular DDR by γH2AX (green), and pan-nuclear content was visualized by DAPI staining (blue). White dashed lines demarcate the nuclear boundaries and white bars represent 10 µm. On the right-hand panels of the respective images in (**F**), the profiles of NS1 (red) and γH2AX staining along the transverse section of the APAR body are shown. (**G**) Schematic of MVM infection for evaluating MVM replication. (**H**) Synchronized A9 cells were infected with MVM for 24 h. Cells were treated with iATR at the indicated concentrations from 12 hpi to 14 hpi before being washed out. Virus replication was evaluated using Western blots for NS1 levels compared with Tubulin as loading control. (**I**) MVM replication at 24 hpi was evaluated in the absence (mock) or presence of iATR at 2 µM using Taqman qPCR assay directed against the plus strand. Statistical analysis was performed by paired Student's *t*-test with p values represented by: * $p < 0.05$, ** $p < 0.01$ and *** $p < 0.001$.

4. Discussion

In this study, we have validated that NS1 is a bona fide marker for parvovirus-induced cellular DNA damage. Additionally, we have systematically perturbed the major cellular DDR signaling pathways, determining that ATM, PARP, and DNA-PK are not involved in regulating NS1 localization to induced cellular DDR sites. Strikingly, ATR inhibition decreases NS1 relocalization to cellular DDR sites, leading to attenuated MVM replication. Taken together, these findings suggest that although ATR signaling is inactivated by MVM infection at late stages, it is required at the early stages of the viral infection to initially establish APAR bodies.

Mass spectrometry studies investigating the host proteins that associate with MVM NS1 have previously discovered that NS1 interacts with the host protein Protein Kinase CK2 (CK2, [41]). In this regard, the NS1 protein of autonomous parvoviruses functions as an adaptor, connecting CK2 with cytoskeletal proteins such as tropomyosin, to cause cytopathic effects in permissive cells [37]. Additionally, since CK2 also has an established role in connecting MDC1 and NBS1 [42], we initially hypothesized that CK2 might serve as a connecting link between NS1 and cellular DDR proteins. However, the CK2 inhibitor did not impact the relocalization of MVM-NS1 to cellular DDR sites. Interestingly, CK2 is made up of two subunits: a catalytic alpha subunit, which interacts with NS1 during MVM infection, and a regulatory beta subunit. While the inhibitor used in this study targeted the function of the alpha subunit, it remains possible that the catalytic function is not required for NS1-CK2α interaction. These findings suggest that the role of CK2's catalytic activity in regulating the MVM life cycle is independent of the localization of NS1 (and by extension MVM) to cellular DDR sites.

Much of our understanding of virus–host interactions comes from transfection of viral proteins ectopically. However, our findings in this study suggest there are phenotypic differences in how viral proteins interact with the host during infection versus ectopic expression. This may be due to the absence of the replicating viral genomes. Alternatively, it is possible that active virus replication causes global changes that modulate NS1-DDR interactions differently. While the inhibition of ATR obliterates NS1 relocalization to sites of DNA damage in overexpression, during infection the presence of increasing MVM DNA molecules and additional viral protein expression presents the potential for redundant pathways to be activated, which can then induce relocalization. This may be contributing to why relocalization is inhibited in cells at early stages of infection but not late stages. One limitation of current laser micro-irradiation studies is the inability to perform synchronous infection assays with U2OS cells, which is the established model system for studying DDR signaling. This makes it difficult to rigorously evaluate how NS1 localization to cellular micro-irradiated sites changes over the course of infection. Time lapse live cell imaging experiments and laser micro-irradiation studies in synchronous MVM infection systems will provide more clues on these aspects of the viral life cycle.

While relocalization was only attenuated during early infection by inhibition of ATR, APAR body formation was still impacted and correlated with decreased overall virus replication. Previous work investigating APAR body formation has shown that while at lower resolutions NS1 appears to be directly associated with γH2AX, at higher resolution, MVM APAR bodies form in distinct pockets surrounded by or directly next to γH2AX [13,14,26]. In the presence of the ATR inhibitor, there is a greater separation of NS1 from that of cellular γH2AX. One possible interpretation for this observation is that MVM localizes inefficiently to cellular sites of DNA damage in the absence of ATR signals. This builds on our observations that NS1-DDR interactions are dependent on ATR signaling. Our observations with the ATR inhibitor also suggest that while NS1 initially associates with γH2AX to form APAR bodies, the inability of NS1 to relocalize and expand to new cellular DDR sites results in smaller APAR bodies. This is further supported by decreased levels of NS1 and viral genome later in infection in the presence of the ATR inhibitor. In stark contrast, the virus-induced cellular DNA damage signals activate the ATM kinase pathways [14]. We have recently discovered that efficient MVM expression and replication depend on

MRE11 in an MRN-complex-independent manner [35]. These findings suggest that MVM utilizes distinct aspects of cellular DDR pathways at different stages of the viral life cycle, establishing a distinction between the signals necessary for expression from those required for localization.

An attractive mechanism by which PIKKs may regulate NS1 localization to cellular DDR sites is via phosphorylation of their SQ/TQ motifs. Cellular Serine/Threonine residues that are associated with glutamine residues on the primary amino acid sequence are phosphorylation targets of ATM and ATR kinases [43]. Further supporting this assertion, the Rep 68/78 protein of AAV2 localizes to cellular DDR sites in an ATM/ATR-dependent manner [44]. In line with these expectations, the MVM NS1 protein contains two SQ and two TQ motifs. We hypothesize that these are the residues that serve as the phosphorylation substrates for ATM and ATR kinases. Our ChIP studies show that ATR associates with the MVM genome. However, based on our findings, it remains unknown why these sites might be specifically targeted by ATR and not ATM. Future studies will focus on dissecting these conundrums on parvovirus–host genome interactions.

Prior studies on MVM pathogenesis established that MVM infection inactivates CHK1 (downstream of ATR) by inhibiting the activation of the transducer TopBP1 [29]. However, our findings suggest that while ATR may be inactivated at late stages, it is required at the early stages of infection to establish viral replication centers in the nuclear compartment. Perhaps ATR interaction at early stages facilitates the opening of the viral genome for access by host replication proteins, whereas at late stages this enhances genome instability and chromosome fragmentation. Alternatively, it is possible that ATR inactivation at the late stages of infection is a mechanism evolved by parvoviruses to evade integration into the host genome. It remains unclear, however, whether this requirement for ATR pathway inactivation is induced on the viral genome or on the host genome. Interestingly, Adenovirus infection induces distinct virus and host-mediated ATM signals [45]. We speculate that MVM, by virtue of being a single-stranded DNA virus, interacts with the host ATR pathway via a similar route. Future studies will elucidate how distinct single-stranded DNA repair pathways on the viral versus cellular genomes drive viral pathogenesis and can be used for oncolytic virotherapies.

Supplementary Materials: The following supporting information can be downloaded at: https://www.mdpi.com/article/10.3390/v15061243/s1, Figure S1: The impact of the respective DDR inhibitor treatments were determined in U2OS cells that were UV irradiated at 100 J/m^2 in a Stratagene crosslinker. Cell were allowed to recover for 30 min in the presence of the indicated inhibitors before being processed for imaging with the respective phospho-specific antibodies that are targeted by the inhibitors. Foci were counted for multiple nuclei (where each nucleus represents one datapoint) and plotted side-by-side with mock-treated samples. Statistical comparisons were performed by Student's *t*-tests as described in the statistical analysis section. The inhibitors/ligands that were tested and validated were: (A) PARP inhibitor Olaparib, (B) RPA inhibitor, (C) Protein Kinase CK2 inhibitor, (D) CHK1 inhibitor, (E) DNAPK inhibitor, (F) pan ATM/ATR inhibitor Caffeine, (G) ATR inhibitor at 1 μM and (H) ATM inhibitor. Figure S2: NS1 intensity over microirradiated stripe normalized to total levels of NS1 during inhibitor treatments show NS1 localization to cellular DDR sites is independent of ATM and DNA-PK signaling but depends on ATR signaling. Ratio of (NS1 intensity on microirradiated stripe)/(total NS1 intensity) was measured for 10 or more nuclei for each inhibitor condition with error bars representing SEM. Statistical comparisons were performed by One-way ANOVA, with ns representing non-significant statistical difference, * represents $p < 0.05$, ** represents $p < 0.001$ and *** represents $p < 0.0001$. Figure S3: Representative grayscale images of NS1 relocalization to laser micro-irradiated stripes from Figures 2H and 3C, where cells were treated with (A) caffeine, (B) ATM inhibitor, (C) ATR inhibitor during ectopic NS1 expression, and with ATR inhibitor at (D, left) 1 μM and (D, right) 2 μM concentrations during MVM infection.

Author Contributions: Conceptualization, C.I.S.L. and K.M.; methodology, C.I.S.L. and K.M.; validation, C.I.S.L. and K.M.; formal analysis, C.I.S.L. and K.M.; investigation, C.I.S.L. and K.M.; data curation, C.I.S.L. and K.M.; writing—original draft preparation, C.I.S.L. and K.M.; writing—review and editing, C.I.S.L. and K.M.; visualization, C.I.S.L. and K.M.; supervision, K.M.; project administration, K.M.; funding acquisition, K.M. All authors have read and agreed to the published version of the manuscript.

Funding: This research was funded by NIH/NIAID K99/R00 Pathway to Independence Award, grant number AI148511 to K.M. and The Wisconsin Partnership Program's New Investigator Award (PERC Grant G-4942) to K.M. The author(s) thank the University of Wisconsin Carbone Cancer Center Flow Cytometry Laboratory, supported by NIH grant P30 CA014520, for use of its facilities and services.

Institutional Review Board Statement: Not applicable.

Informed Consent Statement: Not applicable.

Data Availability Statement: All relevant data supporting the findings of this study are available within the paper and its Supplementary material. All other data are available from the corresponding author on request.

Acknowledgments: We acknowledge members of the Majumder Lab for critical reading of the manuscript.

Conflicts of Interest: The authors declare no conflict of interest. The funders had no role in the design of the study; in the collection, analyses, or interpretation of data; in the writing of the manuscript; or in the decision to publish the results.

References

1. Cotmore, S.F.; Agbandje-McKenna, M.; Chiorini, J.A.; Mukha, D.V.; Pintel, D.J.; Qiu, J.; Soderlund-Venermo, M.; Tattersall, P.; Tijssen, P.; Gatherer, D.; et al. The family parvoviridae. *Arch. Virol.* **2014**, *159*, 1239–1247. [CrossRef] [PubMed]
2. Cotmore, S.F.; Tattersall, P. Parvoviruses: Small does not mean simple. *Annu. Rev. Virol.* **2014**, *1*, 517–537. [CrossRef] [PubMed]
3. Cotmore, S.F.; Tattersall, P. The ns-1 polypeptide of minute virus of mice is covalently attached to the 5′ termini of duplex replicative-form dna and progeny single strands. *J. Virol.* **1988**, *62*, 851–860. [CrossRef] [PubMed]
4. Cotmore, S.F.; Christensen, J.; Nüesch, J.P.; Tattersall, P. The ns1 polypeptide of the murine parvovirus minute virus of mice binds to dna sequences containing the motif [acca]2-3. *J. Virol.* **1995**, *69*, 1652–1660. [CrossRef]
5. Christensen, J.; Tattersall, P. Parvovirus initiator protein ns1 and rpa coordinate replication fork progression in a reconstituted dna replication system. *J. Virol.* **2002**, *76*, 6518–6531. [CrossRef] [PubMed]
6. Cotmore, S.F.; Gottlieb, R.L.; Tattersall, P. Replication initiator protein ns1 of the parvovirus minute virus of mice binds to modular divergent sites distributed throughout duplex viral dna. *J. Virol.* **2007**, *81*, 13015–13027. [CrossRef]
7. Mouw, M.; Pintel, D.J. Amino acids 16-275 of minute virus of mice ns1 include a domain that specifically binds (acca)2-3-containing dna. *Virology* **1998**, *251*, 123–131. [CrossRef]
8. Naeger, L.K.; Cater, J.; Pintel, D.J. The small nonstructural protein (ns2) of the parvovirus minute virus of mice is required for efficient dna replication and infectious virus production in a cell-type-specific manner. *J. Virol.* **1990**, *64*, 6166–6175. [CrossRef]
9. Bashir, T.; Horlein, R.; Rommelaere, J.; Willwand, K. Cyclin a activates the dna polymerase delta -dependent elongation machinery in vitro: A parvovirus dna replication model. *Proc. Natl. Acad. Sci. USA* **2000**, *97*, 5522–5527. [CrossRef]
10. Bashir, T.; Rommelaere, J.; Cziepluch, C. In vivo accumulation of cyclin a and cellular replication factors in autonomous parvovirus minute virus of mice-associated replication bodies. *J. Virol.* **2001**, *75*, 4394–4398. [CrossRef]
11. Tattersall, P.; Ward, D.C. Rolling hairpin model for replication of parvovirus and linear chromosomal dna. *Nature* **1976**, *263*, 106–109. [CrossRef] [PubMed]
12. Young, P.J.; Jensen, K.T.; Burger, L.R.; Pintel, D.J.; Lorson, C.L. Minute virus of mice ns1 interacts with the smn protein, and they colocalize in novel nuclear bodies induced by parvovirus infection. *J. Virol.* **2002**, *76*, 3892–3904. [CrossRef] [PubMed]
13. Ruiz, Z.; Mihaylov, I.S.; Cotmore, S.F.; Tattersall, P. Recruitment of dna replication and damage response proteins to viral replication centers during infection with ns2 mutants of minute virus of mice (mvm). *Virology* **2011**, *410*, 375–384. [CrossRef] [PubMed]
14. Adeyemi, R.O.; Landry, S.; Davis, M.E.; Weitzman, M.D.; Pintel, D.J. Parvovirus minute virus of mice induces a dna damage response that facilitates viral replication. *PLoS Pathog.* **2010**, *6*, e1001141. [CrossRef]
15. Adeyemi, R.O.; Pintel, D.J. Parvovirus-induced depletion of cyclin b1 prevents mitotic entry of infected cells. *PLoS Pathog.* **2014**, *10*, e1003891. [CrossRef]
16. Fuller, M.S.; Majumder, K.; Pintel, D.J. Minute virus of mice inhibits transcription of the cyclin b1 gene during infection. *J. Virol.* **2017**, *91*, e00428-17. [CrossRef]
17. Pancholi, N.J.; Price, A.M.; Weitzman, M.D. Take your pikk: Tumour viruses and dna damage response pathways. *Philos. Trans. R. Soc. B Biol. Sci.* **2017**, *372*, 20160269. [CrossRef]
18. Weitzman, M.D.; Fradet-Turcotte, A. Virus dna replication and the host dna damage response. *Annu. Rev. Virol.* **2018**, *5*, 141–164. [CrossRef]
19. Warburton, A.; Markowitz, T.E.; Katz, J.P.; Pipas, J.M.; McBride, A.A. Recurrent integration of human papillomavirus genomes at transcriptional regulatory hubs. *NPJ Genom. Med.* **2021**, *6*, 101. [CrossRef]

20. Feitelson, M.A.; Lee, J. Hepatitis b virus integration, fragile sites, and hepatocarcinogenesis. *Cancer Lett.* **2007**, *252*, 157–170. [CrossRef]
21. McBride, A.A. Human papillomaviruses: Diversity, infection and host interactions. *Nat. Rev. Microbiol.* **2022**, *20*, 95–108. [CrossRef] [PubMed]
22. Jang, M.K.; Shen, K.; McBride, A.A. Papillomavirus genomes associate with brd4 to replicate at fragile sites in the host genome. *PLoS Pathog.* **2014**, *10*, e1004117. [CrossRef] [PubMed]
23. Canela, A.; Maman, Y.; Jung, S.; Wong, N.; Callen, E.; Day, A.; Kieffer-Kwon, K.R.; Pekowska, A.; Zhang, H.; Rao, S.S.P.; et al. Genome organization drives chromosome fragility. *Cell* **2017**, *170*, 507–521.e518. [CrossRef] [PubMed]
24. Barlow, J.H.; Faryabi, R.B.; Callén, E.; Wong, N.; Malhowski, A.; Chen, H.T.; Gutierrez-Cruz, G.; Sun, H.W.; McKinnon, P.; Wright, G.; et al. Identification of early replicating fragile sites that contribute to genome instability. *Cell* **2013**, *152*, 620–632. [CrossRef] [PubMed]
25. Canela, A.; Maman, Y.; Huang, S.N.; Wutz, G.; Tang, W.; Zagnoli-Vieira, G.; Callen, E.; Wong, N.; Day, A.; Peters, J.M.; et al. Topoisomerase ii-induced chromosome breakage and translocation is determined by chromosome architecture and transcriptional activity. *Mol. Cell* **2019**, *75*, 252–266.e258. [CrossRef]
26. Majumder, K.; Wang, J.; Boftsi, M.; Fuller, M.S.; Rede, J.E.; Joshi, T.; Pintel, D.J. Parvovirus minute virus of mice interacts with sites of cellular dna damage to establish and amplify its lytic infection. *Elife* **2018**, *7*, e37750. [CrossRef]
27. Majumder, K.; Boftsi, M.; Whittle, F.B.; Wang, J.; Fuller, M.S.; Joshi, T.; Pintel, D.J. The ns1 protein of the parvovirus mvm aids in the localization of the viral genome to cellular sites of dna damage. *PLoS Pathog.* **2020**, *16*, e1009002. [CrossRef]
28. Schwartz, R.A.; Carson, C.T.; Schuberth, C.; Weitzman, M.D. Adeno-associated virus replication induces a dna damage response coordinated by dna-dependent protein kinase. *J. Virol.* **2009**, *83*, 6269–6278. [CrossRef]
29. Adeyemi, R.O.; Pintel, D.J. The atr signaling pathway is disabled during infection with the parvovirus minute virus of mice. *J. Virol.* **2014**, *88*, 10189–10199. [CrossRef]
30. Majumder, K.; Etingov, I.; Pintel, D.J. Protoparvovirus interactions with the cellular dna damage response. *Viruses* **2017**, *9*, 323. [CrossRef]
31. Cater, J.E.; Pintel, D.J. The small non-structural protein ns2 of the autonomous parvovirus minute virus of mice is required for virus growth in murine cells. *J. Gen. Virol.* **1992**, *73 Pt 7*, 1839–1843. [CrossRef] [PubMed]
32. Schoborg, R.V.; Pintel, D.J. Accumulation of mvm gene products is differentially regulated by transcription initiation, rna processing and protein stability. *Virology* **1991**, *181*, 22–34. [CrossRef] [PubMed]
33. Majumder, K.; Boftsi, M.; Pintel, D.J. Viral chromosome conformation capture (v3c) assays for identifying trans-interaction sites between lytic viruses and the cellular genome. *Bio-Protoc.* **2019**, *9*, e3198. [CrossRef] [PubMed]
34. Boftsi, M.; Majumder, K.; Burger, L.R.; Pintel, D.J. Binding of ccctc-binding factor (ctcf) to the minute virus of mice genome is important for proper processing of viral p4-generated pre-mrnas. *Viruses* **2020**, *12*, 1368. [CrossRef] [PubMed]
35. Bunke, L.E.; Larsen, C.I.S.; Pita-Aquino, J.N.; Jones, I.K.; Majumder, K. The dna damage sensor mre11 regulates efficient replication of the autonomous parvovirus minute virus of mice. *J. Virol.* **2023**, e00461-23, *online ahead of print*. [CrossRef]
36. Ray Chaudhuri, A.; Nussenzweig, A. The multifaceted roles of parp1 in dna repair and chromatin remodelling. *Nat. Rev. Mol. Cell Biol.* **2017**, *18*, 610–621. [CrossRef]
37. Nüesch, J.P.; Rommelaere, J. Ns1 interaction with ckii alpha: Novel protein complex mediating parvovirus-induced cytotoxicity. *J. Virol.* **2006**, *80*, 4729–4739. [CrossRef]
38. Liu, J.; Luo, S.; Zhao, H.; Liao, J.; Li, J.; Yang, C.; Xu, B.; Stern, D.F.; Xu, X.; Ye, K. Structural mechanism of the phosphorylation-dependent dimerization of the mdc1 forkhead-associated domain. *Nucleic Acids Res.* **2012**, *40*, 3898–3912. [CrossRef]
39. Cotmore, S.F.; Nüesch, J.P.; Tattersall, P. Asymmetric resolution of a parvovirus palindrome in vitro. *J. Virol.* **1993**, *67*, 1579–1589. [CrossRef]
40. Cotmore, S.F.; Nuesch, J.P.; Tattersall, P. In vitro excision and replication of 5′ telomeres of minute virus of mice dna from cloned palindromic concatemer junctions. *Virology* **1992**, *190*, 365–377. [CrossRef]
41. Nüesch, J.P.; Rommelaere, J. A viral adaptor protein modulating casein kinase ii activity induces cytopathic effects in permissive cells. *Proc. Natl. Acad. Sci. USA* **2007**, *104*, 12482–12487. [CrossRef] [PubMed]
42. Spycher, C.; Miller, E.S.; Townsend, K.; Pavic, L.; Morrice, N.A.; Janscak, P.; Stewart, G.S.; Stucki, M. Constitutive phosphorylation of mdc1 physically links the mre11-rad50-nbs1 complex to damaged chromatin. *J. Cell Biol.* **2008**, *181*, 227–240. [CrossRef]
43. Blackford, A.N.; Jackson, S.P. Atm, atr, and dna-pk: The trinity at the heart of the dna damage response. *Mol. Cell* **2017**, *66*, 801–817. [CrossRef] [PubMed]
44. Boftsi, M.; Whittle, F.B.; Wang, J.; Shepherd, P.; Burger, L.R.; Kaifer, K.A.; Lorson, C.L.; Joshi, T.; Pintel, D.J.; Majumder, K. The adeno-associated virus 2 (aav2) genome and rep 68/78 proteins interact with cellular sites of dna damage. *Hum. Mol. Genet.* **2021**, *31*, 985–998. [CrossRef] [PubMed]
45. Shah, G.A.; O'Shea, C.C. Viral and cellular genomes activate distinct dna damage responses. *Cell* **2015**, *162*, 987–1002. [CrossRef]

viruses

MDPI

Article

Self-Assembly of Porcine Parvovirus Virus-like Particles and Their Application in Serological Assay

Yanfei Gao [1,†], Haiwei Wang [1,†], Shanghui Wang [1], Mingxia Sun [1], Zheng Fang [1], Xinran Liu [2], Xuehui Cai [1,*] and Yabin Tu [1,*]

[1] State Key Laboratory of Veterinary Biotechnology, Harbin Veterinary Research Institute, Chinese Academy of Agricultural Sciences, Harbin 150069, China

[2] Regeneron Pharmaceuticals Inc., 777 Old Saw Mill River Road, Tarrytown, New York, NY 10591, USA

* Correspondence: caixuehui@caas.cn (X.C.); tutabin@caas.cn (Y.T.); Tel.: +86-451-51051768 (Y.T.); Fax: +86-451-51997166 (X.C. & Y.T.)

† These authors contributed equally to this work.

Abstract: Porcine parvovirus (PPV) is widely prevalent in pig farms. PPV is closely related to porcine respiratory disease complex (PRDC) and porcine circovirus disease (PCVD), which seriously threatens the healthy development of the pig industry. Although commercial antibody detection kits are available, they are expensive and unsuitable for large-scale clinical practice. Here, a soluble VP2 protein of PPV is efficiently expressed in the *E. coli* expression system. The VP2 protein can be self-assembled into virus-like particles (VLPs) in vitro. After multiple steps of chromatography purification, PPV-VLPs with a purity of about 95% were obtained. An indirect, enzyme-linked immunosorbent assay (I-ELISA), comparable to a commercial PPV kit, was developed based on the purified PPV-VLPs and was used to detect 487 clinical pig serum samples. The results showed that the I-ELISA is a simple, cost-effective, and efficient method for the diagnosis of clinical pig serum and plasma samples. In summary, high-purity, tag-free PPV-VLPs were prepared, and the established VLP-based I-ELISA is of great significance for the sero-monitoring of antibodies against PPV.

Keywords: porcine parvovirus; virus-like particles; diagnostic; I-ELISA

Citation: Gao, Y.; Wang, H.; Wang, S.; Sun, M.; Fang, Z.; Liu, X.; Cai, X.; Tu, Y. Self-Assembly of Porcine Parvovirus Virus-like Particles and Their Application in Serological Assay. *Viruses* **2022**, *14*, 1828. https://doi.org/10.3390/v14081828

Academic Editor: Giorgio Gallinella

Received: 25 July 2022
Accepted: 18 August 2022
Published: 20 August 2022

1. Introduction

Porcine parvovirus (PPV), the common causative agent of reproductive failure associated with swine, belongs to the genus *Parvovirus* within the family *Parvoviridae*. The genotypes of PPV have been characterized to date, including seven strains from classical PPV type 1 (PPV1) to six novel strains (PPV2–PPV7). Among the seven viruses, PPV1, first discovered in cell culture contaminants in Germany in 1965 [1], is the most prevalent and is considered to be one of the main pathogens causing infertility and abortion in sows [2]. PPV2–PPV7 were discovered successively through detection techniques, such as metagenomic sequencing [3–8]. A PPV capsid is a small, non-enveloped, icosahedral, and spherical shell, with a diameter size of about 20~25 nm [9], that contains a single-stranded, linear DNA with a genome size of about 5~6 kilobases (kb) [10,11]. There are two main open reading frames (ORF) in the genome of PPV: ORF1, located at the 5′ end, encodes three nonstructural proteins (NS1, NS2, and NS3); and ORF2, located at the 3′ end, encodes three structural proteins (VP1, VP2, and VP3), among which VP2 is the main capsid component and the protective antigen [12].

PPV disease is widespread and mainly affects fetal pigs. PPV can cross the placental barrier to the fetus, which causes porcine reproductive disorder. In pig farms, sows often have clinical manifestations, such as mummification, reduced litter size, sow dystocia, and repeated mating, suggesting that the disease may break out in pig herds [13]. The disease mostly occurs in the spring, summer, sow parturition, and mating season, and once infected, it will quickly spread to the whole herd, making it challenging to eradicate. When sows are infected in the early stage of pregnancy, the mortality rate of embryos and fetuses can be as high as 80% to 100%. The most susceptible period is the first 30 to 40 days of pregnancy. If infection occurs during this period, fetuses become mummified, or smaller litters should be expected, resulting in substantial economic consequences [14]. If PPV infection occurs after fetal immunity has been acquired, fetuses become subclinical.

Virus-like particles (VLPs) are built from one or more units of viral capsid proteins by self-assembling them into morphological structures, with surface conformations similar to those of natural virus particles. Since VLPs do not contain viral nucleic acid, and their conformational epitopes imitate natural virus particles, VLPs are well known for many biological applications in disease control and prevention and diagnostic virology. For example, a VLP-based vaccine can offer several advantages over traditional vaccine approaches (inactivated whole viruses or attenuated viruses) based on a safe production process, low cost, high yield, a variety of overexpression systems, and robust immune responses. Now, PPV-VLPs can be constructed by genetic engineering, which is of great significance for the prevention of PPV. PPV-VLPs are composed of only the structural protein VP2s that automatically form a structure similar to naïve PPV virions in vitro, thus eliciting protective neutralizing antibodies when inoculated in pigs. Previous studies have shown that the recombinant PPV-VP2 protein can be successfully expressed in insect/baculovirus, yeast, and *E.coil* expression systems [15–18] and retains high immunogenicity.

The other application of VLPs is in the development of serological assays detecting antibodies against their natural pathogens. A high-throughput and reliable, serological assay with high sensitivity and specificity are essential for identifying the infected population and current seroprevalence. VLP-based serological assay naturally benefits from the high specificity of VLPs, thus minimizing cross-activity against other viruses. Serological ELISA coated with VLPs has been widely used to detect antibodies or neutralization epitopes [19,20]. For example, the ELISAs coated with VLPs of porcine circovirus type 2 (PCV2) and porcine circovirus type 3 (PCV3) have been reported and proved to have good sensitivity, specificity, and repeatability [21–23]. Recently, a commercial ELISA using an indirect ELISA (I-ELISA) format was developed to detect PPV1 with an unknown antigen expressed in baculovirus growth in insect cells. It is of great interest to compare this commercial kit with I-ELISA based on PPV1 VLPs expressed in *E. coli*. The *E. coli* expression system has the advantages of being cost-effective, having high growth rate, being easy to scale up, having reduced downstream bioprocesses, and having improved protein quality. The PPV-VLP-based I-ELISA (PPV-VLP-ELISA) assay developed based on the *E. coli* expression system should be ideal for extensively and dynamically monitoring PPV spread in swine herds. Considering there is only one serotype of PPV, the method is expected to detect antibodies against all genotypes. Furthermore, high cost and delayed delivery associated with importing currently available PPV commercial kits in the context of persistent inflation necessitate the need to develop domestic kits for efficient PPV control.

In this study, we described a proof-of-concept study to develop a serological I-ELISA method using recombinant PPV-VLPs expressed in the *E. coli* expression system and purified without the introduction of any fusion tags. The sensitivity and specificity of this I-ELISA assay were characterized. Agreement to the commercial I-ELISA kit and the prevalence of PPV in clinical pig samples using this I-ELISA were investigated.

2. Materials and Methods

2.1. Swine Serum Samples

To ensure the specificity of the assay, serum samples were screened for only PPV infection, excluding other pathogens, such as porcine reproductive and respiratory syndrome virus (PRRSV), pseudorabies virus (PRV), and PCV2 by ELISA and PCR. The samples with the highest concentration were selected as positive serum and employed to coat ELISA plates for the PPV-VLP-ELISA and used for ELISA optimization and Western blot. Negative serum samples were obtained from 55 specified, pathogen-free (SPF) piglets, which were collected from the Experimental Animal Center at the Veterinary Research Institute (Harbin,

China). A total of 487 clinical serum samples were collected from northeastern China in 2020 and 2021 for testing via the PPV-VLP-ELISA.

2.2. Gene Amplification and Optimization

The VP2 sequence of PPV obtained from Genbank (Accession No. MF447833) was used as a reference. Subsequently, the VP2 gene was codon-optimized and synthesized by the Genscript Corporation and ligated into the expression vector pET28a.

2.3. Construction and Expression of Recombinant VP2 Protein in E. coli

The recombinant vector pET28a-PPV-VP2 was transformed into BL21(DE3)-competent cells containing chaperone pTf-16. Monoclonal bacteria were selected on the plate containing kanamycin and chloramphenicol, then activated for 12 h at 37 °C and 220 rpm/min in 5 mL of TB medium, which contained 160 ug/mL of chloramphenicol and 50 ug/mL kanamycin. Subsequently, 4 mL of bacterial solution was transferred to 200 mL of TB culture medium at the ratio of 1:50 at the same temperature and shaking speed for 2 h 30 min, after which the temperature was reduced to 16 °C, and IPTG and L-Arabinose with the final concentration of 0.1 mmol/L and 2 mg/ mL were added to induce VP2 expression for 20 h. Upon completion of protein induction, the bacteria culture was centrifuged at 6000 g/min for 10 min. The cell pellets were weighed (g) and resuspended in a disruption buffer (200 mM NaCl, 20 mM Tris-HCl, 10% glycerol, pH 8.0) at a ratio of 1 (wet bacteria weight (g)): 10 (disruption buffer (mL)). After mixing well, sonication was performed with an ultrasonic cell disruptor (Cole Parmer, Vernon Hills, IL, USA). SDS-PAGE and Western blot were used to check the expression and solubility of the recombinant VP2 protein. After protein electrophoresis, one part was stained with Coomassie brilliant blue, and the other part was transferred to a PVDF membrane in PBST for 2 h. The PVDF membrane was washed three times with PBST for 15 min and probed with the PPV-specific positive serum (1:5000 dilution) for 1 h at RT. The PVDF membrane was washed three times again and detected with fluorescently-labeled anti-pig secondary antibody (Biodragon, Beijing China, 1:10,000) for 40 min at RT. The PVDF membrane was then washed three times again in the dark and then scanned on a near-infrared fluorescence scanning imaging system (Odyssey CLX, USA).

2.4. Purification of PPV-VLPs

The sonicated solution was clarified at 12,000 g/min for 30 min to remove bacterial debris and inclusion bodies. The supernatant was precipitated with PEG6000, and the protein precipitate was centrifuged at 12,000 g/min for 30 min. The pellet was resuspended in resuspension buffer (20 mM Tris, pH 8.0). The resuspended solution was loaded on a DEAE Bestarose Fast Flow column (Bestchrom, Shanghai, China) in an automated FPLC system (AKTA, GE-Healthcare Life Sciences, USA), and the fractions containing effluent from the bulk VLPs were collected. The effluent fractions were subjected to a Sepharose 6FF 16/96 column (Bestchrom, China) equilibrated with equilibration buffer (20 mM Tris-HCl, pH 8.0) at the flow rate of 1.5 mL/min, and the second half of the first peak was collected. The collected protein fractions were further loaded onto a heparin-agarose column (Bestchrom, China) and eluted with elution buffer (500 mM NaCl, 20 mM Tris-HCl). Finally, the eluted fraction was passed through a Sepharose 6FF 16/96 column (Bestchrom, China), which was equilibrated with equilibration buffer (20 mM Tris-HCl, pH 8.0) at a flow rate of 1.5 mL/min. The first peak was collected in separate 15 mL centrifuge tubes, with 10 mL per tube. The protein elutions were analyzed with SDS-PAGE and TEM.

2.5. TEM Procedure of PPV-VLPs

The sample was incubated for 10 min at RT. Subsequently, the PPV-VLPs were fully adsorbed onto the copper mesh and dried at RT. The copper mesh was negatively stained with 2.5% phosphotungstic acid for 1 min after being dried, and the excess stain was blotted off using filter paper and carefully placed on the TEM (HITACHI, Tokyo, Japan) for observation.

2.6. Determination of Hemagglutination of PPV-VLPs

The hemagglutination activity of PPV-VLPs was determined by a hemagglutination assay. In a 96-well V-plate, 25 uL PBS was added to each well, then 25 uL PPV-VLPs were added to the first column of wells and mixed to generate 2-fold dilution. Then, 25 uL of the 2-fold-diluted PPV-VLPs were added to the second column of wells and mixed, repeating the dilution pattern across the plate to complete the 2-fold serial dilutions of antigen PPV-VLPs. A total of 25 uL 1% chicken erythrocyte suspension was added to the plate and shaken for 2 min to mix well. The control group used only 25 uL of PBS and 25 uL of 1% chicken red blood cell suspension. The results were determined 1 h later, and the highest dilution that allowed 100% agglutination of red blood cells was the hemagglutination titer of PPV-VLPs.

2.7. Optimization of the PPV-VLP-ELISA Procedure

Purified PPV-VLPs were used as antigens to develop I-ELISA. The checkerboard method was applied to determine the optimal serum dilution and antigen-coating concentration. The concentration of PPV-VLPs was determined by a BCA kit (Thermo, Waltham, MA, USA). PPV-VLPs were diluted to 0.5 ug/mL, 1 ug/mL, 2.5 ug/mL, 5 ug/mL, 7.5 ug/mL, and 10 ug/mL in carbonate coating buffer (pH 9.6) and then plated on ELISA plates (Biofil, Guangzhou, China) to determine the optimal antigen-coating concentration. Positive and negative sera were diluted at 1:50, 1:100, and 1:150 (*v*/*v*) with PBST to determine the optimal serum dilution. Additionally, the reaction time, temperature, and other conditions were optimized.

2.8. Standardization of PPV-VLP-ELISA Procedure

PPV-VLPs were coated with 100 μL/well, at a concentration of 1 μg/mL, in a 96-well ELISA microplate (Biofil, China) overnight at 4 °C. The coated plates were washed three times with PBST and then blocked with an enzyme plate stabilizer (InnoReagents, China) for 2 h in a 37 °C incubator (Yiheng, Shanghai, China). The blocked plates were washed three times, and 100 μL of the diluted serum samples were added and incubated at 37 °C for 1 h. Then, the plates were washed three times, and 100 μL HRP-SPA dilution (Bosterbio, Wuhan, China, 1:10,000) was added and incubated for 1 h at 37 °C. After the three-time washes, 100 μL of tetramethylbenzidine (TMB, Solarbio, Beijing, China) was added to each well and incubated for 15 min at 37 °C in the dark. Finally, 50 μL of stop solution (1M HCl) was added to stop the reaction, and the OD450nm value was measured with an ELISA plate reader (PE, Corona, CA, USA).

2.9. Determination of Cut-Off Value

Fifty-five negative sera were employed to determine the cut-off value. All sera were analyzed by PPV-VLP-ELISA three times independently to reduce the deviation. The mean OD450nm value (X) and standard deviation (SD) were calculated, and the cut-off value was defined as X + 3SD.

2.10. Reproducibility and Cross-Reactivity Assay

Twelve serum samples were selected to evaluate the reproducibility of the PPV-VLP-ELISA. For each sample, the coefficient of variation (CV) values between plates (inter-assay variation) and within plates (intra-assay variation) were calculated. The results showed that both the inter-assay and intra-assay variation were less than 10%. Four positive sera and one negative serum diluted at 1:50, 1:100, 1:200, 1:400, 1:800, 1:1600, 1:3200, and 1:6400 were applied to evaluate the sensitivity of this method. The specificity of the method was evaluated by comparing the OD450nm values of the standard positive serum with those of the selected, potentially interfering viruses (African swine fever virus (ASFV), Japanese encephalitis virus (JEV), PRRSV, foot-and-mouth disease virus (FMDV), PCV2, simian immunodeficiency virus (SIV), transmissible gastroenteritis virus (TGEV), and porcine epidemic diarrhea virus (PEDV)).

2.11. Cultivation and Proliferation of PPV

Pig kidney (PK-15) cells were obtained and preserved by the Harbin Veterinary Research Institute (Harbin, China). The PK-15 cells were revived in the cell culture flask, and when the bottom of the flask was confluent with PK-15 cells, the cells were digested and transferred to a new flask. PPV was then inoculated into the flask and cultured in a cell incubator (Thermo, USA) at 37 °C and 5% carbon dioxide. When about 80% of the inoculated cells became cytopathic, they were repeatedly incubated. The viruses were fully released by three freeze–thaw cycles and were harvested at 2000 r/min for 10 min to remove cell debris and frozen at −80 °C.

2.12. Comparison of the PPV-VLP-ELISA with the Commercial PPV ELISA Kit for Detection of Anti-PPV Antibodies

Sixty-four samples were randomly selected from 487 serum samples for comparison between commercial ELISA kits (Ingenasa, Spain) and PPV-VLP-ELISA. Sixty-four samples were tested using a commercial kit, according to the instructions, and positive and negative samples were placed and labeled separately. These samples were subsequently tested using PPV-VLP-ELISA. Each serum was analyzed three times independently, using commercial kits and PPV-VLP-ELISA to minimize bias.

2.13. Indirect Immunofluorescence Assay Verification of Five Positive Samples Determined by PPV-VLP-ELISA

The five positive serum samples to be tested were named A, B, C, D, and E, respectively, and then an indirect immunofluorescence assay (IFA) was performed. First, PK-15 cells were infected with PPV for 48 h, after which the cells were fixed with 4% paraformaldehyde for 30 min at RT and then washed with PBS three times. Permeabilization fluid (0.25% Triton-X100) was added at 100 uL/well and was placed on ice for 15 min. After washing three times with PBS, a blocking solution (5% BSA) was added for 1 h. After another three-time wash, the serum samples and SPF serum were diluted at 1:100, added to the wells, and incubated at 37 °C for 2 h. After another three-time wash, a FITC-labeled goat anti-pig secondary antibody (Sigma, Burlington, MA, USA) was added at a dilution of 1:200 and incubated at 37 °C for 1 h. After the last three-time washes, results were measured with an inverted fluorescence microscope (AMG, Denver, CO, USA).

3. Results

3.1. Expression and Purification of PPV-VLPs from E. coli

The recombinant plasmid pET28a-PPV-VP2 was constructed and transformed in *E. coli* BL21 (DE3) competent cells, and cells containing the plasmid were inoculated in TB medium. The recombinant VP2 protein (molecular weight ~64 kDa) was IPTG- and L-Arabinose-induced with or without the co-expression of the chaperone plasmid pTf-16. When expressed in the absence of chaperone pTf-16, the VP2 protein was poorly expressed and less soluble (Figure 1A). When co-expressed with chaperone pTf-16, both the expression and solubility of the VP2 protein significantly increased (Figure 1B). Western blot analysis also confirmed the folding of the VP2 protein obtained from chaperone pTf-16 co-expression, as it reacted with specific positive sera (Figure 2A). As described above, expressed VP2 proteins were purified by three columns: ion-exchange column (IEC), size-exclusion column (SEC), and heparin-agarose column (HP). While self-assembled PPV-VLPs were observed after HP (Figure 2B), a few heterogeneous protein bands and odd-shaped impurity particles around 25 nm could also be clearly observed under SDS-PAGE (Figure 2C) and TEM (Figure 2D). PPV-VP2 proteins were further purified via another SEC (Figure 3A–C). Homogeneous and intact particles without any impurities were observed under TEM (Figure 3D).

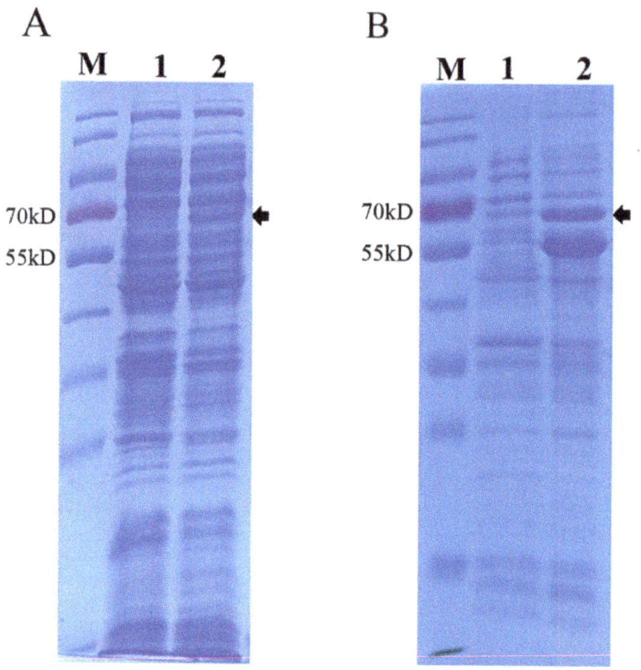

Figure 1. SDS-PAGE analysis of PPV VP2 protein expression in E. coli. (**A**) Coomassie staining of PPV VP2 protein expressed in *E. coli* without chaperone pTf-16. (**B**) Coomassie staining of PPV VP2 protein in *E. coli* co-expressed with chaperone pTf-16. M. Marker. Lane 1, Coomassie staining of PPV VP2 protein before IPTG and L-Arabinose induction. Lane 2, Coomassie staining of PPV VP2 protein after IPTG and L-Arabinose induction.

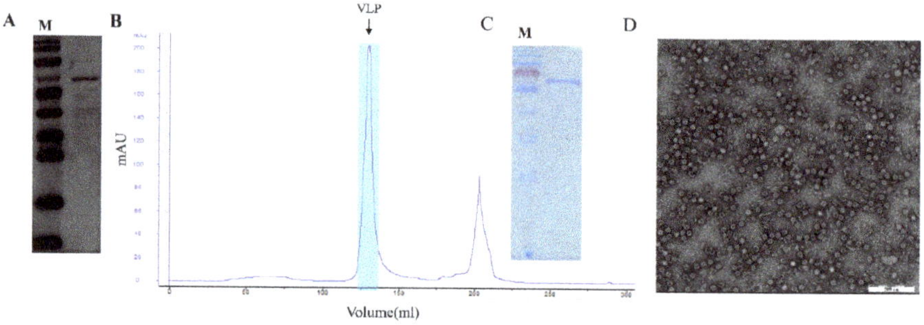

Figure 2. Analysis and purification of PPV VP2 protein and PPV-VLPs after initial HP. (**A**) Western blot analysis of PPV VP2 protein probed with specific positive serum. (**B**) Heparin-affinity profile of self-assembled PPV-VLPs. The peak represents properly-assembled PPV-VLPs. (**C**) Coomassie staining of the PPV VP2 protein. (**D**) The TEM image of the PPV-VLPs.

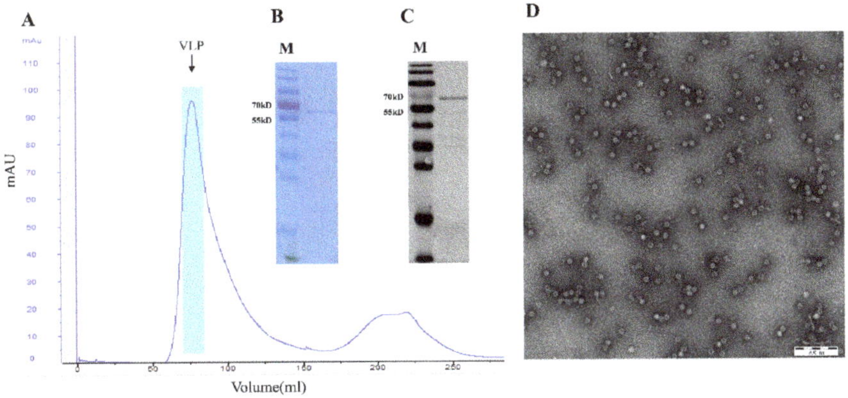

Figure 3. Analysis of PPV VP2 protein and PPV-VLPs after 2nd SEC purification. (**A**) SEC profile of PPV-VLPs. The peak represents properly-assembled PPV-VLPs. (**B**) Coomassie staining of the PPV VP2 proteins after 2nd SEC purification. (**C**) Western blot analysis of the more purified PPV VP2 proteins. (**D**) TEM image of the PPV-VLPs.

3.2. Hemagglutination Activity of PPV-VLPs

The hemagglutination activity of PPV-VLPs was confirmed to be 2^8 (1:256) (Figure 4), indicating that the PPV-VLPs correctly displayed the epitope of PPV required for hemagglutination activity, and the structure was similar to that of the native PPV.

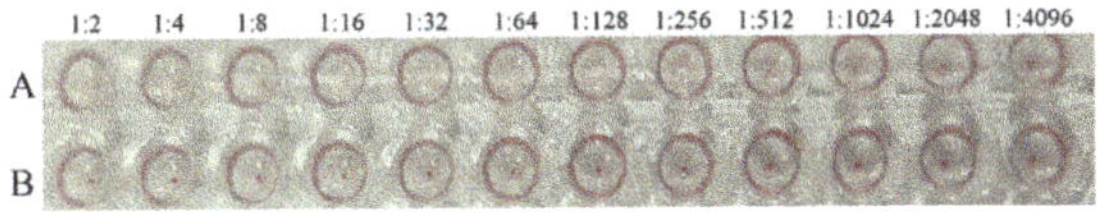

Figure 4. The hemagglutination test of PPV-VLPs. (**A**) Hemagglutination titer of the purified PPV-VLPs. (**B**) The negative control.

3.3. Standardization of the PPV-VLP-ELISA Procedure

The optimization of the VLP-based I-ELISA was guided by OD450nm and P/N values (ratio of the OD value of a test sample to the average OD value of negative control). A total of 50 mM of carbonate-bicarbonate buffer (pH 9.6) and plate stabilizer were selected as the final coating and blocking buffers, respectively. The concentration of purified PPV-VLPs was determined to be 0.1 mg/mL using the BCA protein concentration measurement kit (Thermo, USA). Checkerboard titration experiments showed that when coating concentration for PPV-VLPs was 1 μg/mL and the serum dilution was 1:50, the P/N ratio can be ultimately optimized. All experiments were performed in triplicate (Table 1). Fifty-five negative serum samples were used to determine cut-off values, with the mean OD and SD values of 0.149 and 0.059, respectively (Figure 5A). Therefore, the cut-off value for the PPV-VLP-ELISA was 0.326 (X + 3SD). Serum with an OD450nm value greater than or equal to this threshold was considered positive. Otherwise, it was determined to be negative for PPV antibodies. The experiments showed that this optimized method has good sensitivity and specificity (Figure 5B,C).

Table 1. Optimal sample dilutions and coating antigen for PPV-VLP-ELISA.

Serum Dilution	Concentration of Coating Antigen (X ± SD, ug/mL)					
	10	**7.5**	**5**	**2.5**	**1**	**0.5**
1:50 (+)	1.194 ± 0.0898	1.524 ± 0.0757	1.675 ± 0.0764	1.199 ± 0.0396	1.966 ± 0.0233	1.225 ± 0.0452
1:50 (−)	0.0985 ± 0.002	0.0965 ± 0.002	0.1565 ± 0.023	0.1085 ± 0.013	0.1225 ± 0.011	0.113 ± 0.01
P/N	13.13	15.78	10.70	11.05	17.47	10.84
1:100 (+)	0.517 ± 0.021	0.8335 ± 0.047	1.1095 ± 0.046	0.6395 ± 0.122	1.52 ± 0.1075	0.945 ± 0.006
1:100 (−)	0.1 ± 0.002	0.1185 ± 0.0021	0.149 ± 0.0028	0.0915 ± 0.009	0.119 ± 0.01	0.1105 ± 0.004
P/N	5.10	7.3	7.45	6.99	12.77	8.55
1:150 (+)	0.728 ± 0.11	1.156 ± 0.113	1.1011 ± 0.016	0.754 ± 0.0339	1.268 ± 0.012	0.8925 ± 0.0446
1:150 (−)	0.127 ± 0.037	0.087 ± 0.0212	0.0875 ± 0.013	0.174 ± 0.0368	0.087 ± 0.007	0.1185 ± 0.0629
P/N	5.73	13.29	11.55	5.26	12.22	6.69

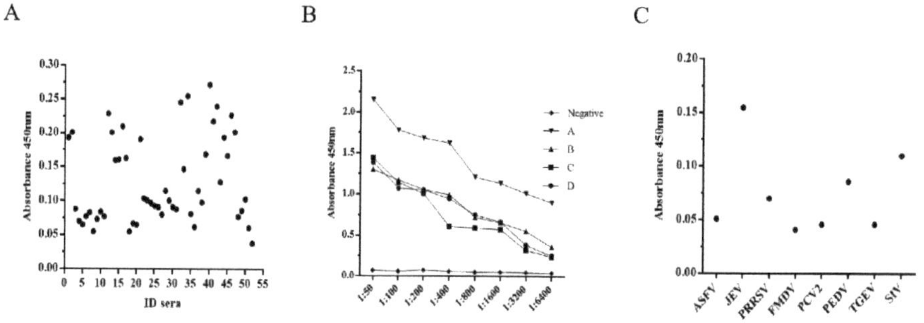

Figure 5. Characterization of PPV-VLP-ELISA. (**A**) Determination of the cut-off value for PPV-VLP-ELISA. (**B**) Determination of the sensitivity of PPV-VLP-ELISA. (**C**) Determination of the specificity of PPV-VLP-ELISA.

3.4. Coincidence Rate with the Ingezim PPV ELISA Kit for Detection of Anti-PPV Antibodies

Clinical pig serum samples (n = 64) were used to determine the reliability of the PPV-VLP-ELISA compared to the commercial PPV-ELISA kit. These sera were randomly selected from 487 serum samples and tested using both commercial ELISA kits and PPV-VLP-ELISA developed in-house. When tested using the commercial ELISA kit, 36 (56.25%) of 64 serum samples were positive and 28 (43.75%) of 64 serum samples were negative. When tested using the PPV-VLP-ELISA method,. 41 (64.1%) of 64 serum samples were positive and 23 (35.9%) of 64 serum samples were negative (Table 2). The results were similar to the commercial ELISA kit, as the overall concordance rate was 92.2% (59/64) between PPV-VLP-ELISA and the commercially available PPV-Ingenasa-ELISA kit. Among 41 samples tested positive by PPV-VLP-ELISA, 36 samples also tested positive in the commercial kit and the other 5 samples tested negative in the commercial kit. The results suggested that the sensitivity and specificity of PPV-VLP-ELISA were at least comparable to those of the commercial kits.

Table 2. Comparison of the PPV-VLP-ELISA with the commercial PPV ELISA kit for detection of anti-PPV antibodies.

PPV-VLP-ELISA	Commercial Kit		
	Positive	**Negative**	**Total**
Positive	36	5	41
Negative	0	23	23
Total	36	28	64

3.5. Confirmation of PPV-VLP-ELISA Tested Positive Samples with Indirect Immunofluorescence Assay

The IFA results agreed with the PPV-VLP-ELISA results. Five positive sera determined by PPV-VLP-ELISA were also confirmed positive by IFA. SPF serum as a negative control was proved to be negative by IFA (Figure 6).

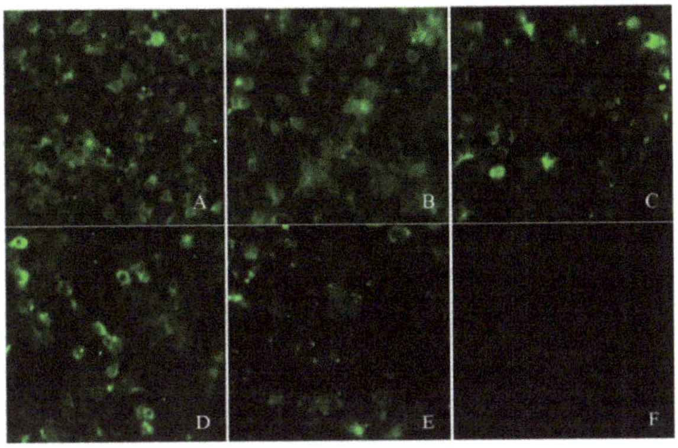

Figure 6. Reactivity of five positive sera with PPV antibodies by IFA. (**A–E**) are the IFA results of the five sera, respectively. (**F**) IFA analysis of SPF pig serum (negative control).

3.6. Application of PPV-VLP-ELISA to Screen Clinical Pig Serum Samples

Swine serum samples collected in northeast China in 2020 and 2021 were tested with PPV-VLP-ELISA. A total of 432 samples (88.7%) tested positive, and 55 samples (11.3%) tested negative. The result showed a high positive rate of PPV antibodies in the tested herd (Figure 7), indicating that PPV is widespread in pig farms and poses a serious threat to the local pig industry. In conclusion, PPV-VLP-ELISA has high application value in the monitoring and eradication of PPV in the future.

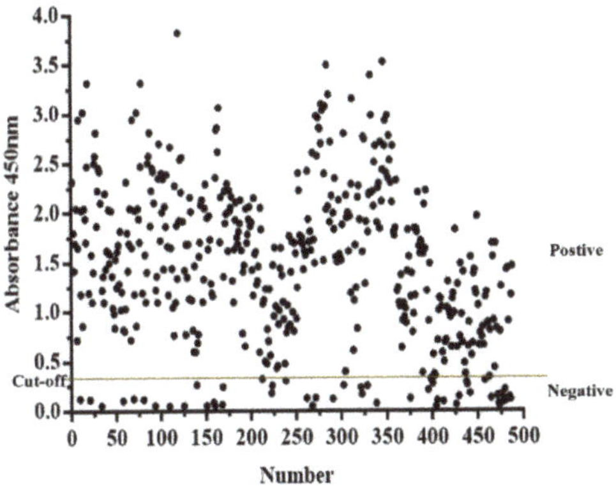

Figure 7. PPV-VLP-ELISA was employed to screen clinical swine serum samples (n = 487).

4. Discussion

Currently, different expression host systems can express VLPs, including bacteria, insect, yeast, mammalian cell, cell-free, and plant expression systems [24]. Recombivax HB, the world's first genetically engineered vaccine for the prevention of hepatitis B, is a VLP vaccine expressed by the *saccharomyces cerevisiae* expression system [25,26]. From then on, multiple VLP vaccines were approved, including human papillomavirus (HPV), hepatitis B virus (HBV), hepatitis E virus (HEV), and H1N1 vaccine, etc. [27]. About 30% of approved VLP vaccines are produced by bacterial expression systems, mainly in *E. coli*. Other VLP bacterial expression systems besides *E. coli*, *Lactobacillus*, and *Pseudomonas aeruginosa* are responsible for vaccines against HPV and cowpea chlorosis mottle virus (CCMV) [28,29]. While bacterial expression systems may have many advantages in expressing VLPs, such as high growth rate, being easy-to-scale up, and low cost, their applications should be evaluated cautiously due to the lack of post-translational modification of proteins. Concerns about endotoxin contamination may further reduce the scope of its application [30]. The yeast expression system is widely used to produce VLPs for HPV and HBV. Insect and mammalian cell expression systems have been used to produce VLPs since the 1980s. The plant cell expression system and cell-free expression system have recently been found capable of producing VLPs.

VLPs only contain viral capsid proteins but no viral genetic material. Their conformational epitopes and morphological structure are similar to those of natural viruses and have good immunogenicity [31,32]. VLPs can induce strong humoral and cellular immune responses and are considered a highly efficient vaccine platform [33]. In recent years, the technologies of expressing PPV VP2 proteins and self-assembly into VLPs have been greatly advanced. These new technologies have been advancing the production and future development of VLP-based vaccines [18]. PPV VP2 is a non-enveloped protein that can self-assemble into VLPs under suitable conditions, without additional modifications. Therefore, compared with other eukaryotic expression systems, the *E. coli* expression system, without protein modifications, is proper and desirable for producing VP2 proteins. Assembled PPV-VLPs are highly likely to form conformation similar to that of natural viral particles. The suitability of the *E. coli* expression system to produce the VP2 protein was verified by both the results from PPV-VLP-ELISA and previous studies regarding VLP-based vaccines [18,34].

In this study, the *E. coli* expression system has been employed successfully to express and purify tag-free PPV-VLPs. PPV-VLPs have many advantages, including cost-effectiveness, high-yield expression, and high-density cultivation. Thus, it is significant for diagnosis and vaccine development.

The VLP has only viral structural proteins without viral genetic material, and its morphological structure is similar to that of natural virus particles [35,36]. It is capable of mimicking external epitopes and conformational epitopes of viruses [37,38]. Therefore, the VLP is more suitable for establishing the ELISA diagnostic method. Recent studies have shown that the PPV is closely related to porcine respiratory diseases, so monitoring and vaccination against the PPV plays an important role in the prevention and treatment of PRDC and PCVD [39,40]. Therefore, establishing a diagnostic method with high sensitivity, high specificity, and suitability for large-scale screening is of great significance for the control of PPV. This paper successfully showed a high-sensitivity, high-specificity, and low-cost PPV-VLP-ELISA method using high-purity PPV-VLPs. Subsequently, the VLP-ELISA method was successfully used for PPV antibody detection in 487 clinical serum samples collected in northeast China in 2020 and 2021. It was found that PPV was widely prevalent in Chinese pig farms, indicating that this method can be widely used in PPV epidemiological studies.

5. Conclusions

The *E. coli* expression system has been employed for the expression and purification of tag-free PPV-VLPs, which could be used for the development of a VLP-based PPV vaccine. In addition, this is the first report of the I-ELISA method based on PPV-VLPs for testing the PPV-specific antibodies in clinical pig serum. The PPV-VLP-ELISA is highly specific, sensitive, and reproducible. It is a valuable tool for monitoring the prevalence of PPV.

Author Contributions: Y.T. and X.C. conceptualized the work and designed the studies; Y.G., H.W., S.W., and M.S. performed the experiments; Y.T., Z.F., and X.C. analyzed the data. Y.G. X.L., and H.W. wrote the manuscript. All authors have read and agreed to the published version of the manuscript.

Funding: This study was supported by a grant from the Open Project of State Key Laboratory of Urban Water Resource and Environment from the Harbin Institute of Technology (No. HC202023).

Institutional Review Board Statement: Not applicable.

Informed Consent Statement: Not applicable.

Data Availability Statement: The data presented in this study are available upon request from the corresponding author.

Acknowledgments: We are greatly indebted to our colleagues for providing technical support and valuable suggestions.

Conflicts of Interest: The authors declare that they have no competing interests.

Disclaimer: Xinran Liu, current employment Regeneron Pharmaceuticals, Inc. Xinran Liu contributed to this article, and the views expressed do not necessarily represent the views of Regeneron Pharmaceuticals Inc.

References

1. Mayr, A.; Bachmann, P.A.; Siegl, G.; Mahnel, H.; Sheffy, B.E. Characterization of a Small Porcine DNA Virus. *Arch. Gesamte Virusforsch.* **1968**, *25*, 38–51. [CrossRef] [PubMed]
2. Cadar, D.; Csagola, A.; Kiss, T.; Tuboly, T. Capsid protein evolution and comparative phylogeny of novel porcine parvoviruses. *Mol. Phylogenet. Evol.* **2013**, *66*, 243–253. [CrossRef] [PubMed]
3. Cheung, A.K.; Wu, G.; Wang, D.; Bayles, D.O.; Lager, K.M.; Vincent, A.L. Identification and molecular cloning of a novel porcine parvovirus. *Arch. Virol.* **2010**, *155*, 801–806. [CrossRef]
4. Hijikata, M.; Abe, K.; Win, K.M.; Shimizu, Y.K.; Keicho, N.; Yoshikura, H. Identification of new parvovirus DNA sequence in swine sera from Myanmar. *Jpn. J. Infect. Dis.* **2001**, *54*, 244. [PubMed]
5. Lau, S.; Woo, P.; Tse, H.; Fu, C.; Au, W.; Chen, X.; Tsoi, H.; Tsang, T.; Chan, J.; Tsang, D.; et al. Identification of novel porcine and bovine parvoviruses closely related to human parvovirus 4. *J. Gen. Virol.* **2008**, *89*, 1840–1848. [CrossRef] [PubMed]
6. Ni, J.; Qiao, C.; Han, X.; Han, T.; Kang, W.; Zi, Z.; Cao, Z.; Zhai, X.; Cai, X. Identification and genomic characterization of a novel porcine parvovirus (PPV6) in China. *Virol. J.* **2014**, *11*, 203. [CrossRef]
7. Schirtzinger, E.; Suddith, A.; Hause, B.; Hesse, R.A. First identification of porcine parvovirus 6 in North America by viral metagenomic sequencing of serum from pigs infected with porcine reproductive and respiratory syndrome virus. *Virol. J.* **2015**, *12*, 170. [CrossRef]
8. Xiao, C.; Giménez-Lirola, L.; Jiang, Y.; Halbur, P.; Opriessnig, T. Characterization of a novel porcine parvovirus tentatively designated PPV5. *PLoS ONE* **2013**, *8*, e65312.
9. Afolabi, K.O.; Iweriebor, B.C.; Okoh, A.I.; Obi, L.C. Increasing diversity of swine parvoviruses and their epidemiology in African pigs. *Infect. Genet. Evol.* **2019**, *73*, 175–183. [CrossRef]
10. Novosel, D.; Cadar, D.; Tuboly, T.; Jungic, A.; Stadejek, T.; Ait-Ali, T.; Csagola, A. Investigating porcine parvoviruses genogroup 2 infection using in situ polymerase chain reaction. *BMC Vet. Res.* **2018**, *14*, 163. [CrossRef]
11. Ranz, A.I.; Manclús, J.J.; Díaz-Aroca, E.; Casal, J.I. Porcine Parvovirus: DNA Sequence and Genome Organization. *J. Gen. Virol.* **1989**, *70*, 2541–2553. [CrossRef] [PubMed]
12. Xu, Y.; Li, Y. Induction of immune responses in mice after intragastric administration of Lactobacillus casei producing porcine parvovirus VP2 protein. *Appl. Env. Microbiol.* **2007**, *73*, 7041–7047. [CrossRef] [PubMed]
13. Meszaros, I.; Olasz, F.; Csagola, A.; Tijssen, P.; Zadori, Z. Biology of Porcine Parvovirus (Ungulate parvovirus 1). *Viruses* **2017**, *9*, 393. [CrossRef] [PubMed]
14. Streck, A.F.; Truyen, U. Porcine Parvovirus. *Curr. Issues Mol. Biol.* **2020**, *37*, 33–46. [CrossRef]
15. Antonis, A.F.; Bruschke, C.J.; Rueda, P.; Maranga, L.; Casal, J.I.; Vela, C.; Hilgers, L.A.; Belt, P.B.; Weerdmeester, K.; Carrondo, M.J.; et al. A novel recombinant virus-like particle vaccine for prevention of porcine parvovirus-induced reproductive failure. *Vaccine* **2006**, *24*, 5481–5490. [CrossRef]
16. Guo, C.; Zhong, Z.; Huang, Y. Production and immunogenicity of VP2 protein of porcine parvovirus expressed in Pichia pastoris. *Arch. Virol.* **2013**, *159*, 963–970. [CrossRef]
17. Yang, D.; Chen, L.; Duan, J.; Yu, Y.; Zhou, J.; Lu, H. Investigation of Kluyveromyces marxianus as a novel host for large-scale production of porcine parvovirus virus-like particles. *Microb. Cell Fact.* **2021**, *20*, 24. [CrossRef]
18. Wang, J.; Liu, Y.; Chen, Y.; Wang, A.; Wei, Q.; Liu, D.; Zhang, G. Large-scale manufacture of VP2 VLP vaccine against porcine parvovirus in Escherichia coli with high-density fermentation. *Appl. Microbiol. Biotechnol.* **2020**, *104*, 3847–3857. [CrossRef]
19. Almanza, H.; Cubillos, C.; Angulo, I.; Mateos, F.; Caston, J.R.; van der Poel, W.H.; Vinje, J.; Barcena, J.; Mena, I. Self-assembly of the recombinant capsid protein of a swine norovirus into virus-like particles and evaluation of monoclonal antibodies cross-reactive with a human strain from genogroup II. *J. Clin. Microbiol.* **2008**, *46*, 3971–3979. [CrossRef]
20. Chao, D.Y.; Whitney, M.T.; Davis, B.S.; Medina, F.A.; Munoz, J.L.; Chang, G.J. Comprehensive Evaluation of Differential Serodiagnosis between Zika and Dengue Viral Infections. *J. Clin. Microbiol.* **2019**, *57*, e01506-18. [CrossRef]

21. Nainys, J.; Lasickiene, R.; Petraityte-Burneikiene, R.; Dabrisius, J.; Lelesius, R.; Sereika, V.; Zvirbliene, A.; Sasnauskas, K.; Gedvilaite, A. Generation in yeast of recombinant virus-like particles of porcine circovirus type 2 capsid protein and their use for a serologic assay and development of monoclonal antibodies. *BMC Biotechnol.* **2014**, *14*, 100. [CrossRef] [PubMed]
22. Wang, Y.; Wang, G.; Duan, W.T.; Sun, M.X.; Wang, M.H.; Wang, S.H.; Cai, X.H.; Tu, Y.B. Self-assembly into virus-like particles of the recombinant capsid protein of porcine circovirus type 3 and its application on antibodies detection. *AMB Express* **2020**, *10*, 3. [CrossRef]
23. Zhang, Y.; Wang, Z.; Zhan, Y.; Gong, Q.; Yu, W.; Deng, Z.; Wang, A.; Yang, Y.; Wang, N. Generation of *E. coli*-derived virus-like particles of porcine circovirus type 2 and their use in an indirect IgG enzyme-linked immunosorbent assay. *Arch. Virol.* **2016**, *161*, 1485–1491. [CrossRef] [PubMed]
24. Santi, L.; Huang, Z.; Mason, H. Virus-like particles production in green plants. *Methods* **2006**, *40*, 66–76. [CrossRef] [PubMed]
25. Ho, J.K.; Jeevan-Raj, B.; Netter, H.J. Hepatitis B Virus (HBV) Subviral Particles as Protective Vaccines and Vaccine Platforms. *Viruses* **2020**, *12*, 126. [CrossRef] [PubMed]
26. Michel, M.L.; Tiollais, P. Hepatitis B vaccines: Protective efficacy and therapeutic potential. *Pathol. Biol.* **2010**, *58*, 288–295. [CrossRef] [PubMed]
27. Shirbaghaee, Z.; Bolhassani, A. Different applications of virus-like particles in biology and medicine: Vaccination and delivery systems. *Biopolymers* **2016**, *105*, 113–132. [CrossRef]
28. Aires, K.A.; Cianciarullo, A.M.; Carneiro, S.M.; Villa, L.L.; Boccardo, E.; Pérez-Martinez, G.; Perez-Arellano, I.; Oliveira, M.L.S.; Ho, P.L. Production of Human Papillomavirus Type 16 L1 Virus-Like Particles by Recombinant Lactobacillus casei Cells. *Appl. Environ. Microbiol.* **2006**, *72*, 745–752. [CrossRef]
29. Phelps, J.P.; Dao, P.; Jin, H.; Rasochova, L. Expression and self-assembly of cowpea chlorotic mottle virus-like particles in Pseudomonas fluorescens. *J. Biotechnol.* **2007**, *128*, 290–296. [CrossRef]
30. Zhao, Q.; Allen, M.J.; Wang, Y.; Wang, B.; Wang, N.; Shi, L.; Sitrin, R.D. Disassembly and reassembly improves morphology and thermal stability of human papillomavirus type 16 virus-like particles. *Nanomedicine* **2012**, *8*, 1182–1189. [CrossRef]
31. Ding, X.; Liu, D.; Booth, G.; Gao, W.; Lu, Y. Virus-Like Particle Engineering: From Rational Design to Versatile Applications. *Biotechnol. J.* **2018**, *13*, e1700324. [CrossRef] [PubMed]
32. Yadav, R.; Zhai, L.; Tumban, E. Virus-like Particle-Based L2 Vaccines against HPVs: Where Are We Today? *Viruses* **2019**, *12*, 18. [CrossRef] [PubMed]
33. Lamarre, B.; Ryadnov, M.G. Self-assembling viral mimetics: One long journey with short steps. *Macromol. Biosci.* **2011**, *11*, 503–513. [CrossRef]
34. Wang, K.; Zhou, L.; Chen, T.; Li, Q.; Li, J.; Liu, L.; Li, Y.; Sun, J.; Li, T.; Wang, Y.; et al. Engineering for an HPV 9-valent vaccine candidate using genomic constitutive over-expression and low lipopolysaccharide levels in Escherichia coli cells. *Microb. Cell Fact.* **2021**, *20*, 227. [CrossRef]
35. He, J.; Cao, J.; Zhou, N.; Jin, Y.; Wu, J.; Zhou, J. Identification and functional analysis of the novel ORF4 protein encoded by porcine circovirus type 2. *J. Virol.* **2013**, *87*, 1420–1429. [CrossRef] [PubMed]
36. Hsu, C.W.; Chang, M.H.; Chang, H.W.; Wu, T.Y.; Chang, Y.C. Parenterally Administered Porcine Epidemic Diarrhea Virus-Like Particle-Based Vaccine Formulated with CCL25/28 Chemokines Induces Systemic and Mucosal Immune Protectivity in Pigs. *Viruses* **2020**, *12*, 1122. [CrossRef] [PubMed]
37. Brune, K.D.; Howarth, M. New Routes and Opportunities for Modular Construction of Particulate Vaccines: Stick, Click, and Glue. *Front. Immunol.* **2018**, *9*, 1432. [CrossRef]
38. Lua, L.H.L.; Connors, N.K.; Sainsbury, F.; Chuan, Y.P.; Wibowo, N.; Middelberg, A.P.J. Bioengineering virus-like particles as vaccines. *Biotechnol. Bioeng.* **2014**, *111*, 425–440. [CrossRef]
39. Nelsen, A.; Lin, C.-M.; Hause, B.M. Porcine Parvovirus 2 Is Predominantly Associated With Macrophages in Porcine Respiratory Disease Complex. *Front. Vet. Sci.* **2021**, *8*, 726884. [CrossRef]
40. Lagan Tregaskis, P.; Staines, A.; Gordon, A.; Sheridan, P.; McMenamy, M.; Duffy, C.; Collins, P.J.; Mooney, M.H.; Lemon, K. Co-infection status of novel parvovirus's (PPV2 to 4) with porcine circovirus 2 in porcine respiratory disease complex and porcine circovirus-associated disease from 1997 to 2012. *Transbound. Emerg. Dis.* **2021**, *68*, 1979–1994. [CrossRef]

viruses

MDPI

Article

Evaluation of Molecular Test for the Discrimination of "Naked" DNA from Infectious Parvovirus B19 Particles in Serum and Bone Marrow Samples

Arthur Daniel Rocha Alves [1], Barbara Barbosa Langella [1], Mariana Magaldi de Souza Lima [1], Wagner Luís da Costa Nunes Pimentel Coelho [1], Rita de Cássia Nasser Cubel Garcia [2], Claudete Aparecida Araújo Cardoso [3], Renato Sergio Marchevsky [4], Marcelo Alves Pinto [1] and Luciane Almeida Amado [1,*]

1 Laboratório de Desenvolvimento Tecnológico em Virologia, Instituto Oswaldo Cruz, FIOCRUZ, Avenida Brasil, 4365, Manguinhos, Rio de Janeiro 21040-900, Brazil; arthuralves@aluno.fiocruz.br (A.D.R.A.); babi.langella@gmail.com (B.B.L.); mari.magaldi13@gmail.com (M.M.d.S.L.); wagnercoelho@aluno.fiocruz.br (W.L.d.C.N.P.C.); marcelop@ioc.fiocruz.br (M.A.P.)

2 Departamento de Microbiologia e Parasitologia, Instituto Biomédico, Universidade Federal Fluminense, Niterói, Rio de Janeiro 24210-230, Brazil; ritacubel@id.uff.br

3 Departamento Materno Infantil, Faculdade de Medicina, Universidade Federal Fluminense, Niterói, Rio de Janeiro 24033-900, Brazil; claudetecardoso@id.uff.br

4 Vice Diretoria de Qualidade, Instituto de Tecnologia em Imunobiológicos, FIOCRUZ, Avenida Brasil, 4365, Manguinhos, Rio de Janeiro 21040-900, Brazil; march@bio.fiocruz.br

* Correspondence: l_amado@ioc.fiocruz.br; Tel.: +55-(21)-2562-1876

Abstract: Low levels of parvovirus B19 (B19V) DNA can be detected in the circulation and in different tissue of immunocompetent individuals for months or years, which has been linked to inflammatory diseases such as cardiomyopathy, rheumatoid arthritis, hepatitis, and vasculitis. However, the detection of B19V DNA does not necessarily imply that infectious virions are present. This study aimed to evaluate the method based on the Benzonase® treatment for differentiation between the infectious virions from "naked" DNA in serum and bone marrow (BM) samples to be useful for the B19V routine diagnosis. In addition, we estimated the period of viremia and DNAemia in the sera and bone marrow of nonhuman primates experimentally infected with B19V. Serum samples from ten patients and from four cynomolgus monkeys experimentally infected with B19V followed up for 60 days were used. Most of the human serum samples became negative after pretreatment; however, only decreased viral DNA loads were observed in four patients, indicating that these samples still contained the infectious virus. Reduced B19V DNA levels were observed in animals since 7th dpi. At approximately 45th dpi, B19V DNA levels were below 10^5 IU/mL after Benzonase® pretreatment, which was not a consequence of active B19V replication. The test based on Benzonase® pretreatment enabled the discrimination of "naked DNA" from B19V DNA encapsidated in virions. Therefore, this test can be used to clarify the role of B19V as an etiological agent associated with atypical clinical manifestations.

Keywords: Benzonase®; parvovirus B19; acute infection; persistent infection; viral DNA load

Citation: Alves, A.D.R.; Langella, B.B.; Lima, M.M.d.S.; Coelho, W.L.d.C.N.P.; Cubel Garcia, R.d.C.N.; Cardoso, C.A.A.; Marchevsky, R.S.; Pinto, M.A.; Amado, L.A. Evaluation of Molecular Test for the Discrimination of "Naked" DNA from Infectious Parvovirus B19 Particles in Serum and Bone Marrow Samples. *Viruses* **2022**, *14*, 843. https://doi.org/10.3390/v14040843

Academic Editor: Giorgio Gallinella

Received: 11 February 2022
Accepted: 5 April 2022
Published: 18 April 2022

1. Introduction

Parvovirus B19 (B19V) is a small (23–28 nm in diameter), nonenveloped icosahedral virus containing a single-stranded DNA genome of 5596 nucleotides [1]. B19V is classified as belonging to the *Parvoviridae* family, *Erythroparvovirus* genus, and *Primate erythroparvovirus 1* species, due to its tropism for erythroid progenitor cells, predominantly in the bone marrow and fetal liver [1,2].

B19V is a common, global pathogen that infects children and adults, and serological studies indicate that over 40–60% of healthy adults have anti-B19V IgG antibodies due to previous exposure [3,4]. B19V is mainly transmitted via the respiratory route. Still, it can also be transmitted vertically from the mother to the fetus via the transfusion of whole blood or pooled blood products or via organ transplantation [3,4].

Viral transmission occurs most often during the viremia period that precedes the clinical presentation [3–5]. Approximately one week after a respiratory infection, a high amount of viral DNA (>10^{12} IU/mL) can persist for 6 to 7 days in the peripheral blood, saliva and respiratory secretions of acutely infected individuals. The classical slapped-cheek rash associated with erythema infectiosum (also known as the fifth disease) and arthralgia develops 17–18 days after infection, at the time of the appearance of IgM- and IgG-specific antibodies [4,5].

B19V infection is usually acute and self-limited and causes no symptoms in most healthy individuals [6]. However, the virus can also induces transient aplastic crisis in patients with underlying hemolytic anemia [7], persistent anemia in immunocompromised patients and hydrops fetalis and fetal loss in pregnant women [8,9]. The wide range of diseases depends on the hematological and immune status of the host [10].

B19V DNA can be detected at low levels (10^4 IU/mL) in the blood and various tissues (bone marrow, skin, tonsils, liver and heart) of immunocompetent individuals for months or years after acute infection, even when B19V antibodies are present [11–13]. However, whether the detection of viral DNA in the blood and tissues of seropositive and asymptomatic individuals reflects the presence of an infectious virus has not been elucidated. This point is of particular concern since B19V is resistant to most inactivation procedures used in manufacturing blood-derived products and can be transmitted by pooled blood products [11–13]. Furthermore, B19V DNA persistence in these tissues may suggest a causal relationship with some clinical conditions, such as myocarditis, chronic arthropathy and acute liver failure (ALF) [3,13–15].

Recently, Molenaar-de Backer and collaborators [16] presented a method for differentiating between B19V DNA in EDTA-plasma samples resulting from active viral replication and B19V viremia. The method is based on plasma pretreatment with Benzonase® prior to nucleic acid extraction. The authors proposed that the remaining B19V DNA can be released from tissues without active replication, suggesting that the role of B19V in clinical syndromes, such as myocarditis and arthritis, based mainly on the detection of B19V DNA in the blood and tissues without further support by serology, clinical signs or epidemiology should be carefully reconsidered [16].

A case of recurrent B19V DNAemia in a patient with hereditary spherocytosis, which was initially interpreted as viral reactivation, was clarified after confirming the absence of infectious viral particles in the patient's blood. The hypothesis was raised that the second episode of DNAemia represented the mass release of B19V DNA from the bone marrow and was, therefore, not the result of active infection [17].

In a previous study, we investigated the presence of B19V in archived liver tissues from patients undergoing liver transplantation for the management of ALF. B19V DNA and viral replication were detected in matched serum and explanted liver samples from 23% of the patients [14]. However, further studies are required to understand the correct meaning of the detection of B19V DNA in their serum and tissues. In this way, differentiating whether genome detection corresponds to an infectious virus could help to clarify the causal relationship between B19V infection and ALF.

These data demonstrate that a laboratory test to establish the nature of B19V DNA (infectious particle or not) can be a tool to interpret the presence of B19V DNA correctly, which would be valuable for determining a causal relationship between B19V and atypical clinical manifestations. Additionally, this simple test could be further utilized to ensure the safety of blood products for transfusion and transplantation purposes.

Thus, this study aimed to evaluate the method based on the Benzonase® treatment for differentiation between the presence of the infectious virions from "naked" DNA in serum and bone marrow samples to be applied in the routine diagnosis of the B19V infection. In addition, we estimated the period of viremia and DNAemia in the sera and bone marrow of nonhuman primates experimentally infected with B19V.

2. Materials and Methods

2.1. Biological Samples and Ethical Aspects

The performance of the assay was evaluated, in duplicate, using different samples types that have been stratified into four panels, as follows:

Panel 1. Includes five archived (−20 °C) serum samples (encoded as H01 to H05) obtained from patients with exanthematic illness, sent to the LADTV/IOC-Fiocruz for B19V diagnostic evaluation. These samples were characterized as B19V DNA and anti-B19V IgM-positive and were used to establish the optimum concentration of endonuclease in serum treatments.

Panel 2. Ten follow-up serum samples were obtained from five patients with exanthematic illness (encoded as H06 to H10) who tested positive for B19V-DNA and anti-B19V IgM.

Panel 3. Ten follow-up serum samples were obtained from five patients with unspecific symptoms (encoded as H11 to H15) who tested positive for B19V-DNA and anti-B19V IgG and negative for B19V IgM.

Panels 2 and 3 included serum samples from patients monitored for up to 30 days, enrolled at the Hospital Antonio Pedro-Federal Fluminense University and Hospital Getúlio Vargas Filho (Niterói, Brazil). Blood samples from each patient were obtained at the onset of the symptoms during the medical consultation [considered as the 0-day post-admission (dpa)], and a second sample was obtained 30 days later (30 dpa) (Figure 1).

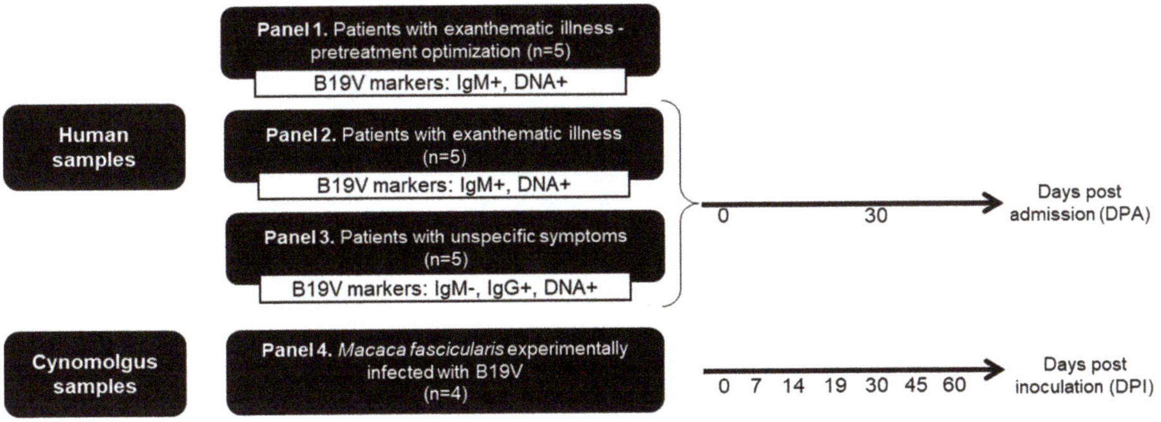

Figure 1. Study population. Serum samples were obtained from patients with B19V markers (IgM, IgG and DNA). Serum and bone marrow (BM) samples were obtained from cynomolgus monkeys experimentally infected with B19V.

Panel 4. Since the timing of infection of the patients is unsure, we included serial serum and bone marrow samples from four cynomolgus monkeys (*Macaca fascicularis*), experimentally infected with B19V (encoded as Cy01 to Cy04) to accurately determine the time of infection and correlate it with B19V DNA levels. These animals were clinically healthy, young adults (weighing 3–5 kg), ranging in age from three to four years old from the Department of Primatology, Institute of Science and Technology in Biomodels (Fiocruz), as described by Leon et al. [18]. These samples collected at 7, 14, 19, 30, 45 and 60 days post B19V inoculation (dpi) were stored at −70 °C in the LADTV-IOC/Fiocruz biorepository until the beginning of this study [18] (Figure 1).

The study protocol was approved by the Ethics Committee of Oswaldo Cruz Institute (protocol # 1.896.353), all partnering health units, and the Animal Use Ethics Committee of Oswaldo Cruz Institute (protocol # P0064-00).

2.2. Diagnostic Criteria of B19V Infection

Serum samples were tested, in duplicate, for anti-B19V IgG and anti-B19V IgM by SERION ELISA classic Parvovirus B19 IgG and IgM® (Virion\Serion, Wurzburg, Germany), according to the manufacturer's instructions. These assays have sensitivity and specificity > 99% and are composed of virus-like particles (VLPs) containing recombinant VP2 protein to detect B19V IgG and IgM [19]. For anti-B19V IgM detection, a previous dilution of the samples with SERION Rheumatoid Factor-Absorbent (Virion\Serion, Wurzburg, Germany) was made to avoid non-specific ligation of IgM-antibodies (rheumatoid factors), that could lead to false-positive results.

Panels 1 and 2 include serum samples from patients with specific symptoms of B19V infection, anti-B19V IgM and IgG positive, and B19V-DNA positive, indicating a profile of acute infection. On the other hand, panel 3 includes serum samples anti-B19V IgM negative, anti-B19V IgG positive and B19V-DNA positive, indicating a profile of past and persistent infection.

2.3. Endonuclease Pretreatment

To investigate whether the B19V DNA detected was encapsidated in viral particles (virions) or not ("naked DNA"), serum and BM samples were pretreated with the Benzonase® enzyme (25 kU; Sigma-Aldrich, San Luis, MO, USA). Benzonase® is a genetically engineered endonuclease obtained from *Serratia marcescens* that degrades all forms of genetic material (DNA and RNA) that are free in the sample (i.e., not encapsidated by protein particles in the case of viruses or protected by the lipid bilayer in the case of cells) [16].

The efficiency of Benzonase® to cleave viral nucleic acids present in the serum samples were evaluated as follows. Each serum sample (200 μL) was divided into two 100 μL aliquots. Benzonase® was added to one aliquot, and the other aliquot was not treated with endonuclease as the control sample to compare the effect of the pretreatment.

Both aliquots (Benzonase®-pretreated and the control) were incubated together while shaking at 120 rpm for 1 h at 37 °C. Then, the samples were kept at room temperature to stop the reaction, as recommended by the manufacturer and FDA guidelines [20], followed by viral DNA extraction and PCR for the specific detection of B19V DNA. To determine the optimal endonuclease concentration and evaluate its effect on different B19V viral loads, a panel of five serum samples (H01 to H05) with different viral loads (10^3 IU/mL to 10^7 IU/mL) were analyzed, in duplicate, with the following concentrations of Benzonase® (25 kU): 0.1 U/μL; 0.5 U/μL; 1.0 U/μL; 1.5 U/μL; 2.0 U/μL; 2.5 U/μL.

Positive and negative virion controls were also included in each experiment. As a positive virion control, a serum (sample H05) from a patient with acute B19V infection (anti-B19V IgM-positive and B19V-DNA of 10^7 IU/mL, genotype 1A) was used. As a negative control of virion, a "naked" B19V-DNA (purified from a serum sample) was used. These controls were pretreated with Benzonase® in the same way as the samples and tested with and without pretreatment with an endonuclease.

We used a modified MAPIA (multi-antigen print immunoassay) to evaluate if there were viral particles in serum samples in which the genome titer remained detectable after benzonase pretreatment. This assay consists of a thin layer of immobilizated antigen or antibody onto nitrocellulose membrane by micro-printing, without denaturing conditions, followed by a standard chromogenic immunoassay [21]. In this case, mouse IgG anti-B19V VP1 monoclonal (1:1.200) (Abcam Inc., Waltham, MA, USA) was micro-printed to a nitrocellulose membrane using semi-automatic printing equipment (CAMAG automatic TLC sample 4, CAMAG, Muttenz, Switzerland). The membranes were incubated (37 °C, 30 min) with 1mL of blocker buffer PBS-milk (0.5% skimmed milk (*w*/*v*) in PBS). After that, the membrane was washed (3-fold) with PBS-Tween 20 (0.05%) (PBST) and incubated

(37 °C, 30 min) with serum, diluted in PBST (1:100), H09 (0 dpa; B19V-DNA negative after benzonase pretreatment) and H10 (0 dpa; B19V-DNA positive after Benzonase® pretreatment). After washing (3-fold, 37 °C, 5 min) with PBST, the membranes were incubated (37 °C, 1 h) with the mouse anti-B19V VP1 monoclonal (1:1.200). After the washing step, the conjugate (Goat IgG anti-mouse with peroxidase; 1:1.200) was added and incubated (37 °C, 30 min). After an additional washing step (3-fold), the immune complex was revealed with diaminobenzidine in citrate/phosphate buffer, pH 5.0, 30% H_2O_2. The membranes were rinsed in purified water at room temperature to stop the reaction. The strips were dried to be analyzed.

2.4. B19V DNA Extraction and qPCR

B19V DNA was extracted from all samples, including the nuclease-treated and non-treated aliquots and the positive and negative controls, using a QIAamp DNA Mini Kit (Qiagen, Hilden, Germany), according to the manufacturer's instructions. DNA was eluted with 200 µL of elution buffer and stored at −70 °C until use.

Real-time PCR (qPCR) was carried out using the TaqMan system (Applied Biosystems 7500 Real-Time PCR System, Applied Biosystems, Waltham, MA, USA) as described previously [22]. For absolute quantification, a synthetic standard curve of the B19V NS1 region [custom synthesized by IDT® (CoralVille, IA)] was designed (nt 1905–1987, GenBank: NC_000883.2). Primers for the NS1 region (nt 1905F and 1987R) and a single labeled 5′ FAM probe (nt 1925–1948, GenBank: NC_000883.2) were used.

2.5. Statistical Analysis

Statistical analyses were performed with GraphPad Prism 8.3.1. software (GraphPad Software, San Diego, CA, USA). Continuous variables were expressed as mean and were compared with the Mann-Whitney U test. All p-values were two-sided, and those <0.05 were considered statistically significant.

3. Results

3.1. Determination of the Optimal Benzonase® Concentration

Serum samples (H01-H05) from five patients with acute B19V infection were pretreated with Benzonase®, and viral DNA was then extracted from these samples and subjected to qPCR analysis.

As shown in Table 1 and Figure 2, the amount of B19V DNA in samples containing 10^5 IU/mL (H01 and H04) was not significantly reduced after Benzonase® pretreatment at concentrations varying from 0.1 to 2.0 U/µL, indicating the presence of infectious virions. However, the viral DNA load exhibited at least one $\log_{10}$ reduction in the other three samples (H02, H03 and H05) containing 10^6 to 10^7 IU/mL after treatment with 2.0 U/µL Benzonase®. The viral DNA loads remained almost the same, using a higher concentration of Benzonase (2.5 U/µL). Thus, we established a concentration of 2.0 U/µL to test the clinical samples.

Table 1. Optimization of Benzonase® concentration among human serum samples.

ID	Serum (IU/mL)							DNA [a] (IU/mL)		
	Nontreated (Mean ± SD)	0.1 (Mean ± SD)	0.5 (Mean ± SD)	1.0 (Mean ± SD)	1.5 (Mean ± SD)	2.0 (Mean ± SD)	2.5 (Mean ± SD)	0.1 (Mean ± SD)	0.5 (Mean ± SD)	1.0 (Mean ± SD)
H01	$3.5 \times 10^5 \pm 3.3 \times 10^5$	$2.1 \times 10^5 \pm 2.0 \times 10^5$	$1.9 \times 10^5 \pm 1.9 \times 10^5$	$1.5 \times 10^5 \pm 1.5 \times 10^5$	$1.0 \times 10^5 \pm 1.4 \times 10^5$	$1.1 \times 10^5 \pm 1.4 \times 10^5$	NT	$9.4 \times 10^3 \pm 8.8 \times 10^3$	Negative	Negative
H02	$6.6 \times 10^6 \pm 5.7 \times 10^6$	$4.6 \times 10^5 \pm 3.8 \times 10^5$	$3.4 \times 10^5 \pm 2.7 \times 10^5$	$2.4 \times 10^5 \pm 1.9 \times 10^5$	$5.6 \times 10^4 \pm 6.2 \times 10^4$	$3.9 \times 10^4 \pm 3.4 \times 10^4$	NT	$6.1 \times 10^3 \pm 2.1 \times 10^3$	Negative	Negative
H03	$2.2 \times 10^6 \pm 2.0 \times 10^6$	$4.9 \times 10^5 \pm 8.9 \times 10^4$	$4.8 \times 10^5 \pm 3.6 \times 10^5$	$8.9 \times 10^5 \pm 7.7 \times 10^5$	$6.4 \times 10^5 \pm 4.8 \times 10^5$	$3.3 \times 10^5 \pm 2.1 \times 10^5$	NT	$5.1 \times 10^4 \pm 6.4 \times 10^3$	$3.4 \times 10^3 \pm 3.2 \times 10^3$	Negative
H04	$8.6 \times 10^5 \pm 8.4 \times 10^5$	$5.8 \times 10^5 \pm 6.5 \times 10^5$	$5.4 \times 10^5 \pm 6.1 \times 10^5$	$4.9 \times 10^5 \pm 5.7 \times 10^5$	$4.7 \times 10^5 \pm 5.2 \times 10^5$	$3.8 \times 10^5 \pm 4.3 \times 10^5$	$2.1 \times 10^5 \pm 4.8 \times 10^4$	$5.6 \times 10^4 \pm 3.4 \times 10^4$	$5.2 \times 10^3 \pm 2.6 \times 10^3$	Negative
H05	$1.3 \times 10^7 \pm 1.7 \times 10^7$	$5.4 \times 10^6 \pm 6.7 \times 10^6$	$5.6 \times 10^5 \pm 5.9 \times 10^5$	$5.4 \times 10^5 \pm 6.0 \times 10^5$	$5.2 \times 10^5 \pm 6.2 \times 10^5$	$1.5 \times 10^5 \pm 3.1 \times 10^4$	$1.1 \times 10^5 \pm 1.0 \times 10^4$	$4.9 \times 10^4 \pm 2.9 \times 10^4$	$3.1 \times 10^4 \pm 1.8 \times 10^4$	Negative

ID: Identification; IU/mL: International Units per milliliter; SD: standard deviation; NT: Non-tested due to insufficient sample volume. [a] Extracted DNA was also treated with Benzonase® to become a negative control and to check the standardized Benzonase® concentration.

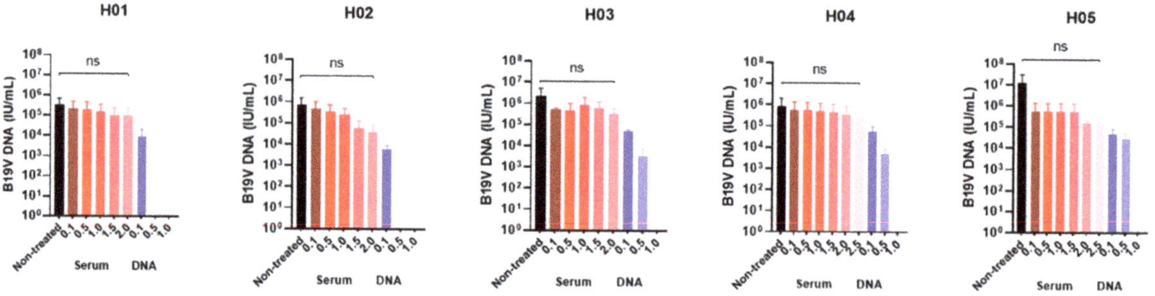

Figure 2. Optimization of Benzonase® concentration among human serum samples. IU/mL: International Units per milliliter. Ns: non-significative.

The effect of Benzonase® pretreatment (1.0 U/µL) on the load of the "naked" DNA controls reduced the genome copy numbers to undetectable levels, signifying that the samples comprised naked DNA.

The positive control (sample H05) was positive in all experiments, so there were virions in this sample. On the other hand, the negative control, which consists of the DNA from the serum sample treated with Benzonase®, was negative in all experiments.

3.2. Effect of Benzonase® Pretreatment on the B19V DNA Levels in Serum Samples from Infected Patients

Serial serum samples were obtained from ten patients that were B19V DNA positive. Among them, five patients had a profile of B19V acute infection (H06-H10; average age of 10 years, ranging from 3 to 39 years), and five had a profile of B19V persistent infection (H11-H15; average age of 9 years, ranging from 6 to 28 years). All sera collected from anti-B19V IgM positive individuals, 30 days post-admission (30 dpa), remained positive for B19V DNA. In contrast, second samples from most of the individuals' anti-B19V IgM negative (3/5) became negative for B19V DNA (Table 2 and Figure 3).

Table 2. Performance of Benzonase® pretreatment among human sera samples from patients B19V DNA positive, according to anti-B19V IgM presence.

	ID	Sera Collected at 0 dpa			Sera Collected at 30 dpa		
		B19V Load (IU/mL) (Mean ± SD)	B19V Load Treated (IU/mL) (Mean ± SD)	p-Value	B19V Load (IU/mL) (Mean ± SD)	B19V Load Treated (IU/mL) (Mean ± SD)	p-Value
Anti-B19V IgM positive	H06	$9.3 \times 10^5 \pm 8.7 \times 10^5$	$1.6 \times 10^4 \pm 1.4 \times 10^4$	<0.01	$1.7 \times 10^5 \pm 1.4 \times 10^5$	Negative	<0.01
	H07	$4.3 \times 10^7 \pm 3.1 \times 10^7$	$6.4 \times 10^4 \pm 4.1 \times 10^4$		$2.1 \times 10^5 \pm 1.9 \times 10^5$	Negative	
	H08	$1.9 \times 10^6 \pm 2.3 \times 10^6$	$2.4 \times 10^4 \pm 1.9 \times 10^4$		$9.0 \times 10^5 \pm 7.8 \times 10^5$	Negative	
	H09	$1.7 \times 10^6 \pm 1.5 \times 10^6$	Negative		$8.4 \times 10^5 \pm 8.2 \times 10^5$	Negative	
	H10	$2.3 \times 10^5 \pm 1.7 \times 10^5$	$1.7 \times 10^5 \pm 1.6 \times 10^5$		$2.2 \times 10^3 \pm 1.6 \times 10^3$	Negative	
Anti-B19V IgM negative	H11	$1.9 \times 10^5 \pm 2.7 \times 10^5$	Negative	<0.01	Negative	Negative	<0.01
	H12	$1.8 \times 10^5 \pm 1.3 \times 10^5$	$1.8 \times 10^5 \pm 1.7 \times 10^5$		$3.7 \times 10^4 \pm 2.9 \times 10^4$	Negative	
	H13	$3.3 \times 10^5 \pm 8.4 \times 10^5$	$1.8 \times 10^5 \pm 1.7 \times 10^5$		Negative	Negative	
	H14	$4.6 \times 10^4 \pm 2.5 \times 10^4$	Negative		Negative	Negative	
	H15	$5.7 \times 10^4 \pm 4.9 \times 10^4$	Negative		$4.0 \times 10^4 \pm 3.9 \times 10^4$	Negative	

D: Identification; B19V: Parvovirus B19; IU/mL: International Units per milliliter; dpa: days post-admission; SD: standard deviation.

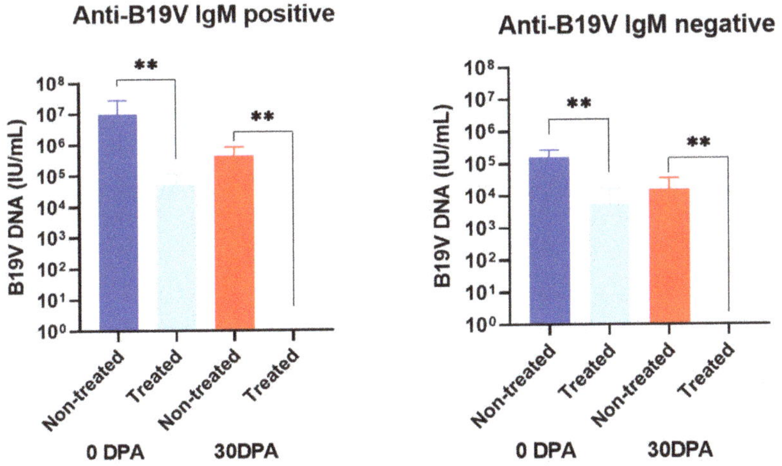

Figure 3. Performance of Benzonase® pretreatment in serial serum samples collected from patients with anti-B19V IgM positive and negative. IU/mL: International Units per milliliter; DPA: Days post-admission; ** p-value < 0.01.

After pretreatment with endonuclease (2.0 U/µL), in most of the samples anti-B19V IgM positive (H06, H07, H08 and H10), the B19 DNA remained detectable, despite the DNA load being partially reduced after pretreatment, suggesting that part of the B19V DNA in these samples was encapsidated in viral particles (Table 2). On the other hand, among patients without anti-B19V IgM, three (H11, H14 and H15) became undetectable, which is compatible with a nonencapsidated state of B19V DNA. However, all the samples collected 30 days after admission were 100% sensitive to endonuclease, confirming the presence of "naked" DNA.

In both groups (anti-B19V IgM positive and negative), the differences in the viral load before and after endonuclease pretreatment were statistically significant in samples collected at 0 and 30 dpa ($p < 0.05$).

The presence of encapsidated B19V DNA in a serum sample (H10) in which the B19V DNA remained detectable after pretreatment with Benzonase® was proven by MAPIA (Figure 4A). The immune complex of anti-B19V/ B19V VP1-VP2 confirmed the occurrence of B19V particles in this sample. In contrast, Figure 4B shows the absence of B19V particles in a serum sample (H09) in which B19V DNA became undetectable after pretreatment with Benzonase®.

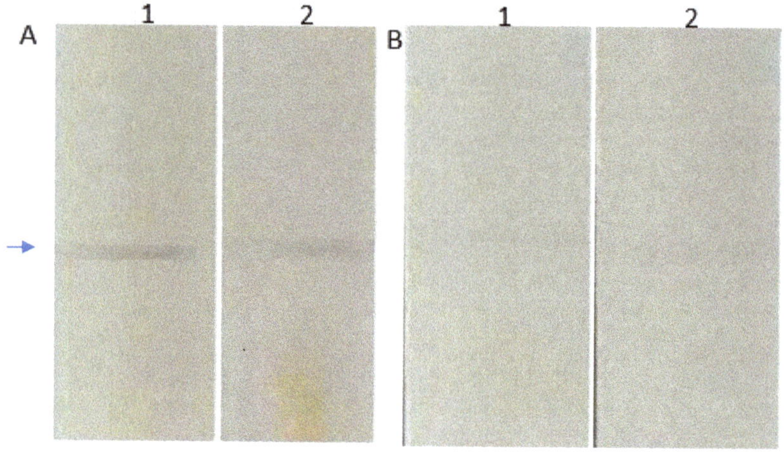

Figure 4. Evaluation of B19V particles' presence in serum samples by MAPIA. In this assay, the immunocomplex of mouse anti-B19V monoclonal antibody/ B19V VP1-VP2 capsid proteins was revealed by goat IgG anti-mouse-peroxidase (arrow). (**A**) Serum sample (H10) with B19V DNA detectable before (**1**) and after benzonase pretreatment (**2**). (**B**) Serum sample (H09) with B19V DNA undetectable before (**1**) and after benzonase pretreatment (**2**).

3.3. Evaluation of B19V DNA in Serum and Bone Marrow Samples from Experimentally Infected Cynomolgus Monkeys

As shown in Figure 5, a correlation between the appearance of anti-B19V IgG in serum and the sensitivity of viral DNA in serum and bone marrow to Benzonase® treatment was observed.

In the Cy01, which showed early seroconversion of IgG at the 7th dpi, B19V DNA remained detectable until the 30th dpi after benzonase® treatment. While, Cy02 and Cy03, in which seroconversions were detected at the 14th dpi, B19V DNA remained detectable until the 45th dpi, indicating a longer presence of encapsidated B19V DNA in these animals with later seroconversion, than that observed in Cy01 (Figure 5).

From 30th dpi, a reduction in viral loads was seen in serum and bone marrow samples after Benzonase® treatment compared with nontreated samples, indicating that "naked" and encapsidated B19V DNA coexist until the 60th dpi. At this point, the DNA from the infectious virions was no longer detectable. For Cy04, as seroconversion occurred only at the 45th dpi, B19V DNA remained detectable after endonuclease treatment, demonstrating the longest presence of infectious virions.

The difference between the treated and nontreated serum samples was not statistically significant ($p > 0.05$).

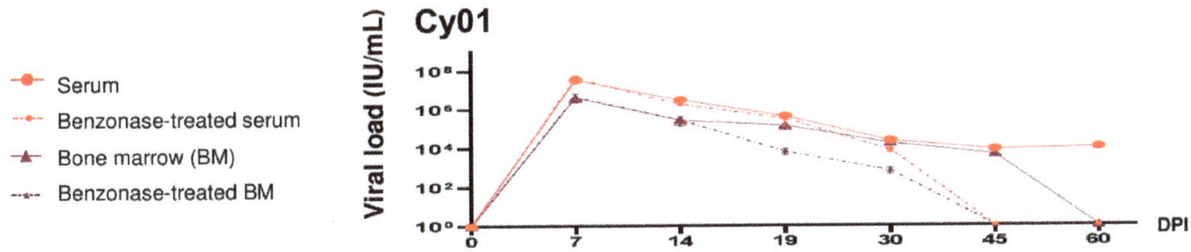

DPI	0	7	14	19	30	45	60
IgG anti-B19V	–	+	+	+	+	+	+
Viral load Serum (non-treated)	Negative	2.69×10^{7}	2.38×10^{6}	4.21×10^{5}	3.01×10^{4}	8.01×10^{3}	1.03×10^{4}
Viral load Serum (treated)	Negative	2.14×10^{7}	2.00×10^{6}	1.83×10^{5}	7.81×10^{3}	Negative	Negative
Viral load BM (non-treated)	Negative	2.38×10^{6}	1.67×10^{5}	1.20×10^{5}	1.14×10^{4}	4.68×10^{3}	Negative
Viral load BM (treated)	Negative	2.02×10^{6}	1.54×10^{5}	6.01×10^{3}	6.68×10^{2}	Negative	Negative

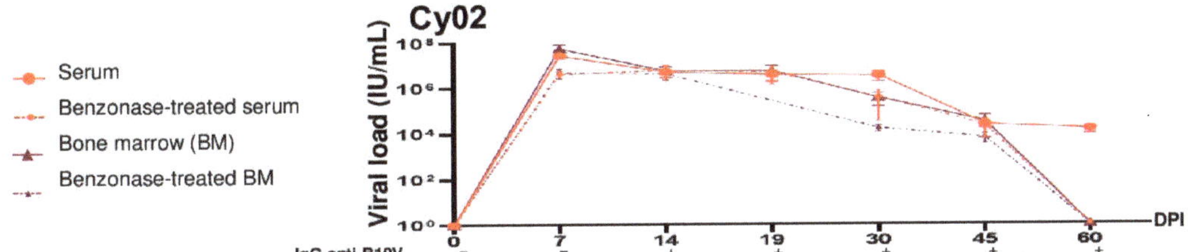

DPI	0	7	14	19	30	45	60
IgG anti-B19V	–	–	+	+	+	+	+
Viral load Serum (non-treated)	Negative	2.00×10^{7}	3.41×10^{6}	3.14×10^{6}	2.00×10^{6}	3.14×10^{4}	1.02×10^{4}
Viral load Serum (treated)	Negative	6.60×10^{6}	2.48×10^{6}	2.11×10^{6}	1.46×10^{5}	1.16×10^{4}	Negative
Viral load BM (non-treated)	Negative	3.13×10^{7}	2.55×10^{6}	2.33×10^{6}	1.60×10^{5}	6.48×10^{4}	Negative
Viral load BM (treated)	Negative	2.53×10^{6}	2.13×10^{6}	NT [a]	1.07×10^{4}	5.34×10^{3}	Negative

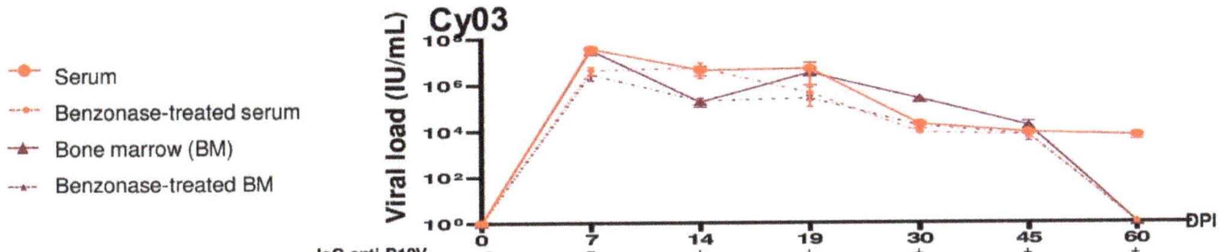

DPI	0	7	14	19	30	45	60
IgG anti-B19V	–	–	+	+	+	+	+
Viral load Serum (non-treated)	Negative	2.40×10^{7}	2.33×10^{6}	2.17×10^{6}	1.09×10^{4}	6.71×10^{3}	8.61×10^{3}
Viral load Serum (treated)	Negative	7.54×10^{6}	2.20×10^{6}	2.00×10^{5}	8.02×10^{3}	6.68×10^{3}	Negative
Viral load BM (non-treated)	Negative	2.85×10^{7}	2.00×10^{5}	2.41×10^{6}	1.70×10^{5}	1.00×10^{4}	Negative
Viral load BM (treated)	Negative	2.53×10^{6}	1.53×10^{5}	2.00×10^{5}	1.20×10^{4}	6.68×10^{3}	Negative

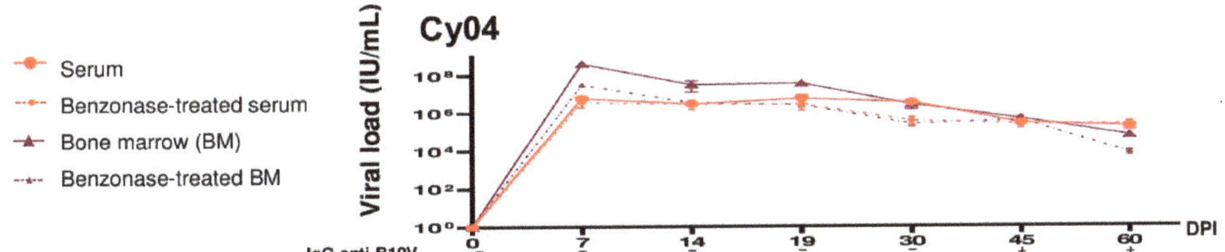

DPI	0	7	14	19	30	45	60
IgG anti-B19V	–	–	–	–	–	+	+
Viral load Serum (non-treated)	Negative	6.61×10^{6}	2.55×10^{6}	2.33×10^{6}	2.35×10^{6}	1.99×10^{5}	1.47×10^{5}
Viral load Serum (treated)	Negative	2.16×10^{6}	2.14×10^{6}	2.14×10^{6}	1.94×10^{5}	1.40×10^{5}	1.34×10^{5}
Viral load BM (non-treated)	Negative	3.37×10^{8}	3.02×10^{7}	2.72×10^{7}	1.83×10^{6}	5.70×10^{5}	6.08×10^{4}
Viral load BM (treated)	Negative	2.73×10^{7}	2.35×10^{6}	2.17×10^{6}	1.93×10^{5}	1.62×10^{5}	8.02×10^{3}

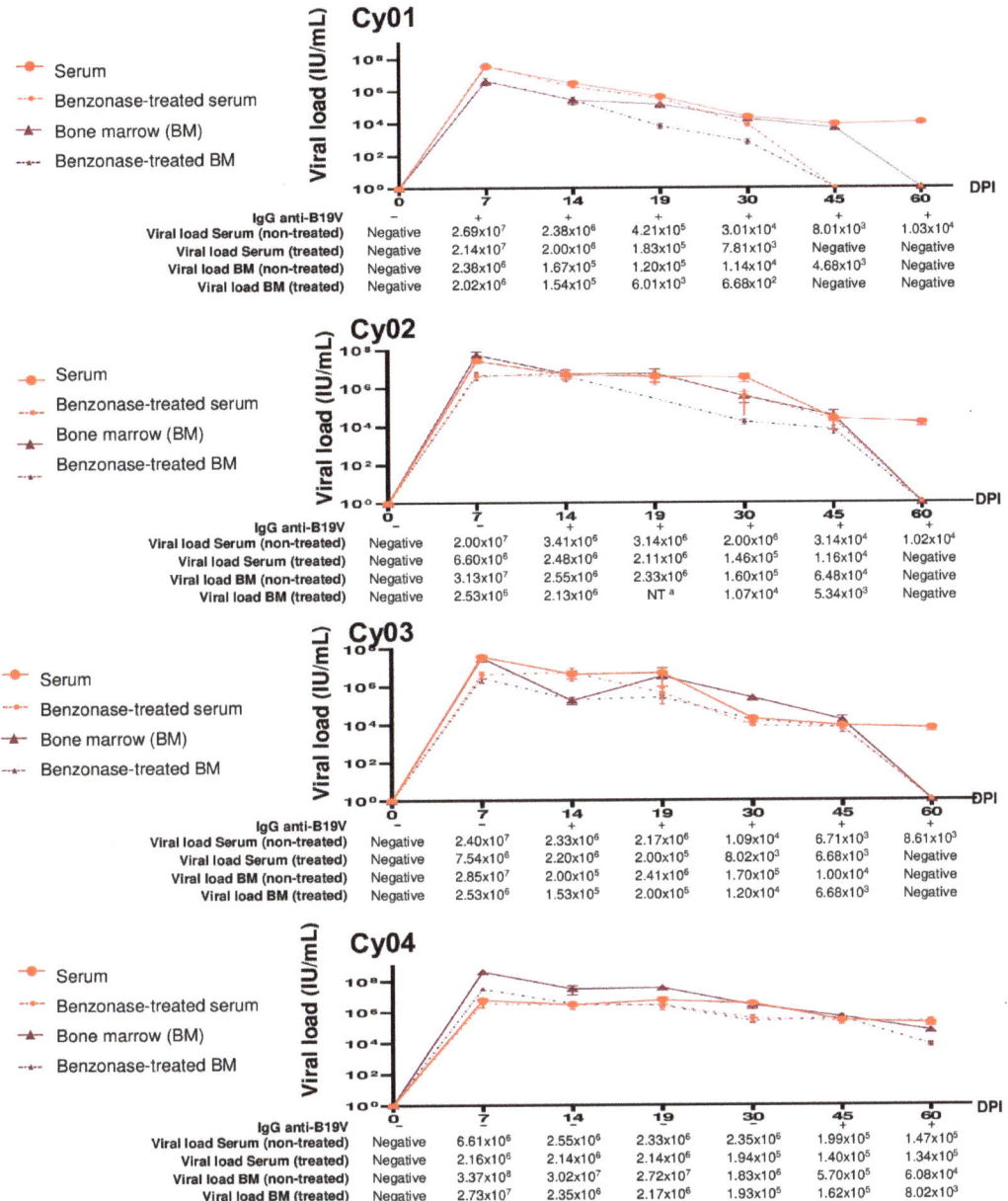

Figure 5. Follow-up of anti-B19V IgG and B19V DNA levels during the experimental infection in cynomolgus monkeys (n = 4). IU/mL: International Units per milliliter; BM: Bone marrow; –: Negative; +: Positive; DPI: Days-post infection; [a] Not tested due to insufficient bone marrow sample.

4. Discussion

In this study, we evaluated the performance of a method based on sample pretreatment with Benzonase® followed by qPCR to detect and quantify B19V infectious viral particles (virions) in serum and in bone marrow. It has been reported that viral DNA can be diagnosed in peripheral blood several days or months after the acute infection [23–25]. To understand the clinical significance of long-term B19V DNA detection, reliable methods are needed to confirm the virions in tissues from these patients and their association with the B19V clinical course, as suggested by other researchers in the context of autoimmune thyroid gland diseases [26], the skin without dermatological injury [27], and myocardial inflammatory injury [28].

Serial samples from naturally B19V-infected individuals and experimentally infected cynomolgus monkeys demonstrated that the presence of B19V DNA in the blood did not necessarily correlate with the presence of infectious viral particles (virions) circulating. This finding is in accordance with a previous study that revealed the presence of virions only at the beginning (approximately 60 days) of the infection. Molenaar-de-Backer and collaborators determined that after five months, only naked-strands B19V DNA was found [16].

The ideal concentration of Benzonase® for use in serum and BM samples was determined. An optimal Benzonase® concentration of 2.0 U/μL was adopted since, using a higher concentration of Benzonase® (2.5 U/μL), the viral loads remained the same. All serum samples from patients with and without anti-B19V IgM showed partially or completely reduced viral loads after Benzonase® pretreatment, which suggested the cooccurrence of viremia and DNAemia in both groups of patients on the first collection day. Most of the patients with a profile of acute infection (H06, H07, H08, H10) remained with the viral DNA detectable, showing a partial reduction of the genome titer, which suggests that during the acute phase of infection, the DNA is predominantly encapsidated. The MAPIA showed that the detection of viral DNA in these samples, even after endonuclease treatment, could be ascribed to the presence of the encapsidated viral DNA.

The viral DNA from three patients with a profile of acute infection (H09) became undetectable after endonuclease treatment on the first collection day. This result suggests that probably this patient was in an advanced period of infection and no longer in an acute infection. This indicates that the Benzonase® pretreatment assay must be used as an additional approach to attest the status of infection. Although IgM, in general, is a sensitive indicator of recent infection, it lacks clinical specificity in many contexts. Furthermore, anti-B19V IgM can remain detectable for approximately 30 days post-infection [29], or it can, in the acute phase, be of very low titer and thus remain below the threshold of detection in a low-sensitive IgM ELISA. Lastly, it can pick up non-specific IgM [30]. Approximately 30 days after the first collection, all samples were negative for B19V DNA after Benzonase® pretreatment, demonstrating that there was only 'naked' B19V DNA. These samples collected approximately 30 days after infection showed viral loads between 10^3–10^5 IU/mL, which suggested that samples with a viral load $\leq 10^4$ IU/mL do not contain infectious virus, as suggested by other groups, European Pharmacopoeia and Food and Drug Administration [29,31,32].

The 60-day follow-up of experimentally infected cynomolgus monkeys (*Macaca fascicularis*) revealed high B19V viremia in most animals even after seroconversion. The results observed in patients and animals were similar, as the endonuclease pretreatment experiments demonstrated that during the first 30 days of B19V infection, the presence of B19V DNA was indicative of infectious virus. Subsequently, B19V DNA was degraded by the endonuclease, indicating that "naked DNA" was predominantly present. B19V "naked DNA" was generally diagnosed under the viral load of 10^5 IU/mL, indicating that samples with this viral load are not potentially infectious.

These results are of great relevance for blood banks, considering that the detection of B19V DNA in blood donor samples with a viral load $\leq 10^4$ IU/mL does not pose a residual risk for blood transfusion transmission [33,34] since these blood donors with low viremia, no longer have B19V virions.

In the persistent infection, there is a lower viral genome expression, possibly contributing to the maintenance of the virus in tissues, that can be relevant to the balance and outcome of the different types of infection associated with B19V [35]. It has been proposed that the persistence of B19V DNA in blood, also known as DNAemia, can result from B19V DNA released from apoptotic or necrotic cells [36,37]. The passive release of viral DNA may likely explain the genome present in the blood in some cases, while in other cases, active viral infection is responsible. Therefore, B19V DNA present in the blood approximately 45 days after acute infection probably derives from a different origin, but it remains unknown hitherto.

B19V infects erythrocyte progenitors binding to the cellular receptor globoside (or P antigen), which induces structural changes in the capsid, leading to the accessibility of the N-terminal region of VP1 (VP1u) that is required for internalization [38]. However, this internalization in cell types that are not permissive to infection does not appear to start a productive infection cycle, leading to an accumulation of B19V DNA [38]. This was confirmed by the presence of B19V DNA in many tissues that are not permissive to the virus [13]. Naked DNA can be released into the circulation by apoptosis or necrosis or when cells are normally renewed and via exocytosis. This release by cells can occur for years or even decades after the initial B19V infection, depending on cell type. Since different cell types have different turnover rates, this can cause an aleatory release of B19V DNA, explaining the gradual decline in viremia after acute infection. [16].

Conventional and real-time molecular assays can detect low quantities of viral DNA because they are extremely sensitive techniques. However, they do not differentiate between infectious virus particles and "naked DNA." Therefore, the treatment method with an endonuclease that cleaves any DNA or RNA present in a sample is quite useful in determining whether B19V DNA is infectious and linked to replication [16].

The availability of a simple and reliable method to distinguish viral particles from naked genetic material could be especially applicable for no cultivable viruses, such as B19V, whose productive infection is highly restricted to erythroid progenitor cells of the bone marrow [4], and for viruses whose isolation procedure requires a high biosafety level, such as SARS-CoV-2. Other future applications of this test include the correct diagnoses of several viral infections, as prolonged periods of viremia have been increasingly observed with the development of highly sensitive molecular techniques for viral genome detection and the detection of viral genomes spread in multiple organs of infected patients. Establishing the relevance of viremia in these cases and the causal relationship of this finding with infection is of paramount importance for the correct laboratory diagnoses of viral infections.

The small human (n = 10) and monkey (n = 4) sample sizes and the differential periods of observation for the collected samples (30 days for humans and 60 days for monkeys) could be considered limitations of this study.

5. Conclusions

The laboratory test based on Benzonase® pretreatment of serum and BM samples enabled the discrimination of "naked DNA" from B19V infectious particles in these clinical specimens. Therefore, this test can be a valuable tool to be used in routine diagnosis to clarify the role of B19V as an etiological agent associated with atypical clinical manifestations and an additional approach to attest the timing of the infection.

Author Contributions: A.D.R.A. and L.A.A. were involved in the conception and design of this study and in the analysis and interpretation of the data. A.D.R.A., B.B.L., M.M.d.S.L. and W.L.d.C.N.P.C. were involved in performing the tests. All authors were involved in the drafting of the paper and agreed to be accountable for all aspects of the work. All authors have read and agreed to the published version of the manuscript.

Funding: We are thankful to the Coordination for the Improvement of Higher Education Personnel–CAPES for the fellowship awarded; MS/Inova Fiocruz—Geração de conhecimento (number: 1825330), FAPERJ-JCNE (number: e-26/201.406/2021) and the Oswaldo Cruz Institute for funding this study.

Institutional Review Board Statement: The study was conducted in accordance with the Declaration of Helsinki, and was approved by the Ethics Committee of Oswaldo Cruz Institute (protocol # 1.896.353), by all partnering health units and by the Animal Use Ethics Committee of Oswaldo Cruz Institute (protocol # P0064-00).

Informed Consent Statement: Informed consent was obtained from all subjects involved in the study.

Data Availability Statement: Not applicable.

Conflicts of Interest: The authors declare no conflict of interest.

References

1. Cotmore, S.F.; Agbandje-McKenna, M.; Canuti, M.; Chiorini, J.A.; Eis-Hubinger, A.M.; Hughes, J.; Mietzsch, M.; Modha, S.; Ogliastro, M.; Pénzes, J.J.; et al. ICTV Virus Taxonomy Profile: *Parvoviridae*. *J. Gen. Virol.* **2019**, *100*, 367–368. [CrossRef] [PubMed]
2. Bua, G.; Manaresi, E.; Bonvicini, F.; Gallinella, G. Parvovirus B19 Replication and Expression in Differentiating Erythroid Progenitor Cells. *PLoS ONE* **2016**, *11*, e0148547. [CrossRef] [PubMed]
3. Heegaard, E.D.; Brown, K.E. Human parvovirus B19. *Clin. Microbiol. Rev.* **2002**, *15*, 485–505. [CrossRef] [PubMed]
4. Qiu, J.; Söderlund-Venermo, M.; Young, N.S. Human Parvoviruses. *Clin. Microbiol. Rev.* **2017**, *30*, 43–113. [CrossRef]
5. Anderson, M.J.; Higgins, P.G.; Davis, L.R.; Willman, J.S.; Jones, S.E.; Kidd, I.M.; Pattison, J.R.; Tyrrell, D.A.J. Experimental parvoviral infection in humans. *J. Infect. Dis.* **1985**, *152*, 257–265. [CrossRef]
6. Woolf, A.D.; Campion, G.V.; Chishick, A.; Wise, S.; Cohen, B.J.; Klouda, P.T.; Caul, O.; Dieppe, P.A. Clinical manifestations of human parvovirus B19 in adults. *Arch. Intern. Med.* **1989**, *149*, 1153–1156. [CrossRef]
7. Pattison, J.R. The pathogenesis of diseases associated with B19 virus. *Behring Inst. Mitt.* **1990**, *85*, 55–59.
8. Brown, K.E.; Green, S.W.; Antunez de Mayolo, J.; Young, N.S.; Bellanti, J.A.; Smith, S.D.; Smith, T.J. Congenital anaemia after transplacental B19 parvovirus infection. *Lancet* **1994**, *343*, 895–896. [CrossRef]
9. White, F.V.; Jordan, J.; Dickman, P.S.; Knisely, A.S. Fetal parvovirus B19 infection and liver disease of antenatal onset in an infant with Ebstein's anomaly. *Pediatr. Pathol. Lab. Med.* **1995**, *15*, 121–129. [CrossRef]
10. Young, N.S.; Brown, K.E. Parvovirus B19. *N. Engl. J. Med.* **2004**, *350*, 586–597. [CrossRef]
11. Cassinotti, P.; Siegl, G. Quantitative evidence for persistence of human parvovirus B19 DNA in an immunocompetent individual. *Eur. J. Clin. Microbiol. Infect. Dis.* **2000**, *19*, 886–887. [CrossRef] [PubMed]
12. Norja, P.; Hokynar, K.; Aaltonen, L.M.; Chen, R.; Ranki, A.; Partio, E.K.; Kiviluoto, O.; Davidkin, I.; Leivo, T.; Eis-Hübinger, A.M.; et al. Bioportfolio: Lifelong persistence of variant and prototypic erythrovirus DNA genomes in human tissue. *Proc. Natl. Acad. Sci. USA* **2006**, *103*, 7450–7453. [CrossRef] [PubMed]
13. Adamson-Small, L.A.; Ignatovich, I.V.; Laemmerhirt, M.G.; Hobbs, J.A. Persistent parvovirus B19 infection in non-erythroid tissues: Possible role in the inflammatory and disease process. *Virus Res.* **2014**, *190*, 8–16. [CrossRef]
14. Alves, A.D.; Melgaço, J.G.; Cássia Nc Garcia, R.; Raposo, J.V.; de Paula, V.S.; Araújo, C.C.; Pinto, M.A.; Amado, L.A. Persistence of Parvovirus B19 in liver from transplanted patients with acute liver failure. *Future Microbiol.* **2020**, *15*, 307–317. [CrossRef]
15. Söderlund, M.; von Essen, R.; Haapasaari, J.; Kiistala, U.; Kiviluoto, O.; Hedman, K. Persistence of parvovirus B19 DNA in synovial membranes of young patients with and without chronic arthropathy. *Lancet* **1997**, *349*, 1063–1065. [CrossRef]
16. Molenaar-de Backer, M.W.; Russcher, A.; Kroes, A.C.; Koppelman, M.H.; Lanfermeijer, M.; Zaaijer, H.L. Detection of parvovirus B19 DNA in blood: Viruses or DNA remnants? *J. Clin. Virol.* **2016**, *84*, 19–23. [CrossRef]
17. Reber, U.; Moser, O.; Dilloo, D.; Eis-Hubinger, A.M. On the utility of the benzonase treatment for correct laboratory diagnosis of parvovirus B19 infection. *J. Clin. Virol.* **2017**, *95*, 10–11. [CrossRef]
18. Leon, L.A.; Marchevsky, R.S.; Gaspar, A.M.; Garcia Rde, C.; Almeida, A.J.; Pelajo-Machado, M.; De Castro, T.X.; Nascimento, J.P.D.; Brown, K.E.; Pinto, M.A. Cynomolgus monkeys (*Macaca fascicularis*) experimentally infected with B19V and hepatitis A virus: No evidence of the co-infection as a cause of acute liver failure. *Mem. Inst. Oswaldo Cruz* **2016**, *111*, 258–266. [CrossRef]
19. Virion\Serion. SERION ELISA Classic Parvovirus B19 IgG/IgM 2022. Available online: https://www.serion-diagnostics.de/index.php?eID=dumpFile&t=f&f=5684&token=7c18512b5138b8f2e5dec0a78e0f8d4edc94ccd4 (accessed on 30 June 2021).
20. Guidance for Industry, Characterization and Qualification of Cell Substrates and Other Biological Materials Used in the Production of Viral Vaccines for Infectious Disease Indications, U.S. Department of Health and Human Services Food and Drug Administration Center for Biologics Evaluation and Research [February 2010]. Available online: https://www.fda.gov/media/78428/download (accessed on 7 April 2022).
21. Lyashchenko, K.P.; Singh, M.; Colangeli, R.; Gennaro, M.L. A multi-antigen print immunoassay for the development of serological diagnosis of infectious diseases. *J. Immunol. Methods* **2000**, *242*, 91–100. [CrossRef]
22. Alves, A.D.R.; Cubel Garcia, R.D.C.N.; Cruz, O.G.; Pinto, M.A.; Amado Leon, L.A. Quantitative real-time PCR for differential diagnostics of parvovirus B19 infection in acute liver failure patients. *Expert Rev. Mol. Diagn.* **2019**, *19*, 259–266. [CrossRef]
23. Juhl, D.; Görg, S.; Hennig, H. Persistence of Parvovirus B19 (B19V) DNA and humoral immune response in B19V-infected blood donors. *Vox Sang.* **2014**, *107*, 226–232. [CrossRef] [PubMed]
24. Kerr, J.R.; Curran, M.D.; Moore, J.E.; Coyle, P.V.; Ferguson, W.P. Persistent parvovirus B19 infection. *Lancet* **1995**, *345*, 1118. [CrossRef]
25. Musiani, M.; Zerbini, M.; Gentilomi, G.; Plazzi, M.; Gallinella, G.; Venturoli, S. Parvovirus B19 clearance from peripheral blood after acute infection. *J. Infect. Dis.* **1995**, *172*, 1360–1363. [CrossRef]
26. Gravelsina, S.; Nora-Krukle, Z.; Svirskis, S.; Cunskis, E.; Murovska, M. Presence of B19V in Patients with Thyroid Gland Disorders. *Medicina* **2019**, *55*, 774. [CrossRef] [PubMed]

27. Santonja, C.; Santos-Briz, A.; Palmedo, G.; Kutzner, H.; Requena, L. Detection of human parvovirus B19 DNA in 22% of 1815 cutaneous biopsies of a wide variety of dermatological conditions suggests viral persistence after primary infection and casts doubts on its pathogenic significance. *Br. J. Dermatol.* **2017**, *177*, 1060–1065. [CrossRef] [PubMed]
28. Van Linthout, S.; Elsanhoury, A.; Klein, O.; Sosnowski, M.; Miteva, K.; Lassner, D.; Abou-El-Enein, M.; Pieske, B.; Kühl, U.; Tschöpe, C. Telbivudine in chronic lymphocytic myocarditis and human parvovirus B19 transcriptional activity. *ESC Heart Fail.* **2018**, *5*, 818–829. [CrossRef] [PubMed]
29. Maple, P.A.; Hedman, L.; Dhanilall, P.; Kantola, K.; Nurmi, V.; Söderlund-Venermo, M.; Brown, K.E.; Hedman, K. Identification of past and recent parvovirus B19 infection in immunocompetent individuals by quantitative PCR and enzyme immunoassays: A dual-laboratory study. *J. Clin. Microbiol.* **2014**, *52*, 947–956. [CrossRef]
30. Bredl, S.; Plentz, A.; Wenzel, J.J.; Pfister, H.; Möst, J.; Modrow, S. False-negative serology in patients with acute parvovirus B19 infection. *J. Clin. Virol.* **2011**, *51*, 115–120. [CrossRef]
31. European Pharmacopoeia (Ph.Eur.). *B19 VIRUS DNA for NAT Testing BRP (Y0000285)*; European Pharmacopoeia: Strasbourg, France, 2019; p. 3.
32. Food and Drug Administration (FDA). *Nucleic Acid Testing (NAT) to Reduce the Possible Risk of Human Parvovirus B19 Transmission by Plasma-Derived Products (HFM-40)*; Outreach and Development (OCOD) (HFM-40): Rockville, MD, USA, 2009; p. 7.
33. Lefrère, J.J.; Maniez-Montreuil, M.; Morel, P.; Defer, C.; Laperche, S. Safety of blood products and B19 parvovirus. *Transfus. Clin. Biol.* **2006**, *13*, 235–241. [CrossRef]
34. Lefrère, J.J.; Servant-Delmas, A.; Candotti, D.; Mariotti, M.; Thomas, I.; Brossard, Y.; Lefreère, F.; Girot, R.; Allain, J.-P.; Laperche, S. Persistent B19 infection in immunocompetent individuals: Implications for transfusion safety. *Blood* **2005**, *106*, 2890–2895. [CrossRef]
35. Bonvicini, F.; Manaresi, E.; Di Furio, F.; De Falco, L.; Gallinella, G. Parvovirus b19 DNA CpG dinucleotide methylation and epigenetic regulation of viral expression. *PLoS ONE* **2012**, *7*, e33316. [CrossRef] [PubMed]
36. Corcioli, F.; Zakrzewska, K.; Rinieri, A.; Fanci, R.; Innocenti, M.; Civinini, R.; De Giorgi, V.; Di Lollo, S.; Azzi, A. Tissue persistence of parvovirus B19 genotypes in asymptomatic persons. *J. Med. Virol.* **2008**, *80*, 2005–2011. [CrossRef] [PubMed]
37. Schenk, T.; Enders, M.; Pollak, S.; Hahn, R.; Huzly, D. High prevalence of human parvovirus B19 DNA in myocardial autopsy samples from subjects without myocarditis or dilative cardiomyopathy. *J. Clin. Microbiol.* **2009**, *47*, 106–110. [CrossRef] [PubMed]
38. Ganaie, S.S.; Qiu, J. Recent Advances in Replication and Infection of Human Parvovirus B19. *Front. Cell. Infect. Microbiol.* **2018**, *8*, 166. [CrossRef]

viruses

MDPI

Case Report

Clinical Presentation of Parvovirus B19 Infection in Adults Living with HIV/AIDS: A Case Series

Daniela P. Mendes-de-Almeida [1,2,3], Joanna Paes Barreto Bokel [1,4], Arthur Daniel Rocha Alves [5], Alexandre G. Vizzoni [1], Isabel Cristina Ferreira Tavares [6], Mayara Secco Torres Silva [6], Juliana dos Santos Barbosa Netto [6], Beatriz Gilda Jegerhorn Grinsztejn [6] and Luciane Almeida Amado Leon [5,*]

1 Hematology Department, Evandro Chagas National Institute of Infectious Diseases, Oswaldo Cruz Foundation (FIOCRUZ), Rio de Janeiro 21040-360, RJ, Brazil; daniela.almeida@ini.fiocruz.br (D.P.M.-d.-A.); joanna.bokel@ini.fiocruz.br (J.P.B.B.); alexandre.vizzoni@ini.fiocruz.br (A.G.V.)
2 Research Center, Instituto Nacional de Câncer (INCA), Rio de Janeiro 20220-430, RJ, Brazil
3 Department of Medical Affairs, Clinical Studies, and Post-Registration Surveillance (DEAME), Institute of Technology in Immunobiologicals/Bio-Manguinhos, Oswaldo Cruz Foundation (FIOCRUZ), Rio de Janeiro 21040-360, RJ, Brazil
4 Onco-Hematology Unit, Clínica São Vicente, Rio de Janeiro 22451-100, RJ, Brazil
5 Laboratory of Technological Development in Virology, Instituto Oswaldo Cruz, Oswaldo Cruz Foundation (FIOCRUZ), Rio de Janeiro 21040-360, RJ, Brazil; arthur.alves@ioc.fiocruz.br
6 Laboratory of Clinical Research on STD/AIDS, Evandro Chagas National Institute of Infectious Diseases, Oswaldo Cruz Foundation (FIOCRUZ), Rio de Janeiro 21040-360, RJ, Brazil; isabel.tavares@ini.fiocruz.br (I.C.F.T.); mayara.secco@ini.fiocruz.br (M.S.T.S.); juliananetto@gmail.com (J.d.S.B.N.); beatriz.grinsztejn@gmail.com (B.G.J.G.)
* Correspondence: l_amado@ioc.fiocruz.br; Tel.: +55-21-2562-1876

Abstract: Parvovirus B19 (B19V) infection varies clinically depending on the host's immune status. Due to red blood cell precursors tropism, B19V can cause chronic anemia and transient aplastic crisis in patients with immunosuppression or chronic hemolysis. We report three rare cases of Brazilian adults living with human immunodeficiency virus (HIV) with B19V infection. All cases presented severe anemia and required red blood cell transfusions. The first patient had low $CD4^+$ counts and was treated with intravenous immunoglobulin (IVIG). As he remained poorly adherent to antiretroviral therapy (ART), B19V detection persisted. The second patient had sudden pancytopenia despite being on ART with an undetectable HIV viral load. He had historically low $CD4^+$ counts, fully responded to IVIG, and had undiagnosed hereditary spherocytosis. The third individual was recently diagnosed with HIV and tuberculosis (TB). One month after ART initiation, he was hospitalized with anemia aggravation and cholestatic hepatitis. An analysis of his serum revealed B19V DNA and anti-B19V IgG, corroborating bone marrow findings and a persistent B19V infection. The symptoms resolved and B19V became undetectable. In all cases, real time PCR was essential for diagnosing B19V. Our findings showed that adherence to ART was crucial to B19V clearance in HIV-patients and highlighted the importance of the early recognition of B19V disease in unexplained cytopenias.

Keywords: Parvovirus B19; HIV infection; hemolysis; hereditary spherocytosis

Citation: Mendes-de-Almeida, D.P.; Bokel, J.P.B.; Alves, A.D.R.; Vizzoni, A.G.; Tavares, I.C.F.; Silva, M.S.T.; Netto, J.d.S.B.; Grinsztejn, B.G.J.; Amado Leon, L.A. Clinical Presentation of Parvovirus B19 Infection in Adults Living with HIV/AIDS: A Case Series. *Viruses* **2023**, *15*, 1124. https://doi.org/10.3390/v15051124

Academic Editor: Giorgio Gallinella

Received: 14 April 2023
Revised: 2 May 2023
Accepted: 4 May 2023
Published: 8 May 2023

1. Introduction

Parvovirus B19 infection (B19V) is often asymptomatic or presents with mild disease. It can present as erythema infectiosum during childhood, a viral exanthem (also known as "slapped cheek" syndrome), hydrops fetalis in pregnant women, which can lead to miscarriages, or with less common symptoms that include painful or swollen joints (polyarthopathy syndrome). The infection is usually self-limited and resolves within one to two weeks. Due to red blood cell (RBC) precursors tropism, B19V might cause the temporary cessation of the bone marrow's RBC production, leading to transient aplastic crisis (TAC), mainly in patients with chronic hemolysis, including hereditary spherocytosis (HS). The overlapping arrest of RBC production and excessive destruction can cause potentially life-threatening anemia, requiring urgent blood transfusions [1].

Pure red cell aplasia (PRCA) has been described in patients living with HIV/AIDS (PLWHA), affecting up to 4.5% of patients [2,3]. Therefore, some authors recommend the prompt consideration of B19V-mediated PRCA for PLWHA with severe isolated anemia [4]. Patients with persistent or recurrent viremia have absent or low levels of specific antibodies. Clinical hallmarks of B19V infection in PLWHA include fatigue and pallor, while immune-mediated symptoms (rash and arthralgia) are generally lacking. The treatment of persistent B19V with intravenous immunoglobulin (IVIG) reduces the viral load and usually results in a marked resolution of anemia [5].

Herein, we report three rare cases of Brazilian PLWHA with B19V-mediated severe anemia. The HIV patients were treated at the Instituto Nacional de Infectologia Evandro Chagas (INI/Fiocruz) and manifested with different clinical presentations. We discuss B19V infection in PLWHA, clinical presentation, diagnostic challenges, and therapeutic responses. These cases highlight the importance of the early recognition of B19V disease in unexplained cytopenias settings.

2. Detailed Case Descriptions

2.1. Case 1

A 27-year-old Black male diagnosed with HIV months after birth in 1994 had a history of multiple infections, including pneumocystosis, tuberculosis (TB), and bacterial pneumonia. Due to poor adherence to antiretroviral therapy (ART), the patient had an extensively drug-resistant viral infection and was taking lamivudine (3TC), tenofovir (TDF), darunavir/ritonavir (DRV/r), dolutegravir (DTG), etravirine (ETR), and fostemsavir, and presented with anemia and mild leukopenia in November 2020. A bone marrow biopsy showed 70% cellularity, normoblastic erythroid series, reduced granulocytic series, and megakaryocytes with preserved morphology, absence of granulomas, and negative special stains for fungi and mycobacteria. Malignancies were ruled out. In April 2021, he complained of vertigo, headache, vomiting, and fever, and was admitted with a deterioration of the anemic condition, mild hepatitis, and no adenopathy. He exhibited hemoglobin (Hb) 1.7 g/dL, hematocrit (Ht) 6.5%, white blood cells (WBC) 2.33 $\times$ 10^9/L, neutrophils 0.204 $\times$ 10^9/L, and platelets 354,000/mm^3, with corrected reticulocytes 0%, aspartate aminotransferase 251 U/L, alanine aminotransferase 351 U/L, HIV viral load 40,305 copies/mL, and a $CD4^+$ count of 6 cells/µL (Table 1). During hospitalization, he received a transfusion of six packed RBCs. He returned in October 2021 with complaints of dyspnea on minor exertion and intense prostration and reported chest pain the night before. He presented tachycardia and hepatosplenomegaly and received multiple blood transfusions. The myelogram was reviewed, showing giant proerythroblasts with nuclear inclusions (Figure 1A), which raised suspicions of B19V infection. B19V screening included nested PCR for the VP1/VP2 genome region [6], with viral load determined by real-time polymerase chain reaction (qPCR) for the NS1 genome region [7]. In October 2021, B19V PCR was positive in serum with 4.3 $\times$ 10^{10} IU/mL, while anti-B19V IgM and IgG were negative. Genotype 1a was defined based on a B19V phylogenetic tree (Figure 2). He received IVIG 400 mg/kg/day for three consecutive days and showed a complete response with stabilized RBC counts. In July 2022, the patient remained non-adherent to ART but without anemia, maintaining a low $CD4^+$ count (11 cells/µL) and high HIV viral load (27,642 copies/mL). B19V DNA remained detectable (1.8 $\times$ 10^6 IU/mL), and IgM and IgG were indeterminate. As he was asymptomatic with normal blood cell counts, a new course of IVIG was not indicated.

Table 1. Laboratory findings' evolution of three HIV-positive patients with Parvovirus B19 infection.

Laboratory Analysis	Test Method	Reference Value	Case 1			Case 2			Case 3		
			April/21 *	October/21	July/22	April/21	August/21 *	June/22	January/22	February/22 *	July/22
Hemoglobin (g/dL)	Flow Cytometry	(10.5–14.8)	1.7	5.2	13.9	12.5	5.6	16.4	9.4	6.5	11.6
Hematocrit (%)	Flow Cytometry	(40–54)	6.5	15.6	40.3	34.8	15.2	46.5	29.1	18.7	35.3
MCV (μm^3)	Flow Cytometry	(80–96)	85.0	82.0	85.4	111.5	104.8	101.3	82.4	77.3	82.7
MCHC (g/dL)	Flow Cytometry	(32–36)	26.0	33.0	34.5	35.9	36.8	35.3	26.6	26.9	27.2
Platelet counts (per mm^3)	Flow Cytometry	(155,000–409,000)	354,000	255,000	143,000	119,000	41,000	135,000	245,000	175,000	241,000
WBC (per mm^3)	Flow Cytometry	(4500–11,000)	2330	2790	3950	4780	1480	5890	2510	1190	2880
Neutrophil counts (per mm^3)	Flow Cytometry	(1470–6750)	204	1850	2528	3435	577	3239	1832.3	654.4	2163
Direct antiglobulin	Gel Test	Negative	Negative	Negative	Positive	NA	Negative	Negative	NA	NA	Negative
G6PD phenotype	Brewer	Normal	NA	NA	Normal	NA	Normal	Normal	NA	NA	NA
Reticulocytes **	Flow Cytometry	(0.5–1.5%)	0.0	0.0	1.1	NA	NA	0.2	0.8	ND	ND
Lactate desidrogenase (UI/L)	Enzymatic	(85–227)	243	448	218	209	6204	179	962	830	518
Ferritin (ng/mL)	Immunoassay	(26–388)	1215	1302	701	NA	611	596	3078	4037	ND
C-reactive protein (mg/dL)	Turbidimetric	(<0.3)	5.2	23.73	2.52	0.63	1.27	NA	1.0	3.45	0.6
Aspartat aminotransferase (U/L)	Enzymatic	(15–37)	251	26	22	114	190	26	93	455	74
Alanine aminotransferase (U/L)	Enzymatic	(12–78)	302	51	31	62	38	25	159	414	99
Total bilirrubin (mg/dL)	Jendrassik and Grof	(0.0–1.0)	0.85	1.36	0.6	0.93	3.07	1.38	0.65	1.21	0.80
Indirect bilirrubin (mg/dL)	Jendrassik and Grof	(0.0–0.7)	0.47	0.91	0.14	0.69	2.27	0.97	0.33	0.38	0.36
GGT (U/L)	Enzymatic	(15–85)	122	118	37	80	40	152	368	626	628
Alkaline phosphatase (U/L)	Enzymatic	(46–116)	1140	133	104	69	61	64	665	1529	326
HIV viral load (copies/mL)	qPCR	ND	40,305	NA	27,642	ND	ND	ND	345,605	130	72
CD4+ T lymphocytes (cells/μL)	Flow Cytometry	(40.4–1612)	6	65	11	NA	127	200	69	138	299
PCR VP1VP2	PCR	-	Positive	NA	Positive	NA	Positive	Negative	NA	Positive	Negative
qPCR NS1 (IU/mL)	qPCR	-	4.3×10^{10}	NA	1.8×10^6	NA	8.9×10^3	Negative	NA	5.9×10^4	Negative
IgM anti-B19V	ELISA	-	Negative	NA	ID	NA	ID	ID	NA	Negative	Negative
IgG anti-B19V	ELISA	-	Negative	NA	ID	NA	Positive	Positive	NA	Positive	Positive

Abbreviations: WBC: White blood cell; MCV: Mean Corpuscular Volume; MCHC: Mean corpuscular hemoglobin concentration; B19V: Parvovirus B19; G6PD: Glucose-6-phosphate dehydrogenase; GGT: Gamma-glutamyl transpeptidase; ND: Not detectable; NA: Not available; ID: indeterminate; PCR: Polymerase chain reaction; qPCR: Real time polymerase chain reaction; ELISA: Enzyme Linked Immuno-Sorbent Assay; * B19V detection; ** Reticulocytes corrected by the level of anemia.

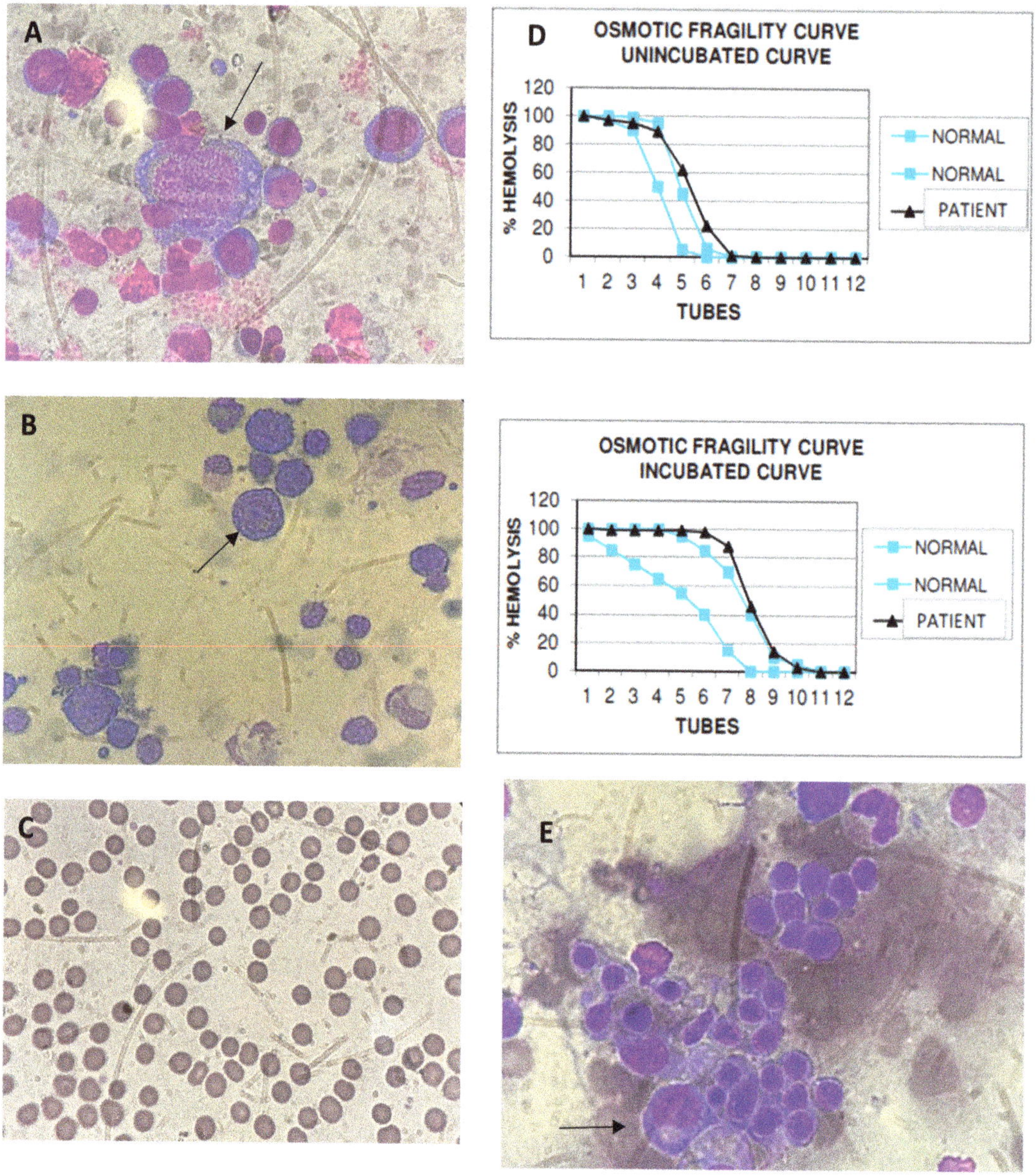

Figure 1. Myelogram, peripheral blood smear, and osmotic fragility test curve findings in patients with B19V and HIV. B19V inclusion in abnormally large pronormoblast with basophilic and vacuolated cytoplasm in bone marrow aspirate (arrows) (×400) is shown for Cases 1 (**A**) and 2 (**B**). Small-sized, spherical-shaped, deep-staining red blood cells (RBC) are shown to lack an area of central pallor at peripheral blood film, accounting for more than 50% of RBC in Case 2 (**C**). (**D**) The osmotic fragility test curve (black) for Case 2 is shown; slightly right-skewed curves suggest that RBCs hemolyze more quickly than usual (blue curves as range reference) both in unincubated and in incubated curves. B19V inclusion in abnormally large pronormoblast with basophilic and vacuolated cytoplasm in bone marrow aspirate is shown for Case 3 (arrow) (×400) (**E**).

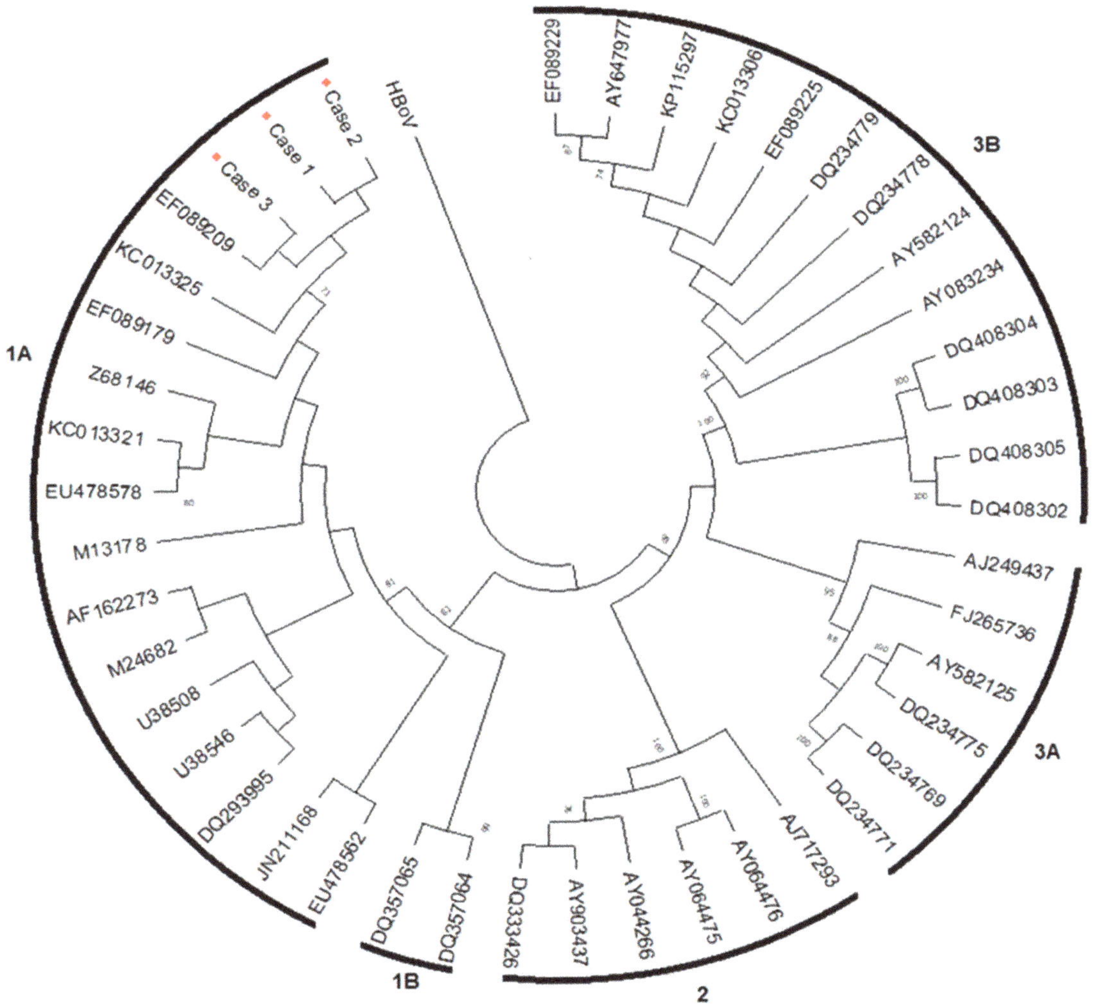

Figure 2. Parvovirus B19 phylogenetic tree.

A phylogenetic tree of Parvovirus B19 (VP1/VP2 gene; among 420 bp) in patients with HIV and anemia (red diamonds), defined as genotype 1a, inferred by using the Maximum Likelihood method and Tamura-Nei model [8]. Evolutionary analyses were conducted in MEGA X [9]. A human bocavirus (HBoV; GQ243610) sequence was used to root the tree. Sequences were analyzed using the Bio-Edit sequence alignment editor, v. 7.2.5 (mbio.ncsu.edu/BioEdit/bioedit.html, accessed on 17 July 2022) and they were compared with the following sequences available in GenBank (Hall 1999): Genotype 1a: EF089179 and EF089209 (Brazil/PA), KC013321 and KC013325 (Brazil/SP), Z68146-Stu and EU478578-EU478562 (Germany), M13178-Au (USA), AF162273-Hv (Finland), M24682-Wi (UK), U38508 (Ireland), U38546-BrIII (Brazil/RJ), DQ293995 (Belgium), JN211168 (The Netherlands); Genotype 1b: DQ357064 and DQ357065 (Vietnam); Genotype 2: DQ333426, AY903437 and AJ717293-Berlin (Germany), AY064475-A6 and AY064776 (Italy), AY044266-LaLi (Finland); Genotype 3a: AJ249437-V9 (France), AY582125, DQ234775, DQ234769 and DQ234771 (Ghana); and Genotype 3b: AY083234-D91.1 (France), DQ408302-DQ408305 (Germany), AY582124, DQ234778-DQ234779 (Ghana). The three samples from this study were deposited in the GenBank database under accession numbers OQ917657, OQ917658, and OQ917659.

2.2. Case 2

A 61-year-old White male of Spanish origin living with HIV since 2009 with regular use of TDF, 3TC, and DTG since 2017 presented an undetectable HIV viral load and historically low $CD4^+$ counts below 200 cells/mm^3. He sought medical consultation in August 2021 after four weeks of malaise, lethargy, and an acute incident of dizziness, diarrhea, and syncope. He had hypothyroidism and no history of hematologic disorders, but his mother suffered from chronic anemia. The patient was submitted to a full blood workup that showed pancytopenia (Hb 5.6 g/dL, Ht 15.2%, WBC 1.48 $\times$ 10^9/L, neutrophils 0.547 $\times$ 10^9/L, and platelets 41,000 per mm^3), mildly elevated serum ferritin (611 µg/L), and anemic hemolytic features (Table 1). He also presented a negative direct antiglobulin test and did not show evidence of renal dysfunction, iron, or glucose-6-phosphate dehydrogenase deficiency. Reticulocyte counts were not available. During the physical examination, he exhibited jaundice and a palpable spleen. He was admitted for further investigation and received three transfusions of packed RBCs. The HIV viral load at admission was undetectable, and the $CD4^+$ count was 127 cells/mm^3. As he sustained pancytopenia, a bone marrow aspirate and a biopsy were performed. The myelogram showed giant proerythroblasts with nuclear inclusions (Figure 1B). The bone marrow histology disclosed 95% cellularity, mild erythroid hyperplasia, megaloblastic findings, and no hemophagocytic lymphohistiocytosis. Furthermore, the bone marrow sample showed negative results in the acid-alcohol-fast-bacilli (AFB) test, cultures for fungi, and mycobacteria. Analyses of anti-B19V IgM were indeterminate, and anti-IgG antibodies were positive. Results from the PCR included the detection of 8.92 $\times$ 10^3 IU/mL B19V, and genotype 1a was identified (Figure 2). The patient received IVIG 500 mg/kg/d for four days after 37 days from the onset of symptoms. The patient had no significant symptoms, and the RBC count stabilized immediately after treatment. Ten months later, his laboratory results showed a resolution of the pancytopenia but the maintenance of a mild elevation of indirect bilirubin, indicative of chronic hemolysis. B19V PCR was no longer detected in peripheral blood. Abdominal ultrasonography excluded gallstones or the maintenance of splenomegaly. A blood smear analysis was performed, which revealed spherocytes in more than 50% of RBCs (Figure 1C), and an osmotic fragility test (OFT) was suggestive of RBC membranopathy. In addition, hemoglobin electrophoresis showed no changes. We concluded that this case was B19V-induced pancytopenia in an immunocompromised patient presenting with HS. He continued receiving folate supplementation and had no clinical symptoms.

2.3. Case 3

A 27-year-old Black man was newly diagnosed with HIV in December 2021 during admission due to respiratory symptoms and pancytopenia. He also presented disseminated TB and had increased transaminase levels after starting treatment with rifampicin, isoniazid, pyrazinamide, and ethambutol. Thus, doctors suspected TB-related hepatotoxicity and switched treatment to levofloxacin, amikacin, and ethambutol, while he tolerated the reintroduction of the first-line scheme over three weeks. The patient presented with 345,605 copies/mL HIV viral load and 69 cells/mm^3 $CD4^+$ counts. After four weeks of TB treatment, ART was initiated with a negative AFB in the sputum. Eighteen days after starting ART, he presented with a new asymptomatic elevation of transaminases associated with a pattern of a cholestatic lesion, anemia (Hb 9.4 d/dL and Ht 29.1%), and leukopenia (WBC 2510 cells/mm^3) and average platelet counts. One month after ART initiation—on February 2022—the patient was hospitalized with anemia aggravation requiring RBC transfusion and cholestatic hepatitis, leading to a new suspension of tuberculostatic drugs. The HIV viral load decreased to 130 copies/mL, and $CD4^+$ counts improved to 138 cells/mm^3 (Table 1). The patient was re-screened for opportunistic infections, with a negative investigation for histoplasmosis and cryptococcosis. A myelogram showed enlarged erythroblasts with nuclear inclusions (Figure 1E). Bone marrow histopathologic analysis showed serous stromal degeneration and a reactive lymphoid aggregate. Abdominal ultrasonography evidenced hepatosplenomegaly and the thickening of the gallbladder wall with no signs of lithiasis. To address the TB-associated inflammatory reconstitution inflammatory syndrome (IRIS-TB) hypothesis, he received systemic corticosteroid therapy (prednisone 1 mg/kg/day for seven days with posterior waning) and presented a resolution of laboratory abnormalities. He tolerated the reintroduction of anti-TB treatment. A retrospective analysis from a serum sample collected in February 2022 revealed B19V DNA detectable at 5.9×10^4 IU/mL, B19V genotype 1a, and anti-B19V IgG positivity, corroborating bone marrow findings and confirming the B19V infection (Table 1 and Figure 2). No additional measures were adopted for B19V, as the patient's DNA became undetectable, and symptoms resolved after IRIS-TB treatment.

3. Discussion

The relationship between anemia and B19V infection is well known [4,10–12]. B19V DNA was detected by dot blot hybridization in sera from 5 of 30 (17%) PLWHA with Ht <24% and 4 of 13 (31%) patients with Ht < 20% in a study published in 1997, suggesting that B19V was a substantial contributor to severe anemia in HIV infection in the pre-high-potency ART era [13]. A recent study that enrolled 158 HIV-infected children in Nigeria showed a low prevalence of B19V among HIV-positive children (~2%). Nevertheless, a significant relationship was established between B19V infection and the severity of anemia ($p = 0.015$) [14]. A Brazilian study conducted ten years ago estimated a frequency of B19V seroconversion of 31.8% in a cohort of 88 HIV-infected patients, and showed that patients who seroconverted were 5.40 times more likely to have anemia than those who did not [15]. There is a lack of more recent data on the frequency of B19V and HIV coinfection in Brazil.

Adherence to medication is one of the most critical factors for a successful ART. Poor medication adherence can lead to treatment failure and the development of drug-resistant strains of HIV. Several studies have shown that adherence to antiretroviral medication is associated with better health outcomes in HIV-positive individuals [16,17]. Hematological changes are common findings in PLWHA, particularly in poor adherent individuals. Anemia and thrombocytopenia have been demonstrated to be independent predictors of morbidity and mortality [18]. Although cytopenias often respond to ART, in some patients they can persist. Our case series confirmed that the B19V course depends on the host's immunologic status, as DNA detection only lasted in the first case, who was a patient not adherent to ART.

Several case reports describe B19V infection in patients with HS, with patient's findings usually including fever, fatigue, a family history of HS in most patients (59%), and in some cases liver dysfunction [19]. Although HS diagnosis usually occurs in childhood and young adult life, HS may be diagnosed at any time, including in old age [20]. B19V infection can cause TAC in patients with increased destruction or loss of RBCs, as it occurs in HS. Patients may also have congestive heart failure, hypo flow stroke, and acute splenic sequestration [21]. Our second case's clinical presentation and evolutive findings after IVIG suggested TAC with an underlying chronic hemolytic anemia. HS was confirmed after investigation.

HS is the most common RBC membrane disorder worldwide, and the most common hereditary hemolytic anemia in people with Northern European ancestry, with a prevalence of 1 in 1000 to 2500 [22]. The abnormal spherocytes' shape is due to inadequate vertical linkages between the cytoskeleton and the lipid bilayer [22]. RBCs exhibit increased osmotic fragility and deformability, resulting in extravascular hemolysis due to the increased destruction of RBCs when passing through the spleen. The eosin-5′-maleimide binding test is the most accurate screen for HS diagnosis because it binds to specific erythrocyte membrane molecules [23]. However, it is scarcely offered in Brazil and is only required in complex cases. The diagnosis here was straightforward based on clinical history, physical examination, and laboratory data. Although TAC specifically affects RBC lines, WBCs and platelets may also decline. Despite high suspicion, we could not characterize TAC in our second patient due to the lack of reticulocyte counts and typical histologic bone marrow findings during the pancytopenia episode.

Bone marrow potentially suffers from the combined effects of HIV, inflammatory mediators released during infection, nutritional deficiency, and opportunistic pathogens [24]. B19V should be considered part of the differential diagnosis of severe hypoproliferative anemia in PLWHA. B19V diagnosis is not obvious, and clinicians should search for bone marrow abnormalities and molecular virological findings. Due to immunosuppression, PLWHA usually lack IgM production, leading to the prolonged destruction of RBC progenitors [25]. B19V might have played a role in our third case's presentation, despite the patient having other possible causes for anemia and hepatitis, such as HIV myelopathy, opportunistic infections, TB-related hepatotoxicity, and IRIS-TB.

Nevertheless, the diagnosis of B19V-induced anemia in PLWHA is rare, possibly due to underdiagnosing [25,26]. Molecular diagnosis through qPCR was decisive in establishing B19V diagnosis in our cases because of the low serologic sensitivity. Genotype 1a was found in all samples of this study, and there was no apparent relationship between the infecting genotype and the clinical course. Genotype 1 is the most common B19V genotype detected globally [27,28] and among HIV patients [14]. In a Brazilian study among five HIV-positive patients receiving ART who had B19V infections confirmed by qPCR, four exhibited genotype 1a strain, and the remaining patient presented a genotype 3b strain [29]. Ferry et al. found that the detection of B19V genotypes 2 or 3 was infrequent in a large cohort of immunocompromised, HIV-infected anemic patients, despite the use of highly sensitive qPCR methods [30]. Although these three genotypes have been reported in Brazil, genotype 1 is the most common [31–33]. The B19V sequences obtained from three cases were closely related to sequences EF089179, EF089209, and KC013325, isolated from Brazilian patients (from Rio de Janeiro, São Paulo and Pará states, respectively) with compromised immunological and/or hematological status [31,34].

Despite the low $CD4^{+}$ counts, our patients did not experience a worse prognosis than immunocompetent individuals. The treatment of B19V infection depends on the clinical burden and the host's immune response. Spontaneous resolution can occur if the immune system reconstitutes; no further treatment is needed in these cases. Still, IVIG is a fundamental source of neutralizing antibodies for persistently symptomatic individuals. Usually, only one course of IVIG is required for long-term remission [5]. The coronavirus disease 2019 (COVID-19) resulted in interruptions in HIV diagnosis and virological control, impacting ART supply chains and negatively affecting PLWHA's treatment adherence and quality of care [35]. We hypothesize that the COVID-19 pandemic may have influenced B19V's incidence in PLWHA. Further studies regarding B19V frequency in PLWHA are needed in Brazil to understand factors associated with severity and disease evolution, particularly after the COVID-19 pandemic.

4. Conclusions

Our three cases descriptions highlight the importance of B19V diagnosis in PLWHA. Cytopenias are often multifactorial, and performing a comprehensive clinical evaluation is essential to prevent delayed diagnosis and morbidity. Persistent B19V infection in PLWHA is challenging to differentiate from other opportunistic infections or IRIS. Therefore, a high index of suspicion for B19V should be of concern for HIV patients with cytopenias and advanced immunosuppression. The decision to treat B19V should always be clinically guided. Although IVIG therapy is the primary treatment to clear viremia in PLWHA, ART compliance is essential to normalize blood cell counts and prevent B19V relapse.

Author Contributions: D.P.M.-d.-A., J.P.B.B. and L.A.A.L. designed the study; J.P.B.B., J.d.S.B.N., M.S.T.S., I.C.F.T. and D.P.M.-d.-A. attended the patient; D.P.M.-d.-A., J.P.B.B. and A.G.V. analyzed the clinical data; A.D.R.A. performed the serological and molecular analysis; D.P.M.-d.-A., J.P.B.B., J.d.S.B.N., A.D.R.A., M.S.T.S., I.C.F.T. and L.A.A.L. wrote the original draft; L.A.A.L. provided funding; J.d.S.B.N., B.G.J.G. and L.A.A.L. revised and edited the manuscript and supervised the study. All authors have read and agreed to the published version of the manuscript.

Funding: We are thankful to the Coordination for the Improvement of Higher Education Personnel—CAPES for the fellowship awarded, and FAPERJ-JCNE (number: e-26/201.406/2021) and the Oswaldo Cruz Institute for funding this study. Instituto Nacional de Infectologia Evandro Chagas was in charge of the publication fee.

Institutional Review Board Statement: The study was conducted in accordance with the Declaration of Helsinki and was approved by the Ethics Committee of Oswaldo Cruz Institute (CAAE number: 16918919.7.0000.5248, protocol #3.627.364).

Informed Consent Statement: Written informed consent was obtained from all subjects involved in the study.

Data Availability Statement: The data that support the findings of this study are available from the National Center for Biotechnology Information (NCBI) at https://www.ncbi.nlm.nih.gov/.

Acknowledgments: We thank the patients for providing consent, Paula Detepo and Fernando Loureiro Maior for the clinical discussion, Filipe V. Santos-Bueno for technical support, and all the members of the Laboratory of Clinical Analysis of the School of Pharmacy (LACFar, UFRJ, Brazil) for performing the Osmotic Fragility Curve.

Conflicts of Interest: The authors declare no conflict of interest.

References

1. Broliden, K.; Tolfvenstam, T.; Norbeck, O. Clinical Aspects of Parvovirus B19 Infection. *J. Intern. Med.* **2006**, *260*, 285–304. [CrossRef] [PubMed]
2. Crabol, Y.; Terrier, B.; Rozenberg, F.; Pestre, V.; Legendre, C.; Hermine, O.; Montagnier-Petrissans, C.; Guillevin, L.; Mouthon, L.; Groupe d'experts de l'Assistance Publique-Hopitaux de Paris; et al. Intravenous Immunoglobulin Therapy for Pure Red Cell Aplasia Related to Human Parvovirus B19 Infection: A Retrospective Study of 10 Patients and Review of the Literature. *Clin. Infect. Dis.* **2013**, *56*, 968–977. [CrossRef] [PubMed]
3. Vaz, S.O.; Guerra, I.C.; Freitas, M.I.; Marques, L. Pure Red Cell Aplasia and HIV Infection: What to Suspect? *BMJ Case Rep.* **2018**, bcr-2018-224625. [CrossRef]
4. Wylde, J.; Berneri, M.A.; Malherbe, J.A.J.; Davel, S. Isolated Anemia in a 69-Year-Old Man with HIV-1: Features of Pure Red Cell Aplasia Mediated by Chronic Parvovirus-B19 Infection. *Am. J. Case Rep.* **2022**, *23*, e936445-1. [CrossRef] [PubMed]
5. Heegaard, E.D.; Brown, K.E. Human Parvovirus B19. *Clin. Microbiol. Rev.* **2002**, *15*, 485–505. [CrossRef]
6. Durigon, E.L.; Erdman, D.D.; Gary, G.W.; Pallansch, M.A.; Torok, T.J.; Anderson, L.J. Multiple Primer Pairs for Polymerase Chain Reaction (PCR) Amplification of Human Parvovirus B19 DNA. *J. Virol. Methods* **1993**, *44*, 155–165. [CrossRef]
7. Alves, A.D.R.; Cubel Garcia, R.D.C.N.; Cruz, O.G.; Pinto, M.A.; Amado Leon, L.A. Quantitative Real-Time PCR for Differential Diagnostics of Parvovirus B19 Infection in Acute Liver Failure Patients. *Expert Rev. Mol. Diagn.* **2019**, *19*, 259–266. [CrossRef]
8. Tamura, K.; Nei, M. Estimation of the Number of Nucleotide Substitutions in the Control Region of Mitochondrial DNA in Humans and Chimpanzees. *Mol. Biol. Evol.* **1993**, *10*, 512–526. [CrossRef]
9. Kumar, S.; Stecher, G.; Li, M.; Knyaz, C.; Tamura, K. MEGA X: Molecular Evolutionary Genetics Analysis across Computing Platforms. *Mol. Biol. Evol.* **2018**, *35*, 1547–1549. [CrossRef]
10. Tun, M.M.; Chowdhury, T.; Nway, N.; Noel, P.; Gousy, N.; Roy, A.; Htet, S.Y. Parvovirus Infection Leading to Severe Anemia in an Adult Patient With HIV Disease. *Cureus* **2022**, *14*, e29148. [CrossRef]
11. Gor, D.; Singh, V.; Gupta, V.; Levitt, M. A Persistent Parvovirus Infection Causing Anemia in an HIV Patient Requiring Intravenous Immunoglobulin Maintenance Therapy. *Cureus* **2022**, *14*, e24627. [CrossRef] [PubMed]
12. Thibile, S.; Barrett, C.; Potgieter, S.; Joubert, G.; Malherbe, J. Adult Pure Red Cell Aplasia at Universitas Academic Hospital, Bloemfontein, South Africa: A 9-Year Review. *S. Afr. Med. J.* **2022**, *112*, 753–759. [CrossRef]
13. Abkowitz, J.L.; Brown, K.E.; Wood, R.W.; Kovach, N.L.; Green, S.W.; Young, N.S. Clinical Relevance of Parvovirus B19 as a Cause of Anemia in Patients with Human Immunodeficiency Virus Infection. *J. Infect. Dis.* **1997**, *176*, 269–273. [CrossRef] [PubMed]
14. Aleru, B.O.; Olusola, B.A.; Faneye, A.O.; Odaibo, G.N.; Olaleye, D.O. Prevalence and Genotypes of Parvovirus B19 Among HIV Positive Children in Ibadan, Oyo State, Nigeria. *Arch. Basic Appl. Med.* **2018**, *6*, 113–117.
15. De Azevedo, K.M.L.; Setúbal, S.; Camacho, L.A.B.; de Cássia Nasser Cubel Garcia, R.; Siqueira, M.M.; Pereira, R.F.A.; de Oliveira, S.A. Parvovirus B19 Seroconversion in a Cohort of Human Immunodeficiency Virus-Infected Patients. *Mem. Inst. Oswaldo Cruz* **2012**, *107*, 356–361. [CrossRef] [PubMed]
16. Nachega, J.B.; Uthman, O.A.; Anderson, J.; Peltzer, K.; Wampold, S.; Cotton, M.F.; Mills, E.J.; Ho, Y.-S.; Stringer, J.S.A.; McIntyre, J.A.; et al. Adherence to Antiretroviral Therapy during and after Pregnancy in Low-Income, Middle-Income, and High-Income Countries: A Systematic Review and Meta-Analysis. *AIDS* **2012**, *26*, 2039–2052. [CrossRef]

17. Wittkop, L.; Günthard, H.F.; De Wolf, F.; Dunn, D.; Cozzi-Lepri, A.; De Luca, A.; Kücherer, C.; Obel, N.; Von Wyl, V.; Masquelier, B.; et al. Effect of Transmitted Drug Resistance on Virological and Immunological Response to Initial Combination Antiretroviral Therapy for HIV (EuroCoord-CHAIN Joint Project): A European Multicohort Study. *Lancet Infect. Dis.* **2011**, *11*, 363–371. [CrossRef]
18. Mocroft, A.; Kirk, O.; Barton, S.E.; Dietrich, M.; Proenca, R.; Colebunders, R.; Pradier, C.; Monforte, A.A.; Ledergerber, B.; Lundgren, J.D. Anaemia Is an Independent Predictive Marker for Clinical Prognosis in HIV-Infected Patients from across Europe. *AIDS* **1999**, *13*, 943–950. [CrossRef]
19. Kobayashi, Y.; Hatta, Y.; Ishiwatari, Y.; Kanno, H.; Takei, M. Human Parvovirus B19-Induced Aplastic Crisis in an Adult Patient with Hereditary Spherocytosis: A Case Report and Review of the Literature. *BMC Res. Notes* **2014**, *7*, 137. [CrossRef]
20. Bolton-Maggs, P.H.B.; Langer, J.C.; Iolascon, A.; Tittensor, P.; King, M.-J. Guidelines for the Diagnosis and Management of Hereditary Spherocytosis—2011 Update: Guideline. *Br. J. Haematol.* **2012**, *156*, 37–49. [CrossRef]
21. Saarinen, U.M.; Chorba, T.L.; Tattersall, P.; Young, N.S.; Anderson, L.J.; Palmer, E.; Coccia, P.F. Human Parvovirus B19-Induced Epidemic Acute Red Cell Aplasia in Patients with Hereditary Hemolytic Anemia. *Blood* **1986**, *67*, 1411–1417. [CrossRef] [PubMed]
22. Risinger, M.; Kalfa, T.A. Red Cell Membrane Disorders: Structure Meets Function. *Blood* **2020**, *136*, 1250–1261. [CrossRef] [PubMed]
23. Wu, Y.; Liao, L.; Lin, F. The Diagnostic Protocol for Hereditary Spherocytosis-2021 Update. *J. Clin. Lab. Anal.* **2021**, *35*, e24034. [CrossRef]
24. Marchionatti, A.; Parisi, M.M. Anemia and Thrombocytopenia in People Living with HIV/AIDS: A Narrative Literature Review. *Int. Health* **2021**, *13*, 98–109. [CrossRef]
25. Koduri, P.R. Parvovirus B19-Related Anemia in HIV-Infected Patients. *AIDS Patient Care STDs* **2000**, *14*, 7–11. [CrossRef] [PubMed]
26. Watanabe, D.; Taniguchi, T.; Otani, N.; Tominari, S.; Nishida, Y.; Uehira, T.; Shirasaka, T. Immune Reconstitution to Parvovirus B19 and Resolution of Anemia in a Patient Treated with Highly Active Antiretroviral Therapy. *J. Infect. Chemother.* **2011**, *17*, 283–287. [CrossRef]
27. Ivanova, S.K.; Mihneva, Z.G.; Toshev, A.K.; Kovaleva, V.P.; Andonova, L.G.; Muller, C.P.; Hübschen, J.M. Insights into Epidemiology of Human Parvovirus B19 and Detection of an Unusual Genotype 2 Variant, Bulgaria, 2004 to 2013. *Eurosurveillance* **2016**, *21*, 30116. [CrossRef]
28. Hübschen, J.M.; Mihneva, Z.; Mentis, A.F.; Schneider, F.; Aboudy, Y.; Grossman, Z.; Rudich, H.; Kasymbekova, K.; Sarv, I.; Nedeljkovic, J.; et al. Phylogenetic Analysis of Human Parvovirus B19 Sequences from Eleven Different Countries Confirms the Predominance of Genotype 1 and Suggests the Spread of Genotype 3b. *J. Clin. Microbiol.* **2009**, *47*, 3735–3738. [CrossRef]
29. Pereira, R.F.A.; Cássia Nasser Cubel Garcia, R.; de Azevedo, K.M.L.; Setúbal, S.; de Siqueira, M.A.M.T.; de Oliveira, S.A. Clinical Features and Laboratory Findings of Human Parvovirus B19 in Human Immunodeficiency Virus-Infected Patients. *Mem. Inst. Oswaldo Cruz* **2014**, *109*, 168–173. [CrossRef]
30. Ferry, T.; Hirschel, B.; Dang, T.; Meylan, P.; Delhumeau, C.; Rauch, A.; Weber, R.; Elzi, L.; Bernasconi, E.; Schmid, P.; et al. Infrequent Replication of Parvovirus B19 and Erythrovirus Genotypes 2 and 3 among HIV-Infected Patients with Chronic Anemia. *Clin. Infect. Dis.* **2010**, *50*, 115–118. [CrossRef]
31. Freitas, R.B.; Melo, F.L.; Oliveira, D.S.; Romano, C.M.; Freitas, M.R.C.; Macêdo, O.; Linhares, A.C.; De A Zanotto, P.M.; Durigon, E.L. Molecular Characterization of Human Erythrovirus B19 Strains Obtained from Patients with Several Clinical Presentations in the Amazon Region of Brazil. *J. Clin. Virol.* **2008**, *43*, 60–65. [CrossRef] [PubMed]
32. Keller, L.W.; Barbosa, M.L.; Melo, F.L.; Pereira, L.M.; David-Neto, E.; Lanhez, L.E.; Durigon, E.L. Phylogenetic Analysis of a Near-Full-Length Sequence of an Erythrovirus Genotype 3 Strain Isolated in Brazil. *Arch. Virol.* **2009**, *154*, 1685–1687. [CrossRef] [PubMed]
33. Garcia, S.D.O. O Significado das Variantes do Eritrovírus em Pacientes com Citopenias de Origem Desconhecida. Master's Thesis, Universidade de São Paulo, São Paulo, Brazil, 2010.
34. Da Costa, A.C.; Bendit, I.; De Oliveira, A.C.S.; Kallas, E.G.; Sabino, E.C.; Sanabani, S.S. Investigation of Human Parvovirus B19 Occurrence and Genetic Variability in Different Leukaemia Entities. *Clin. Microbiol. Infect.* **2013**, *19*, E31–E43. [CrossRef] [PubMed]
35. Brazier, E.; Ajeh, R.; Maruri, F.; Musick, B.; Freeman, A.; Wester, C.W.; Lee, M.; Shamu, T.; Crabtree Ramírez, B.; d'Almeida, M.; et al. Service Delivery Challenges in HIV Care during the First Year of the COVID-19 Pandemic: Results from a Site Assessment Survey across the Global IeDEA Consortium. *J. Int. AIDS Soc.* **2022**, *25*, e26036. [CrossRef] [PubMed]

viruses

MDPI

Brief Report

First Report of Skunk Amdoparvovirus (Species *Carnivore amdoparvovirus* 4) in Europe in a Captive Striped Skunk (*Mephitis mephitis*)

Franziska K. Kaiser [1,†], Madeleine de le Roi [2,†], Wendy K. Jo [1,‡], Ingo Gerhauser [2], Viktor Molnár [3], Albert D. M. E. Osterhaus [1], Wolfgang Baumgärtner [2] and Martin Ludlow [1,*]

1 Research Center for Emerging Infections and Zoonoses, University of Veterinary Medicine Hannover, Foundation, 30559 Hannover, Germany
2 Department of Pathology, University of Veterinary Medicine Hannover, Foundation, 30559 Hannover, Germany
3 Hannover Adventure Zoo, 30175 Hannover, Germany
* Correspondence: martin.ludlow@tiho-hannover.de; Tel.: +49-51-1953-6112
† These authors contributed equally to this work.
‡ Current Address: Institute of Virology, Charité-Universitätsmedizin Berlin, Corporate Member of Freie Universität Berlin, Humboldt Universität zu Berlin, 12203 Berlin, Germany.

Abstract: Skunk amdoparvovirus (*Carnivore amdoparvovirus 4*, SKAV) is closely related to Aleutian mink disease virus (AMDV) and circulates primarily in striped skunks (*Mephitis mephitis*) in North America. SKAV poses a threat to mustelid species due to reported isolated infections of captive American mink (*Neovison vison*) in British Columbia, Canada. We detected SKAV in a captive striped skunk in a German zoo by metagenomic sequencing. The pathological findings are dominated by lymphoplasmacellular inflammation and reveal similarities to its relative *Carnivore amdoparvovirus 1*, the causative agent of Aleutian mink disease. Phylogenetic analysis of the whole genome demonstrated 94.80% nucleotide sequence identity to a sequence from Ontario, Canada. This study is the first case description of a SKAV infection outside of North America.

Keywords: skunk amdoparvovirus; parvovirus; striped skunk; next generation sequencing; virus surveillance

Citation: Kaiser, F.K.; de le Roi, M.; Jo, W.K.; Gerhauser, I.; Molnár, V.; Osterhaus, A.D.M.E.; Baumgärtner, W.; Ludlow, M. First Report of Skunk Amdoparvovirus (Species *Carnivore amdoparvovirus 4*) in Europe in a Captive Striped Skunk (*Mephitis mephitis*). *Viruses* **2023**, *15*, 1087. https://doi.org/10.3390/v15051087

Academic Editor: Giorgio Gallinella

Received: 22 March 2023
Revised: 25 April 2023
Accepted: 27 April 2023
Published: 28 April 2023

1. Introduction

The genus *Amdoparvovirus* in the family *Parvoviridae* is currently comprised of five species each containing a single virus, *Carnivore amdoparvovirus 1* (Aleutian mink disease virus, AMDV), *Carnivore amdoparvovirus 2* (gray fox amdovirus, GFAV), *Carnivore amdoparvovirus 3* (raccoon dog and fox amdoparvovirus, RFAV), *Carnivore amdoparvovirus 4* (skunk amdoparvovirus, SKAV), and *Carnivore amdoparvovirus 5* (red panda amdoparvovirus, RpAPV) [1,2]. Amdoparvoviruses are small, non-enveloped virus particles that contain a single-stranded, negative-sense DNA genome of approximately 4.8 kb [3,4]. This contains two gene cassettes, which encode for multiple proteins via alternative splicing for the non-structural proteins NS1, NS2, NS3, and the more conserved capsid proteins VP1 and VP2, respectively [5]. Amdoparvoviruses are known for genetic plasticity with frequent recombination events [6] and a wide host range within the order *Carnivora* including different mink species (*Mustela* spp.), arctic, gray, and red foxes (*Vulpes* spp.), lynx (*Lynx rufus*), raccoon dogs (*Nyctereutes procyonoides*), red panda (*Ailurus fulgens*), otters (*Lutrinae*), badgers (*Meles meles*), and marten species (*Martes* spp.) [7–12].

The prototypical representative of this genus, AMDV can cause high economic losses in mink farms [13] and has also been associated with rare diseases in humans [14,15]. It is assumed that AMDV originated in North America and was transported to Europe as a result of transcontinental animal trading [16,17]. Genomic investigations have demonstrated transmission of AMDV between wild and farmed mink and have highlighted the role of wild animals as a possible long-term virus reservoir [18,19]. The severity of amdoparvovirus-associated disease ranges from subclinical, persistent infections in healthy carriers to lethal systemic disease, depending on the virus strain and host species [4,20]. A fatal outcome is particularly noted in farmed mink possessing the Aleutian coat color gene, responsible for grey fur, upon infection by AMDV.

Skunk amdoparvovirus (SKAV) is widespread in North America, with an unknown genetic diversity [21]. SKAV infection has been reported in free-ranging skunks (*Mephitis mephitis*) in British Columbia and California with an incidence of 86% and 65%, respectively [22,23], and in a captive skunk [24]. SKAV is not host restricted with infection also reported in mink and ferrets (*Mustela putorius furo*) [16,25]. However, in common with other amdoparvoviruses, the potential of SKAV to infect different carnivore species remains largely uncharacterized. In general, the most common lesions observed in animals infected with amdoparvoviruses comprise splenomegaly and lymphoplasmacellular inflammation in various organ systems with reports of nephritis, myocarditis, encephalitis, and pneumonia [5,10,26,27].

In this study, we have identified the first case of SKAV infection in Europe in a captive striped skunk in Germany and have analyzed the pathology and evolutionary relationship of this strain to previously described amdoparvoviruses.

2. Materials and Methods

2.1. Gross Pathology and Histopathology

A 7-year-old male striped skunk was submitted to the Department of Pathology (University of Veterinary Medicine Hannover, Foundation) in 2016. Initially, the animal was in private possession in Germany (North Rhine-Westphalia) and subsequently transferred to a zoo in Germany (Lower Saxony), where it was kept until euthanasia. During a comprehensive post-mortem examination, organ samples were harvested and stored at −80 °C for molecular diagnostic assays, as well as in 10% neutral-buffered formalin for 24 h prior to embedding in paraffin wax for the purpose of histological investigations. Sections (2–4 μm) of formalin-fixed and paraffin-embedded (FFPE) tissues were mounted on SuperFrost® Plus slides (Glasbearbeitungswerke GmbH & Co. KG, Braunschweig, Germany) and stained with hematoxylin and eosin. Furthermore, iron deposits (hemosiderin) and collagen fibers were detected on selected slides using Turnbull's blue and Azan staining, respectively.

2.2. Genome Sequencing and Analysis

Spleen, liver, and kidney samples from a diseased striped skunk (sample number S521/16) were processed for metagenomic sequencing. Tissue preparation included three freeze/thaw cycles of homogenized sample material and OmniCleave endonuclease treatment (Epicenter Biotechnologies, Madison, WI, USA). Nucleic acids were extracted with a guanidinium thiocyanate-phenol-chloroform extraction using TRIzol (Qiagen, Hilden, Germany). Viral sequences were enriched within these samples by use of a sequence-independent single-primer amplification (SISPA) protocol [28] modified with non-ribosomal hexamers [29]. Preparation of cDNA libraries was achieved using a Nextera XT DNA Sample Preparation Kit (Illumina, San Diego, CA, USA) prior to sequencing on an Illumina MiSeq sequencer (MiSeq Reagent Kit v3, 2 × 300 cycles, Illumina, San Diego, CA, USA). For downstream analysis, raw reads were mapped against the SKAV reference genome (GenBank accession no. NC_034445.1) using Geneious Prime (Biomatters, Ltd., Auckland, New Zealand). In addition, we confirmed the exact sequence of a G-rich region of the SKAV genome between nucleotide positions 2503–2516 (GenBank accession no. OQ294046), by PCR using Phusion® High-Fidelity PCR kit (NEB, Ipswich, MA, USA) with the forward primer 5′-GTTCCTCAGCACTATCCTG-3′ and reverse primer 5′-GTATCAGTAGTTCTACCAGC-3′ prior to Sanger sequencing. This region has a variable length in different published *Carnivore amdoparvovirus* 4 genomes. The complete genome sequence of the SKAV strain was deposited on GenBank (GenBank accession no. OQ294046).

2.3. Phylogenetic Analysis

The evolutionary relationship between carnivore amdoparvovirus representatives was investigated for whole genome sequences, and NS1 and VP2 genes. A multiple sequence alignment of amdoparvoviruses was generated with sequences downloaded from GenBank using MAFFT version 7 [30]. The general time reversible model with a discrete gamma distribution (+G) and some evolutionarily invariable sites (+I) was calculated as the best fit with MEGA X for all alignments and used for the maximum likelihood method with 1000 bootstraps [31]. MEGA X was used to perform the analysis with 40 sequences each [32]. Branch lengths illustrate the number of nucleotide substitutions per site as indicated by the scale bar. Recombination analyses were performed with the integrated software package RDP4 [33], which included the algorithms RDP, GeneConv, Bootscan, MaxChi, Chimera, SiScan, and 3Seq with an initial cut-off p-value of 0.01. The criteria for selection of recombination events for further analyses was detection by at least three of the algorithms and with $p < 0.05$.

2.4. Statistics

For calculating the divergence between available complete NS1 and VP2 coding sequences of SKAV, means and standard deviation were calculated and a two samples t-test was conducted to test the null hypothesis $\mu 1 - \mu 2 = 0$. The sample size for the comparison of 31 NS1 sequences was $n = 465$ and $n = 528$ for all 33 VP2 sequences.

3. Results

3.1. Macro- and Histopathology Findings

The skunk with a 2.09 kg body weight showed elevated liver and kidney parameters, mild ascites, and ataxia of the hind limbs and was euthanized due to poor general condition. Symptoms were observed for at least four months prior to euthanasia. Ultrasonographic and radiological examination revealed calcifications of the renal pelvis, thickened and calcified vessels of the liver as well as thickened bile ducts. At necropsy, the animal was in a good to moderate nutritional condition and showed severe jaundice. The amount of urea determined in the anterior eye chamber fluid exceeded the maximum detection limit and was greater than 300 mg/dL substantiating uremia [34]. The entire liver showed miliary yellowish-white to greyish-red nodules throughout the parenchyma and on the capsule. Further findings included a marked splenomegaly and an irregular surface of both kidneys accompanied by a striated cortex. The vessels in the renal pelvis, renal artery and vein, abdominal aorta, vena cava, and mesenteric and coronary vessels were markedly thickened, hardened, and whitish in color. Both parathyroid glands were mildly to moderately enlarged. The lung displayed multiple up to 5 mm in diameter, whitish, subpleural nodules.

Histopathological lesions of the liver were characterized by severe inter- and intralobular septating fibrosis partly replacing the original parenchyma, dilated and multifocally capillarized sinusoids accompanied by an intrasinusoidal fibrosis, a mild lymphoplasmacellular portal inflammation, a mild biliary duct hyperplasia and a mild multifocal hemosiderin deposition (Figure 1A). Both kidneys showed severe multifocal to coalescing non-suppurative interstitial nephritis with moderate interstitial fibrosis (Figure 1B). The tunica media and tunica adventitia of the abdominal aorta, vena cava, coronary arteries, mesenteric blood vessels, serosal blood vessels of the urinary bladder and colon as well as blood vessels of the kidney and tongue showed a severe multifocal to coalescing calcification associated with granulomatous inflammation and occasionally cholesterol crystal deposition (Figure 1C). In addition, calcifications were also noted within the gastric submucosa. Furthermore, mild to moderate multifocal lymphoplasmacellular gastroenteritis was observed. Central nervous system lesions included a mild multifocal vacuolization of the subcortical white matter and moderate meningeal fibrosis with mild calcifications in the cerebrum as well as a mild diffuse vacuolization of cerebellar white matter accompanied by moderate vacuolization of cerebellar neurons (Figure 1D). A mild gliosis, several dilated myelin sheaths with myelinophages, and few spheroids were detected in the cervical and thoracic spinal cord. The lumbar spinal cord displayed mild neuronal vacuolization and moderate lymphoplasmacellular meningitis. Additional lesions comprised mild to moderate lymphoplasmacellular to suppurative rhinitis and a severe vacuolization of the adrenal cortex. The pulmonary and mesenteric lymph nodes showed mild to moderate follicular hyperplasia and moderate plasmocytosis. The spleen was characterized by marked extramedullary hematopoiesis and mild to moderate hyperplasia of both red and white pulp. Multiple foam cell granulomas, atelectasis, alveolar edema, and mild hemorrhages were found in the lung.

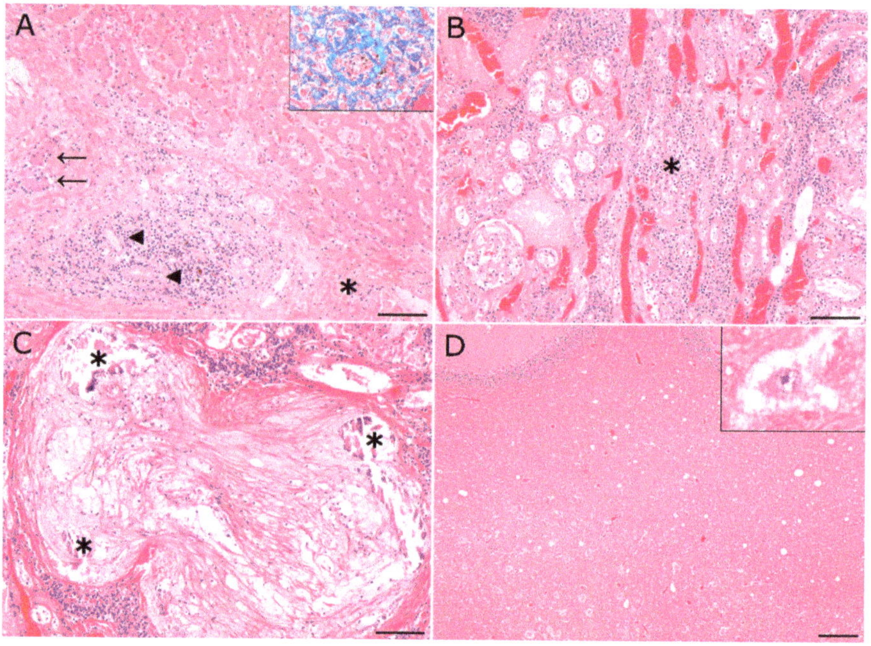

Figure 1. Histopathologic findings. (**A**) Mild lymphoplasmacellular inflammation, moderate fibrosis (asterisk), and mild biliary duct hyperplasia (arrowheads) in portal triads. Fibrosis extended into the adjacent parenchyma surrounding islands of intact hepatocytes (arrows, scale bar: 100 µm, hematoxylin and eosin). Insert: Fibrosis is characterized by increased numbers of bluish collagen fibers (Azan stain). (**B**) Severe multifocal to coalescing non-suppurative interstitial nephritis (asterisk) with moderate interstitial fibrosis (scale bar: 100 µm, hematoxylin and eosin). (**C**) Severe multifocal calcification (asterisks) of a renal vessel associated with granulomatous inflammation (scale bar: 100 µm, hematoxylin and eosin). (**D**) Mild diffuse vacuolization of the cerebellar white matter (scale bar: 200 µm, hematoxylin and eosin). Insert: Moderate vacuolization of cerebellar neurons (hematoxylin and eosin).

3.2. *Virus Detection and Phylogenetic Analysis*

Given that the pathological analyses of tissues from the skunk were indicative of a chronic carnivore amdoparvovirus virus infection, and the well-documented sequence diversity of members of the genus Amdoparvovirus, next-generation sequencing (NGS) was performed to confirm this hypothesis. Mapping of recovered reads to a reference *Carnivore amdoparvovirus 4* sequence derived from a skunk (GenBank accession no. NC_034445.1) enabled the assembly of a 4583 bp genome, which contained an additional 166 bp and 172 bp at the 5′ and 3′ genomic ends, respectively, compared to the reference sequence. Phylogenetic analyses based on whole genome sequences and NS1 and VP2 coding sequences were performed to determine the evolutionary relationship of this SKAV genome sequence to other SKAV strains. Based on analysis of the complete genome sequence, the German SKAV strain groups with sequences from Ontario, Canada (Figure 2). It is most closely related to a strain characterized in 2022 from Ontario (OL889876.1), sharing 94.80% nucleotide identity. Due to frequently observed recombination events among amdoparvoviruses and associated differential evolutionary dynamics in both ORFs, the phylogenetic relationships of both NS1 and VP2 sequences were analyzed separately. A sequence identity of 94.82% was observed in the NS1 coding sequence with a SKAV strain from British Columbia, Canada in 2022 (GenBank accession no. OL889857.1) (Figure 3A). The highest nucleotide identity of the VP2 coding sequence was with a strain also characterized in 2022 from Ontario, Canada (GenBank accession no. OL889876.1) (Figure 3B). Given the discordant geographical clustering displayed by the German SKAV strain in the phylogenetic trees constructed using NS1 and VP2 sequences, recombination analysis was performed using the software package RDP4 on full-length SKAV genome sequences. However, no evidence could be detected of a potential recombination event in the German SKAV genome sequence, which met the criteria for a positive event. A comparison of sequence similarity from all available VP2 coding sequences revealed an average nucleotide sequence identity of 95.16% (1.82 SE). Nucleotide sequences of NS1 coding sequences share an average nucleotide similarity of 92.60% (1.56 SE). This demonstrates a significantly ($p < 0.05$) higher degree of conservation on the nucleotide level of VP2 coding sequences compared to NS1 coding sequences.

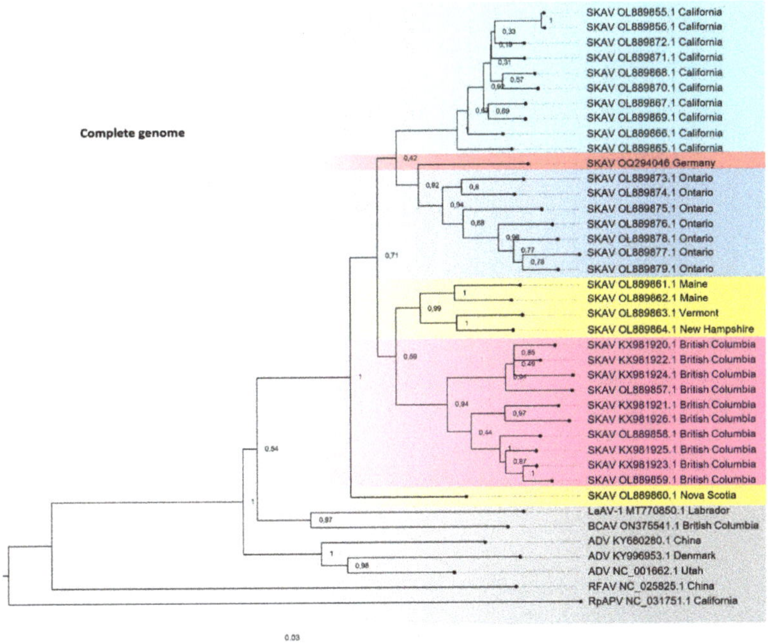

Figure 2. Evolutionary analysis of different amdoparvoviruses based on the complete genome sequences. SKAV genomes from similar geographical areas are highlighted in the same color and SKAV-related amdoparvoviruses are highlighted in grey. A total of 1000 bootstraps, GTR + G + I; +G, parameter = 0.3359; +I, 31.80% sites; log likelihood of presented tree −32,286.07. ADV, Aleutian mink disease parvovirus (*Carnivore amdoparvovirus 1*); BCAV, British Columbia amdoparvovirus (unclassified); SKAV, skunk amdoparvovirus (*Carnivore amdoparvovirus 4*); LaAV-1, Labrador amdoparvovirus 1 (*Carnivore amdoparvovirus 6*); RFAV, racoon dog and fox amdoparvovirus (*Carnivore amdoparvovirus 3*); RpAPV, red panda amdoparvovirus (*Carnivore amdoparvovirus 5*).

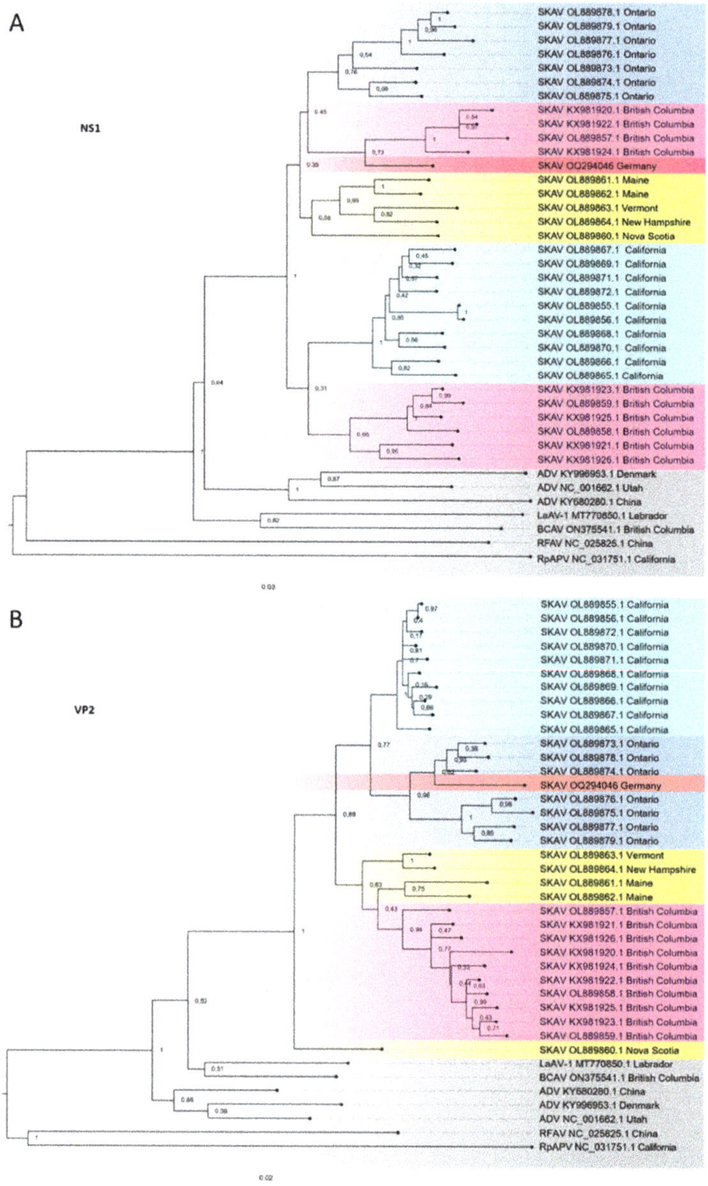

Figure 3. Phylogenetic analysis of the German SKAV strain. (**A**) Maximum likelihood tree based on forty complete 2008 bp NS1 nucleotide sequences. A total of 1000 bootstraps, GTR + G + I; +G, parameter = 0.5105); +I, 26.63% sites; log likelihood of presented tree −17,203.40. (**B**) Maximum likelihood tree based on forty complete 1941 bp VP2 nucleotide sequences (1000 bootstraps, GTR + G + I; +G, parameter = 0.2312; +I, 35.66% sites; log likelihood of presented tree −10,250.79. (**A**,**B**) SKAV genomes from similar geographical areas are highlighted in the same color and SKAV-related amdoparvoviruses are highlighted in grey. ADV, Aleutian mink disease parvovirus (*Carnivore amdoparvovirus 1*); BCAV, British Columbia amdoparvovirus (unclassified); SKAV, skunk amdoparvovirus (*Carnivore amdoparvovirus 4*); LaAV-1, Labrador amdoparvovirus 1 (*Carnivore amdoparvovirus 6*); RFAV, racoon dog and fox amdoparvovirus (*Carnivore amdoparvovirus 3*); RpAPV, red panda amdoparvovirus (*Carnivore amdoparvovirus 5*).

4. Discussion

Skunk amdoparvovirus (species *Carnivore amdoparvovirus 4*; SKAV) is endemic in North American skunk populations. However, little is known about the prevalence and sequence diversity of SKAV outside of Canada and the USA. In this study, we have pathologically and molecularly characterized a case of SKAV infection in a captive striped skunk in Germany. Although this case represents the first description of SKAV outside of North America, the German strain was found to be closely related to a clade of SKAV sequences identified previously in Ontario, Canada. The animal investigated in this study had resided in a zoo in Lower Saxony, Germany, and was previously in private possession in Germany, but further epidemiological information concerning the origin, travel history, and contact species was unfortunately unavailable. However, the phylogenetic analyses suggest that this virus strain was introduced to Germany from North America.

The macroscopic findings of the present case, characterized by splenomegaly, ataxia, and jaundice, are consistent with observations described for AMDV infection in wild and domestic striped skunks [26,27]. Histopathological lesions observed in this study were dominated by multisystemic lymphoplasmacellular inflammation in various organs, including the liver, kidney, stomach, intestine, and central nervous system. Since lymphoplasmacellular inflammatory alterations in various organ systems were already reported in other species infected with amdoparvoviruses, the observed changes are probably directly related to the viral infection [5,10,23,26,27]. The fibrosis in the kidney and liver, the bile duct hyperplasia, and the hyperplasia detected in the spleen and lymph nodes are secondary to the inflammatory processes. Vascular lesions might have been induced by the deposition of antigen–antibody complexes in vessel walls resulting in vasculitis due to a type III hypersensitivity reaction as well as consecutive dystrophic calcification, insudation of lipids, and cholesterol crystal formation (atherosclerosis). Nevertheless, atherosclerosis might have developed independently from virus infection in the present case. Furthermore, calcifications in blood vessels and other organs can be caused by renal insufficiency due to the retention of phosphate, secondary hyperparathyroidism, and precipitation of mineral complexes on endothelia damaged by uremia. The present white matter spongiform degeneration (uremic encephalopathy) also represents a characteristic finding of uremia. The suppurative rhinitis has most likely been induced by secondary bacterial infection and represents an incidental finding similar to vacuolization of adrenal glands, extramedullary hematopoiesis in the spleen, and foam cell granulomas in the lung. Atelectasis, alveolar edema, and hemorrhages within the lung were interpreted as agonal changes.

For AMDV and related carnivore amdoparvoviruses, it has been demonstrated that the structural VP2 gene is genetically more conserved than the non-structural NS1 gene [7,21]. We were able to confirm that SKAV also shows increased conservation of the VP2 gene sequence. This may explain why we were unable to detect evidence of a recombination event in the genome of the German SKAV strain, despite the discordant geographical clustering observed in the NS1 and VP2 phylogenetic trees. Alternatively, the number of available SKAV full genome sequences may not currently be sufficient to enable the detection of a recombinant event in this strain. However, the observation that AMDV strains lack clear geographical clustering [12,35] could not be confirmed for SKAV. The better-defined geographical separation of subclades for SKAV sequences might be due to lower levels of artificial virus spread mediated by animal trading in contrast to the extensive worldwide spread of AMDV due to the movement of mink for the purpose of commercial fur farming activities.

SKAV has been previously shown to cross species barriers and infect American mink (*Neovison vison*) [18]. Based on this information and on the similarity to its close relative AMDV, SKAV can be assumed to be a potential threat to endangered carnivore species in Europe [36,37]. The establishment of endemicity of SKAV strains in wild species of mustelid species in Europe could be mediated by feral American minks that live in many European countries as an invasive species and have been proven to be susceptible to SKAV infection. Furthermore, due to the high mutation rate of carnivore amdoparvoviruses and the potential to recombine, more pathogenic variants could arise, or variants could become adapted to new species following host switches. Zoo animals present a special risk for the introduction of novel infectious diseases, as the close proximity between animals from different geographical areas facilitates interspecies virus transmission or transmission to reside wildlife species. Given the absence of previous reports documenting SKAV in wild mustelid species in Europe and underlined by the potential threat posed to endemic fauna, better controls and monitoring of the health status of imported mustelids should be considered to avoid the introduction of novel species of carnivore amdoparvovirus by acutely or persistently infected animals.

Knowledge of the diversity of amdoparvoviruses has been greatly expanded in recent years, with several new species reported and the host range being possibly extended to bats and rodents [38]. This highlights the necessity for increased surveillance of potential reservoir species and further investigations into the diversity of amdoparvoviruses. In summary, this study describes the first detection of SKAV outside North America, indicating the intercontinental spread of SKAV via the transportation of wildlife animals.

Author Contributions: Conceptualization, M.L.; methodology, F.K.K., M.d.l.R., W.K.J., I.G. and M.L.; software, F.K.K., M.d.l.R. and W.K.J.; validation, F.K.K., M.d.l.R. and W.K.J.; formal analysis, F.K.K., M.d.l.R., W.K.J., I.G. and M.L; investigation, F.K.K., M.d.l.R., W.K.J., I.G., V.M. and M.L.; resources, V.M., A.D.M.E.O., W.B. and M.L.; data curation, F.K.K., W.K.J. and M.d.l.R.; writing—original draft preparation, F.K.K. and M.d.l.R.; writing—review and editing, M.L.; visualization, F.K.K. and M.d.l.R.; supervision, M.L. and W.B.; project administration, M.L. and W.B.; funding acquisition, W.B. and A.D.M.E.O. All authors have read and agreed to the published version of the manuscript.

Funding: This research was funded by the Deutsche Forschungsgemeinschaft (DFG, German Research Foundation)-398066876/GRK 2485/1-VIPER-GRK. This open access publication was funded by the Deutsche Forschungsgemeinschaft (DFG, German Research Foundation)-491094227 "Open Access Publication Funding" and the University of Veterinary Medicine Hannover, Foundation.

Institutional Review Board Statement: These samples were processed at the Research Center for Emerging Infections and Zoonoses, University of Veterinary Medicine Hannover under permit number DE 03 201 0043 21 obtained from the Fachbereich Öffentliche Ordnung, Gewerbe- und Veterinärangelegenheiten, Landeshauptstadt Hannover.

Informed Consent Statement: Not applicable.

Data Availability Statement: The sequencing data presented in this study are available in GenBank, accession no. OQ294046.

Acknowledgments: The authors thank Julia Baskas, Caroline Schütz, and Jana-Svea Harre for their excellent technical assistance. We also thank the Genomics Lab at the Institute of Animal Breeding and Genetics, University of Veterinary Medicine Hannover, Hannover, Germany, for the operation of the MiSeq system.

Conflicts of Interest: The authors declare no conflict of interest. The funders had no role in the design of the study; in the collection, analyses, or interpretation of data; in the writing of the manuscript, or in the decision to publish the results.

References

1. Penzes, J.J.; Soderlund-Venermo, M.; Canuti, M.; Eis-Hubinger, A.M.; Hughes, J.; Cotmore, S.F.; Harrach, B. Reorganizing the family Parvoviridae: A revised taxonomy independent of the canonical approach based on host association. *Arch. Virol.* **2020**, *165*, 2133–2146. [CrossRef] [PubMed]
2. Cotmore, S.F.; Agbandje-McKenna, M.; Canuti, M.; Chiorini, J.A.; Eis-Hubinger, A.M.; Hughes, J.; Mietzsch, M.; Modha, S.; Ogliastro, M.; Penzes, J.J.; et al. ICTV Virus Taxonomy Profile: Parvoviridae. *J. Gen. Virol.* **2019**, *100*, 367–368. [CrossRef] [PubMed]
3. Schuierer, S.; Bloom, M.E.; Kaaden, O.R.; Truyen, U. Sequence analysis of the lymphotropic Aleutian disease parvovirus ADV-SL3. *Arch. Virol.* **1997**, *142*, 157–166. [CrossRef] [PubMed]
4. Bloom, M.E.; Alexandersen, S.; Perryman, S.; Lechner, D.; Wolfinbarger, J.B. Nucleotide sequence and genomic organization of Aleutian mink disease parvovirus (ADV): Sequence comparisons between a nonpathogenic and a pathogenic strain of ADV. *J. Virol.* **1988**, *62*, 2903–2915. [CrossRef] [PubMed]

5. Canuti, M.; Whitney, H.G.; Lang, A.S. Amdoparvoviruses in small mammals: Expanding our understanding of parvovirus diversity, distribution, and pathology. *Front. Microbiol.* **2015**, *6*, 1119. [CrossRef] [PubMed]
6. Franzo, G.; Legnardi, M.; Grassi, L.; Dotto, G.; Drigo, M.; Cecchinato, M.; Tucciarone, C.M. Impact of viral features, host jumps and phylogeography on the rapid evolution of Aleutian mink disease virus (AMDV). *Sci. Rep.* **2021**, *11*, 16464. [CrossRef]
7. Canuti, M.; McDonald, E.; Graham, S.M.; Rodrigues, B.; Bouchard, E.; Neville, R.; Pitcher, M.; Whitney, H.G.; Marshall, H.D.; Lang, A.S. Multi-host dispersal of known and novel carnivore amdoparvoviruses. *Virus Evol.* **2020**, *6*, veaa072. [CrossRef]
8. Li, L.; Pesavento, P.A.; Woods, L.; Clifford, D.L.; Luff, J.; Wang, C.; Delwart, E. Novel amdovirus in gray foxes. *Emerg. Infect. Dis.* **2011**, *17*, 1876–1878. [CrossRef]
9. Shao, X.Q.; Wen, Y.J.; Ba, H.X.; Zhang, X.T.; Yue, Z.G.; Wang, K.J.; Li, C.Y.; Qiu, J.; Yang, F.H. Novel amdoparvovirus infecting farmed raccoon dogs and arctic foxes. *Emerg. Infect. Dis.* **2014**, *20*, 2085–2088. [CrossRef]
10. Alex, C.E.; Kubiski, S.V.; Li, L.; Sadeghi, M.; Wack, R.F.; McCarthy, M.A.; Pesavento, J.B.; Delwart, E.; Pesavento, P.A. Amdoparvovirus Infection in Red Pandas (*Ailurus fulgens*). *Vet. Pathol.* **2018**, *55*, 552–561. [CrossRef]
11. Bodewes, R.; van der Giessen, J.; Haagmans, B.L.; Osterhaus, A.D.; Smits, S.L. Identification of multiple novel viruses, including a parvovirus and a hepevirus, in feces of red foxes. *J. Virol.* **2013**, *87*, 7758–7764. [CrossRef] [PubMed]
12. Leimann, A.; Knuuttila, A.; Maran, T.; Vapalahti, O.; Saarma, U. Molecular epidemiology of Aleutian mink disease virus (AMDV) in Estonia, and a global phylogeny of AMDV. *Virus Res.* **2015**, *199*, 56–61. [CrossRef] [PubMed]
13. Christensen, L.S.; Gram-Hansen, L.; Chriel, M.; Jensen, T.H. Diversity and stability of Aleutian mink disease virus during bottleneck transitions resulting from eradication in domestic mink in Denmark. *Vet. Microbiol.* **2011**, *149*, 64–71. [CrossRef] [PubMed]
14. Jepsen, J.R.; d'Amore, F.; Baandrup, U.; Clausen, M.R.; Gottschalck, E.; Aasted, B. Aleutian mink disease virus and humans. *Emerg Infect Dis* **2009**, *15*, 2040–2042. [CrossRef] [PubMed]
15. Chapman, I.; Jimenez, F.A. Aleutian-Mink Disease in Man. *N. Engl. J. Med.* **1963**, *269*, 1171–1174. [CrossRef]
16. Nituch, L.A.; Bowman, J.; Wilson, P.J.; Schulte-Hostedde, A.I. Aleutian mink disease virus in striped skunks (*Mephitis mephitis*): Evidence for cross-species spillover. *J. Wildl. Dis.* **2015**, *51*, 389–400. [CrossRef]
17. Macdonald, D.W.; Harrington, L.A. The American mink: The triumph and tragedy of adaptation out of context. *N. Z. J. Zool.* **2003**, *30*, 421–441. [CrossRef]
18. Nituch, L.A.; Bowman, J.; Wilson, P.; Schulte-Hostedde, A.I. Molecular epidemiology of Aleutian disease virus in free-ranging domestic, hybrid, and wild mink. *Evol. Appl.* **2012**, *5*, 330–340. [CrossRef]
19. Virtanen, J.; Zalewski, A.; Kolodziej-Sobocinska, M.; Brzezinski, M.; Smura, T.; Sironen, T. Diversity and transmission of Aleutian mink disease virus in feral and farmed American mink and native mustelids. *Virus Evol.* **2021**, *7*, veab075. [CrossRef]
20. Gorham, J.R.; Leader, R.W.; Henson, J.B. The Experimental Transmission of a Virus Causing Hypergammaglobulinemia in Mink: Sources and Modes of Infection. *J. Infect. Dis.* **1964**, *114*, 341–345. [CrossRef]
21. Canuti, M.; Doyle, H.E.; Britton, P.A.; Lang, A.S. Full genetic characterization and epidemiology of a novel amdoparvovirus in striped skunk (*Mephitis mephitis*). *Emerg. Microbes Infect.* **2017**, *6*, e30. [CrossRef] [PubMed]
22. Britton, A.P.; Redford, T.; Bidulka, J.J.; Scouras, A.P.; Sojonky, K.R.; Zabek, E.; Schwantje, H.; Joseph, T. Beyond Rabies: Are Free-Ranging Skunks (*Mephitis mephitis*) in British Columbia Reservoirs of Emerging Infection? *Transbound. Emerg. Dis.* **2017**, *64*, 603–612. [CrossRef]
23. Glueckert, E.; Clifford, D.L.; Brenn-White, M.; Ochoa, J.; Gabriel, M.; Wengert, G.; Foley, J. Endemic Skunk amdoparvovirus in free-ranging striped skunks (*Mephitis mephitis*) in California. *Transbound. Emerg. Dis.* **2019**, *66*, 2252–2263. [CrossRef]
24. Allender, M.C.; Schumacher, J.; Thomas, K.V.; McCain, S.L.; Ramsay, E.C.; James, E.W.; Wise, A.G.; Maes, R.K.; Reel, D. Infection with Aleutian disease virus-like virus in a captive striped skunk. *J. Am. Vet. Med. Assoc.* **2008**, *232*, 742–746. [CrossRef] [PubMed]
25. Alex, C.E.; Canuti, M.; Schlesinger, M.S.; Jackson, K.A.; Needle, D.; Jardine, C.; Nituch, L.; Bourque, L.; Lang, A.S.; Pesavento, P.A. Natural disease and evolution of an Amdoparvovirus endemic in striped skunks (*Mephitis mephitis*). *Transbound. Emerg. Dis.* **2022**, *69*, e1758–e1767. [CrossRef] [PubMed]
26. LaDouceur, E.E.; Anderson, M.; Ritchie, B.W.; Ciembor, P.; Rimoldi, G.; Piazza, M.; Pesti, D.; Clifford, D.L.; Giannitti, F. Aleutian Disease: An Emerging Disease in Free-Ranging Striped Skunks (*Mephitis mephitis*) From California. *Vet. Pathol.* **2015**, *52*, 1250–1253. [CrossRef] [PubMed]
27. Pennick, K.E.; Latimer, K.S.; Brown, C.A.; Hayes, J.R.; Sarver, C.F. Aleutian disease in two domestic striped skunks (*Mephitis mephitis*). *Vet. Pathol.* **2007**, *44*, 687–690. [CrossRef]
28. Allander, T.; Emerson, S.U.; Engle, R.E.; Purcell, R.H.; Bukh, J. A virus discovery method incorporating DNase treatment and its application to the identification of two bovine parvovirus species. *Proc. Natl. Acad. Sci. USA* **2001**, *98*, 11609–11614. [CrossRef]
29. Endoh, D.; Mizutani, T.; Kirisawa, R.; Maki, Y.; Saito, H.; Kon, Y.; Morikawa, S.; Hayashi, M. Species-independent detection of RNA virus by representational difference analysis using non-ribosomal hexanucleotides for reverse transcription. *Nucleic Acids Res.* **2005**, *33*, e65. [CrossRef]
30. Katoh, K.; Rozewicki, J.; Yamada, K.D. MAFFT online service: Multiple sequence alignment, interactive sequence choice and visualization. *Brief Bioinform.* **2019**, *20*, 1160–1166. [CrossRef]
31. Nei, M.; Kumar, S. *Molecular Evolution and Phylogenetics*; Oxford University Press: Oxford, UK, 2000.
32. Kumar, S.; Stecher, G.; Li, M.; Knyaz, C.; Tamura, K. MEGA X: Molecular Evolutionary Genetics Analysis across Computing Platforms. *Mol. Biol. Evol.* **2018**, *35*, 1547–1549. [CrossRef] [PubMed]

33. Martin, D.P.; Murrell, B.; Golden, M.; Khoosal, A.; Muhire, B. RDP4: Detection and analysis of recombination patterns in virus genomes. *Virus Evol.* **2015**, *1*, vev003. [CrossRef] [PubMed]
34. Heidt, G.A.; Hargraves, J. Blood chemistry and hematology of the spotted skunk, Spilogale putorius. *J. Mammal.* **1974**, *55*, 206–208. [CrossRef] [PubMed]
35. Zaleska-Wawro, M.; Szczerba-Turek, A.; Szweda, W.; Siemionek, J. Seroprevalence and Molecular Epidemiology of Aleutian Disease in Various Countries during 1972–2021: A Review and Meta-Analysis. *Animals* **2021**, *11*, 2975. [CrossRef]
36. Fournier-Chambrillon, C.; Aasted, B.; Perrot, A.; Pontier, D.; Sauvage, F.; Artois, M.; Cassiede, J.M.; Chauby, X.; Dal Molin, A.; Simon, C.; et al. Antibodies to Aleutian mink disease parvovirus in free-ranging European mink (*Mustela lutreola*) and other small carnivores from southwestern France. *J. Wildl. Dis.* **2004**, *40*, 394–402. [CrossRef] [PubMed]
37. Manas, S.; Cena, J.C.; Ruiz-Olmo, J.; Palazon, S.; Domingo, M.; Wolfinbarger, J.B.; Bloom, M.E. Aleutian mink disease parvovirus in wild riparian carnivores in Spain. *J. Wildl. Dis.* **2001**, *37*, 138–144. [CrossRef] [PubMed]
38. Canuti, M.; Penzes, J.J.; Lang, A.S. A new perspective on the evolution and diversity of the genus Amdoparvovirus (family *Parvoviridae*) through genetic characterization, structural homology modeling, and phylogenetics. *Virus Evol.* **2022**, *8*, veac056. [CrossRef]

MDPI
St. Alban-Anlage 66
4052 Basel
Switzerland
www.mdpi.com

Viruses Editorial Office
E-mail: viruses@mdpi.com
www.mdpi.com/journal/viruses

www.ingramcontent.com/pod-product-compliance
Lightning Source LLC
LaVergne TN
LVHW070143100526
838202LV00015B/1883
* 9 7 8 3 0 3 6 5 9 4 4 8 4 *